FOURTH EDITION

Urogynecology and Urodynamics

Theory and Practice

FOURTH EDITION

Urogynecology and Urodynamics

Theory and Practice

Edited by

DONALD R. OSTERGARD, M.D., F.A.C.O.G.

Professor of Obstetrics and Gynecology
Director, Division of Urogynecology
University of California, Irvine
Associate Medical Director of Gynecology
Women's Hospital, Long Beach Memorial Medical Center
Long Beach, California

ALFRED E. BENT, M.D., F.R.C.S.(C), F.A.C.O.G.

Head, Division of Urogynecology
Greater Baltimore Medical Center
Clinical Associate Professor
University of Maryland Medical Center
Baltimore, Maryland

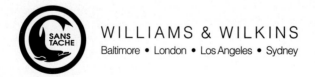

WILLIAMS & WILKINS
Baltimore • London • Los Angeles • Sydney

Editor: Charles W. Mitchell
Managing Editor: Grace E. Miller
Production Coordinator: Linda C. Carlson
Copy Editor: Pamela Thomson
Designer: Norman W. Och
Illustration Planner: Mario Fernández
Cover Designer: Wilma Rosenberger
Typesetter: Graphic World, Inc.
Printer: R.R. Donnelley and Sons, Co. Crawfordsville, IN

Library of Congress Cataloging-in-Publication Data
Urogynecology and urodynamics : theory and practice / edited by Donald R. Ostergard, Alfred E. Bent.—4th ed.
     p.   cm.
   Includes bibliographical references and index.
   ISBN 0-683-06648-X
   1. Urogynecology. 2. Urodynamics. I. Ostergard, Donald R., 1938- . II. Bent, Alfred E.
   [DNLM: 1. Urologic Diseases. 2. Genital Diseases, Female. 3. Urinary Incontinence. 4. Urodynamics.
WJ 190U78 1996]
RG484.U76 1996
616.6—dc20
DNLM/DLC
for Library of Congress   95-47708
                                                                                          CIP

                                            96 97 98 99 00
                              1 2 3 4 5 6 7 8 9 10

ISBN 0-683-06648-X

SPECIAL DEDICATION

This special dedication is given to my wife and friend, Constance, for her encouragement in organizing and editing this fourth edition, and for her unselfish support in my academic pursuits and in the time commitments those involve. For these I am grateful.

Donald R. Ostergard

APPRECIATION

To my Dad—poet, preacher, outdoorsman, humanitarian; equally at home discussing correct English grammar as he was setting up camp in the middle of the woods.

To my Mom—teacher, homemaker; always there for us, and still is; thanks Mom.

To my wife, Callie—provides a loving home and always understanding and supportive of my work; my best fan.

To my sons, Nick and Nate—a continuing source of energy and joy as we watch them grow, and grow with them. It is not what we inherit at birth, or what we have at death, but it is the journey that makes the man. May your blessings be bountiful.

A.E. Bent

PREFACE

The multiplicity of procedures, operations, concepts, and evaluations relating to female urinary incontinence bespeaks the complexity of this problem. In spite of the "80%" surgical cure rate reported by various writers, all too often the physician must care for the patient who is still incontinent after more than one operative procedure. There is genuine uneasiness by all who are confronted by the patient's question: "Will this operation cure my incontinence?" Failures of operative treatment may be due to the lack of proper assessment of the lower urinary tract before surgery.

The goal of this text is to promote a more active role for the obstetrician-gynecologist, urologist, and other physicians in the evaluation of the lower urinary tract regardless of how obvious the patient's symptoms of stress incontinence may seem. Office procedures are available to adequately screen the lower urinary tract. More sophisticated techniques are available to accurately diagnose alterations of vesicourethral physiology. The physician is able to perform an adequate examination to determine which patients require referral. He or she will understand the types of testing required in these complicated patients and how to explain the results of their evaluation.

The medical literature of the past few years contains information concerning gross and functional neurophysiology, maturation of micturition, new techniques for evaluation of the lower urinary tract, urodynamics, endoscopy, and imaging. Most of this material is in publications that physicians do not regularly review. This text collates the relevant medical literature in a readily comprehensive format. The contributors to this text are experts in such diverse areas of medicine as neurology, urology, gynecology, geriatrics, psychiatry, and nursing.

Their collective clinical experience, with a sound basis in the medical literature, leads to the formulation of a logical, orderly, practical evaluation of the patient's lower urinary tract. The thoroughness of this evaluation ensures the likelihood of clinical success. Clinical evaluation and triage provide a clinical diagnosis and treatment program that are unique for each individual patient.

This text brings together the known facets of lower urinary tract physiology and pathophysiology that are needed for an in-depth understanding of the basis of the urinary complaints of the individual patient. The "anatomy of failure" in the past has largely been a failure to apply the correct treatment to the specific urinary malfunction and to a preoccupation with incontinence as the only symptom of the female urinary tract. The availability of modern urodynamic evaluation equipment and imaging techniques now allows us to alter this myopic view of the lower urinary tract. The physician then treats specific problems either medically or surgically. Surgical procedures are applied only when indicated for the patient with true anatomical stress incontinence. The education of the physician in the establishment of specific therapies based on appropriate diagnosis is the goal of this text.

This fourth edition has undertaken an explanation for the grading of genital prolapse. Diagnostic evaluations now include cystoscopy, ambulatory monitoring, ultrasound update, and neuro and electrodiagnostic testing for urinary and fecal incontinence.

The pathology section includes collagen disorders and a major revision of the interstitial cystitis section. The treatment section includes discussions on periurethral bulking agents and laparoscopic Burch urethropexy.

With the text distinctly divided into sections, the reader will be able to follow easily from the normal lower urinary tract and epidemiology, to evaluation, lower urinary tract abnormalities, detrusor instability, and genuine stress incontinence.

CONTRIBUTORS

Sherif R. Aboseif
Assistant Professor
Department of Urology
University of California School of Medicine
San Francisco, California

Rodney A. Appell, M.D., F.A.C.S.
Head, Section of Voiding Dysfunction and Female
   Urology
Department of Urology
The Cleveland Clinic Foundation
Cleveland, Ohio

J. Thomas Benson, M.D., F.A.C.S., F.A.C.O.G.
Clinical Professor of Obstetrics/Gynecology
Indiana University School of Medicine
Director, Obstetrics/Gynecology Education
Methodist Hospital of Indiana
Indianapolis, Indiana

Alfred E. Bent, M.D.
Clinical Associate Professor
University of Maryland Medical Center
Head, Division of Urogynecology
Greater Baltimore Medical Center
Baltimore, Maryland

Arieh Bergman, M.D.
Professor
Department of Obstetrics and Gynecology
University of Southern California School of
   Medicine
Los Angeles, California

Narender N. Bhatia, M.D.
Professor of Obstetrics and Gynecology
UCLA School of Medicine
Head, Division of Urogynecology
Harbor/UCLA Medical Center
Los Angeles, California

Larry W. Bowen, M.D.
Assistant Clinical Professor
Department of Obstetrics and Gynecology
University of California, Davis
Sacramento, California

Stanley A. Brosman, M.D.
Clinical Professor of Surgery/Urology
University of California, Los Angeles
John Wayne Cancer Institute
St. John's Hospital
Santa Monica, California

Richard C. Bump, M.D.
Associate Professor and Chief
Division of Gynecologic Specialties
Duke University Medical Center
Durham, North Carolina

Kathryn L. Burgio, Ph.D.
Associate Professor
Department of Medicine
Director, Continence Program
University of Alabama at Birmingham
Birmingham, Alabama

Linda Cardozo, M.D., F.R.C.O.G.
Professor of Urogynecology
Department of Obstetrics and Gynecology
King's College Hospital
London, United Kingdom

Hilary J. Cholhan, M.D., F.A.C.O.G.
Assistant Professor, Obstetrics and Gynecology
Director, Division of Urogynecology and Pelvic
   Reconstructive Surgery
University of Rochester Medical Center
Rochester, New York

Kimberly W. Coates, M.D.
Associate, Division of Gynecologic Specialties
Department of Obstetrics and Gynecology
Duke University Medical Center
Durham, North Carolina

Jeffrey L. Cornella, M.D.
Assistant Professor
Division of Gynecologic Surgery
Mayo Clinic and Mayo Foundation
Scottsdale, Arizona

Patrice Artress Cruise, Ph.D., R.N.
Associate Director for Community Research
Borun Center for Gerontological Research
University of California, Los Angeles
Reseda, California
Assistant Research Professor
Division of Geriatric Medicine and Gerontology
University of California, Los Angeles
Los Angeles, California

Geoffrey W. Cundiff, M.D.
Assistant Professor
Department of Obstetrics & Gynecology
Duke University Medical Center
Durham, North Carolina

John O.L. DeLancey, M.D.
Associate Professor of Obstetrics and Gynecology
Chief, Division of Gynecology
University of Michigan Medical School
Ann Arbor, Michigan

Philip J. DiSaia, M.D.
Dorothy Marsh Chair in Reproductive Biology
Professor, Department of Obstetrics and
    Gynecology and Radiation Oncology
University of California, Irvine
Irvine, California

John S. Dixon, Ph.D.
Senior Lecturer
Department of Anatomy
The Chinese University of Hong Kong
Shatin, Hong Kong

Scott A. Farrell
Associate Professor
Department of Obstetrics and Gynecology
Dalhousie University
Halifax, Nova Scotia, Canada

Michelle M. Germain, M.D.
Clinical Instructor, Urogynecology and Pelvic
    Reconstruction Surgery
Department of Obstetrics and Gynecology
University of California, Irvine
Long Beach, California

John A. Gosling, M.B., Ch.B., M.D., F.R.C.S.
Professor, Department of Anatomy
The Chinese University of Hong Kong
Shatin, Hong Kong

David E. Hald, M.D.
Chief Resident
Division of Urology
University of California, Irvine
Irvine, California

Sherrie A. Hald, M.D.
Resident
Department of Obstetrics and Gynecology
Kaiser Permanente Medical Center
Los Angeles, California

Nicolette S. Horbach, M.D.
Associate Professor
Director, Division of Gynecology
The George Washington University
Washington, D.C.

W. Glenn Hurt, M.D.
Professor
Department of Obstetrics and Gynecology
Medical College of Virginia
Virginia Commonwealth University
Richmond, Virginia

Janine K. Jensen, M.D., F.A.C.O.G.
Assistant Professor Obstetrics and Gynecology
University of California, Irvine
College of Medicine
Irvine, California

Mickey M. Karram, M.D., F.A.C.O.G.
Director of Urogynecology
Good Samaritan Hospital
Associate Professor of Obstetrics and Gynecology
University of Cincinnati
Cincinnati, Ohio

Vik Khullar, B.Sc., M.B.B.S.
Research Fellow
Department of Obstetrics and Gynecology
King's College Hospital
London, United Kingdom

John J. Klutke, M.D.
Assistant Professor
Department of Obstetrics and Gynecology
University of Southern California School
    of Medicine
Los Angeles, California

Heinz Koelbl, M.D.
Assistant Professor
Department of Gynecology
University of Vienna
Vienna, Austria

Božo Kralj, M.D., Ph.D.
Professor and Director
Department of Obstetrics and Gynecology
University Medical Center
Slovenia, Yugoslavia

Raymond A. Lee, M.D.
Professor
Department of Obstetrics and Gynecology
Mayo Medical School
Rochester, Minnesota

Lawrence R. Lind, M.D.
Clinical Instructor
Department of Obstetrics and Gynecology
Harbor/UCLA Medical Center
Torrance, California

Robert W. Lobel, M.D.
Senior Fellow
Division of Urogynecology
Evanston Hospital
Northwestern University Medical School
Evanston, Illinois

Julie L. Locher, M.A.
Research Associate
Department of Medicine
University of Alabama at Birmingham
Birmingham, Alabama

Mary T. McLennan, M.B.B.S.
Urogynecology Fellow
Gynecology Division
Greater Baltimore Medical Center
Baltimore, Maryland

Joseph M. Montella, M.D.
Assistant Professor
Department of Obstetrics and Gynecology
Jefferson Medical College
Philadelphia, Pennsylvania

Peggy A. Norton, M.D.
Associate Professor
Department of Obstetrics and Gynecology
University of Utah School of Medicine
Salt Lake City, Utah

Donald R. Ostergard, M.D., F.A.C.O.G.
Professor of Obstetrics and Gynecology
Director, Division of Urogynecology
University of California, Irvine
Associate Medical Director of Gynecology
Women's Hospital, Long Beach Memorial
   Medical Center
Long Beach, California

Joseph G. Ouslander, M.D.
Associate Director
Borun Center for Gerontological Research
University of California, Los Angeles
Reseda, California
Associate Professor
Division of Geriatric Medicine and Gerontology
University of California, Los Angeles
Los Angeles, California

C. Lowell Parsons, M.D.
Professor of Surgery/Urology
Division of Urology
University of California, San Diego Medical
   Center
San Diego, California

Eckhard Petri, M.D.
Department of Obstetrics and Gynecology
Schwerin Medical School
Schwerin, Federal Republic of Germany

Charon A. Pierson, R.N., M.S., G.N.P.
Instructor, Family Nurse Practitioner Graduate
   Program
School of Nursing
Doctoral Candidate, Department of Sociology
University of Hawaii, Manoa
Honolulu, Hawaii

David A. Richardson, M.D.
Assistant Professor
Department of Obstetrics and Gynecology
Hutzel Hospital/Wayne State University
Detroit, Michigan

Jack Rodney Robertson, M.D.
Professor of Clinical Obstetrics and Gynecology
Chief of Urogynecology
University of Nevada School of Medicine
Las Vegas, Nevada

Bruce A. Rosenzweig, M.D.
Associate Professor
Department of Obstetrics and Gynecology,
   and Urology
University of Illinois at Chicago
Chicago, Illinois

Peter K. Sand, M.D.
Associate Professor of Obstetrics and Gynecology
Director, Division of Urogynecology
Evanston Hospital
Northwestern University Medical School
Evanston, Illinois

Richard J. Scotti, M.D.
Chief, Obstetrics and Gynecology
Montefiore Medical Center
Bronx, New York

Allan M. Shanberg, M.D., F.A.C.S., F.A.A.P.
Director of Pediatric Urology
Professor of Surgery-Urology
University of California, Irvine
Irvine, California
Director, Reider Laser Center
Long Beach Memorial Medical Center
Long Beach, California

Bob L. Shull, M.D.
Professor
Department of Obstetrics and Gynecology
Scott & White Clinic and Hospital
Texas A&M University Health Science Center
Temple, Texas

Stuart L. Stanton, F.R.C.S., M.R.C.O.G.
Consultant and Director
Urogynecology Unit
St. George's Hospital Medical School
University of London
London, United Kingdom

Charles B. Stone, M.D.
Associate Clinical Professor
Department of Psychiatry
University of California, Los Angeles
School of Medicine
Los Angeles, California

Robert L. Summitt, Jr., M.D.
Associate Professor and Chief
Section of Urogynecology
Department of Obstetrics and Gynecology
The University of Tennessee, Memphis
Memphis, Tennessee

Steven E. Swift, M.D.
Assistant Professor
Department of Obstetrics and Gynecology
Medical University of South Carolina
Charleston, South Carolina

Emil A. Tanagho, M.D.
Professor and Chairman
Department of Urology
University of California School of Medicine
San Francisco, California

Eboo Versi, M.D., Ph.D., M.R.C.O.G.
Chief of Urogynecology
Department of Obstetrics and Gynecology
Brigham and Women's Hospital
Associate Professor
Department of Obstetrics and Gynecology
Harvard Medical School
Boston, Massachusetts

Alison C. Weidner, M.D.
Clinical Fellow
Department of Obstetrics, Gynecology and
  Reproductive Biology
Brigham and Women's Hospital
Boston, Massachusetts

Michael W. Weinberger, M.D.
Assistant Professor
Department of Obstetrics and Gynecology
Director of Urogynecology
University of Wisconsin School of Medicine
Madison, Wisconsin

J. Christian Winters, M.D.
Clinical Assistant Professor
Department of Urology
Louisiana State University Medical Center
New Orleans, Louisiana

Cindy J. Wordell, B.S., Pharm.D.
Assistant Director
Department of Pharmacy
Thomas Jefferson University Hospital
Clinical Associate Professor
Philadelphia College of Pharmacy and
  Science
Philadelphia, Pennsylvania

CONTENTS

SECTION I

NORMAL URINARY TRACT

SECTION II

EPIDEMIOLOGY OF INCONTINENCE

SECTION III

EVALUATION OF THE LOWER URINARY TRACT AND PELVIC FLOOR

SECTION VI

GENUINE STRESS INCONTINENCE

APPENDICES

Introduction and Historical Perspectives

The Time Has Come

Philip J. DiSaia

*There is no more distressing
lesion than urinary incontinence—
A constant dribbling of the repulsive urine soaking
the clothes which cling wet and cold to the thighs,
making the patient offensive to herself and her
family and ostracizing her from society.*
Howard A. Kelly, M.D., 1928

It is somewhat paradoxical that it has taken so long for the field of gynecological urology, which gave birth to the greater discipline of gynecology, to become a science in its own right. In his book *Genitourinary Problems in Women*, Robertson discusses the ancient writing of the Kahun papyrus, written approximately 200 years B.C., which is devoted to diseases of women and includes a discussion of diseases of the urinary bladder. Indeed, the Ebers papyrus in 1550 B.C. classified diseases by systems and organs. Robertson states that in Section 6 of this latter papyrus, there was a description of the cure for a woman who suffered from a disease of her urine, as well as her womb. Henhenit was one of six women attached to the court of Menuhotep II, of the 11th dynasty, who reigned in Egypt about 2050 B.C. Her mummified body was found in 1955; radiographs of this mummy revealed that she had an extensive urinary fistula.

It was one of our own, Marion Sims, who is credited with the birth of modern gynecology through his pioneer work in the treatment of obstetrical urinary fistulas. Robertson writes that Marion Sims chose to study medicine, much to his father's disgust, as the elder had only contempt for the medical profession. Sims' father believed that there was no sci-

ence in medicine and there was no longer honor to be achieved by going from house to house with a box of pills in one hand and a squirt in the other. However, Marion Sims did enter the field of medicine and started his practice in Lancaster, South Carolina. His first two patients were infants who died from cholera. He was so disturbed that he moved to Mount Meigs, Alabama, where he earned the reputation as a great surgeon and married his childhood sweetheart, Eliza Theresa Jones, in December 1836. His practice had flourished at that point and his income was a wholesome $3000 per year.

Robertson tells us of the birth of gynecology with a specific case. Evidently, Sims' settled life was changed by an event that eventually led to his great medical achievement. A Mrs. Merril was thrown from a horse, which resulted in an impacted retroverted uterus. She was brought to Sims after many other physicians had failed to help her. Although Sims did not like to examine women, he did recall the advice of one of his professors from medical school. He placed her in a knee-chest position and reluctantly applied pressure to the vagina. The impacted uterus suddenly yielded and Mrs. Merril had immediate relief. His success with this particular patient led him to consider examining several slave women with vesicovaginal fistulas, using the same rather advantageous knee-chest position. He found this position allowed careful examination of the vagina, which had hitherto been very difficult. When examining patients with a fistula, he was able to clearly see the opening, and he began thinking of methods for repair. As is well known, his first attempts at fistula repair used silk sutures, but the attempts failed.

His first success was with a slave girl named Anarcha, whose fistula repair was accomplished with silver wire sutures. Her fistula first occurred at the age of 17 after childbirth, and she seemed doomed forever to be a disgusting object to herself and to everyone who came near her. It was this that motivated her to submit to so many surgeries. Sims had convinced his jeweler to make the wire out of unalloyed silver drawn out as thin as a horse hair. It was in May of 1849 when he prepared Anarcha for her 13th operation. He brought the edges of the fistula close together with four of his five flexible new silver wires, passing them through little strips of lead to keep them from cutting into the tissue and fastening them tightly by using, once again, his perforated lead shot. Then he introduced the essential catheter into the bladder and readied himself for the tedious week of waiting. On a score or more earlier occasions, he had been sure that when the week was over, he would witness a successful cure; this time he was filled with anxiety. He thought he had played his last trump; if he failed to win now, the game was really lost. Even with this fanatical devotion, he could not keep on forever. At the week's end, almost 4 years to the day when he had first seen those gaping, mocking holes that were Anarcha's souvenirs of childbirth, he had Anarcha placed again on the operating table. With pounding heart and fearful mind, he introduced the speculum. There lay the suture apparatus just as he had fixed it, quite undisturbed by swelling and inflammation. There was no longer any fistula. Its edges had joined close in a perfect union. Anarcha's recovery with the silver sutures in place was uncomplicated, and she remained dry for the rest of her life. This was a great relief for this particular patient because her fistula not only opened into the bladder but into the rectum as well.

In 1852, Sims reported the cure of 252 fistulas out of 320 attempts. It was apparently the use of silver wire sutures that turned repeated failures into predictable successes. Shortly thereafter, Sims left Alabama for New York where he became one of the founders of the Women's Hospital in that city. He toured Europe and operated successfully on patients throughout the continent.

His success did not end with his accomplishments in fistula surgery. The Internal Medical Congress in London in 1881 was perhaps the most satisfactory medical meeting in the life of Marion Sims, where he delivered his thesis and his valedictory address as "Progress in Peritoneal Surgery." Dr. Sims prefaced his remarks by saying that he was prompted to discuss the subject as a result of what he had seen and heard in the surgical and obstetric sections at the International Medical Congress. His object was to lay before the Academy a synopsis of the progress of peritoneal surgery in his own pioneer practice. In his address, the physically afflicted 68-year-old pioneer surgeon was ardent in his plea for surgeons to adopt the new methods, aseptic technique in particular, in dealing with any wound that invaded the peritoneal cavity. He pleaded for the adoption of Lister's principle for preventing infection in all wounds, particularly with the abdomen. "Ovariotomy is the parent of peritoneal surgery," said Sims, and he gave credit to Ephraim McDowell and Washington Atlee, whom he called the "great ovariodomists."

Marion Sims died quietly in 1883 while working on his autobiography entitled *The Story of My Life*, a book that was to be released by his son, Harry Marion Sims, a year after his father's death.

The spirit of Marion Sims was to be assumed by Howard A. Kelly, who was appointed the first professor of gynecology at the Johns Hopkins Medical School. Like Sims, Kelly believed that gynecology and urology were so closely related that they could not be separated. The new Gynecologic Urology Society is the fulfillment of the beliefs of Marion Sims and Howard Kelly.

In 1893, Kelly invented the cystoscope. According to Robertson, he used the so-called air cystoscope with the patient in the knee-chest position. Robertson relates that the cystoscope originally was a hollow tube with a handle and a glass partition that prevented water from running out of the bladder. The bladder had been distended with the installation of water before the insertion of the cystoscope and light was reflected from a head mirror. One day, an assistant to Dr. Kelly dropped the scope and the glass shattered. Kelly had noticed that the vagina ballooned with air when the patient was in the knee-chest position. He concluded that the bladder might be distended with air in a similar manner. He inserted the broken cystoscope, and when he removed the obturator, the bladder ballooned with air and he was able to satisfactorily inspect the bladder mucosa. Kelly's interest in urologic problems of the female intensified, and in 1919, he and Burnam coauthored a text entitled *Disease of the Kidney, Ureters and Bladder.* Kelly wrote, "The commonest form of incontinence is the result of childbirth, entailing an injury to the neck of the bladder; it is occasionally seen in elderly nullipara and is most common after the age of 40. It is usually progressive, beginning with an occasional dribble, later becoming more frequent and occurring on slight provocation. In its incipiency, a strain, cough, sneeze or stepping up to get on a tram car starts a little spurt of urine which, in the course of time, initiates the act which empties the bladder. The list of operations devised to overcome the incontinence is legion; most unsuccessful, but occasionally, temporarily at least, affording some control. The best plan, often successful, is to set free the thickened musculature (sphincter) at the neck of the bladder (Bell's muscle) and to suture it so as to overlap its ends, forming a good internal sphincter." This was to be the forerunner of the Kelly plication as a component of the anterior colporrhaphy.

The individuals at the Johns Hopkins Medical School that followed Kelly were similarly interested in female urology. Guy Hunner described the Hunner's ulcer, which today is called interstitial cystitis. Houston Everett succeeded Hunner; his important contribution was the relationship of the urinary tract to cervical cancer. His concepts are fundamental in modern concepts of gynecological oncology. He is the author of *Gynecologic and Obstetrical Urology* and coauthor of *Female Urology.*

In 1914, Latzko described a new operation for closure of the posthysterectomy vesicovaginal fistula. His simple method consisted of an upper vaginectomy and was easily applicable to a large number of patients in the United States with small fistula posthysterectomy. Many modifications of this technique have been proposed during the last several decades, but the fundamental methodology remains unchanged.

As stated earlier, a surgical approach to stress incontinence was begun by Howard A. Kelly, who reported on the successful outcome in 16 of 20 patients with incontinence who were treated by plication of the vesical neck. In 1949, Marshall, Marchetti, and Krantz reported on a new operation in which they treated 50 patients with stress incontinence; 25 of these patients had previous unsuccessful surgical procedures for incontinence. Their overall success rate was 82%. This retropubic suspension of the bladder neck has been modified by many individuals over the past three decades. The procedure described by Burch in 1968 received great acceptance. This procedure accomplishes the retropubic suspension by suturing of the periurethral tissue to Cooper's ligament.

Most recently, the evaluation of bladder dynamics has been more carefully and scientifically approached. This began with the report by Robertson of the use of the culdoscope modified to accommodate the physician in his inspection of the bladder and urethra. The standard culdoscope, used for many years in gynecology, could not be used to visualize the vesical neck or the urethra because of the right angle of the lens and the heat from the bulb. Robertson modified the Kelly air cystoscope to overcome these obstacles. The new urethroscope had optical glass fibers enclosed between double walls of a stainless steel barrel. An electric source in the handle transmitted cold light around the circumference at the distal end. This allowed magnification at the proximal end. An air vent allowed a closed system by placement of a fingertip over the vent. The development of fiberoptic telescopes revolutionized endoscopy and has made many changes in the practice of gynecology. Robertson developed a new female urethroscope with a direct view telescope that looks into an open barrel tube. The fiberoptic cord and the gas tubing are attached to the head. Carbon dioxide is used for distention of the urethra and bladder. This flexible system allows both thorough inspection of the urinary tract mucosa and the beginnings of analysis of bladder and urethral function. Recently, by utilization of this instrument and modifications thereof, a more sophisticated system for dynamic assessment of bladder and urethral function has been pioneered that has resulted in a more thorough understanding of the process of micturition.

It would appear that the discipline of urogynecology, which gave birth to the larger specialty of gynecology, has finally come of age. Many of us have been frustrated by the paucity of concrete knowledge in the area of stress incontinence and related problems. The number of surgical procedures that have been devised over the last century to accommodate and improve these afflicted patients is legion. Undoubtedly, the fundamental problem was a serious lack of understanding of the etiology. Developments in the last few years would suggest that our understanding of the mechanisms involved in the proper function of the healthy and diseased bladder and urethra are at hand, and appropriate procedures are forthcoming to improve the well-being of this large group of afflicted patients.

The American Board of Obstetrics and Gynecology currently has a task force studying the feasibility of creating a subspecialty in urogynecology and reconstructive pelvic floor surgery. The process by which one would achieve subspecialty status would be analogous to that currently in place for gynecologic oncology, maternal fetal medicine, and reproductive endocrinology and infertility. The objective of this new entity would run parallel to the other subspecialties and would hopefully create a cadre of academic teachers to educate young generalists and specialists in obstetrics and gynecology. The creation of formal fellowship programs and certification processes should encourage solidification of current centers of excellence and propagation of enhanced research activities in a field often neglected in the recent past. In addition, the creation of a subspecialty status will underscore the fact that the historical roots for research and therapy into diseases of the female lower urinary tract truly rest in the field of gynecology.

SECTION I

Normal Urinary Tract

CHAPTER 1

Anatomy of the Female Bladder and Urethra

John O.L. DeLancey

Introduction

Understanding the structure of the lower urinary tract's constituent parts, how they are assembled, and how they function is fundamental to understanding the physiology and pathophysiology of this region. The following discussion of the urethra, bladder, and pelvic floor is intended to cover those aspects of the anatomy that are important to understanding dysfunctions of the lower urinary tract.

Many biologists have remarked upon the intimate connection between form and function, and this is certainly true in the lower urinary tract. Its structure mirrors the dual activities of urine storage and evacuation. The bladder acts as a reservoir, relaxing to receive urine during the filling phase and contracting to evacuate it during the emptying phase. The urethra acts reciprocally by contracting during filling to maintain urine within the bladder and relaxing during voiding to allow for micturition. Both the bladder and urethra contain several separate components within their walls, and these parts are each described to the extent that they are functionally important.

The environment of the pelvic floor, where the urethra is located, is important to lower urinary tract function. One way in which the pelvic floor influences the bladder and urethra is in the support it provides for the vesical neck and proximal urethra. Although we usually think of parts of the urethra as above or below the pelvic floor, in fact it is a part of this structural unit. It was the relationship between genital support and urinary incontinence that was the genesis of the gynecologist's involvement with problems of lower urinary tract function. This remains one of the strongest arguments for our continued management of patients with lower urinary tract dysfunction.

Anatomy of the Lower Urinary Tract

Several terms have been applied to parts of the lower urinary tract. Clinicians have traditionally divided it into the bladder, vesical neck, and urethra. The bladder consists of the detrusor musculature and its underlining mucosa; it also contains the vesical trigone on its dorsal wall. The urethra is a multilayered muscular tube that extends below the bladder and has a specialized mucosal and vascular lining. The vesical neck represents that region of the bladder base where the urethral lumen traverses the wall of the bladder. In this area, therefore, the urethral lumen actually exists in a location surrounded by the bladder. Because the vesical neck has special functional characteristics, it is considered as a separate entity.

BLADDER

The bladder is a hollow viscus whose wall consists of coarse bundles of smooth muscle.

It is lined by a mucosa of transitional epithelium that rests upon a loose submucosa. It can be further subdivided into a dome and a base roughly at the level of the ureteral orifices. The dome is a relatively thin portion of the bladder and is quite distensible, whereas the base has a thicker musculature and undergoes less distention during filling.

Detrusor Muscle

Although separate layers of the detrusor musculature are sometimes described, these are not nearly as well defined as the separate layers in the gut. This reflects the fact that the bladder needs to contract only periodically to increase intravesical pressure to evacuate urine, whereas the gut must work in a coordinated manner to propel its contents in a forward direction. In the dome, the layers are relatively indistinct, but near the base of the bladder they become better defined. The outermost layer is primarily longitudinal in orientation. On the anterior surface of the bladder, longitudinal fibers continue past the vesical neck into the pubovesical muscles and insert into the tissues of the pelvic wall near the pubic symphysis (vide infra).

Within this outer longitudinal layer is an intermediate layer of oblique and circular fibers. The actual fiber directions in this portion of the dome are less well defined than those in the outer layer. The innermost layer is plexiform as can be seen from the pattern of trabeculations visible during cystoscopy. A predominance of longitudinal fibers is usually described in this layer, but this is not striking when the bladder is viewed from its lumen.

In the region of the vesical neck, there are two U-shaped bands of fibers (with each "U" opening in opposite directions). The more prominent Heiss's loop (detrusor loop) passes anterior to the internal meatus and opens posteriorly. The second, which consists of that portion of the intermediate circular layer of the detrusor that lies under the trigone, opens anteriorly. The urethral lumen passes through the openings in these muscular loops (1). This arrangement may provide a sphincteric action when the two straps of muscle pull in opposite directions to close the urethral lumen. However, this is somewhat illogical, because these detrusor fibers

are the very ones that contract during micturition. This would therefore act to close the internal meatus and retard efficient emptying. If this area had a different autonomic innervation, however, reciprocal activity of the dome and base would be possible, and there is evidence that this is the case (2). Nevertheless, these fibers, along with the urinary trigone, form the thickened musculature described as the bladder base.

Trigonal Muscle

There is a separate trigonal primordium within the fetus. It leads to a specialized smooth muscle body that exists in the base of the bladder and in the vesical neck and also extends down into the urethra (Fig. 1.1). It consists of three portions (3, 4): the urinary trigone, the trigonal ring, and the trigonal plate. The urinary trigone is a triangular-shaped body of smooth muscle that has its apices at the internal urinary meatus and the two ureteral orifices. It is slightly elevated above the rest of the detrusor musculature and can be seen cystoscopically, a fact that aids in locating the internal orifices. At the level of the internal urinary meatus, this trigonal musculature spreads out to form a ring at the level of the internal urinary meatus. This ring can be seen surrounding the urethral lumen in the area of the vesical neck. Extending below the level of the trigonal ring is the trigonal plate, which is a column of trigonal tissue extending along the length of the urethra in its dorsal aspect. It lies between the ends of the striated urogenital sphincter.

The urinary trigone and trigonal ring lie within the area where alpha-adrenergically innervated muscle within the bladder base and vesical neck have previously been identified (2). It is anatomically plausible that this may be the alpha-adrenergically innervated tissue believed to be important to vesical neck closure, although large section histochemistry has not been done to localize these receptors. That the trigonal ring might function to close the proximal urethra is suggested by its anatomic location in that area of the vesical neck that relaxes after denervation of this region. Such relaxation is seen in cases of myelodysplasia. This structure needs further study to confirm this functional association.

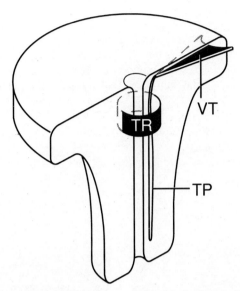

Figure 1.1.   Schematic diagram of the trigonal musculature within the bladder base and urethra (cut in sagittal section). TP, trigonal plate; TR, trigonal ring; VT, vesical trigone. (From DeLancey JOL. Anatomy and embryology of the lower urinary tract. Obstet Gynecol Clin North Am 1989;16:717–729.)

URETHRA

The urethra is a complex muscular tube, and its structure has been described in detail by a number of authors (4–6). It extends below the lower border of the bladder base. As mentioned previously, the wall of the urethra begins some 15% of total urethral length below the beginning of the urethral lumen (7).

The urethra is a hollow tube, approximately 3–4 cm in length, whose wall comprises a series of layers (Fig. 1.2). The outermost layer is the striated urogenital sphincter muscle, which has sometimes been called the striated circular muscle, striated sphincter, or rhabdosphincter. This striated muscle surrounds a thin circular layer of smooth muscle that in turn surrounds a longitudinal layer of smooth muscle. Lying between the smooth muscle and the mucosa of the urethra is a submucosa that is unusually rich in its vascular supply.

Striated Urogenital Sphincter Muscle

Descriptions of the striated urogenital sphincter muscle in the female have frequently been in error because the urethra had been removed to examine it. Studies by Oelrich (8), however, have corrected many previous misconceptions about this area and agree with functional observations of this region.

The striated urogenital sphincter has two different portions: an upper sphincteric portion and a lower arch-like pair of muscular bands (Fig. 1.3). Fibers in the sphincteric portion are circular in orientation and occupy the upper two thirds of the body of this muscle, surrounding the urethral lumen in the region from approximately 20% to 60% of its length. This portion is called the sphincter urethrae and corresponds to the rhabdosphincter described by previous authors (9). Fibers in this region do not form a complete circle, and the gap between its two ends is bridged by the trigonal plate, which completes the circle. The defect in the muscular ring does not impair contraction because the trigonal ring functions as a tendon, bridging the gap between the muscles on its two ends.

The second portion of the striated urogenital sphincter occupies its distal one third, lying adjacent to the urethral lumen approximately 60–80% of its length. It consists of two strap-like bands of striated muscle, which arch over the ventral surface of the urethra. One of these bands originates in the vaginal wall and is called the urethrovaginal

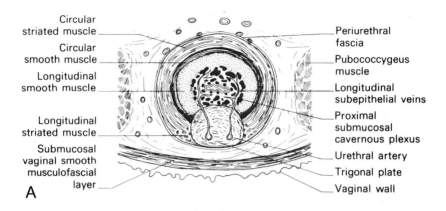

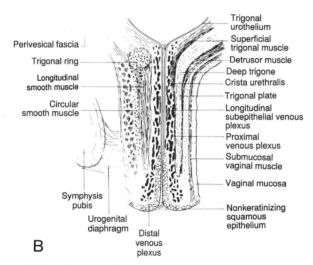

Figure 1.2. Cross sectional (**A**) and sagittal (**B**) schematic diagrams of the urethral structures (From Asmussen M, Miller A. Clinical gynaecological urology. Oxford: Blackwell Scientific Publications, 1983:9.)

sphincter muscle. The other band of muscle, which originates near the ischiopubic ramus, is called the compressor urethrae. These two bands overlap around the ventral surface of the urethra and are separate only in their more lateral projections. It is this muscle that has previously been referred to as the deep transverse perineal muscle, and previous illustrations of this muscle have frequently been inaccurate, leading to confusion about its role in continence.

All three portions of the striated urogenital sphincter muscle are part of the same muscle group and function as a unit. There has been considerable controversy over whether they are somatically or autonomically innervated, and evidence suggests that

their innervation is complex. The fibers within this muscle are primarily slow-twitch muscle (10) and therefore are well suited to maintain constant tone while retaining the ability to contract when additional occlusive force is needed.

Contraction of the striated urogenital sphincter muscle would constrict the lumen of the urethra in its upper portion and compress its ventral wall in the lower one third. The importance of this muscle is that it provides the backup continence mechanism in 50% of continent women with an incompetent vesicle neck (11). It probably also functions during times when the bladder is full and detrusor pressure rises when a woman must contract her pelvic floor until she can urinate. The importance of this muscle is demonstrated by the occurrence of stress urinary incontinence after radical vulvectomy, when the distal urethra containing the compressor urethra and urethrovaginal sphincter is excised. These individuals have no change in resting urethral pressure or urethral support, but they develop stress or total incontinence after excision that includes this musculature (12).

Smooth Muscle

As previously mentioned, the smooth muscle of the urethra arises as a separate embryologic primordium (3). Although contiguous with the detrusor muscle, it is not, as is sometimes described, simply a downward extension of bladder muscle.

There are two distinct smooth muscle layers in the urethra (Fig. 1.4). The circular

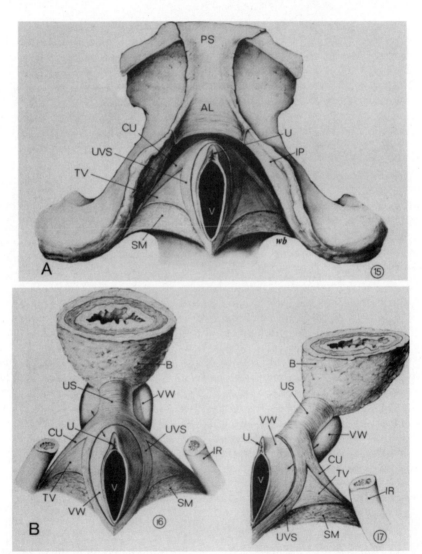

Figure 1.3. Drawings of the striated urogenital sphincter muscle after removal of the perineal membrane. **A.** Pubic bones intact. **B.** Pubic bones removed. AL, arcuate pubic ligament; B, bladder; CU, compressor urethrae; IP, ischiopubic ramus; IR, ischial ramus; PS, pubic symphysis; SM, smooth muscle; TV, transverse vaginae muscle; U, urethra; US, urethral sphincter; UVS, urethrovaginal sphincter; V, vaginal orifice; VW, vaginal wall. (From Oelrich TM. The striated urogenital sphincter muscle in the female. Anat Rec 1983;205:223–232. Copyright © 1983 John Wiley & Sons, Inc. Reprinted with permission.)

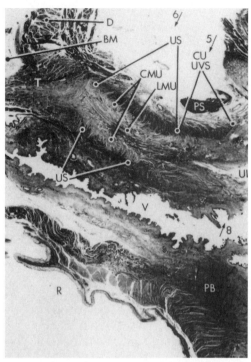

Figure 1.4. Sagittal section from a 29-year-old cadaver. Cut just lateral to the midline and not quite parallel to it. The section contains tissue nearer the midline in the distal urethra, where the lumen can be seen, than at the vesical neck. BM, bladder mucosa; CMU, circular smooth muscle of the urethra; CU, compressor urethrae; D, detrusor muscle; LMU, longitudinal smooth muscles of the urethra; PB, perineal body; PS, pubic symphysis; R, rectum; T, trigonal ring; UL, urethral lumen; US, urethral sphincter; UVS, urethrovaginal sphincter; V, vagina. (From the American College of Obstetricians and Gynecologists. Obstet Gynecol 1986;68:91.)

muscle of the urethra is poorly developed and difficult to identify. It is adjacent to the trigonal ring and extends below it, but as previously mentioned, the embryologic derivations of these two tissues seem different. The longitudinal muscle that lies inside this, however, is well developed and has considerable bulk. It is not continuous with the detrusor musculature per se as is sometimes described but does extend to the level of the trigonal ring (4). It probably functions to shorten the urethra during micturition.

Submucosal Vasculature

The prominence of the submucosal urethral vasculature is remarkable (13). This has been studied by Huisman (4), who found it to be a highly organized arteriovenous complex capable of specific filling and emptying. Although it is difficult to study so small a vascular plexus, Rud et al. (14) found that clamping the arterial supply to the urethra

significantly decreases resting urethral pressure. This vascular bed empties when the urethral pressure rises, and its function, therefore, might be to act as an "inflatable cushion," filling the area within the urethral wall and the mucosa at rest and helping to form a hermetic seal. When the urethral musculature contracts, constricting the lumen, the vascular bed may empty as a result. At these times of increased muscular activity, the vasculature would be of less importance.

Glands

A series of glands is found in the submucosa, primarily along the dorsal (vaginal) surface of the urethra (15) (Fig. 1.5). They are concentrated mainly in the lower and middle thirds and vary in number. The location of urethral diverticula, which are derived from cystic dilation of these glands, follows this distribution, being most common distally and usually originating along the dorsal surface of the urethra. In addition, their origin within the submucosa indicates that the fascia of the urethra must be stretched and attenuated over a diverticulum. Reapproximation of this layer after removal of these lesions is therefore necessary.

Epithelium

The urethra is lined by hormonally sensitive epithelium (4, 16). In the distal urethra, there is a stratified squamous epithelium; in the bladder, as previously mentioned, the epithelium is a transitional type. The line of demarcation between these two epithelia varies depending on the hormonal status of the individual and other undefined factors. It can occur in the midurethra as it does postmenopausally or may extend well up into the bladder during the reproductive years. It is not uncommon during the reproductive years to have an area of stratified squamous epithelium covering the urinary trigone.

Topography

The continence mechanism consists of several structures, and their overall arrangement is displayed in Figure 1.6. The first 15% of the urethra is that portion of the urethral

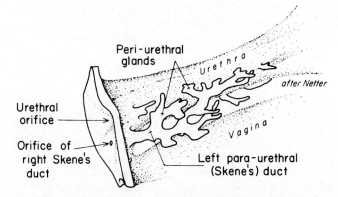

Figure 1.5.   The urethra and periurethral glands. (Redrawn with permission from The Ciba Collection of Medical Illustrations, Vol. 6, Copyright 1973.)

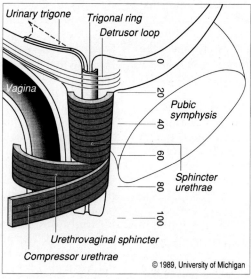

© 1989, University of Michigan

Figure 1.6.   Diagramatic representation showing the component parts of the internal and external sphincteric mechanisms and their locations. The sphincter urethrae, urethrovaginal sphincter, and compressor urethrae are all parts of the striated urogenital sphincter muscle.

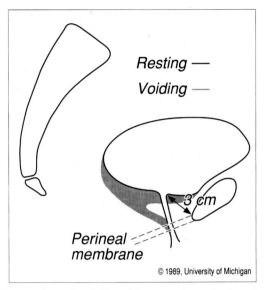

Figure 1.7. Topography and mobility of the normal proximal urethra and vesical neck based on resting and voiding radiographs in normal women (2, 20).

lumen that passes through the bladder base. As previously mentioned, it is surrounded in this region by the trigonal ring and also by the detrusor musculature. Below this intramural region lies the midportion of the urethra that extends from 20% to 60% of the total urethral length. In this location is found the sphincteric portion of the striated urogenital sphincter muscle and the circular and longitudinal smooth muscle. Below this area (from 60–80%), the urethra encounters a region just above the perineal membrane (urogenital diaphragm) where the compressor urethrae and urethrovaginal sphincter portions of the striated urogenital sphincter are found. The distal urethra includes the distal one fifth of the total urethral length, ending at the external urinary meatus. It is primarily fibrous and includes the urethral labia. It functions to aim the urine stream and therefore acts as a nozzle rather than as part of the continence mechanism.

Pelvic Floor

VESICAL NECK SUPPORT AND MOBILITY

The previous sections of this chapter dealt with the components of the lower urinary tract. Studies of patients with stress incontinence reveal that this system cannot function optimally unless it is supported by the pelvic floor. The muscles and connective tissue of the pelvic floor must create an environment in which the urethra, vesical neck, and bladder can function effectively. Conversely, normal support alone is not enough to ensure continence. A woman's ability to remain continent, therefore, results from a combination of normal activity of the vesical neck and urethra and normal function of the pelvic floor. Neither of these two components alone can maintain continence. It has been shown that there is no one-to-one relationship between urethral support and stress continence (17) and that a patient with a poorly functioning vesical neck may have stress incontinence despite normal urethral support (18). Thus, urethral support is not the only factor involved in continence.

Previous studies based on anatomic dissection have emphasized an inert fibrous attachment of the urethra to the lower portion of the pubic bones, usually termed the posterior pubourethral ligaments (19). Such a ligamentous connection would imply that the urethra is firmly and immovably attached to the pubic bones. Further studies of the broader relationship between the urethra and the pelvic floor have shown, however, that it is only the distal one third of the urethra that is fixed in position; the upper two thirds are mobile. This distal portion is where the urethra is attached to the pubic bones by the perineal membrane (urogenital diaphragm) and by the lower portions of the striated urogenital sphincter.

Additionally, in normal standing individuals (20), the vesical neck lies significantly above the level at which the fibrous attachments referred to as the posterior pubourethral ligaments insert into the pubic bones (Fig. 1.7), indicating that it would not be possible for these tissues to support the proximal urethra and vesical neck. Women are able to allow their vesical neck to descend at the onset of micturition by relaxing their levator ani muscles (21), thereby obliterating the posterior urethrovesical angle (2) and demonstrating that the position of the lower urinary tract is under voluntary control. Furthermore, recent electrophysiological studies demonstrated that patients with stress incontinence have evidence of neuromuscular damage, again suggesting that the pelvic floor musculature plays a role in maintaining continence (22–25). Therefore, our under-

standing of urethral support must encompass more than the endopelvic fascia's attachment to bone.

URETHRA AND PELVIC FLOOR

As previously mentioned, fluoroscopic examination of the urethra reveals that the distal portion is fixed in position and the proximal urethra is mobile (26). The point of inflection between these areas has been called the knee of the urethra. It lies at 56% of urethral length, at the point where the urethra comes into relation to the perineal membrane (7).

Perineal Membrane

The fixation of the distal urethra occurs because of its attachment to the pubic bones through the perineal membrane (urogenital diaphragm). The perineal membrane is a sheet of connective tissue that spans the region between the ischiopubic rami. It con-

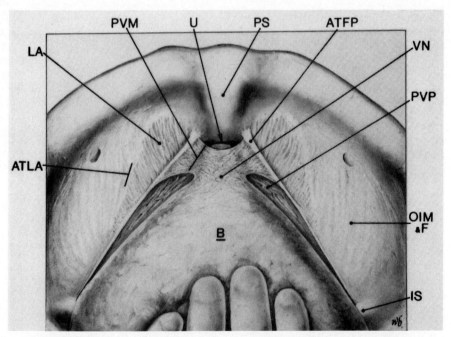

Figure 1.8. Space of Retzius (drawn from cadaver dissection). Pubovesical muscle (PVM) can be seen going from vesical neck (VN) to arcus tendineus fasciae pelvis (ATFP) and running over the paraurethral vascular plexus (PVP). ATLA, arcus tendineus levator ani; B, bladder; IS, ischial spine; LA, levator ani muscles; OIM&F, obturator internus muscle and fascia; PS, pubic symphysis; U, urethra. (From DeLancey JOL. Pubovesical ligament: a separate structure from the urethral supports (pubo-urethral ligaments). Neurourol Urodynam 1989;8:53–61. Copyright © 1989 John Wiley & Sons, Inc. Reprinted with permission of Wiley-Liss, Inc., a division of John Wiley & Sons, Inc.)

sists primarily of a sheet of fibrous connective tissue. The compressor urethrae and urethrovaginal sphincter muscles lie just above it, as does a variable amount of smooth muscle (8). The important attachments of the distal urethra occur immediately adjacent to the urethra and not posteriorly from the rest of the perineal membrane, as can be appreciated from the fact that the pubic bones can be easily palpated on either side of the urethra without any intervening connective tissue membrane. The pictures commonly used to illustrate the "urogenital diaphragm," which show two fascial layers separated by a transverse layer of muscle, are unfortunately incorrect. They have been copied without confirmation from a source over 100 years old (27), despite a previous description that is more accurate (28).

Support of the Proximal Urethra

Because a woman can voluntarily control the position of her proximal urethra above

the perineal membrane, one would expect that the support of the urethra involves voluntary muscle as well as inert connective tissue elements. This is, in fact, what examination of this region reveals. To understand this area, one must remember that the urethra and vagina are not separate structures. Because of their common derivation from the urogenital sinus (5), they are fused in the distal two thirds of the urethra. In this region, they are bound together by the endopelvic connective tissue so that the support of the urethra depends not only on the attachments of the urethra itself to adjacent structures but also on the connection of the vagina and periurethral tissues to the muscles and fasciae of the pelvic wall.

Some review of the anatomy of the space of Retzius is helpful in understanding urethral support (29). On either side of the pelvis there is a band of fibers attached at one end to the lower one sixth of the pubic bone, 1 cm from the midline, and at the other to the ischial spine (Figs. 1.8 and 1.9). This is the

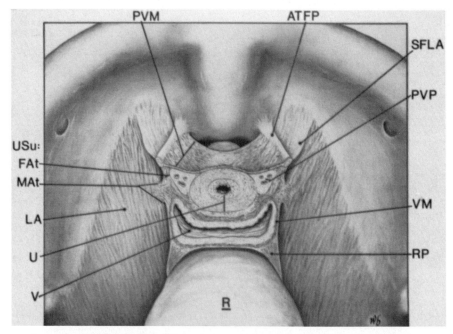

Figure 1.9. Cross-section of the urethra (U), vagina (V), arcus tendineus fasciae pelvis (ATFP), and superior fascia of levator ani (SFLA) just below the vesical neck (drawn from cadaver dissection). Pubovesical muscles (PVM) lie anterior to urethra and anterior and superior to paraurethral vascular plexus (PVP). The urethral supports (USu) (the pubo-urethral ligaments) attach the vagina and vaginal surface of the urethra to the levator ani muscles (MAt, muscular attachment) and to the superior fascia of the levator ani (FAt, fascial attachment). R, rectum; RP, rectal pillar; and VM, vaginal wall muscularis. (From DeLancey JOL. Pubovesical ligament: a separate structure from the urethral supports (pubo-urethral ligaments). Neurourol Urodynam 1989;8:53–61. Copyright © 1989 John Wiley & Sons, Inc. Reprinted with permission of Wiley-Liss, Inc., a division of John Wiley & Sons, Inc.)

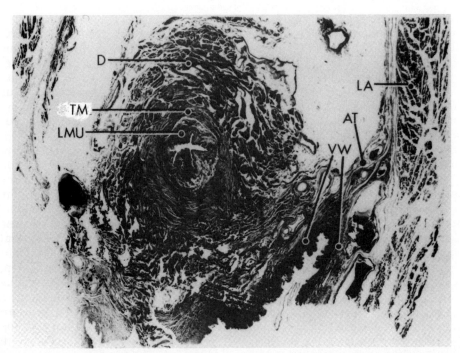

Figure 1.10. Cross section of the vesical neck and pelvic wall showing the connection of the vaginal wall (VW) and its surrounding endopelvic fascia to the arcus tendineus and thereby to the fascia over the levator ani (LA). AT, arcus tendineus fasciae pelvis; D, detrusor muscles; LMU, logitudinal smooth muscle; TM, trigonal muscle (trigonal ring portion).

arcus tendineus fasciae pelvis. In its anterior portion, this band lies on the inner surface of the levator ani muscles, which arise some 3 cm above the arcus tendineus fasciae pelvis. Posteriorly, the levator ani arises from a second arcus, the arcus tendineus fasciae levatoris ani, which fuses with the arcus tendineus fasciae pelvis near the spine. It is the lateral attachment of the endopelvic fascia that supports the urethra and bladder (pubocervical fascia). This structure, which has previously been described under the name "posterior pubourethral ligament," represents the most ventral portion of the arcus tendineus fasciae pelvis and the fascial attachment of the endopelvic fascia. It is also an attachment of the perineal membrane (30).

A number of structures, therefore, including both striated muscle and connective tissue, are important to urethral support. Because of this, we refer to the group of structures that collectively determine the position of the vesical neck as the urethral support system. This system includes the medial portion of the levator ani muscles, the arcus tendineus fasciae pelvis, and the endopelvic fascia.

The endopelvic fascia, in which the urethra and anterior vaginal wall are embedded, has two lateral attachments that participate in urethral support (Fig. 1.10), a fascial attachment and a muscular attachment. The fascial attachment of the urethral support connects the periurethral tissues and anterior vaginal wall to the arcus tendineus fasciae pelvis (Fig. 1.11) and has been called the paravaginal fascial attachment by Richardson et al. (31). The muscular attachments, on the other hand, connect this same periurethral endopelvic fascia to the medial border of the levator ani muscle (Fig. 1.11) (29). This attachment is primarily to the endopelvic fascia of the vagina, and that portion of the levator ani muscle between the pubic bone and vagina is called the pubovaginalis. (It has also been referred to as the vaginolevator attachment in the author's previous work [7].)

This connection of the levator ani muscles to the endopelvic fascia surrounding the vagina and urethra allows the normal resting tone of the levators (32) to maintain the retropubic position of the vesical neck. When the muscle relaxes at the onset of micturition, this allows the vesical neck to rotate downward to the limit of the elasticity of the fascial attachments. Contraction at the end of urination allows the vesical neck to resume its normal position.

The way in which the urethral support system contributes to stress continence can be understood best by viewing the supportive mechanism from the side (Fig. 1.12). The urethra can be seen to lie in a hammock-like layer composed of the endopelvic fascia and anterior vaginal wall. This layer is stabilized by its lateral attachments to the arcus tendineus fascia pelvic and to the medial margin of the levator ani muscles.

During increases in abdominal pressure, the downward force created by increased abdominal pressure on the ventral surface of the urethra compresses the urethra closed against the hammock-like supportive layer (Fig. 1.13). The stability of the fascial layer determines the effectiveness of this closure mechanism in opposing rises in abdominal pressure. If the layer is unyielding, it forms a

firm backstop against which the urethra can be compressed closed, but if it is unstable, the effectiveness of this closure is compromised. The integrity of the attachment to the arcus tendineus and to the levator ani are critical to the stress continence mechanism. Kinesthesiologic EMG recordings of pelvic floor muscle timing show that the levator ani muscles contract during a cough. This contraction would elevate the urethral supports, not only stabilizing the supportive hammock against abdominal pressure but actually adding to the forces favoring urethral closure during times of increased abdominal pressure.

The muscular attachment between the levator ani muscle and the endopelvic fascia is responsible for the voluntary control of vesical neck position visible on vaginal examination or fluoroscopic visualization when the pelvic muscles are contracted and relaxed. Relaxation of these muscles with descent of the vesical neck is associated with the initiation of urination and contraction

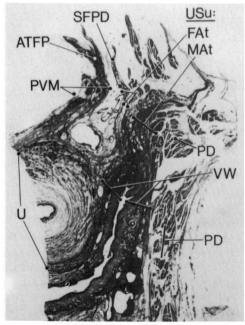

Figure 1.11. Cross-section of the urethra (U), vaginal wall (VW), and pelvic diaphragm (levator ani) (PD) from the right half of the pelvis taken just below the vesical neck at approximately the same level shown in Figure 1.9. The pubovesical muscles (PVM) can be seen anterior to the urethra and attach to the arcus tendineus fasciae pelvis (ATFP). Urethral supports (USu) run underneath (dorsal to) the urethra and vessels. Some of its fibers (MAt) attach to the muscle of the levator ani (LA), whereas others (FAt) are derived from the vaginal wall (VW) and vaginal surface of the urethra (U) and attach to the superior fascia of the levator ani (SFLA). (From Milley PS, Nichols DH. Relationship between the pubo-urethral ligaments and the urogenital diaphragm in the human female. Anat Rec 1971;170:281–283. Copyright © 1983 John Wiley & Sons, Inc. Reprinted with permission.)

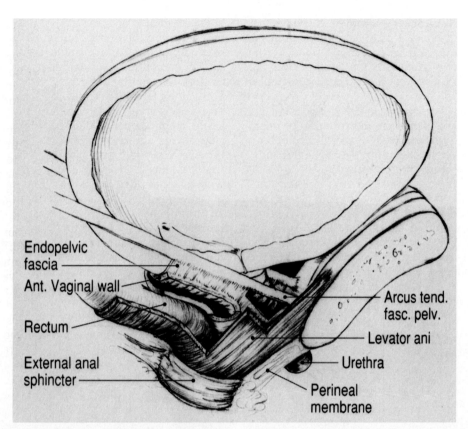

Figure 1.12. Lateral view of the urethral supportive mechanism transected just lateral to the midline. The lateral wall of the vagina and a portion of the endopelvic fascia have been removed to see deeper structures. (From DeLancey JOL. Structural support of the urethra as it relates to stress urinary incontinence: the hammock hypothesis. Am J Obstet Gynecol 1994;170: 1713–1720.)

with arrest of the urinary stream. The limit of downward vesical neck motion is determined by the limit of connective tissue elasticity in the attachments to the arcus tendineus fasciae pelvis.

Also embedded within the endopelvic connective tissue in this region are the pubovesical muscles, which are extensions of the detrusor muscle (Figs. 1.9 and 1.11) (29, 33, 34). They lie within some connective tissue, and when both muscular and fibrous elements are considered together, they are called the pubovesical ligaments in much the same way that the smooth muscle and connective tissue of the ligamentum teres is referred to as the round "ligament." Although the terms pubovesical ligament and pubourethral ligament are sometimes considered to be synonymous, the pubovesical ligaments are only one aspect of the connective tissue and muscle that may influence continence,

and they lie in a separate location from the rest of the urethral supportive tissues (29). It is not surprising, therefore, that these detrusor fibers found in the pubovesical muscles are no different in stress incontinent patients than in those without this condition (35). The actual supportive tissues of the urethra, as described above, are easily separated from the pubovesical ligament by a prominent vascular plexus. Rather than supporting the urethra, the pubovesical muscles may be responsible for assisting in vesical neck opening, as some have suggested (36).

The relationship between urethral support and sphincteric function is a complex one. Miniaturized pressure transducers have permitted us to record highly localized pressures both at rest and during the rapid sequence of events that occur during a cough. A number of authors have noted that these recordings vary depending on which direction the transducer is oriented. Although this is usually considered to be artifact, it reflects the unequal forces that are applied by the supportive tissues of the urethra and the distal portion of the striated urogenital sphincter (37).

These pressure recordings also reveal a significant increase in intraurethral pressure during a cough. These urethral pressure responses have been ascribed to the transmission of abdominal pressure to the intraabdominal portion of the urethra. Anatomically, it is not clear what separates the abdominal from the extraabdominal urethra. Examination of sagittal sections of the urethra (Fig. 1.4) reveals no structure that the urethra pierces to exit the abdomen, and the entire length of the urethra is separated from the visible lumen of the vagina only by the vaginal wall.

The several structures of the pelvic floor that surround the urethra and attach it to its surrounding bony and muscular supports are the active contracting floor that creates the environment of the urethra and vesical neck. Rather than an inert bottom of the abdominal cavity, they are a functioning unit that plays a role in continence. If the passive transmission of intraabdominal pressure to the urethra were the only factor involved in incontinence, then pressures during a cough would be maximal in the proximal urethra. Measurements, however, reveal that the distal urethra has the highest pressure elevations (38, 39). This occurs from 60% to 80% of urethral length in the region where the compressor urethrae and urethrovesical sphincter are located, suggesting that contraction of these muscles during a cough augments urethral pressure in this region.

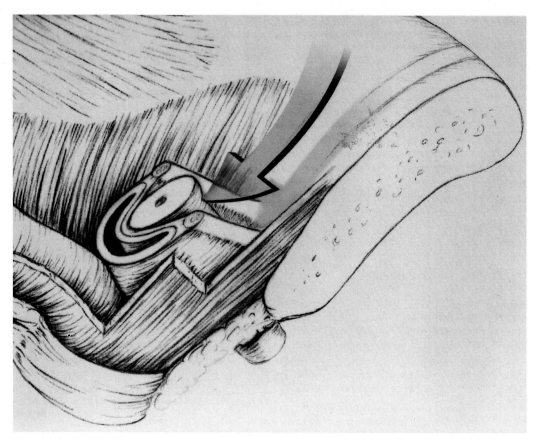

Figure 1.13. The urethral support system seen after the urethra and vagina have been transected just below the vesical neck. The arrow represents the force generated by increased abdominal pressure. (From DeLancey JOL. Structural support of the urethra as it relates to stress urinary incontinence: the hammock hypothesis. Am J Obstet Gynecol 1994;170:1713–1720.)

Table 1.1. Hypotheses Concerning Function of the Urinary Continence Mechanism Elements

Structure	Hypothetical Function
Proximal urethral support	
Connection to levator ani	Tonic contraction maintains high position of vesical neck and contracts during cough to support vesical neck. Relaxes to change position of vesical neck to facilitate micturition.
Connection to arcus tendineus	Assists levators in support and limits the downward excursion of the vesical neck when the levators are relaxed or overcome during cough.
Pubovesical muscles	May facilitate vesical neck opening by pulling on vesical neck when levators relax.
Perineal membrane	Fixes distal urethra to pubic bones.
Internal sphincteric mechanism	
Trigonal ring, detrusor loop, and elastic tissue	Maintains vesical neck closure at rest and is necessary in addition to normal support for continence during cough.
Extrinsic sphincteric mechanism	
Striated urogenital sphincter and circular smooth muscle	Resting tone contributes to resting urethral pressure, and contraction prevents incontinence when marginally compensated proximal mechanism leaks.
Longitudinal smooth muscle	Contracts during micturition to shorten the urethra.
Submucosal vasculature	Fills the space within the muscular tube to maintain a watertight seal.

These pressures frequently exceed intraabdominal pressure, indicating that factors other than abdominal pressure play a role (40). In addition, these pressure rises precede the rise in cough pressure, demonstrating that the pelvic floor muscles are contracting in preparation for the cough (40). This does not imply that abdominal pressure is an unimportant influence on urethral pressure during a cough, but it does raise the question of how the pelvic floor causes this to occur. The fact that stress incontinence persists in some patients despite adequate suspension of the urethra further supports the need to expand our concept of the urethra's response to a cough. Furthermore, recent studies demonstrated the importance of denervation of the pelvic floor to the problem of stress urinary incontinence and genital prolapse (23–25). This opens a new area of investigation that may prove helpful in further understanding the relationship of structure and function in the mechanism of urinary continence.

In summary, evolution has placed a number of structures in and around the lower urinary tract. Each may play some role in either storage or evacuation of urine (Table 1.1). Our understanding of lower urinary tract function depends on knowing the structure and function of each of these individual parts. No one structure is solely responsible for the proper functioning of this region, and future progress in better defining the exact nature of diseases of the lower urinary tract will come from examination of both the structures of this region and their function.

REFERENCES

1. Jeffcoate TNA, Roberts H. Observations on stress incontinence of urine. Am J Obstet Gynecol 1952; 64:721–738.
2. Elbadawi A. Neuromuscular mechanisms of continence. In: Yalla SV, McGuire EJ, Elbadawi A, Blaivas JG, eds. Neurourology and urodynamics. New York: Macmillan, 1989;3–35.
3. Droes JTPM. Observations on the musculature of the urinary bladder and urethra in the human foetus. Br J Urol 1974;46:179–185.
4. Huisman AB. Aspects on the anatomy of the female urethra with special relation to urinary

continence. Contrib Gynecol Obstet 1983;10: 1–31.

5. Krantz KE. The anatomy of the urethra and anterior vaginal wall. Am J Obstet Gynecol 1951;62: 374–386.

6. Ricci J, Lisa JR, Thom CH. The female urethra: a histologic study as an aid in urethral surgery. Am J Surg 1950;79:499–505.

7. DeLancey JOL. Correlative study of paraurethral anatomy. Obstet Gynecol 1986;68:91–97.

8. Oelrich TM. The striated urogenital sphincter muscle in the female. Anat Rec 1983;205: 223–232.

9. Gosling JA. The structure of the female lower urinary tract and pelvic floor. Urol Clin North Am 1985;12:207–214.

10. Gosling JA, Dixon JS, Critchley HOD, Thompson SA. A comparative study of the human external sphincter and periurethral levator ani muscles. Br J Urol 1981;53:35–41.

11. Versi E, Cardozo LD, Studd JWW, Brincat M, O'Dowd TM, Cooper DJ. Internal urinary sphincter in maintenance of female continence. Br Med J 1986;292:166–167.

12. Reid GC, DeLancey JOL, Hopkins MP, et al. Urinary incontinence and radical vulvectomy. Obstet Gynecol 1990;75:852–858.

13. Berkow SG. The corpus spongiosum of the urethra: its possible role in urinary control and stress incontinence in women. Am J Obstet Gynecol 1953;65:346–351.

14. Rud T, Anderson KE, Asmussen M, Hunting A, Ulmsten U. Factors maintaining the intraurethral pressure in women. Invest Urol 1980;17: 343–347.

15. Huffman J. Detailed anatomy of the paraurethral ducts in the adult human female. Am J Obstet Gynecol 1948;55:86–101.

16. Smith P. Age changes in the female urethra. Br J Urol 1972;44:667–676.

17. Fantl AJ, Hurt WG, Bump RC, et al. Urethral axis and sphincteric function. Am J Obstet Gynecol 1986;155:554–558.

18. McGuire EJ. Urodynamic findings in patients after failure of stress incontinence operations. Prog Clin Biol Res 1981;78:351–360.

19. Zacharin RF. The anatomic supports of the female urethra. Obstet Gynecol 1968;21:754–759.

20. Noll LE, Hutch JA. The SCIPP line—an aid in interpreting the voiding lateral cystourethrogram. Obstet Gynecol 1969;33:680–689.

21. Muellner SR. Physiology of micturition. J Urol 1951;65:805–810.

22. Snooks SJ, Swash M. Abnormalities of the innervation of the urethral striated sphincter in incontinence. Br J Urol 1984;56:401–406.

23. Snooks SJ, Badenoch DF, Tiptaft RC, Swash M. Perineal nerve damage in genuine stress urinary incontinence: an electrophysiological study. Br J Urol 1985;57:422–426.

24. Smith ARB, Hosker GL, Warrell DW. The role of pudendal nerve damage in the aetiology of genuine stress urinary incontinence of urine. Br J Obstet Gynaecol 1989;96:29–32.

25. Smith ARB, Hosker GL, Warrell DW. The role of partial denervation of the pelvic floor in the etiology of genitourinary prolapse and stress incontinence of urine: a neurophysiological study. Br J Obstet Gynaecol 1989;96:24–28.

26. Westby M, Asmussen M, Ulmsten U. Location of maximum intraurethral pressure related to urogenital diaphragm in the female subject as studied by simultaneous urethrocystometry and voiding urethrocystography. Am J Obstet Gynecol 1982;144:408–412.

27. Henle J. Handbuch der systematischen Anatomie des Menschen. Bd. II. Braunschweig: Friedrich Vieweg und Sohn, 1883.

28. Luschka H. Die Anatomie des menschlichen Beckens. Tubingen: Laupp and Siebeck, 1864.

29. DeLancey JOL. Pubovesical ligament: a separate structure from the urethral supports (pubourethral ligaments). Neurourol Urodynam 1989; 8:53–61.

30. Milley PS, Nichols DH. Relationship between the pubo-urethral ligaments and the urogenital diaphragm in the human female. Anat Rec 1971;170: 281–283.

31. Richardson AC, Edmonds PB, Williams NL. Treatment of stress urinary incontinence due to paravaginal fascial defect. Obstet Gynecol 1981; 57:357–362.

32. Parks AG, Porter NH, Melzak J. Experimental study of the reflex mechanism controlling muscles of the pelvic floor. Dis Colon Rectum 1962;5:407–414.

33. Gil Vernet S. Morphology and function of the vesico-prostato-urethral musculature. Treviso: Edizioni Canova, 1968.

34. Woodburne RT. Anatomy of the bladder and bladder outlet. J Urol 1968;100:474–487.

35. Wilson PD, Dixon JS, Brown ADG, Gosling JA. Posterior pubo-urethral ligaments in normal and genuine stress incontinent women. J Urol 1983; 130:802–805.

36. Power RMH. An anatomical contribution to the problem of continence and incontinence in the female. Am J Obstet Gynecol 1954;67:302–314.

37. DeLancey JOL. Structural aspects of the extrinsic continence mechanism. Obstet Gynecol 1988;72: 296–301.

38. Constantinou CE. Resting and stress urethral pressures as a clinical guide to the mechanism of continence in the female patient. Urol Clin North Am 1985;12:247–258.

39. Hilton P, Stanton SL. Urethral pressure measurement by microtransducer: the results in symptom-free women and in those with genuine stress incontinence. Br J Obstet Gynaecol 1983; 90:919–933.

40. Constantinou CE, Govan DE. Spatial distribution and timing of transmitted and reflexly generated urethral pressures in healthy women. J Urol 1982;127:964–969.

CHAPTER 2

Embryology and Ultrastructure of the Female Lower Urinary Tract

John A. Gosling and John S. Dixon

This chapter provides a concise account of the development and structure of the lower urinary tract in humans, with special emphasis on the female. Although there is general agreement about the embryology of the region, some aspects of the adult structure are still the subject of debate. The present description of the morphology of the adult female is based on the personal observations of the authors carried out over the last decade.

Embryology of the Female Lower Urinary Tract

DEVELOPMENT OF BLADDER, URETERS, AND URETHRA

Approximately 15 days after fertilization, cells differentiate from the primitive streak and migrate between the ectoderm and endoderm, thus forming the intraembryonic or secondary mesoderm. In most regions, the bilaminar embryonic plate is converted into a trilaminar structure, except in the caudal part of the embryo adjacent to the attachment of the connecting stalk where the mesoderm fails to penetrate. The persistence of this bilaminar region results in the formation of the cloacal membrane (Fig. 2.1), which separates the amniotic cavity from the cloaca. The cloaca is a cavity common to both urogenital and alimentary systems and into which open the allantois, the mesonephric ducts, and the hindgut in their early stages of development. The allantois is a blind-ended diverticulum of endoderm that projects into the mesoderm of the body stalk (Fig. 2.2). As the tail fold enlarges, the connecting stalk and contained allantois are displaced onto the ventral aspect of the embryo. Similar positional changes affect the cloacal membrane, which moves to a more ventral location at the base of the tail fold and connecting stalk. Mesoderm adjacent to the cloacal membrane produces bilateral elevations called the urethral folds, which border a midline surface depression, the external cloaca or proctodeum (Fig. 2.3).

DIVISION OF THE CLOACA

At about 28 days after fertilization (4–5 mm crown rump length [CRL]), the cloaca begins to be divided into smaller dorsal and larger ventral compartments. This partitioning process is produced by growth of a "spur" of mesoderm from the rostral limit of the allantois. As this mesodermal growth extends caudally, it approaches the cloacal membrane and will eventually completely separate the hindgut from the primitive urogenital sinus. It is therefore known as the urorectal septum (Fig. 2.4). As the urorectal septum extends toward the cloacal membrane, the growth of the lateral attachments of the septum to the side walls of the cloaca outstrip its central part. Thus, the caudal part of the septum forms a free margin, the concave edge of which is directed toward the

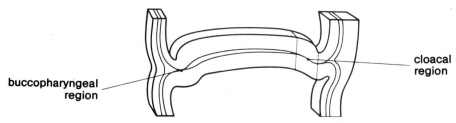

Figure 2.1. Trilaminar embryonic plate. An intermediate layer of secondary mesoderm separates endoderm and ectoderm except in the buccopharyngeal and cloacal regions.

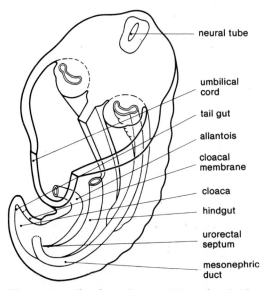

Figure 2.2. The cloaca (4.5-mm CRL embryo). The cloacal membrane is located at the base of the connecting stalk. The mesonephric duct opens into the cloaca ventral to the urorectal septum.

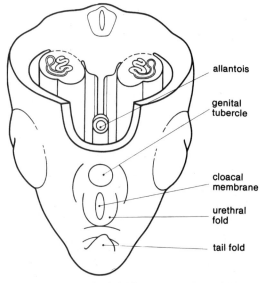

Figure 2.3. Urethral folds (5.5-mm CRL embryo). The relationship between the genital tubercle, the urethral folds, and the cloacal membrane is illustrated.

cloacal membrane. By the 10-mm CRL stage, the lateral sides of the urorectal septum have reached the cloacal membrane. Complete partitioning of the cloaca into primitive urogenital sinus ventrally and rectum dorsally is normally established by 12 mm CRL (Fig. 2.5). Immediately before complete septation, the rectum and primitive urogenital sinus are interconnected by a channel (the cloacal duct) situated on the cranial aspect of the cloacal membrane. This channel may persist due to failure of further growth by the urorectal septum, thus resulting in a fistula between the rectum and urethra. On reaching the cloacal membrane, the urorectal septum divides it into a ventral urogenital membrane and a dorsal anal membrane. The anal and urogenital openings are formed by the independent involution of these membranes, a process that is usually completed by the 18-mm CRL stage. The direction of growth of

the urorectal septum lies dorsal to the opening of the mesonephric ducts, so that by the 8-mm CRL stage, the ducts already terminate in the urogenital sinus portion of the partially divided cloaca.

FORMATION OF THE BLADDER AND URETHRA

As described above, the urorectal septum separates the gut from the developing urogenital system. Once formed, the urogenital membrane extends as far forward and cranially as the attachment of the umbilical cord so that at this stage, it faces forward and there is no infraumbilical abdominal wall. The primitive urogenital sinus now begins to undergo a change in shape, becoming subdivided into a rather cylindrical vesicourethral canal above the level of the openings of the mesonephric ducts and a definitive urogenital sinus below these openings (Fig. 2.5). The urogenital sinus is subdivided into a short narrow cylindrical portion, the pelvic part, and a more extensive phallic part, which is flattened from side to side. The subsequent fate of the latter is intimately related to the development of the external genitalia. In the female, the vesicourethral canal gives rise to the bladder and urethra. The contribution of

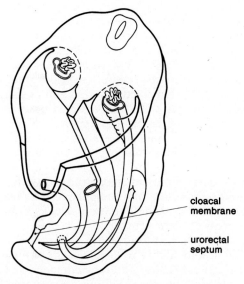

Figure 2.4.   Septation of cloaca (9-mm CRL embryo). The cloacal membrane faces caudally and is approached by the urorectal septum.

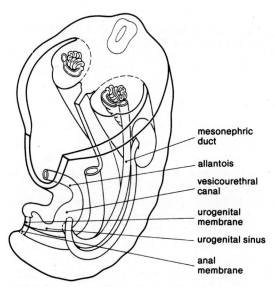

Figure 2.5.   Formation of bladder. The vesicourethral canal becomes dilated to form the bladder and female urethra.

the definitive urogenital sinus is confined to the formation of the vestibule.

As previously described, the mesonephric ducts open into the ventral part of the lateral cloacal wall. At about 28 days after fertilization, cells in the dorsomedial wall of the mesonephric duct begin to proliferate and give rise to a diverticulum, the ureteric bud. The portion of the mesonephric duct that lies between the ureteric bud and the cloaca is renamed the common excretory duct. The position of attachment of the ureteric bud to the mesonephric duct gradually changes, moving first dorsally and then dorsolaterally so that it eventually lies on the lateral aspect of the duct. Concomitant with these positional changes, the common excretory duct shortens because of the absorption of its distal extremity into the wall of the vesicourethral canal. Continuation of this process results in the ureter opening separately into the vesicourethral canal through an orifice situated lateral to that of the mesonephric duct (Fig. 2.6). By the 17-mm CRL stage, further separation of the ureters and mesonephric ducts has occurred and a well-defined trigone may be distinguished (Fig. 2.7). The ureters open into the bladder at the craniolateral angles of the trigone; the mesonephric ducts remain closely apposed to one another and open into the definitive urethra.

After the ureteric orifices have reached their final position, they remain closed by a double-layered membrane (of Chwalla). The lower layer of this membrane is composed of epithelial cells similar to those of the bladder; the upper layer is continuous with the ureteric epithelium. This membrane ruptures between the 25- and 30-mm CRL stage. Thus, the trigone is of mesodermal origin and

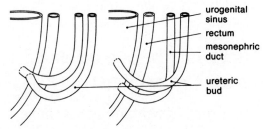

Figure 2.6.   The fate of the common excretory duct. Differential growth results in the incorporation of the common excretory duct into the urogenital sinus. Thus, the ureter gains a separate opening into the sinus, cranial and lateral to that of the mesonephric duct.

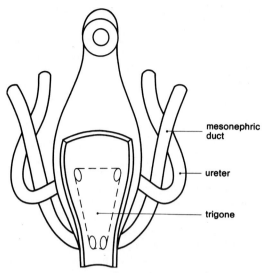

Figure 2.7. Trigone (17-mm CRL embryo). The separation of the mesonephric ducts and ureters produces the trigone, which forms an integral part of the urogenital sinus.

the rest of the bladder is endodermal. This difference probably explains the structural differences between the trigone and the remainder of the bladder.

The apex of the urogenital sinus is continuous with the allantois, the lumen of which becomes obliterated in the umbilical region at an early stage. However, the vesicourethral canal extends up to this region to form the primitive bladder. Continued obliteration of the cranial part causes the bladder apex to gradually descend into the lower abdomen, leaving a fibrous band, the urachus, extending from the apex of the bladder to the umbilicus. This may retain part or all of its lumen into adult life. It is lined by transitional epithelium, and its lower end often communicates with the bladder lumen (1).

Morphology and Ultrastructure of the Female Lower Urinary Tract

STRUCTURE OF THE URINARY BLADDER

The urinary bladder is a hollow muscular organ lined by a mucous membrane and covered on its outer aspect partly by peritoneal serosa and partly by fascia. The muscle coat of the urinary bladder is composed of bundles of smooth muscle cells, which collectively form the detrusor muscle.

Detrusor Muscle

The muscle coat of the bladder is often described as consisting of three layers. The muscle bundles of the outer and inner layers tend to be oriented longitudinally and those of the thicker middle layer are circularly disposed. However, the constituent muscle bundles frequently branch to form an interlacing meshwork. Therefore, discrete muscle layers are not easily discernible. Thus, functionally, the detrusor comprises an integrated unit of interconnected muscle bundles that, on contraction, will cause a reduction in all dimensions of the bladder lumen.

Posteriorly, some of the outer longitudinal muscle bundles extend over the bladder base and merge with the anterior vaginal wall. Anteriorly, some outer longitudinal muscle bundles continue into the pubovesical ligaments and contribute to the muscular components of these structures.

The body and fundus of the bladder are mobile and highly distensible and are capable of expansion into the abdomen to accommodate increased volumes of contained urine. In contrast, the bladder base is relatively indistensible, being closely related to the cervix.

Fine Structure of Detrusor Smooth Muscle Cells

In the electron microscope, detrusor smooth muscle cells appear spindle shaped, varying in length from 150 to 300 μm and from 5 to 10 μm in diameter (Fig. 2.8). An elongated nucleus occupies the widest part of each muscle cell. The sarcoplasm is packed with myofilaments among which numerous electron-dense bodies are scattered at random. Organelles such as mitochondria, Golgi membranes, and granular endoplasmic reticulum are relatively sparse and tend to cluster at either pole of the elongated cell nucleus. The smooth muscle cell membrane (or sarcolemma) is characterized by rows of flask-shaped caveolae interspersed with subsarcolemmal accumulations of electron-dense material (Fig. 2.9). An electron-dense basal lamina covers the outer aspect of each smooth muscle cell except at certain junctional regions. The most frequently observed type of junction between detrusor smooth muscle cells is the region of close approach at which there is a narrowed intercellular separation, 10–20 nm in width, that can sometimes extend for distances in excess of 1 μm (Fig. 2.10). Junctions of the "peg and socket" (Fig. 2.11) and "intermediate" types (Fig. 2.12) are observed occasionally, but gap junctions (or nexuses) are absent. Because electrotonic spread of excitation is believed to occur in the detrusor

muscle, the regions of close approach probably represent the morphological feature that enables this physiological event to take place. The individual cells within a muscle bundle are often so closely packed together that the basal lamina of one cell may become confluent with that of neighboring cells.

Intrinsic Innervation of the Urinary Bladder

The urinary bladder is richly innervated by autonomic nerves that form a dense plexus

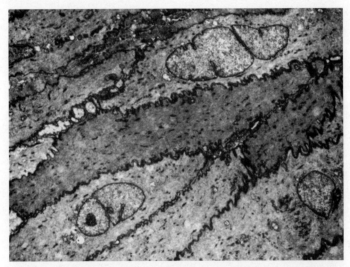

Figure 2.8.   Electron micrograph of closely packed detrusor smooth muscle cells. Magnification ×4500.

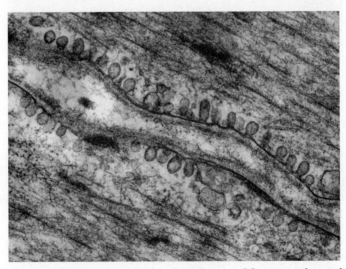

Figure 2.9.   Flask-shaped caveolae are seen at the plasmalemma of these smooth muscle cells, whereas a basal lamina covers their outer surface. Magnification ×52,400.

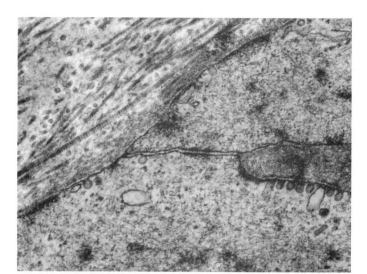

Figure 2.10. A region of close approach between adjacent detrusor smooth muscle cells. A gap of 10–20 nm separates the apposing membranes. Magnification ×42,000.

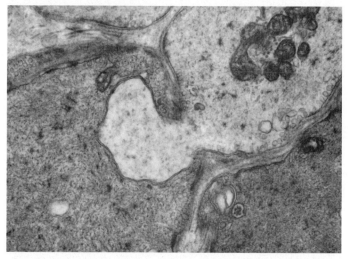

Figure 2.11. A "peg and socket" junction between adjacent detrusor muscle cells. Magnification ×42,000.

within the detrusor muscle. Most of these nerve fibers contain acetylcholinesterase (2–8). Although they occur in profusion throughout the muscle coat of the bladder, some muscle bundles appear to be better innervated than others. Using electron microscopy, the ratio of nerve axons to detrusor smooth muscle cells has been estimated at approximately 1:1 (9). Most axonal varicosities lying adjacent to detrusor smooth muscle cells have fine structural features typical of presumptive cholinergic nerve terminals, that is, they contain clusters of small (40–60 nm diameter) agranular vesicles together with occasional large (80–160 nm diameter) granulated vesicles and small rounded mitochondria (Fig. 2.13). Such terminal regions are generally only partially surrounded by neurilemmal cell cytoplasm, the naked axolemma approaching to within 20 nm of the muscle cells' surface. Thus, most of the autonomic nerves innervating the detrusor muscle are believed to be excitatory cholinergic in type.

The human detrusor muscle is relatively poorly innervated by sympathetic noradrenergic nerves (10), unlike certain other species such as the cat. Noradrenergic nerves and their terminal regions have been shown to accompany the vascular supply to the bladder, but they rarely extend among the smooth muscle bundles of the detrusor.

Immunohistochemical studies have shown that various neuropeptides are present in the autonomic nerve fibers supplying the human lower urinary tract and include neuropeptide Y, vasoactive intestinal polypeptide, substance P, and calcitonin gene-related peptide (11–14). These neu-ropeptides may act as neuromodulators, neurotransmitters, or trophic factors. More recently it has been shown that some nerves supplying the urinary bladder and ureters in humans have the capacity to synthesize the inhibitory neurotransmitter nitric oxide (15), which is synthesized on demand within nerve terminals by the enzyme nitric oxide synthase. Nitrergic nerves are thought to be responsible for nerve-mediated smooth muscle relaxation in the lower urinary tract.

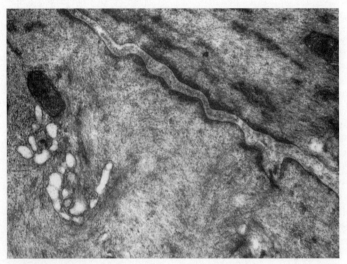

Figure 2.12.   An intermediate junction between adjacent detrusor muscle cells. The apposing membranes are separated by a minimum gap of 50 nm, and the intervening space is occupied by a single basal lamina. Magnification ×84,000.

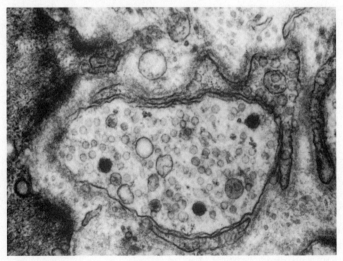

Figure 2.13.   A typical cholinergic nerve terminal among detrusor muscle cells. The axonal varicosity contains numerous small agranular vesicles together with some larger vesicles, some of which possess a central dense granule. Magnification ×56,000.

Intramural Ganglia

Small collections of autonomic ganglion cells occur throughout all regions of the human bladder wall and are especially numerous in the adventitia of the bladder base. These intramural ganglia contain up to 20 or more acetylcholinesterase-positive presumptive cholinergic neurons, similar to those occurring in the vesical plexus (16). Such neurons receive a preganglionic input from both cholinergic (excitatory) and noradrenergic (possibly inhibitory) nerve terminals (17).

In the electron microscope, the intramural ganglion cells appear similar to other parasympathetic neurons that occur elsewhere. However, a number of unusual features have been reported in the intramural ganglia of the human bladder wall (18). First, the investing layer of satellite cell cytoplasm is often incomplete, leaving large areas of the nerve cell surface in direct contact with connective tissue. Second, clusters of three or four neurons have been observed in close proximity to one another without an intervening layer of satellite cell cytoplasm (Fig. 2.14). Nerve cells in this type of configuration thus form ephaptic relationships with their neighbors over extensive areas of their surface. There does not appear to be, however, any specialization of the opposing membranes as would occur at a synapse. The functional significance of this unusual arrangement is not clear. Third, many of the intraganglionic blood capillaries are fenestrated so that adjacent nerve cells may be directly influenced by circulating hormones (e.g., noradrenaline).

Electron microscopy has confirmed the presence of occasional, small, intensely fluorescent cells in the intramural ganglia of the human urinary bladder. Cells of this type are characterized by the presence of numerous, large, membrane-limited granules that are believed to represent amine storage sites.

Submucosal Nerves

In addition to the nerve plexus associated with the detrusor muscle, autonomic nerve fibers also occur immediately beneath the epithelial lining of the urinary bladder, forming the so-called submucosal or suburothelial nerve plexus (19). The constituent nerves are acetylcholinesterase positive. Some clearly accompany submucosal blood vessels, but others lie free in the connective tissue and occasionally penetrate between the basal urothelial cells. The suburothelial plexus is relatively sparse in the bladder dome, but it becomes progressively denser as the bladder neck is approached and is particularly prominent in the trigone.

In the electron microscope, the submucosal nerves are seen to consist of small bundles of axons, most of which are nonmyelinated. Many single axons occur immediately adjacent to the basal urothelial cells. Some of these axons are either completely or partially invested in neurilemmal cell cytoplasm, but others are completely devoid of such a covering (Fig. 2.15). The suburothelial axons possess varicose regions that are packed with axonal vesicles and thus appear rather electron dense at low magnification. The vesicles are of two types, namely small (approximately 50 nm diameter) agranular vesicles and large (approximately 100 nm diameter) vesicles, most of which possess a central dense granule (20). Occasionally, an

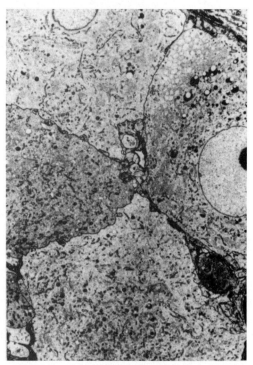

Figure 2.14. Electron micrograph of a group of four intramural neurons lying in close apposition without intervening satellite cell cytoplasm. Magnification ×4500.

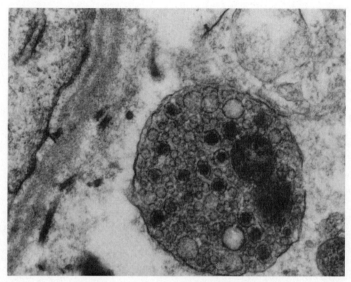

Figure 2.15. A naked axon packed with vesicles lies adjacent to the base of the bladder urothelium. Magnification ×56,000.

axon penetrates the urothelial basal lamina and is found between the basal urothelial cells.

The suburothelial axon terminals have been shown to possess a higher proportion of large granulated vesicles than "typical" cholinergic varicosities.

These vesicles may contain substance P, which has been shown to occur in the subepithelial nerves of the human bladder and which is a well-recognized constituent of primary afferent sensory fibers (21). Thus, many of the submucosal nerves of the bladder are believed to subserve a sensory function, although the possibility that they also exert a trophic influence upon the transitional epithelial cells should not be discounted (22).

Structure of the Trigone and the Ureterovesical Junctions

The trigone is defined as a triangular area of the posterior bladder wall that lies between the ureteric orifices and the internal urethral meatus. The smooth muscle of this region consists of two distinct layers, often termed the superficial and deep trigonal muscles. The latter is continuous with detrusor muscle, but the superficial trigone represents a morphologically distinct component, being composed of relatively small-diameter muscle bundles that are continu-

ous proximally with those of the intramural ureters. The superficial trigone is a relatively thin sheet of muscle but becomes thickened along its superior border to form the interureteric crest (Mercier's bar). Similar thickenings occur along the lateral edges of the superficial trigone (Bell's muscle). Distally, the superficial trigone becomes continuous with the smooth muscle of the proximal urethra.

The distal 1 cm of each ureter is surrounded by an incomplete sleeve of detrusor muscle that forms a sheath (of Waldeyer), separated from the ureteric muscle coat by connective tissue. The ureters pierce the posterior aspect of the bladder and extend obliquely through its wall for a distance of about 2 cm before terminating at the ureteric orifices. Increase in bladder pressure thus occludes the intramural ureters and prevents ureteric reflux of urine. The longitudinally oriented muscle bundles of the intramural ureters become continuous distally with superficial trigonal muscle. Lying between the muscle coat of the intramural ureter and the surrounding detrusor muscle, a third incomplete layer of muscle has recently been described (23). The constituent cells of this intermediate component of the ureterovesical junction possess specific histological and histochemical features that distinguish them from those of the ureter and detrusor. Although the origin and functional significance of this intermediate component remain uncertain, it has been suggested that it may represent a remnant of the mesonephric duct from which the ureter originates during fetal development (23).

Innervation of Ureterovesical Junction and Trigone

The inner ureteric smooth muscle component of the ureterovesical junction receives a dual innervation by cholinergic (parasympathetic) and noradrenergic (sympathetic) nerves. Both types of nerve ramify among the muscle bundles that form this intramural component of the ureter. In contrast, the surrounding detrusor muscle bundles are almost exclusively innervated by cholinergic nerves as described above. The density of the nerves supplying the detrusor is such that its innervation is richer than the combined dual innervation of the adjacent ureteric muscle coat. As with the ureteric component, the intermediate muscle layer of the ureterovesical junction is richly supplied by noradrenergic nerves.

From a functional viewpoint, the ureterovesical junction is a crucially important component of the muscular apparatus of micturition. During the storage phase, the distal ureter and its orifice allow intermittent efflux of urine into the bladder while preventing reflux. Throughout the voiding phase, the ureterovesical junction normally remains closed, thus preventing both reflux and efflux during the rise in bladder pressure that occurs during micturition. To achieve these functions consistently, the muscular activity of the ureterovesical junction must be coordinated with that of the detrusor muscle during both bladder filling and voiding. This coordination is presumably achieved by means of the intrinsic innervation of the ureterovesical junction.

Superficial trigonal muscle is associated with relatively few cholinergic nerves, whereas those of the noradrenergic (sympathetic) variety occur frequently. However, it should be emphasized that the superficial trigonal muscle forms a very minor part of the total muscle mass of the bladder neck and proximal urethra in both sexes and is probably of little significance in the physiological mechanisms that control these regions.

Bladder Neck

The smooth muscle of the bladder neck is histologically, histochemically, and pharmacologically distinct from that of the detrusor muscle proper (7, 19, 24) and should therefore be considered a separate functional unit. A distinct structural difference occurs between males and females in this region. At the male bladder neck, smooth muscle forms a complete circular collar, which extends distally to surround the preprostatic urethra and is continuous with the muscular components of the genital tract. This smooth muscle sphincter is supplied by a rich plexus of sympathetic nerves that on stimulation cause the sphincter to contract, thereby preventing retrograde flow of semen into the urinary bladder at the time of ejaculation.

At the female bladder neck, there is no comparable anatomical sphincter of smooth muscle. The muscle of this region is morphologically distinct; the large-diameter muscle bundles that characterize the detrusor are replaced by muscle bundles of much smaller diameter. However, unlike the circularly orientated preprostatic smooth muscle of the male, most muscle bundles in the female bladder neck extend obliquely or longitudinally into the urethral wall. Thus, it seems unlikely that active contraction of this region plays a significant part in the maintenance of urinary continence in females. However, the bladder neck and proximal urethra contain large quantities of elastic fibers within their walls. These produce occlusion of the urethral lumen, and it has been suggested that the passive elastic resistance offered by the urethral wall is the most important single factor responsible for the closure of the bladder neck and proximal urethra in the continent woman.

STRUCTURE OF THE FEMALE URETHRA

The adult female urethra is approximately 4 cm long and 6 mm in diameter. Beginning at the internal urethral orifice of the bladder, it extends anteroinferiorly behind the symphysis pubis and lies embedded in the anterior wall of the vagina. It traverses the perineal membrane and terminates at the external urethral orifice. Except during the passage of urine, the anterior and posterior walls of the

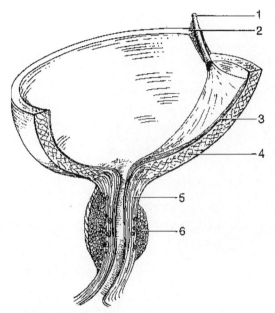

Figure 2.16. A diagram to illustrate the ureterovesical junction, bladder, and urethra in the female. *1*, juxtavesical segment of ureter; *2*, Waldeyer's sheath; *3*, superficial trigone; *4*, trigonal detrusor muscle; *5*, urethral smooth muscle; *6*, rhabdosphincter.

urethra are in close apposition with the urethral epithelium, forming extensive longitudinal folds.

The wall of the female urethra consists of an outer muscle coat and an inner mucous membrane that lines the lumen and is continuous with that of the bladder. The urethral muscularis consists of an incomplete outer sleeve of striated muscle (the rhabdosphincter) and an inner layer of smooth muscle fibers. The rhabdosphincter is separated from adjacent periurethral striated muscle of the anterior pelvic floor by a layer of connective tissue. The constituent fibers of the rhabdosphincter are circularly disposed and form a collar that is thickest in the middle third of the urethra (Fig. 2.16). In this region, the striated muscle completely surrounds the urethra, although the posterior portion lying between the urethra and vagina is relatively thin. Striated muscle extends into the anterior wall of both the proximal and distal thirds of the urethra but is deficient posteriorly in these regions.

The striated muscle cells that comprise the rhabdosphincter are unusually small in cross-section, with diameters of only 15–20 μm (25). Most fibers are histochemically of the slow-twitch type and are therefore ideally suited to maintain tone around the urethral lumen over prolonged periods of time, thus maintaining urinary continence. In contrast, the periurethral striated muscle of the pelvic floor (pubococcygeus) consists of a heterogenous mixture of slow- and fast-twitch fibers of larger diameter (26), similar to other voluntary muscles. The pelvic floor musculature plays an important part in the continence mechanism by providing an additional occlusive force on the urethral wall, particularly during events that are associated with an increase in intraabdominal pressure such as coughing and sneezing. In females, this additional urethral occlusive force is maximal at a level immediately distal to the maximum urethral pressure generated by the rhabdosphincter (the external urethral sphincter).

The smooth muscle component of the urethral wall extends throughout the length of the urethra and consists of slender muscle bundles, most of which are orientated obliquely or longitudinally. A few circularly arranged muscle fibers occur in the outer part of the smooth muscle layer and intermingle with striated muscle cells on the inner aspect of the rhabdosphincter. Proximally, the urethral smooth muscle is continuous with that of the bladder neck, whereas distally the urethral muscle bundles terminate in the subcutaneous adipose tissue surrounding the external urethral meatus.

Close to the midline, a pair of fibromuscular ligaments appear to anchor the anterior aspect of the female urethra to the posteroinferior surface of the symphysis pubis. These so-called pubourethral ligaments are continuous superiorly with the pubovesical ligaments and contain a number of smooth muscle bundles (27) that receive a rich presumptively cholinergic innervation (28) similar to that of the detrusor muscle.

However, according to DeLancey (29), these pubourethral ligaments do not firmly attach the female urethra to the pubic bones as was once believed nor do they provide support for the vesical neck that comes from the pubocervical fascia and its attachment to the arcus tendineus fascia pelvis (29, 30).

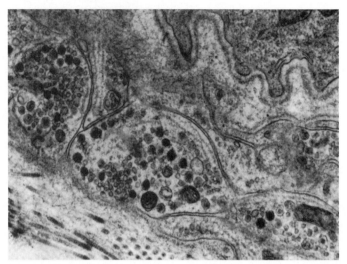

Figure 2.17. Electron micrograph of subepithelial axons from the female urethra. The presumptive sensory axons contain numerous small agranular vesicles and a few of the large granulated type. Magnification ×42,000.

Innervation of the Female Urethra and Levator Ani

The smooth muscle coat of the female urethra is associated with relatively few noradrenergic nerves but receives an extensive presumptive cholinergic innervation identical in appearance to that supplying the detrusor muscle (4). This fact, together with the oblique or longitudinal orientation of the urethral smooth muscle bundles, suggests that the latter may be active during micturition, serving to shorten and widen the urethral lumen.

In addition, relaxation mediated by nonadrenergic and noncholinergic nerves has been demonstrated in the human urethra (31) and may possibly involve nitric oxide (32).

The motor cell bodies of the nerves supplying the rhabdosphincter lie in a discrete area of the anterior horns of the second, third, and fourth sacral segments of the spinal cord collectively known as Onuf's nucleus. The nerve fibers are believed to travel via the pelvic splanchnic nerves and not the pudendal nerves as is often described.

The innervation of the periurethral levator ani muscle is provided by the pudendal nerve, and consequently, electromyographic recordings obtained from this muscle should not be assumed to represent the activity of the adjacent less accessible and differently innervated striated muscle of the rhabdosphincter.

Submucosal Nerves of the Urethra

A dense plexus of acetylcholinesterase-positive nerve fibers occurs immediately beneath the urethral epithelium, similar to that described for the bladder. This submucosal nerve plexus extends throughout the entire length of the female urethra and is thought to perform a sensory function, making the urethral mucosa sensitive to touch, thermal stimulation, distension, and pain (33).

In the electron microscope, small clusters of axons or, more commonly, single axons are observed in close proximity to the basal aspect of the urethral epithelium (Fig. 2.17). Many appear varicose and are packed with axonal vesicles of two main types. Most have diameters of 40–60 nm and have an empty appearance, being referred to as agranular vesicles. The second type of vesicle is larger, with diameters of 80–120 nm, and is characterized by the presence of a central dense granule. The axonal varicosities are generally only partially surrounded by neurilemmal cell cytoplasm. Specialized sensory endings similar to those in the dermis of the skin have not been reported to occur in the wall of the urethra.

REFERENCES

1. Hinman F. Urologic aspects of the alternating urachal sinus. Am J Surg 1961;102:339–343.
2. Mobley TL, Elbadawi A, McDonald DF, Schenk EA. Innervation of the human urinary bladder. Surg Forum 1966;27:505–506.
3. Nyo MM. Innervation of the bladder and urethra. J Anat 1969;105:210.
4. Ek A, Alm P, Andersson K-E, Persson CGA. Adrenergic and cholinergic nerves of the human urethra and urinary bladder: a histochemical study. Acta Physiol Scand 1977;99:345–352.
5. Alm P. Cholinergic innervation of the human urethra and urinary bladder. Acta Pharmacol Toxicol (Kbh) 1978;43(Suppl 2):56–62.
6. Gosling JA. The structure of the bladder and urethra in relation to function. Urol Clin North Am 1979;6:31–38.
7. Kluck P. The autonomic innervation of the human urinary bladder, bladder neck and urethra: a histochemical study. Anat Rec 1980;198: 439–447.
8. McConnell J, Benson GS, Wood JG. Autonomic innervation of the urogenital system: adrenergic and cholinergic elements. Brain Res Bull 1982;9: 679–694.
9. Daniel EEL, Cowan W, Daniel VP. Structural bases for neural and myogenic control of human detrusor muscle. Can J Physiol Pharmacol 1983;61: 1247–1273.
10. Sundin T, Dahlstrom A, Norlen L, Svedmyr N. The sympathetic innervation and adrenoreceptor function of the human lower urinary tract in the normal state and after parasympathetic denervation. Invest Urol 1977;14:322–328.
11. Gu J, Blank MA, Huang WM, et al. Peptide-containing nerves in human urinary bladder. Urology 1984;24:353–357.
12. Mundy AR. Neuropeptides in lower urinary tract function. J Urol 1984;211–218.
13. Polak JM, Bloom SR. Localization and measurement of VIP in the genitourinary system of man and animals. Peptides 1984;5:225–230.
14. Maggi CA. The role of peptides in the regulation of the micturition reflex. An update. Gen Pharmacol 1991;22:1–24.
15. Smet PJ, Edyvane KA, Jonavicius J, Marshall VR. Colocalization of nitric oxide synthase with vasoactive intestinal peptide, neuropeptide Y and tyrosine hydroxylase in nerves supplying the human ureter. J Urol 1994;152:1292–1296.
16. Dixon JS, Gilpin SA, Gilpin CJ, Gosling JA. Intramural ganglia of the human urinary bladder. Br J Urol 1983;55:195–198.
17. Lincoln J, Burnstock G. Autonomic innervation of the urinary bladder and urethra. In: Maggi CA, ed. Nervous control of the urogenital system. Chur, Switzerland: Harwood Academic Publishers, 1993:33–68.
18. Gilpin CJ, Dixon JS, Gilpin SA, Gosling JA. The fine structure of autonomic neurons in the wall of the human urinary bladder. J Anat 1983;137: 705–713.
19. Gosling JA, Dixon JS, Humpherson JA. Functional anatomy of the urinary tract: an integrated text and colour atlas. Edinburgh: Churchill Livingstone, 1983.
20. Dixon JS, Gilpin CJ. Presumptive sensory axons of the human urinary bladder: a fine structural study. J Anat 1987;151:199–207.
21. Wakabayashi Y, Tomoyoshi T, Fujimiya M, Arai R, Maeda T. Substance P-containing axon terminals in the mucosa of the human urinary bladder: pre-embedding immunohistochemistry using cryostat sections for electron microscopy. Histochemistry 1993;100:401–407.
22. Alm P, Alumets J, Brodin E, et al. Peptidergic (substance P) nerves in the genito-urinary tract. Neuroscience 1978;3:419–425.
23. Gearhart JP, Canning DA, Gilpin SA, Lam E, Gosling JA. A histologic and histochemical study of the ureterovesical junction in infancy and childhood. Br J Urol 1993;72:648–654.
24. Nergardh A, Boreus LO. Autonomic receptor function in the lower urinary tract of man and cat. Scand J Urol Nephrol 1972;6:32–36.
25. Von Hayek H. Die Muskulatur des Beckenbodens. In: Alken CE, Dix VW, Goodwin WE, Wildbolz E, eds. Handbuch der Urologie, Vol I. Berlin Heidelburg: Springer, 1969:279–288.
26. Parks AG, Swash M, Urich H. Sphincter denervation in anorectal incontinence and rectal prolapse. Gut 1977;18:656–665.
27. Zacharin RF. The suspensory mechanism of the female urethra. J Anat 1963;97:423–427.
28. Wilson PD, Dixon JS, Brown ADG, Gosling JA. Posterior pubourethral ligaments in normal and genuine stress incontinent women. J Urol 1983; 130:802–805.
29. DeLancey JOL. Structural aspects of the extrinsic continence mechanism. Obstet Gynecol 1988;72: 296–301.
30. Richardson AC, Edmonds PB, Williams NL. Treatment of stress urinary incontinence due to paravaginal fascial defect. Obstet Gynecol 1981; 57:357–362.
31. Anderson K-E, Mattiason A, Sjogren C. Electrically induced relaxation of the noradrenaline contracted isolated urethra from rabbit and man. J Urol 1983;129:210–214.
32. Andersson K-E, Pascual AG, Persson K, Forman A, Tottrup A. Electrically-induced, nerve mediated relaxation of rabbit urethra involves nitric oxide. J Urol 1992;147:253–259.
33. Nathan PW, Smith MC. The centripetal pathway from the bladder and urethra within the spinal cord. J Neurol Neurosurg Psychiatry 1951;14: 262–280.

CHAPTER 3

Physiology of Micturition

Alison C. Weidner and Eboo Versi

Introduction

The urinary bladder is an organ ideally suited for storage and timely expulsion of urine. The kidneys produce urine throughout the day and night, and continuous leakage would be both socially unacceptable and damaging to the skin. During the storage phase, continence is thus maintained by an interplay of structural and neurophysiological factors despite large fluctuations in intraabdominal pressure. During voiding, coordinated expulsion of urine via the opening of the urethra and propulsion forward of urine by detrusor contraction is further evidence of a complex neurophysiological mechanism of reflex pathways and volitional control. The exact mechanisms of continence and voiding function are not fully understood; however, a working knowledge of anatomy, neuroanatomy, physiology, and neurophysiology is crucial to understanding both normal and pathological function of the lower urinary tract. This chapter therefore focuses on neuroanatomy, neurophysiology, vesicourethral physiology, and mechanisms of continence. For each section, the summary is presented in italics followed by the detailed text.

Neuroanatomy: The Basics

The nervous system is divided anatomically into central (brain and spinal cord) and peripheral (nerves) systems that receive sensory input and mediate motor response. Functionally, it is divided into the autonomic and somatic systems. The former receives visceral sensation and regulates smooth muscle and therefore mediates unconscious and involuntary functions, and the latter receives somatic sensation and controls striated voluntary muscle. The peripheral autonomic system is comprised of a two-neuron chain: the neural (ganglionic) synapses for the sympathetic system are usually thought to be remote from the end organ, but the parasympathetic ganglionic synapses are intimate with the end organ, a distinction that has implications for function. In contrast, somatic motor signals are mediated by a single neuron that synapses directly on the striated muscle fiber.

The nervous system is divided into central and peripheral components: central comprised of the brain and spinal cord and peripheral of the cranial and spinal nerves and their ganglia. The peripheral nervous system consists of both autonomic afferents and efferents and somatic reflex systems. Smooth muscle receives autonomic innervation, and striated muscle receives somatic nerve input.

AUTONOMIC

Autonomic efferent function is generally subconscious and organized in a standard system of two neurons: the preganglionic, which has cell bodies in the intermediolateral cell column of the brainstem or spinal cord and axons that synapse onto the ganglion cells, and the postganglionic, consisting of the ganglion cells with axons synapsing on the end organ. Autonomic supply of the lower urinary tract has different origins:

the total sympathetic outflow is from T1–L2 and that of the parasympathetic from S2–S4. The complexity arises in arrangement of spinal nerve roots and ganglia that house this synaptic sequence. Each vertebral level contains a pair of segmental nerves, formed by the union of a dorsal (sensory) and ventral (motor) root. This union is called the mixed spinal nerve, which soon divides into the dorsal and ventral rami. Sympathetic preganglionic fibers run briefly in the ventral ramus and then separate from it to create the white ramus communicans, which leads to one of the paired chains of paravertebral ganglia (Fig. 3.1). The sympathetic preganglionic fibers synapse in these ganglia, and the postganglionic neuron travels through the pararectal (or parasaggital) plexuses to reach the target pelvic organ. The parasympathetic fibers originate in the sacral intermediolateral cell columns and exit via the ventral rami of S2–S4 nerve roots. They form parasympathetic bundles called the pelvic splanchnic nerves that enter nerve plexuses and proceed without synapsing to ganglia in or near the end organ. Thus, they have very short postganglionic fibers.

The visceral afferent (sensory) neural supply passes retrograde along the autonomic pathways, although it is not usually considered part of the autonomic system. These neurons arise within the bladder wall and epithelium of the proximal urethra and convey sensations of filling, stretch, and irritation (nociception). Fibers traveling in parasympathetic pathways to pelvic splanchnic nerves and to sacral spinal levels convey all three types of sensory signals. Those that travel with the sympathetic fibers to the lumbar splanchnic nerves and ultimately the lumbar spinal nerves convey only nociceptive signals (1, 2).

SOMATIC

The somatic portions of the nervous system convey and process conscious sensory information and motor control of voluntary muscle. In the lower urinary tract, the dominant sensory system is the autonomic. Two sets of neurons produce somatic motor (efferent) activity in the pelvis: upper motor neurons, whose cell bodies lie in the gray matter of motor areas of the cortex and brainstem,

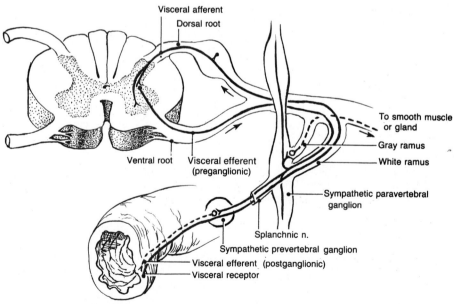

Figure 3.1. Presynaptic sympathetic neurons with cell bodies in the intermediolateral cell column of the spinal cord pass via the ventral root of the spinal nerve to the white ramus communicans to reach the sympathetic paravertebral chain. Here they either synapse or pass along a splanchnic nerve to a prevertebral ganglion. The postsynaptic neuron contacts the end organ. Visceral afferents travel via the dorsal root. The dotted line represents reflex signals elicited in the paravertebral ganglion by the efferent signal. (From April EW. The nervous system. In: Anatomy. New York: Wiley, 1984:33–42.)

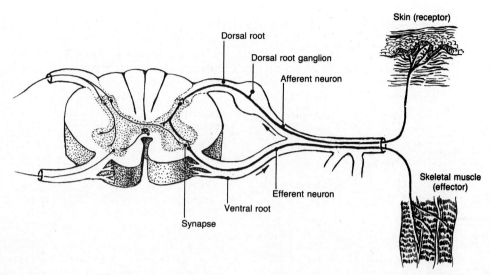

Figure 3.2. The somatic reflex arc. Somatic afferent neurons with cell bodies in the dorsal root ganglion convey sensory information from stretch receptors in the bladder to the spinal cord. The information is passed through small internuncial neurons to the motor neuron. The somatic reflex inhibits the efferent neurons with cell bodies in the ventral horn of the spinal cord, ultimately inhibiting detrusor contraction. (From April EW. The nervous system. In: Anatomy. New York: Wiley, 1984:33–42.)

and lower motor neurons, with cell bodies in the ventral horns of the spinal gray matter of S2–S4. Axons course from the lower motor neuron through spinal nerves to make synaptic connections with motor end plates on skeletal muscle fibers.

Sensory afferent somatic input from the periphery of the pelvis travels back to the spinal cord via the dorsal root and synapses in the sacral gray matter to form a reflex arc with efferent neurons. These reflex arcs can be simple, with one sensory and one motor neuron, or more complex, with various interneurons intercalated between them. The spinal region containing these complicated and poorly understood reflex systems is called the sacral micturition center, described below (Fig. 3.2).

Central Neuroanatomy: Central Modulation of Peripheral Control

The pyramidal detrusor area is the uppermost region of the central nervous system devoted to control of the lower urinary tract. Efferent axons travel down the white matter of the spinal cord to their specific destina- *tions: axons for the detrusor muscle control descend to cell bodies in the intermediolateral cell column and those for the periurethral muscle control to cell bodies in the ventromedial cell column. Ascending afferents travel to the nucleus ventralis posterolateralis of the thalamus. Various regions of the brain exert specific types of control and modulation of lower urinary tract function, generally in the form of tonic inhibition. Central nervous system disease thus generally results in detrusor hyperactivity.*

Cortical control of the detrusor muscle rests in the supramedial portion of the frontal lobes and in the genu of the corpus callosum, the region known as the pyramidal detrusor area (Fig. 3.3). Fibers arising from cell bodies of this region travel with other cortical axons in the corticobulbar tract via the basal ganglia and selectively terminate in the pons on the detrusor motor nuclei of the nucleus lateralis dorsalis. Efferents from each division of the neurological system then travel according to the principles described above. For instance, detrusor muscle control is via efferent autonomic fibers that descend to detrusor motor neurons in the intermediolateral cell column of the spinal cord from T10 to L2 and S2 to S4 (3, 4). Correspondingly, the cortical pathways controlling periurethral striated muscle (somatic motor innervation) origi-

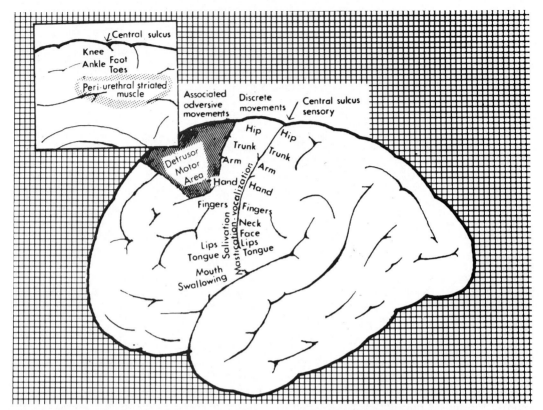

Figure 3.3. Central nervous system representation of peripheral structures in the cerebrum. (From Bhatia NN. Neurophysiology of micturition. In: Os- tergard DR, Bent AE, eds. Urogynecology and urody- namics: theory and practice, 3rd ed. Baltimore: Wil- liams & Wilkins, 1991:31–54.)

nate in the central vertex of the pudendal cerebral cortical area (Fig. 3.3) and descend to pudendal nuclei in the ventromedial por- tion of the ventral gray matter of S1–S3.

Sensory afferents from the pelvis ascend in specialized tracts: proprioception in the pos- terior columns and exteroception (pain, tem- perature, and touch) in the lateral spinotha- lamic tracts. Input from both sources runs to the cortex via the anterior vermis of the cerebellum (5). Ascending afferent fibers from the periurethral striated muscle travel via the nucleus ventralis posterolateralis in the thalamus to the pudendal cortical area, described above.

The net balance of frontal signals to the lower urinary tract is inhibitory, that is, these higher centers of the brain provide tonic inhibition of detrusor contraction. Frontal lobe lesions therefore chiefly cause loss of voluntary control of micturition and thus loss of suppression of the detrusor reflex and uncontrolled voiding. Similarly, the internal capsule is strategically located as the path- way of all cortical fibers to the brainstem, and the compact nature of the pyramidal tract there is susceptible to systemic occlusive vascular disease that can then result in de- trusor hyperreflexia due to loss of tonic inhi- bition (Table 3.1).

Most sensory afferent pathways from the detrusor and the periurethral striated mus- cles end in the cerebellum, which coordi- nates micturitional muscular activity and uses γ-amino butyric acid as a neurotrans- mitter. Disease in the cerebellum causes loss of coordination and therefore spontaneous high-amplitude bladder hyperreflexia (3, 6, 7). The limbic system is a common site for epileptiform activity and a known center for autonomic and emotional input. Although neither the role of the latter nor the neuroana- tomic pathways are clear, seizure activity in the limbic region may be responsible for the urinary incontinence that often accompanies such attacks.

PONTINE MICTURITION CENTER

Earlier neuroanatomic description of the micturition reflex suggested that the main relay center for afferent and efferent signals was the sacral spinal cord. Current understanding is based on multiple lines of experimental evidence that indicate that coordination of voiding function requires intact neurological anatomy in the pons and the sacral spinal cord nuclei as well as their connections through the long tracts of the spinal cord. Lesions above the pontine center cause release of normal tonic detrusor inhibition and lead to detrusor contraction and incontinence, whereas lesions between the pons and sacral cord generally cause voiding discoordination or dyssynergia. Other neuroanatomically distinct regions around this center may be active in modulating and transmitting the micturition reflex.

It was once believed that micturition was coordinated purely in the sacral spinal cord; however, various experimental data now suggest that the bulk of control is exerted in the rostral brainstem, in an area known as the nucleus locus coeruleus, also called pontine mesencephalic reticular formation (3, 6–10). This area represents the final common pathway for normal bladder filling and voiding. It has subsequently been designated the pontine micturition center, and the supportive sacral reflex system is the sacral micturition center. When the neural pathways between the pontine and sacral micturition centers are intact, micturition is achieved by activation of the micturition reflex, which results in a coordinated series of events consisting of relaxation of the striated urethral musculature, detrusor contraction, and hence opening of the bladder neck and urethra. This system is dependent on norepinephrine as the primary neurotransmitter as demonstrated by Yoshimura et al. (9) in cats using electrical stimulation of the nucleus locus coeruleus to produce a bladder contraction that was augmented by L-dopa, a norepinephrine precursor, and abolished by prazocin, an α-1 adrenergic receptor antagonist.

Lesions that interrupt these pathways have various effects dependent on the level of interruption. For instance, studies in cats show that neurons at the level of the inferior colliculus (the level of the pontine micturition center) are critical to the integration of the micturition reflex. Lesions above this point abolish input from more cephalad brain formations and facilitate detrusor contraction and hence incontinence by removing the inhibitory control (Fig. 3.4). The result is involuntary voiding that is coordinated in the sense that detrusor contraction and urethral relaxation happen together. A classic clinical example is seen in patients with Parkinson's disease. These patients lack the dopamine needed for neurotransmission in the basal ganglia, and the result is gait disturbance, tremor, and, frequently, incontinence

Table 3.1. Clinical Manifestation of Upper Motor Neuron Defects (Brain and Spinal Cord Lesions)

Lesion	EMG Findings	Urodynamic Findings
Multiple sclerosis (scattered demyelination)	Often markedly prolonged SRL, suggesting occult sacral demyelination. Delayed or absent evoked potentials, indicating lesions of ascending or descending spinal cord tracts	Variable, dependent on location of lesion. Range from detrusor hyperreflexia and detrusor sphincter dyssynergia to hypotonic bladder
Parkinson's disease (basal ganglia degeneration)	Normal	Marked hyperreflexia and pelvic floor spasticity
Cerebrovascular accidents (loss of cortical input to pontine micturition center)	Normal	Normal coordination of voiding but low bladder volume and lack of conscious control
Trauma (any spinal trauma between the pons and level S2–S4)	Normal	Detrusor sphincter dyssynergia

SRL, sacral reflex latency.

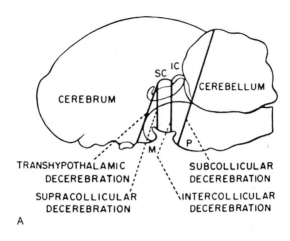

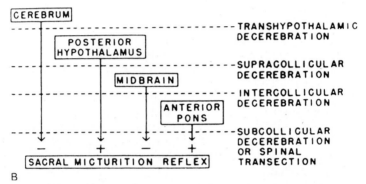

Figure 3.4. **A.** Drawing of a sagittal section of the cat brain showing various levels of brain transections made in the study of the supraspinal control of micturition. SC, superior colliculus; IC, inferior colliculus; M, midbrain; P, pons. (From Tang PC. Levels of the brainstem and diencephalon controlling the micturition reflex. J Neurophysiol 1955;18:583.) **B.** Diagram indicating the net facilitatory and inhibitory actions of the various levels of the brain identified by the transection procedures shown in **A**. (From Tang PC, Ruch TC. Localization of brainstem and diencephalic areas controlling the micturition reflex. J Comp Neurol 1956;106:213.)

from detrusor hyperreflexia (5, 6). More recent data suggest that this characterization may, however, be erroneous and that the changes seen in patients suffering from Parkinson's disease are age related and not disease specific (11).

Transsections below the pons but above the sacral cord, however, can cause partial urinary retention. These infrapontine/suprasacral lesions generally result in voiding that is uncoordinated with striated urethral activity in that the detrusor and urethra contract simultaneously. This clinically manifests as detrusor striated sphincter dyssynergia, a diagnosis that has been misused but technically requires a neurological lesion that interrupts the pontine/sacral axis (Table 3.1). Further evidence that the center for initiating micturition is seated in the rostral pons

rather than the sacral region is found in multiple cat experiments where interruption of the bladder afferent pathways by bilateral section of the L7–S3 dorsal roots abolished spontaneous bladder contractions but left intact bladder contraction and external urethral sphincter relaxation when these were elicited by electrical stimulation in the dorsal pontine tegmentum (9, 10, 12). One explanation of this data is that the rostral pons processes sensory input from the bladder and activates micturition.

This pontine reticular formation needs to be activated by a critical level of afferent input from stretch receptors in the bladder wall (1) and is modulated by areas above the pons such as the cerebral cortex but also other regions within the pons. For example, pelvic nerve afferent evoked potentials in the periaqueductal gray matter of the pons increased in magnitude with increasing bladder volume, but electrical stimulation of this area did not evoke a bladder contraction (10). This indicates that the periaqueductal gray receives afferent information from the bladder but does not itself initiate efferent signals for bladder contraction. Instead, it has a modulatory role on pontine function.

SACRAL REFLEX MICTURITION CENTER

The sacral spinal cord houses the detrusor motor nucleus and the pudendal motor nucleus that mediate local reflex arcs that further modulate the micturition response. Various models have been proposed outlining these reflexes in different animal systems, and it is unclear precisely which are most active in humans.

The sacral micturition reflex center of the spinal cord discussed above is actually located at T11–L1 vertebral level in the adult. Disparity in the growth of the spinal cord and vertebral column during adolescence causes the end of the spinal cord (the conus medullaris) to lie near the L1 or L2 vertebral body. Therefore, the roots of segmental nerves in this region emerge from the spinal cord at a point higher than that nerve's intervertebral foramen, through which the nerve leaves the vertebral canal. The conus medullaris in the adult is actually very short but houses the entire S1–S5 cord segments, within which are the important nuclei for micturition: the detrusor motor nucleus of the autonomic system in the intermediolateral gray matter and the pudendal motor nucleus of the somatic system in the ventromedial gray matter (Fig. 3.5). These nuclei are the loci of the proposed spinal reflex arcs of micturition that were first described by Mahoney et al. in 1977 (13).

These are a series of storage, initiation of voiding, and micturition reflexes proposed as a method of understanding the experimental events in cats where the sacral detrusor nucleus is divided into a dorsal and a lateral band, with innervation to the bladder in the lateral band (14). Strikingly characteristic of this region is the extensive collateral neural

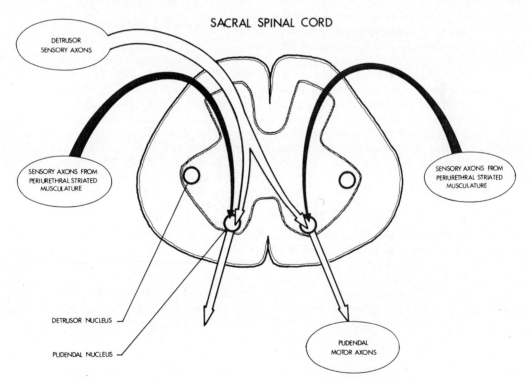

Figure 3.5. Diagram of sacral micturition center. (From Bhatia NN. Neurophysiology of micturition. In: Ostergard DR, Bent AE, eds. Urogynecology and urodynamics: theory and practice, 3rd ed. Baltimore: Williams & Wilkins, 1991:31–54.)

Table 3.2. Clinical Manifestation of Lower Motor Neuron Defects

Lesion	EMG Findings	Urodynamic Findings
Diabetes mellitus (peripheral neuropathy)	Prolonged SRL, suggesting denervation	Detrusor hyporeflexia and increased postvoid residual
Pelvic nerve damage (i.e., after simple or radical hysterectomy)	Same	Detrusor areflexia
Pudendal nerve damage (after vaginal delivery)	May have prolonged spinal, perineal, and pudendal NTML	Poor distal urethral sphincter tone, suggesting perineal nerve damage
Spina bifida occulta (variable, often profound denervation of pelvic floor)	Absent or weakly detectable SRL	Weak distal urethral sphincter with unstable detrusor contractions
Trauma to nerve level S2–S4 (location of sacral micturition center)	Normal	Detrusor areflexia

SRL, sacral reflex latency; NTML, nerve terminal motor latency.

projections that extend dorsally, ventrally, and even rostrocaudally in both gray and white matter (15). These collaterals may help mediate intraspinal integration of signals such as those controlling the sphincter reflexes (1). Three reflex pathways have been consistently shown in experimental animal models and probably have clinical significance in humans. A detrusor-urethral stimulating reflex exists in which increased detrusor tension stimulates urethral smooth muscle contraction to help maintain continence. In humans this is seen as rising intraurethral pressure in response to bladder filling. Periurethral striated muscle activity causes a feedback inhibition of detrusor contraction, and this has given impetus to the notion that pelvic floor exercises can, via this reflex, help to treat patients with detrusor instability. An increase in bladder pressure also triggers reflex ganglionic inhibition of the detrusor via visceral afferent fibers in the pelvic nerve, thus allowing the bladder to accommodate a larger volume (3, 14). Clinical evidence in humans of these local reflex pathways is easily demonstrated by the success of functional electrical stimulation (FES) techniques that use reflex responses to treat conditions such as detrusor instability. Controlled electrical impulses are sent over pudendal afferent pathways to sacral nerve roots, eliciting a reflex inhibition of detrusor contraction and improving cystometric findings in patients with detrusor instability (16). Reflex pathways must be essentially intact if FES treatment is to be successful. The importance of intact reflex systems is evident in a variety of clinical conditions involving lower motor neuron defects and urinary abnormalities (Table 3.2).

Peripheral Circuitry: The Lower Urinary Tract

The autonomic nervous system provides the bulk of neural control of the lower urinary tract. Dominant tone is via the parasympathetic system, which affects detrusor contraction primarily through cholinergic transmission. The parasympathetics travel via the pelvic nerve and arise in S2–S4. Sympathetic transmission arises in T10–L2 to form the inferior hypogastric nerves that join parasympathetic fibers to form the pelvic plexus. Adrenergic synapses predominate in the postganglionic sympathetic system, where stimulation produces both detrusor inhibition and excitation of the trigone and urethral smooth muscle. The distribution of postsynaptic receptors corresponds to the dominant regional muscular function: cholinergic receptors are dense in the detrusor, whereas adrenergic receptors predominate in the bladder base and proximal urethra. A number of related substances such as peptides, ATP, and prostanoids also act as neurotransmitters and neuromodulators.

The somatic neural supply is divided into motor and sensory fibers. Motor efferents arise in the anterior horn of S3 and S4 and supply striated muscle via both the pelvic and pudendal nerves. Somatic sensory afferents travel in the same pathways in the opposite direction to synapse in the intermediolateral column of S2–S4.

As noted previously, nervous input to the lower urinary tract is via three general pathways: parasympathetic, arising from S2–4 and traveling via the pelvic nerve; sympathetic, via white rami communicans, paravertebral sympathetic chain, and the hypogastric nerve; and somatic, via the pudendal and pelvic nerves from the anterior horn of the sacral cord.

PARASYMPATHETIC

Parasympathetic tone dominates the lower urinary tract during voiding and provides the primary excitatory input. Efferent cholinergic preganglionic fibers arise in the intermediolateral gray matter of the sacral spinal cord (S3, S4, and often S2) and exit the ventral roots as the pelvic splanchnic nerves (also called nervi erigentes). These bundles of parasympathetic fibers enter the paired (left and right) inferior hypogastric plexuses, extending to the pelvic plexus that is formed at the base of the hypogastric artery. These two plexuses merge into the pelvic plexus and travel on as the pelvic nerve to synapse in the wall of the bladder, a location susceptible to disruption by infection or stretch (Fig. 3.6). Transmission at these ganglia is by acetylcholine, the postsynaptic receptor being cholinergic, but modulated by purinergic and enkephalinergic influences (1, 8, 14). The ganglion cells on the surface of the bladder

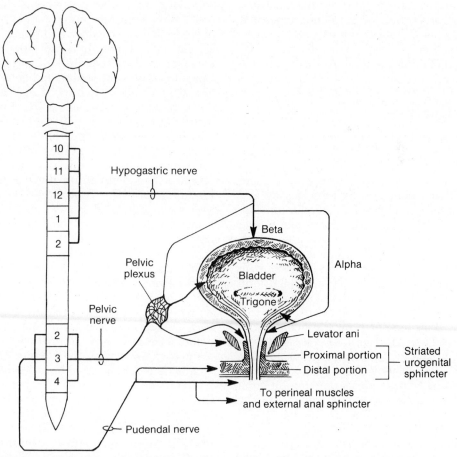

Figure 3.6. Peripheral innervation of the female lower urinary tract. (From Benson JT, Walters MD. Neurophysiology of the lower urinary tract. In: Walters MD, Karram MM, eds. Clinical urogynecology. St. Louis: Mosby, 1993:17–28.)

FILLING/STORAGE

Inhibition of
parasympathetics

Stimulation of
sympathetics:
alpha-contraction
beta-relaxation

Stimulation of
somatic nerves to
striated urogenital
sphincter

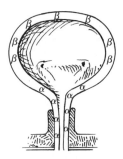

VOIDING

Stimulation of
parasympathetics

Inhibition of
sympathetics

Inhibition of
somatic nerves to
striated urogenital
sphincter

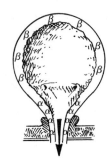

Figure 3.7. Actions of the autonomic and somatic systems during bladder filling/storage and voiding. (From Benson JT, Walters MD. Neurophysiology of the lower urinary tract. In: Walters MD, Karram MM, eds. Clinical urogynecology. St. Louis: Mosby, 1993: 17–28.)

send short axons to detrusor smooth muscle, which responds to the synaptic release of acetylcholine by contracting. This cholinomimetic effect on the neuromuscular junction is mediated by muscarinic receptors, indicated by histochemical studies that show a large proportion of ganglionic cells that contain acetylcholinesterase (1, 7). The overall function is to stimulate detrusor contraction and inhibit urethral smooth muscle (Fig. 3.7).

SYMPATHETIC

Sympathetic fibers, in contrast, emerge via ventral rami from the intermediolateral nuclei of T10–L2 to form the white rami communicans and synapse in sympathetic chain ganglia and then pass through the left and right prevertebral ganglia, lateral to the spinal cord. These postganglionic fibers form the superior hypogastric plexus from which flow caudally the right and left inferior hypogastric nerves. These nerves (together with parasympathetic outflow from S2–S4) form the above noted pelvic plexus at the base of the hypogastric artery. Neurons from this plexus then terminate on the bladder and urethra. Their function is to release norepinephrine and excite the smooth muscle of the urethra and bladder base and to reflexly inhibit the detrusor muscle and inhibit input to vesical parasympathetic ganglia (14) by suppressing presynaptic cholinergic release (Fig. 3.7).

End organ autonomic anatomy is intricate, as receptor types are distributed preferentially according to neural input and poten-

tial organ function. For instance, cholinergic muscarinic receptors predominate in the detrusor and are less commonly present in the muscle of the trigone and urethra. Acetylcholine diffusion across these synapses stimulates muscular contraction. In contrast, adrenergic receptors predominate in the muscle of the trigone and urethra. These are subdivided into alpha receptors, which are stimulated by high doses of norepinephrine and cause contraction, and beta receptors, which respond to lower doses and produce smooth muscle relaxation (3). The distribution of adrenergic receptors is such that beta receptors are prominent on the detrusor to provide relaxation of the detrusor with sympathetic discharge and alpha receptors predominate on the trigone and urethra to mediate contraction (Fig. 3.8). Thus, sympathetic discharge results in relaxation of the bladder dome and contraction of the proximal urethra—a continence action. The bladder neck itself is sexually differentiated. In the male, the muscle is more pronounced, has an adrenergic supply, and acts as a genital sphincter to prevent retrograde ejaculation. In the female, the bladder neck muscle is a continuation of the detrusor muscle and arranged in such a manner so as to open the bladder neck on contraction—a voiding action (17). Interplay between the sympathetic and parasympathetic input provides the balance of muscular tone for the detrusor. In contrast, the trigone and urethra are separate embryologically from the detrusor and have almost exclusively adrenergic innervation (Table 3.3).

SOMATIC

Somatic (striated) motor efferent innervation to the lower tract is mostly via the pudendal nerve. The cell bodies of the pudendal nerve originate in Onuf's nucleus in the anterior horn of S2–S4 (7), a region more resistant to degenerative processes that afflict other anterior horn cells such as amylotropic lateral sclerosis and multiple sclerosis. This may explain the often observed disparity between neurological manifestations of these diseases with regards to the bladder and striated muscles (12). These neurons exit the

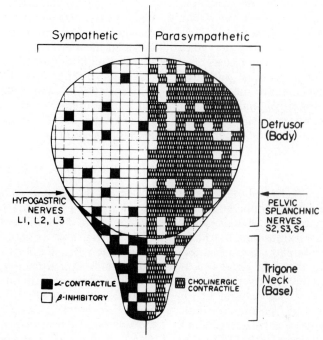

Figure 3.8. Distribution of cholinergic and adrenergic receptors in the bladder and urethra. (From Rohner TJ. In: Hinman F, ed. Benign prostatic hypertrophy. New York: Springer-Verlag, 1983;361–372.)

Table 3.3. Receptors for Putative Transmitters in the Lower Urinary Tract

Tissue	Cholinergic	Adrenergic	Other
Bladder body	+ (M_2)	– (β_2)	+ Purinergic (P_2) – VIP + Substance P – Neuropeptide Y
Bladder base	+ (M_2)		– VIP – Neuropeptide Y
Ganglia	+ (N) + (M_1)	+ (α_1) – (α_2) + (β)	– Enkephalinergic – Purinergic (P_1) + Substance P
Urethra	+ (M)	+ (α_1) + (α_2) – (β_2)	+ Purinergic (P_2) – VIP – Neuropeptide Y – Nitric oxide
Sphincter striated muscle	+ (N)		

Letters in parentheses indicate receptor type: M = muscarinic; N = nicotinic. + and – indicate excitatory and inhibitory effects, respectively. VIP = vasoactive intestinal polypeptides.
Adapted from deGroat WC. Anatomy and physiology of the lower urinary tract. Urol Clin North Am 1993;20:383–401.

spinal cord via ventral rami of S2 through S4 to form the pudendal nerve, which gives off the inferior rectal nerve before dividing into the perineal nerve and the dorsal nerve of the clitoris. The perineal nerve then supplies the urethral sphincter, the anterior levator ani, and the superficial perineal muscles.

The striated sphincter urethrae may have dual innervation by both the pudendal nerve and branches of the pelvic nerve via the pelvic plexus, but this is controversial. Data from an anatomic study indicate innervation via the pelvic nerve (17), whereas electrophysiological techniques suggest pudendal innervation (18). More distally, the compressor urethrae and urethrovaginal sphincter receive their innervation via the pudendal nerve (3, 8).

VISCEROSENSORY

Viscerosensory innervation of the detrusor consists of proprioceptive fibers in the muscle wall that transmit signals when stimulated by bladder fullness and free nerve endings in the mucosa and submucosa that transmit pain and temperature signals (1–3). These detrusor afferent fibers run in the pelvic nerve to the dorsal column of the S2–S4 spinal segments. Some afferents probably also run in the hypogastric nerve, which may explain why patients with T10 lesions can sense catheter passage and distension (3, 19, 20). In contrast, urethral sensory fibers travel mostly in the pudendal nerve to synapse in the dorsal sacral cord.

Sensory afferents are of two major types: myelinated (Aδ) and unmyelinated (C) fibers (1, 5, 19). Aδ fibers increase firing in a linear fashion in response to bladder distention within normal range of volume (21, 22). Higher threshold C fibers have been detected in cats and are postulated in humans. They are termed "silent C-fibers" because they do not fire until activated by chemical irritation, cold, or other noxious stimuli (23–25). Capsaicin is a neurotoxin that can be instilled intravesically where it causes an irritation that prompts the micturition reflex and diminishes bladder capacity. Research with human subjects suffering from detrusor overactivity indicates that intravesical capsaicin causes an initial detrusor contraction but subsequent improvement in bladder capac-

ity lasting weeks to months (14, 19, 25, 26). This effect is via a selective activation of receptors on the cell membrane of unmyelinated C fiber sensory neurons. This initially leads to membrane depolarization and signal transmission, but prolonged exposure has a selective neurotoxic effect of axonal damage and depletion of neuropeptides, which blocks signal transmission (25). Interestingly, urinary retention was not noted in the above experiments but could be induced at high doses in newborn rats, indicating a qualitative and quantitative difference in toxic effect on sensory afferents at different developmental stages (19, 27, 28). Probably, the C fibers act as modulators of the micturition reflex but are not necessary for normal voiding (14, 29, 30).

NONADRENERGIC NONCHOLINERGIC

Despite the predominance of muscarinic receptors in the bladder, it is well known that even massive doses of atropine cannot obliterate all detrusor contractile activity. This observation has led to the search for the postulated nonadrenergic noncholinergic (NANC) parasympathetic neurotransmitter system (1, 2, 7, 19, 30). By strict definition, a neurotransmitter is a substance released by a presynaptic neuron in response to a neural stimulus and acts on the postsynaptic membrane. Few of these NANC substances have been shown to meet criteria as neurotransmitters. However, a number apparently act in a modulatory fashion (Table 3.3). For instance, ATP is released by electrical stimulation of the pelvic nerve (1, 31) and has a concentration-dependent contractile effect on the detrusor (1, 19, 31) but probably acts as an inhibitory transmitter at the ganglion (7). ATP may release prostaglandins $PGF_2\alpha$, PGE_2, and prostacyclin, which may play a role in modulation of the micturition reflex by sensitizing sensory nerves and lowering the threshold bladder volume required to stimulate afferent signals to the brain (32, 33). These prostanoids probably contribute more to resting tone rather than directly influencing detrusor contraction (34).

Several peptides have demonstrable activity in the lower urinary tract. Neuropeptide Y (NY), substance P, vasoactive intestinal polypeptide (VIP), and nitric oxide have all been identified in efferent pathways in humans (1, 19, 35). Exogenous NY can inhibit release of norepinephrine and acetylcholine from postganglionic nerves and therefore block contraction, whereas substance P and VIP have smooth muscle relaxant effects (1). VIP is found in particularly high concentrations in the trigone and in pelvic ganglion cells (36) but is reduced in patients with detrusor instability or hyperreflexia, suggesting that loss of VIP may be either a part of the etiology or a consequence of this disorder (36). A large percentage of sensory afferent neurons also contain peptides implicated in the NANC network: enkephalins, somatostatin, cholecystokinin, and galanin are all detectable in submucosal and subepithelial layers of the bladder (14, 37, 38). Capsaicin administration causes release of these peptides from nerve terminals, suggesting a modulatory role in afferent nerves as well (14).

Clinical Applications of Neurophysiology

Current standardization of the technique for subtraction urethral cystometry and urethral pressure profile measurement makes their clinical and experimental measurements relevant. Microtransducers precisely spaced in flexible catheters allow measurement of pressures under conditions of rest and stress at various points in the lower urinary tract. Calculations are then possible that further describe the relationship of various anatomic points. The transmission pressure ratio is one such calculation that is used to describe the impact of intraabdominal pressure on various portions of the urethra. It is extrapolated into a description of the functional capacity of the urethra in maintaining continence.

Electromyography, evoked potentials, and other studies of pudendal nerve conduction provide another approach to the clinical evaluation of the lower urinary tract. Denervation resulting in suboptimal muscular function can be quantified with these methods. Obstetrical trauma is traditionally implicated as the cause of pudendal nerve injury, but controversy exists as to the extent of its role in the ultimate manifestation of incontinence.

SUBTRACTED URETHRAL CYSTOMETRY

The technique of subtraction urethral cystometry (SUCM) measures the intravesical and intraurethral pressures under periods of rest and stress. These measurements in normal patients and in abnormal patients, such as those with spina bifida occulta, can provide new insights into the management of lower urinary tract pathology. Various techniques involving balloon catheters and constant infusion methods have been used in the past; however, a brief review of the current terms and techniques is presented here.

Standardized SUCM uses highly accurate solid-state microtransducers as force measurement devices placed in specially designed urethral catheters as described by Asmussen and Ulmsten (39). The small size of the transducer (0.75 mm^2) ensures that these forces, interpreted as pressures, are measured over a small area. A urethral catheter with two microtransducers mounted, for example, 6 cm apart allows for simultaneous measurement of urethral and bladder pressure. Another catheter is placed at the vaginal fornix or in the rectum, allowing intraabdominal measurement. By measuring abdominal and bladder pressure, the clinician can distinguish between those events that are unique to the bladder and those that are common to all intraabdominal structures (40, 41).

The transducer does not measure hydrostatic pressure but rather the stress component at right angles to its surface. This results in a slight difference in the force measured depending on the orientation, with greatest force being measured when the receptor is placed anteriorly and the lowest when the receptor is facing posteriorly. Lateral orientation at 9 o'clock in the urethra provides an average measurement that is most reproducible at rest (42). For practical purposes, these force measurements can be interpreted as pressure measurements. The catheters are connected to an amplifier and to a paper recorder or to a computerized system. The output of the paper recorder or image on the computer screen can show traces of bladder, urethral, abdominal, and subtraction pressures, allowing easier evaluation of the re-

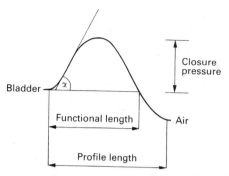

Figure 3.9. The resting profile. This profile is obtained by pulling the catheter through the urethra so that the proximal sensor passes through the bladder neck and passes out through the external meatus while the distal sensor remains in the bladder throughout. From this profile measures can be made of the maximal urethral pressures, the rate of increase of pressure in the proximal urethra, and also the profile lengths. (From Versi E, et al. Br J Obstet Gynaecol 1988;95:147–152.)

sults, especially during a rapidly occurring event such as a cough (43). During actual cystometry, the bladder is filled by a constant infusion of warmed or room temperature normal saline or contrast medium at slow (<10 mL/min), medium (50–100 mL/min), or rapid (>100 mL/min) filling rates. The infusion is either via a filling catheter placed alongside the measuring catheter or via an extra port in the measuring catheter itself. SUCM is carried out with the catheter static in the urethra and care is taken to avoid movement to ensure that the urethral sensor is always at the point of maximum urethral pressure.

URETHRAL PRESSURE PROFILOMETRY

By withdrawing the catheter through the urethra at a constant speed, a urethral pressure profile can be obtained. During such a withdrawal, the transducer passes the full length of the urethra from the urethrovesical junction to the external urethral meatus. This produces the urethral pressure profile, a recording that measures the urethral pressure at every point in its functional length, either at rest (Fig 3.9) or as the patient coughs repeatedly, creating a stress profile (Fig. 3.10, A–C). Recordings of resting and stress profiles are regarded as satisfactory if two consecutive profiles are the same. Measurements can also be taken with the urethral sensor at the point of maximum urethral pressure. The

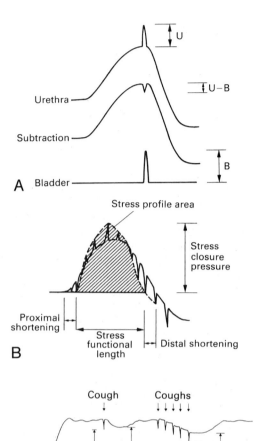

Figure 3.10. A. This shows how a stress profile is recorded. The top line shows the pressures at the proximal sensor as it passes through the urethra and the bottom line shows the pressures at the distal sensor that remains in the bladder throughout. The middle trace is the electronic subtraction. A cough spike is shown on the urethral and bladder trace. Note the notch in the subtraction trace due to the cough impulse being greater in the bladder than the urethra. (From Versi E, et al. Br Med J 1986;292:166–167.) **B.** The stress profile. This is the subtraction trace and the dotted line defines the profile. From it can be measured proximal shortening, stress functional urethral length, distal shortening and the stress maximum urethral closure pressure, and the shaded area under the profile. (From Versi and Cardozo. Prog Obstet Gynaecol 1990;8:193–218.) **C.** This shows recordings taken as the catheter is pulled out to the maximum urethral pressure point and then stopped. The effects of a single cough and multiple coughs are demonstrated at the point of maximum pressure. (From Versi E, et al. Br J Obstet Gynaecol 1988;95:147–152.)

patient lies still for 2–3 minutes while a pressure trace is obtained, and she is asked to cough once and then provide a series of coughs. The response to a single cough and to multiple coughs is measured on the subtraction trace by noting the instantaneous minimum pressure during the cough, the sustained urethral closure pressure after the cough(s), and the recovery time to the maximal urethral pressure (44, 45). Care should be taken to standardize bladder volume and patient position.

Transmission pressure ratios (TPR) are a measure of the differential transmission of the cough impulse to the urethra and bladder and are calculated as shown (Fig. 3.11). The functional urethral length can be divided into four equal lengths and the mean TPR computed for each quartile for each patient. The maximum TPR (TPRmax) can be noted for each patient (Fig. 3.12) as can the point on the urethra where it occurs (TPRmode) (46). In this way, 30 variables can be assessed per urethral pressure profile study (46, 47), but the most commonly used variables are the functional urethral length, the total urethral length, the maximum urethral pressure, urethral closure pressure, and bladder pressure. The clinical applications of these measurements and the related calculations are easily appreciated and are covered in Chapter 10.

ELECTROMYOGRAPHY

A second and complementary approach in the evaluation of lower urinary tract function uses electromyography (EMG), a technique that records electrical activity arising in muscle fibers during voluntary contractions and at rest. The fundamental concept of this technique is the "motor unit": the anterior horn cell, its axon, the axonal branches,

motor end plates, and the muscle fibers innervated (48–50). EMG allows the recording of action potentials derived from motor units in a contracting muscle.

Excitation of a single lower motor neuron normally leads to activation of all the muscle fibers that it innervates, that is, those that comprise the given motor unit. The recorded potential is a sum of the individual action potentials, and its duration relates to the anatomic distribution of end plates of those muscle fibers in the units under study. When partial denervation occurs, the intact axons that remain reinnervate the adjacent quiescent fibers, with the net result of higher motor unit fiber density (51). The EMG signal manifests this increase in the number of fibers, a finding indicative of denervation.

Three general techniques have traditionally been used to study EMG activity from pelvic floor muscles and urethral sphincters. First, surface electrodes are mounted on urethral, vaginal, or anal catheters and are placed adjacent to the muscle under study. The noninvasive nature of this technique inherently limits its assurance that the activity measured is in fact of the muscle under study and not a signal from adjacent muscle. Surface measurements are therefore particularly useful for motor nerve conduction velocity and terminal motor latency measurements, both involving initiation of muscular

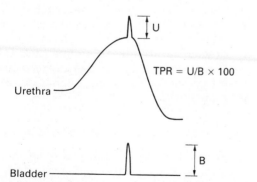

Figure 3.11. Calculation of the transmission pressure ratio (TPR) of the cough impulse to the urethra and bladder. (From Versi E, et al. Br J Obstet Gynaecol 1988;95:147–152.)

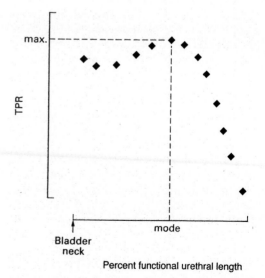

Figure 3.12. Distribution of transmission pressure ratios (TPR) with respect to functional urethral length. (From Versi E. Br J Obstet Gynaecol 1990;97:251–259.)

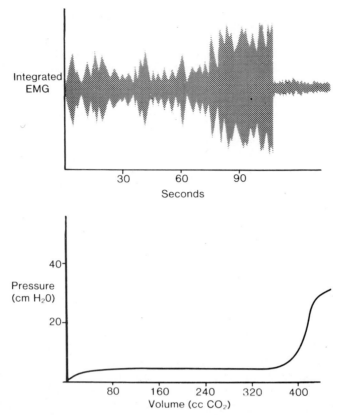

Figure 3.13. Normal combined tracing of urethral EMG done during a cystometrogram. There is a gradual increase in EMG activity reflecting urethral closure. This is suppressed before the detrusor contraction as the urethral sphincter relaxes. (From Bhatia NN. Neurourology and urodynamics: sphincter EMG and electrophysiological testing. In: Ostergard DR, Bent AE, eds. Urogynecology and urodynamics: theory and practice, 3rd ed. Baltimore: Williams & Wilkins, 1991:143–163.)

activity by direct stimulation of the nerve supply of the muscle under study (48). When done concurrently with urethrocystometry, however, surface EMG can accurately time sphincteric activity during detrusor contractions (Fig. 3.13) (49). Second, needle electrodes can be inserted directly into the anal sphincter, pelvic floor muscles, or urethral striated sphincter. These can measure local discharges, which is not possible with surface electrodes. However, needle electrodes can only provide information about a very localized region of muscular activity and cannot represent the sum activity of a given sphincter or muscle. Third, single-fiber EMG can minimize the limitations of needle electrodes by recording activity from only one muscle fiber in an individual motor unit (52). Single-fiber EMG by convention involves recording the mean number of single muscle fiber action potentials recorded by a single electrode in 20 different positions in the

same muscle (48). Under normal conditions, the average number of fiber potentials recorded for a given motor unit (or fiber density) is 1.4–1.5 (49, 53) (Fig. 3.14). Muscle damage will result in regeneration, but these new muscle fibers will require a nerve supply that they obtain from adjacent branches of a single axon. This new arrangement changes the amplitude and pattern of EMG signals in a characteristic fashion. This is interpreted as an increase in fiber density that has become a useful parameter by which to characterize prior denervation.

PUDENDAL NERVE LATENCY STUDIES

Evoked potentials and pudendal and perineal nerve terminal motor latencies offer related techniques that more directly assess the distal motor innervation of the pelvic floor muscles. The pudendal nerve has the inferior rectal branches that innervate the external anal sphincter and perineal branches that innervate the periurethral striated muscles. Conduction in the spinal cord, spinal nerves, and motor nerve fibers can be assessed by electrical stimulation at various sites and measurement of the latency of onset of response of muscles innervated by the pudendal nerve and its branches. Normal ranges exist for comparison (Fig. 3.15). The location and type of stimulus determines the neural pathway studied by evoked potentials, ranging from visual stimuli of the occipital cortex to detect retrobulbar neuritis in patients suspected of having multiple sclerosis despite normal neurourological findings (49) to transcutaneous needle stimulation of the motor cortex or sacral spinal nerve roots to detect abnormalities of pelvic floor innervation (48). Pudendal nerve terminal motor latency (PNTML) measurement works on the same principle as evoked potentials but is accomplished by electrical stimulation applied rectally to the pudendal nerve near the ischial spine and recording electrodes placed near the anal sphincter. Perineal nerve conduction measurements are done via an analogous intraurethral catheter.

Multiple studies of nulliparous and multiparous women using techniques of single-fiber EMG and PNTML have implicated ob-

stetrical trauma in the development of genuine stress incontinence, citing evidence of partial denervation of pelvic floor muscles (53–57). The populations included in these studies and the extrapolation inherent in EMG technique has made interpretation of clinical data somewhat controversial, however. For example, Smith et al. (54) performed single-fiber EMG of the pubococcygeus muscle of both normal women and patients with stress incontinence and/or prolapse. They found significantly more reinnervation in the incontinent group and concluded that denervation from birth injury likely contributed to prolapse (54). Barnick and Cardozo (58), on the other hand, argue that reinnervation might be considered a favorable outcome for muscle function and noted that more precise techniques of concentric needle EMG of the external urethral sphincter itself showed no difference in their study between incontinent women and continent controls, but unfortunately they did not study obstetrical variables. Direct comparisons of patients with respect to parity and number of vaginal deliveries found no difference between clinically continent and incontinent patients but did note an association between increased number of vaginal deliveries and distal urethral sphincter dysfunction in the normal group (59). In contrast, Sultan et al. (60) prospectively studied PNTML prolongation in primiparous and multiparous patients both before and after vaginal delivery and noted significant changes in PNTML and perineal descent, most strikingly after the first delivery. It is unclear whether perineal descent is the cause or effect of pudendal nerve damage. Furthermore, the role of the latter in the genesis of genuine stress incontinence needs to be defined. Nonetheless, the techniques described here do provide an important insight into mechanisms of continence even if their clinical role remains to be established.

Maintenance of Continence

NORMAL STORAGE PHASE MECHANISM

The urinary bladder is a high capacitance system that adapts easily to increasing volume without an increase in pressure until a threshold volume is reached. At that point,

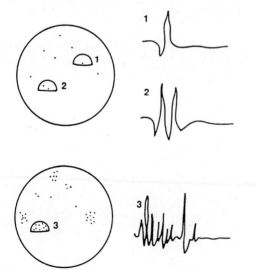

Figure 3.14.   Single fiber EMG. Areas of pickup (*1, 2,* and *3*) with associated recorded responses. *1* and *2* indicate normal muscle, and *3* indicates muscle with reinnervation. (From Benson JT. Pelvic floor neuropathy, electrodiagnosis. In: Benson JT, ed. Female pelvic floor disorders: investigation and management. New York: WW Norton & Co., 1992:157–165.)

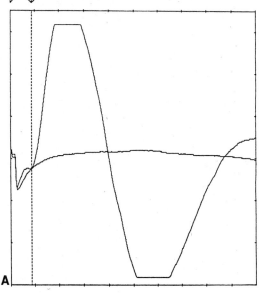

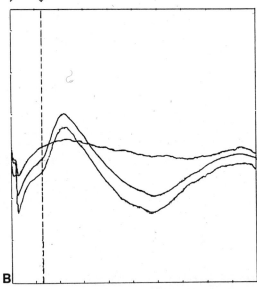

Figure 3.15. Pudendal nerve terminal motor latency. **A.** Before vaginal delivery. **B.** After delivery. Normal mean and standard deviation is 2.1 ± 0.2 ms. G, gain; H, high frequency filter setting; L, low frequency filter setting; PW, pulse width of stimulus; S, sweep speed; RR, repetition rate per second; SC, scale; AVE, number of averaged stimuli; T, time to receptor of L1 or cortex; DELTA, difference in the two times. (From Benson JT. Pelvic floor neuropathy, electrodiagnosis. In: Benson JT, ed. Female pelvic floor disorders: investigation and management. New York: WW Norton & Co., 1992:157–162.)

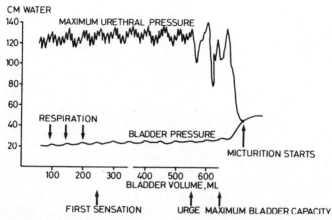

Figure 3.16. Simultaneous urethrocystometry (SUCM) during slow bladder filling. (From Rud T, Asmussen M. Neurophysiology of the lower urinary tract as measured by simultaneous urethral cystom-etry. In: Ostergard DR, Bent AE, eds. Urogynecology and urodynamics: theory and practice, 3rd ed. Baltimore: Williams & Wilkins, 1991:55–80.)

stretch receptors in the bladder wall initiate afferent signals via the pelvic nerve that reach the pontine micturition center. Central inhibitory signals override the reflex to void until overcome by increasing volume, voiding is initiated, the detrusor contracts, and micturition ensues.

The viscoelastic bladder wall is a structure with considerable capacitance, and during natural filling at the average low rate of infusion of urine via renal production, there is no bladder pressure rise. This is called accommodation and is a function of the passive elastic and viscoelastic properties of the smooth muscle and connective tissue of the bladder wall. The normal female bladder will hold between 100 and 300 mL of urine before the first sensation of fullness reaches consciousness. The bladder adapts, and pressure increases only slightly when the volume increases until at least 600 mL (Fig. 3.16). It is commonly observed that maximum urethral pressure increases slowly as bladder pressure increases (49, 50); however, some evidence exists that urethral pressure actually declines with bladder filling, and this decline is associated with stress incontinence (61). It is unclear whether this reduction of urethral pressure has functional importance or is an artifact of urethral pressure measurement technique.

Bladder filling also activates mechanoreceptors in the bladder wall and action potentials can be detected in the pelvic nerve in the parasympathetic pathway leading to S2–S4 (3, 4). Even after this point, however, further filling of the bladder will not cause a detrusor contraction if central inhibition is intact. With increased filling, the desire to void will increase but can still be inhibited with cortical signals descending on the pontine micturition center. At some critical volume (which is dependent on age, pathology, and psychogenic factors), it is no longer possible to suppress the pontine input, and voiding ensues. The normal functional bladder capacity of between 400 and 600 mL is well below the threshold at which inhibition is overcome (43).

MICTURITION

Actual voiding is a series of events of relaxation of the pelvic floor, inhibition of urethral sphincter contraction, followed by a rise in bladder pressure. Detrusor contraction results in opening of the bladder neck, and micturition continues until bladder pressure declines below urethral pressure and flow is interrupted. This usually occurs when the bladder is empty. The submucosal venous plexus surrounding the urethra aids in restoration of urethral pressure.

When the desire to void is felt and the social circumstances are appropriate, the micturition reflex is voluntarily elicited. Cortical signals act on the pontine center, causing its efferents to first inhibit somatic puden-

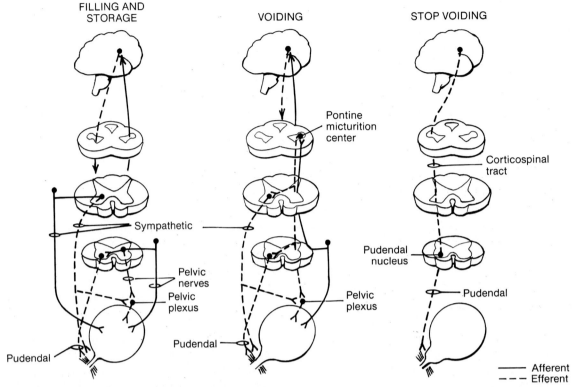

Figure 3.17. Summary of major neurological pathways involved in bladder function. *Storage,* bladder distention results in afferent pelvic nerve discharge. After synapse in pudendal nucleus efferent, pudendal nerve impulses result in contraction of external urethral sphincter. At the same time, afferent sympathetic discharges traverse the hypogastric nerve. After synapse in sympathetic nuclei, efferent firing causes inhibition of transmission of postganglionic parasympathetic neuron, which inhibits detrusor contraction, and increased tone in the proximal urethra. Net effect is that urethral pressure remains greater than detrusor pressure, facilitating urine storage. *Voiding,* afferent pelvic nerve discharges ascend in spinal cord and synapse in pontine micturition center. Descending efferent pathways cause inhibition of pudendal firing, which relaxes external sphincter; inhibition of sympathetic firing, which permits postganglionic para- sympathetic transmission; and pelvic parasympathetic firing, which causes detrusor contraction. Net result is that relaxation of external sphincter causes decrease in urethral pressure followed almost immediately by detrusor contraction and voiding ensues. *Stop,* voluntary interruption of urinary stream. Descending corticospinal pathways emanating from motor cortex synapse in pudendal nucleus, resulting in contraction of external urethral sphincter. Urethral pressure increases above detrusor pressure, interrupting stream. Subsequent to this, the parasympathetic-induced detrusor contraction ceases and detrusor pressure declines. (From Benson JT, Walters MD. Neurophysiology of the lower urinary tract. In: Walters MD, Karram MM, eds. Clinical urogynecology. St Louis: Mosby, 1993:17–28. Modified from Blavias JG. J Urol 1982;127:958.)

dal firing, thus relaxing the pelvic floor and external urethral sphincter, and then to stimulate parasympathetic S2–S4 fibers, causing detrusor contraction (Fig. 3.17). The sequence of events is first a relaxation of striated muscle, followed by a slow increase in bladder pressure. This shifts the balance of intraurethral versus intravesical pressure and allows urine to escape the bladder. The bladder neck is opened by the contraction of smooth muscle fibers at that location that are a continuation of the detrusor muscle (17). The trigone and vesicourethral junction drop caudally at the same time that the intraurethral pressure falls (Fig. 3.16). This indicates that the pelvic floor muscles cease to support the urethra and by this process facilitate funneling of the bladder outlet. It is interesting to note that bladder pressure during micturition does not need to exceed the maximum intraurethral pressure in the individual at rest except when a Valsalva maneuver is performed (43) (Fig. 3.18). In fact, cystometrics can demonstrate that in some women, especially older women, a decrease in the intraurethral pressure is the only change occurring at the time of initiation of micturition. This can be achieved by pelvic floor and urethral relaxation, resulting in loss of outflow resistance. Consequently, urine can run out sufficiently fast to empty the bladder within a short period of time without any significant detectable rise in detrusor pressure (43). This does not, however, mean that detrusor force does not contribute to voiding. Voiding pressure is a function of detrusor contractility and outflow resistance. Under normal circumstances, outflow resistance during micturition is low or zero, yielding a functional voiding pressure of the same. If, however, the patient interrupts voiding (the stop test) and outflow resistance rises, an isometric detrusor pressure is measurable. Some women routinely use intraabdominal pressure via the Valsalva maneuver to increase bladder pressure and thereby initiate or maintain flow or increase flow rate (Fig. 3.19). This is often unnecessary because the detrusor is functional, but in some cases, especially the elderly, such a Valsalva maneuver is used to augment a failing detrusor contraction. During normal voiding, however, the bladder pressure remains relatively constant. Periurethral striated muscles are reflexly relaxed as long as urine is running in the urethra (62). Micturition is continuous

and the bladder is completely emptied, and then the bladder pressure decreases and urethral pressure increases over the premicturition level and settles to a normal resting level.

When asked to interrupt urinary flow, some women can contract their pelvic floor musculature such that intraurethral pressure rapidly increases to a level that is adequate to interrupt the urinary stream (43). After this point, the increase occurs more slowly, and gradually urethral pulsations return as maximum urethral pressure is reached. The return of pulsations suggests that the submucosal venous plexus is being filled by blood and indicates its prominence in maintaining continence at rest.

It is known, however, from EMG studies that the striated muscle relaxes before the urethral vascular pulsations disappear and the latter only reappear when voiding is stopped (43) (Fig. 3.20). The vascular refilling takes approximately 10–20 seconds. This is the same period of time that it takes the urethral pressure to increase and stabilize. The synchrony of these events bolsters the critical importance of the vascular cushion in maintaining urethral seal and closure pressure at rest.

URETHRAL AND SUPPORT STRUCTURES: ANATOMY AND HISTOLOGY

The female urethra is a structurally tenuous organ that nonetheless contributes to

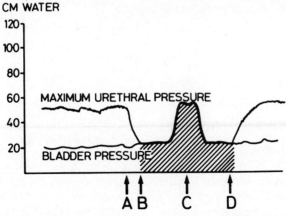

Figure 3.18. Micturition without detrusor contraction. **A,** urethral pressure falls; **B,** micturition starts; **C,** flow is increased by the Valsalva maneuver; and **D,** micturition is stopped voluntarily. (From Rud T, Asmussen M. Neurophysiology of the lower urinary tract as measured by simultaneous urethral cystometry. In: Ostergard DR, Bent AE, eds. Urogynecology and urodynamics: theory and practice, 3rd ed. Baltimore: Williams & Wilkins, 1991:55–80.)

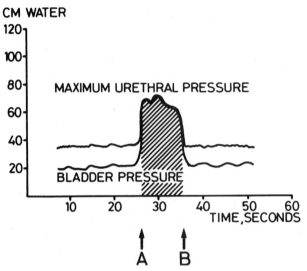

Figure 3.19. Valsalva micturition in an elderly woman. No pulsations of maximum urethral pressure are noted. **A** and **B** define the extent of the Valsalva maneuver. (From Rud T, Asmussen M. Neurophysiology of the lower urinary tract as measured by simultaneous urethral cystometry. In: Ostergard DR, Bent AE, eds. Urogynecology and urodynamics: theory and practice, 3rd ed. Baltimore: Williams & Wilkins, 1991:55–80.)

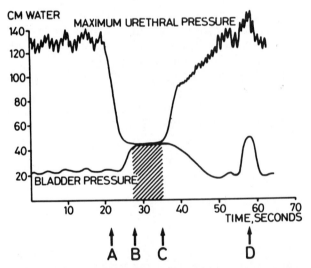

Figure 3.20. Micturition at a bladder volume lower than maximum capacity. **A,** Urethral pressure falls; **B,** micturition starts; **C,** micturition is stopped voluntarily; and **D,** pressure rises due to the patient's change of position, which is artifactual. (From Rud T, Asmussen M. Neurophysiology of the lower urinary tract as measured by simultaneous urethral cystometry. In: Ostergard DR, Bent AE, eds. Urogynecology and urodynamics: theory and practice, 3rd ed. Baltimore: Williams & Wilkins, 1991:55–80.)

continence via a variety of physiological mechanisms. A thick mucosa supported by a cushion of highly vascular submucosa provides a watertight seal and uses the cardiac cycle to maintain this seal without striated muscular energy expenditure. Collagen and elastin fibers in the submucosa provide an estrogen-dependent framework of support. Smooth and striated muscle fibers add a variable degree of closure pressure depending on their location in the urethra. Longitudinal smooth muscle contributes a constant portion of urethral tone. Selective anesthetic or operative block of either striated or smooth muscle disrupts a measurable portion of urethral closure pressure, indicating a contribution from both.

The female urethra is a short (3–4 cm) tube with an actual lumen only during micturition or in pathological states. Urethral closure pressure, therefore, is what provides coaptation and closure and is a critical element of the continence mechanism. Urethral anatomic structures provide much of the total urethral contribution to continence: the urethral mucosal epithelium, the submucosal vascular plexus, submucosal connective tissues, smooth muscle fibers in the urethral wall, and periurethral striated muscle are all integral to urethral function. The tension exerted by the smooth and striated muscle around and within the urethral wall compresses the connective and vascular tissues that form the inner part of the urethral wall and molds these tissues to form a watertight seal of the epithelium. The sum total of these components provides urethral continence (Fig. 3.21).

Complete apposition of the urethral mucosa is dependent first on its compressibility. Normal premenopausal mucosa is a thick highly folded surface. It is supported by a thick, spongy, submucosal cavernous vascular plexus. This plexus acts like a cylindrical cushion that helps maintain a hermetic closure along the length of the urethra by approximating mucosa to mucosa. Under normal circumstances, the urethral pressure demonstrates oscillations that correspond to the cardiac rate (Fig. 3.22) and the prominence of the pulsations changes with patient age, periurethral vascular integrity, and sex hormone status (63). In younger women, the urethral pressure oscillations can be as large as 25 cm H_2O, but with increasing age, the vessels become more thick walled and less elastic and the pulses diminish to less than 5 cm in the postmenopausal period (64). Estro-

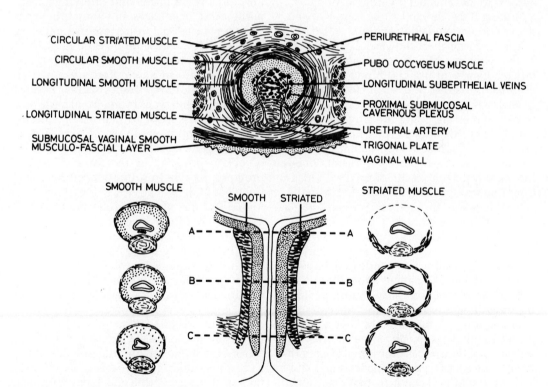

Figure 3.21. Urethral anatomy. The submucosal vascular plexus matures after puberty but undergoes great changes after menopause. Smooth and especially striated muscles decrease with age. The striated components become almost rudimentary. These changes in anatomy correspond well with the pressure changes presented in Figure 3.19. (From Rud T, Asmussen M. Neurophysiology of the lower urinary tract as measured by simultaneous urethral cystometry. In: Ostergard DR, Bent AE, eds. Urogynecology and urodynamics: theory and practice, 3rd ed. Baltimore: Williams & Wilkins, 1991:55–80.)

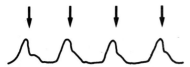

Figure 3.22. Pulsations at maximum urinary pressure. The arrows indicate occlusion of the aortic valve, which indicates a close connection to the arterial system. (From Rud T, Asmussen M. Neurophysiology of the lower urinary tract as measured by simultaneous urethral cystometry. In: Ostergard DR, Bent AE, eds. Urogynecology and urodynamics: theory and practice, 3rd ed. Baltimore: Williams & Wilkins, 1991:55–80.)

gen replacement therapy reverses this postmenopausal decline, but the effect is antagonized by progestogen supplementation (64). Maximum urethral pressure correspondingly declines with age from a maximum of approximately 120 cm at age 20 to an average of 40 cm at age 60 (65). This age-related decline begins around age 25 and does not appear to be affected by the menopause, a finding that detracts from an estrogen deprivation-related etiology (66).

The importance of the vascular plexus is further confirmed by observations of the effect of changes of urethral blood supply on urethral pressures. Raz et al. (67) demonstrated a one third reduction in urethral pressure after clamping the urethral blood supply in female dogs. Furthermore, reestablishment of the blood supply after bilateral common iliac artery occlusion results in an increase in the amplitude of urethral pulsations that was greater than expected from the actual increase in urethral pressure (68). Similarly, pharmacological treatment with alpha blockers decreases pulsations significantly just as alpha agonists cause a marked increase in pulsation amplitude (69). Experiments in the awake patient show that interruption of micturition causes an immediate increase in urethral pressure via external compression of the urethra by striated muscles, followed quickly by a return of a pulsation pattern as baseline tonus of smooth muscle once again predominates (Fig. 3.20). This is a similar pattern to that seen after reestablishment of the aortic blood flow in the study described above. Thus, it is obvious that the submucosal vascular plexus is of significant importance for regulation of urethral pressure at rest.

Of slightly more controversial role is the submucosal collagen and elastic tissues that occupy the deeper layers of the urethra. The walls of the female urethra are rich in collagen and smooth muscle fibers, which are arranged predominantly longitudinally and in parallel to each other. Collagen predominates over the bulk of the urethral length, but near the bladder neck elastin fibers are more numerous (70). The effect of estrogen here is thought to be similar to that noted in the skin of other parts of the body. In general, estrogen replacement therapy thickens skin by reducing collagen breakdown (71) and increasing water and hyaluronic acid content (72). Estrogen replacement after menopause reverses the normal decline in skin thickness by increasing collagen in a similar fashion (73). Urethral pressure profile changes, however, correlate with skin collagen content but not with skin thickness, suggesting that the mechanism of observed estrogen effect on the urethra is via collagen and implying an important role of collagen in maintaining continence at rest (74). Furthermore, recent work with relative expression of various types of collagen in normal and abnormal conditions suggests a role in pelvic floor dysfunction. Individuals with recurrent inguinal hernias express collagen types in abnormal ratios and defective cross-linkages that may create inherent structural weakness of tissues (75). Although this correlation holds true for loss of pelvic integrity in the form of genital prolapse, its role in urinary incontinence is not clear (76).

Urethral smooth muscle consists of a thick inner longitudinal layer and a thin outer circular layer. The function of the inner longitudinal layer is uncertain. Although it is difficult to explain morphologically how a longitudinal layer could act in maintaining continence, there is a variety of data that indicates a role for smooth muscle in urethral closure. Intravenous injection with phentolamine, a smooth muscle blocker, results in a 36–65% reduction in urethral pressure noted in various studies (77–79). It is reasonable to believe that part of this effect may have also been mediated by other vascular or striated muscle factors; however, studies of anesthesia administration bolsters the role of smooth muscle. Pudendal anesthesia, which blocks striated muscle activity, does not create incontinence (70, 80). McGuire and Wagner (81) performed bilateral rhizotomy, which denervates striated muscle, and did not find incontinence until the addition of (smooth muscle-blocking) spinal anesthesia. The role of smooth muscle in the urethra is probably also influenced by sexual differentiation. The detrusor muscle of the bladder consists of a complex meshwork of interlacing large smooth muscle bundles embedded in connective tissue. This layer continues into the bladder neck where it is more prominent in men than in women (82). In men, it acts as a genital sphincter to prevent retrograde ejaculation, but in women, on contraction of the detrusor muscle, it seems to open the bladder neck before micturition. Bladder neck closure is probably a function of elastin fibers (46, 83, 84). Csapo (85) demonstrated a relationship between actinomycin content of the uterus and estrogen status, and it is known that smooth muscle can be profoundly affected by estrogens (86). More recent work involves connexins, which compose gap junctions in smooth muscle. The expression of connexins seems to be controlled by sex hormones (87).

The exact contribution of striated muscle to continence is also not clearly understood. According to the work of DeLancey (88), the proximal portion of the striated urethral muscle fibers surround the smooth muscle layer described above. These striated fibers are incomplete ventrally and lie at variable position (usually 18–64%) along the length of the urethra (88) (Fig. 3.23). The distal striated sphincter lies in the so-called urogenital diaphragm and is of maximum strength at 54–76% of the total urethral length. Some fibers of the distal sphincter encircle both urethra and vagina (urethrovaginal sphincter), whereas others pass

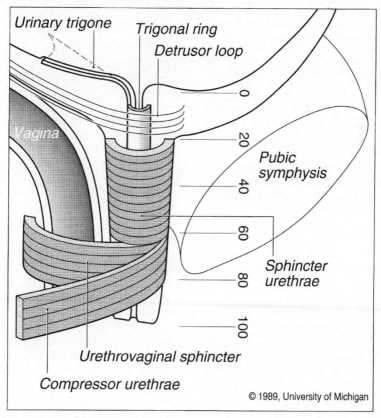

Figure 3.23. Diagrammatic representation showing the component parts of the internal and external sphincteric mechanisms and their locations. The sphincter urethrae, urethrovaginal sphincter, and compressor urethrae are all parts of the striated urogenital sphincter muscle. (From Wall LL, Norton PA, DeLancey JOL, eds. Practical urogynecology. Baltimore: Williams & Wilkins, 1993:17.)

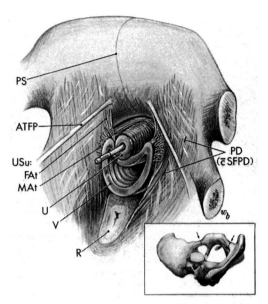

Figure 3.24. Proximal urethra and its surrounding structures, with the urethra (*U*), vagina (*V*), and rectum (*R*), transected at the level of the vesical neck. Shown with catheter in place for orientation. ATFP, arcus tendineus fascia pelvis; PD, pelvic diaphragm; PS, pubic symphysis; SFPD, superior fascia of the pelvic diaphragm; USu, urethral supports; FAt, fascial attachment; MAt, muscular attachment. (From DeLancey JOL. Obstet Gynecol 1988;72:296–301.)

out laterally and insert into the urogenital diaphragm near the pubic rami (compressor urethrae). The urethra and vagina are attached to the levator ani muscles through the pubourethral ligaments (30, 88, 89). Evidence of the supportive role of these ligaments is shown in early magnetic resonance imaging (MRI) research, which indicated visualization of disruption of these ligaments in patients with stress incontinence (90). During a voluntary contraction in an effort to hold urine, urethral pressure measurements show the greatest peak of pressure at two points: proximally, where the attachment to the vagina exists, and even greater distally, at the greatest concentration of urethral striated muscle (88). DeLancey theorized that the proximal peak is formed when the urethra is compressed during contraction of the levator ani between the vagina and a precervical arch running in front of the urethra between the arcus tendinei—the "horsebow" configuration (Fig. 3.24). The distal peak occurs in a region at 60–80% of urethral length, where the compressor urethrae and urethrovaginal

sphincter are located. This suggests that these muscles are active in creating the urethral pressure rise during "stress" and contributing to urethral closure pressure, as this peak is distal to the intraabdominal zone (89).

These views are nonetheless consistent with observations of pressure transmission to the bladder and urethra. Enhorning (91) was the first to describe that urethral pressure exceeded bladder pressure during cough in continent women but not in those who were incontinent. Further work emphasized the role of abdominal pressure increases in maintaining continence under stress, but there remains a role for striated muscle contraction. Importantly, Constantinou et al. (92) observed increased urethral EMG activity preceding the urethral pressure increase commonly noted during a cough. This EMG activity implies an active skeletal muscular contraction, which aids urethral closure during stress.

MECHANISM OF CONTINENCE

Local structural mechanisms that aid in maintaining continence are complex and poorly understood. A series of recent theories propose a variety of anatomic defects to explain clinical incontinence, but more recent research indicates that many of these "defects" are equally prevalent in continent women. Studies of the transmission of intraabdominal pressure to the bladder neck provide an alternative approach, proposing that the bladder neck itself must be subject to changes in intraabdominal pressure to create a pressure differential that maintains continence. These theories are best integrated with that of compelling cadaveric research on the ligamentous and soft tissue structural support of the bladder neck and surrounding structures. Future research will need to focus on the synthesis of physiological and anatomic data to accurately understand the function of this complex anatomic region.

Research in this area has been hampered because understanding of continence mechanisms is poor. Many early theories emphasized anatomic etiologies for failure to maintain continence. Lapides (83) and Lapides et al. (93) proposed one of the first theories of incontinence to blame the presence of an extremely short urethra, but this has not been supported by subsequent reports in which no difference was found in urethral length between continent and stress incontinent women (91, 94–98), and success of corrective surgery could not be correlated with changes in the functional urethral length (97, 99–101). This is hardly surprising as the mechanism of surgical correction apparently involves many factors and is not purely a matter of restoration of normal anatomy (98, 102). In a large study of 102 urodynamically normal women and 70 patients with genuine stress incontinence, there was a 10% ($P <$ 0.001) reduction in the functional urethral length in the incontinent group (47). However, the clinical significance of this finding is not clear, and the difference was not found to have diagnostic relevance due to the large degree of overlap between the normal and incontinent women. Jeffcoate and Roberts (103) suggested that loss of the posterior urethrovesical angle caused stress incontinence, and this proposition was strengthened by Green (99). This idea took hold for years, and cystography became often mis-

used as a diagnostic technique. However, in Jeffcoate and Robert's original description, about a fifth of the incontinent patients did not have loss of this posterior angle. This was subsequently reiterated when Kitzmiller et al. (104) showed that 26% of stress incontinent women had normal angles and 28% of continent women had an abnormal posterior angle. Similarly, Fantl et al. (105) showed loss of this angle in 98% of stress incontinent women, but they also demonstrated it in 94% of patients with detrusor instability. Hodgkinson (106) then proposed that if the bladder neck was at a higher level than the bladder base, continence would be maintained due to kinking of the urethra during stress, but subsequent observation revealed that only 30–70% of continent women exhibited this anatomic arrangement (104, 105). Hutch (107) proposed that if the internal urethral sphincter (bladder neck) was flat, continence would be maintained, but if there was funneling, then stress incontinence would ensue. However, Versi et al. (84) showed in a large study of 147 patients that

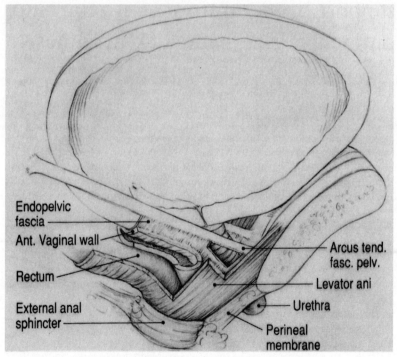

Figure 3.25. Structures involved in urethral supports drawn from dissection and three-dimensional reconstruction made from serial sections. Note connection of endopelvic fascia and vaginal wall that lie under urethra to arcus tendineus fascia pelvis and its connection to levator ani muscle. (From DeLancey JOL. Am J Obstet Gynecol 1994;170:1713–1723.)

19% of continent women had an open bladder neck at rest on fluoroscopy, and Chapple et al. (108) found a prevalence of 24%
in a smaller series of young asymptomatic
women. Furthermore, 51% of normal continent women in a population with a median
age of 50.4 years has been shown to have
bladder neck opening during coughing; these
women managed to maintain continence via
distal urethral sphincter mechanisms (84).

The complexity of the anatomic arrangement has led to more recent focus on pressure
differences between the bladder and urethra.
Enhorning (91) proposed that incontinence
will occur when intravesical pressure exceeds the intraurethral pressure. At rest, the
intraurethral pressure is greater than the intravesical pressure, and this relationship is
maintained during an increase in intraabdominal pressure if the pressure is transmitted equally to the bladder and proximal
urethra. It has been suggested that loss of
such transmission to the proximal urethra
results in genuine stress incontinence because of its displacement outside the intraabdominal position (81, 91, 94, 106, 109, 110).

This passive mechanism of incontinence
cannot explain all experimental findings.
Analysis of urethral pressure transmission
ratios reveals that before the cough impulse is
detected in the bladder, an active contraction
occurs in the urethra (111, 112), suggesting
the presence of an active mechanism. More
recently, DeLancey (89) suggested that continence is maintained because the vagina supports the bladder neck much as a hammock
and that the lateral vaginal supports at the
level of the bladder neck act like guy ropes
(Fig. 3.25). This hypothesis is fueled by information from cadaveric dissections (90,
113) and MRI studies (114). However, in both
cases the subject has been supine. If the
DeLancey hypothesis is correct, MRI images
in the erect position should reveal connective tissue discontinuities in this region. This
research is ongoing at the time of this publication.

Conclusion

An appreciation of the neural circuitry is
essential for understanding the function of
the lower urinary tract. Although knowledge
of this and neurophysiological mechanisms
allow us to understand the cause of incontinence in patients with nervous system disease, the etiology in most (neurologically
intact) remains obscure. Overall, detrusor
instability is the most important cause, but
we do not know its etiology in the neurologically intact female. The fault may lie at the
level of the detrusor, but if so, why does
behavior modification work? Most patients
presenting to the gynecologist have loss of
urethral support (genuine stress incontinence due to hypermobility) and yet we
know so little about its etiology. Is it due to
fascial disruption or pudendal nerve damage? Until we have a better understanding of
the pathophysiology, we and our patients
will continue to suffer from complications of
surgery or high failure rates of nonsurgical
management.

REFERENCES

1. de Groat WC. Anatomy and physiology of the
   lower urinary tract. Urol Clin North Am 1993;
   20:383–401.
2. Swash M. Innervation of the bladder, urethra
   and pelvic floor. In: Drife JO, Hilton T, Stanton
   SL, eds. Micturition. New York: Springer-Verlag,
   1990:17–39.
3. Benson JT, Walters MD. Neurophysiology of the
   lower urinary tract. In: Walters MD, Karram
   MM, eds. Clinical urogynecology. St. Louis:
   Mosby, 1993:17–28.
4. Kulseng-Hanssen S, Klevmark B. Continence
   mechanism. In: Drife JO, Hilton T, Stanton SL,
   eds. Micturition. New York: Springer-Verlag,
   1990:41–55.
5. Benson JT. Neurophysiologic control of the
   lower urinary tract. Obstet Gynecol Clin North
   Am 1989;16:733–752.
6. Bhatia NN. Neurophysiology of micturition. In:
   Ostergard DR, Bent AE, eds. Urogynecology and
   urodynamics: theory and practice, 3rd ed. Baltimore: Williams and Wilkins, 1991:31–54.
7. Chancellor MB, Blaivas J. Physiology of the
   lower urinary tract. In: Kursh ED, McGuire EJ,
   eds. Female urology. Philadelphia: JB Lippincott, 1994:39–53.
8. Mundy AR, Stevenson DP, Wein AJ, eds. Clinical
   physiology of the bladder, urethra and pelvic
   floor. In: Urodynamics: principles, practice, and
   application. New York: Churchill-Livingstone,
   1984:14–25.
9. Yoshimura N, Sasa M, Yoshida O, Takaori S.
   Mediation of micturition reflex by central norepinephrine from the locus coeruleus in the cat.
   J Urol 1990;143:840–843.
10. Noto H, Roppolo JR, Steers WD, de Groat WC.
    Electrophysiological analysis of the ascending
    and descending components of the micturition

reflex pathway in the rat. Brain Res 1991;549: 95–105.

11. Malone-Lee JG, Sa'adu A, Lieu PK. Evidence against the existence of a specific parkinsonian bladder. Neurourol Urodynam 1993;12: 341–343.

12. Blaivas JG. The neurophysiology of micturition: a clinical study of 550 patients. J Urol 1982;127: 958–963.

13. Mahoney DT, Laberte RO, Blais DJ. Integral storage and voiding reflexes: neurophysiologic concept of continence and micturition. Urology 1977;10:95–106.

14. de Groat WC, Booth AM, Yoshimura N. Neurophysiology of micturition and its modification in animal models of human disease. In: Maggi CA, ed. The autonomic nervous system: nervous control of the urogenital system, vol 3. London: Harwood Academic Publishers, 1993;227–240.

15. Morgan CW, de Groat WC, Felkins LA, et al. Axon collaterals indicate broad intraspinal role for sacral preganglionic neurons. Proc Natl Acad Sci USA 1991;88:6888–6892.

16. Sundin T, Carlsson CA, Kock NG. Detrusor inhibition induced from mechanical stimulation of the anal region and from electrical stimulation of pudendal nerve afferents. Invest Urol 1974;11:374–378.

17. Gosling J. Structure of the lower urinary tract and pelvic floor. In: Raz S, ed. Clinics in obstetrics and gynecology. Philadelphia: WB Saunders, 1985:285–294.

18. Vodusek DB. Individual motor unit analysis in the diagnosis of urethral sphincter innervation. J Neurol Neurosurg Psychiatry 1989;52: 812–813.

19. Maggi CA. The role of peptides in the regulation of the micturition reflex: an update. Gen Pharmacol 1991;1:1–24.

20. Sutherst JR, Frazer MI, Richmond DH, Haylen BH, eds. Basic neurophysiology and pharmacology of the lower urinary tract. In: Introduction to clinical gynaecological urology. London: Butterworth-Heineman, 1990:21–30.

21. Jänig W, Koltzenberg M. Pain arising from the urogenital tract. In: Maggi CA, ed. The autonomic nervous system: nervous control of the urogenital system, vol 3. London: Harwood Academic Publishers, 1992:525–536.

22. Torrens M, Morrison JFB. The physiology of the lower urinary tract. Berlin: Springer-Verlag, 1987.

23. Fall M, Lindström S, Mazieres L. A bladder-to-bladder cooling reflex in the cat. J Physiol 1990; 427:281–300.

24. Häbler HJ, Jänig W, Koltzenburg M. Activation of unmyelinated afferent fibres by mechanical stimuli and inflammation of the urinary bladder in the cat. J Physiol 1990;425:545–562.

25. Fowler CJ, Beck RO, Gerrard S, Betts CD, Fowler CG. Intravesical capsacin for treatment of detrusor hyperreflexia. J Neurol Neurosurg Psychiatry 1994;57:169–173.

26. Birder La, de Groat WC. Increased c-fos expression in spinal neurons after chemical irritation of the lower urinary tract of the rat. J Neurosci 1992;12:4878–4889.

27. Jancso' G, Kiraly E, Such G, Joo F, Nagy A. Neurotoxic effect of capsaicin in mammals. Acta Physiol Hung 1987;69:295–313.

28. Szolcsányi J, Anton F, Reeh PW, Handwerker HO. Selective excitation by capsacin of mechano-heat sensitive nociceptors in rat skin. Brain Res 1988;446:262–268.

29. Maggi CA. The dual sensory and efferent function of capsaicin-sensitive sensory nerves in the bladder and urethra. In: The autonomic nervous system: nervous control of the urogenital system, vol 3. London: Harwood Academic Publishers, 1993:383–401.

30. Cheng C-L, Ma C-P, de Groat WC. The effects of capsaicin on micturition and associated reflexes in the rat. Am J Physiol 1993;265:R132–R138.

31. Husted S, Sjögren C, Andersson K-E. Direct effects of adenosine and adenine nucleotides on isolated human urinary bladder and their influence on electrically induced contractions. J Urol 1983;130:392–398.

32. Jeremy JY, Tsang V, Mikhailidis DP, Rogers H, Morgan RJ, Dandona P. Eicosanoid synthesis by human urinary bladder mucosa: pathological implications. Br J Urol 1987;59:36–39.

33. Maggi CA, Evangelista S, Grimaldi G, Santicioli P, Gioletti A. Meli A. Evidence of the involvement of arachidonic acid metabolites in spontaneous and drug-induced contractions of rat urinary bladder. J Pharmacol Exp Ther 1984;230: 500–513.

34. Andersson K-E, Sjögren C. Aspect on the physiology and pharmacology of the bladder and urethra. Progr Neurobiol 1882;19:71–81.

35. Wall LL, Norton PA, DeLancey JOL, eds. Pelvic anatomy and the physiology of the lower urinary tract. In: Practical urogynecology. Baltimore: Williams and Wilkins, 1993:6–40.

36. Van Arsdalen K, Wein AJ. Physiology of micturition and continence. In: Krane RJ, Siroky M, eds. Clinical neuro-urology, vol 2. New York: Little, Brown, 1991:63–89.

37. de Groat WC. Neuropeptides in pelvic afferent pathways. Experientia 1987;43:801–813.

38. Keast JR, de Groat WC. Segmental distribution and peptide content of primary afferent neurons innervating the urogenital organs and colon of male rats. J Comp Neurol 1992;319:615–623.

39. Asmussen M, Ulmsten U. A new technique for measurements of the urethra pressure profile. Acta Obstet Gynecol Scand 1976;55:167–173.

40. Brubaker L, Sand PK. Cystometry, urethrocystometry, and videocystourethrography. Clin Obstet Gynecol 1990;33:315–323.

41. Versi E, Cardozo L. Urodynamics. In: Studd J, ed. Progress in obstetrics and gynecology, vol 8. New York: Churchill Livingstone, 1990: 193–218.

42. Hilton P. Urethral pressure profile at rest: an analysis of variance. Neurourol Urodyn 1983;1: 303–311.

43. Rud T, Asmussen M. Neurophysiology of the lower urinary tract as measured by simultaneous urethral cystometry. In: Ostergard DR, Bent AE, eds. Urogynecology and urodynamics: theory and practice, 3rd ed. Baltimore: Williams and Wilkins, 1991:55–80.

44. Versi E. Relevance of urethral pressure profilometry to date. In: Drife JO, Hilton T, Stanton SL, eds. Micturition. New York: Springer-Verlag, 1990:81–109.
45. Rai RS, Versi E. Urethral pressure profilometry. Int Urogynecol J 1991;2:222–227.
46. Versi E. The significance of an open bladder neck in women. Br J Urol 1991;68:42–43.
47. Versi E. Discriminant analysis of urethral pressure profilometry data for the diagnosis of genuine stress incontinence. Br J Obstet Gynaecol 1990;97:251–259.
48. Swash M, Snooks SJ. Electromyography in pelvic floor disorders. In: Henry MM, Swash M, eds. Coloproctology and the pelvic floor: pathophysiology and management. London: Butterworths, 1985:88–103.
49. Bhatia NN. Neurourology and urodynamics: sphincter electromyography and electrophysiological testing. In: Ostergard DR, Bent AE, eds. Urogynecology and urodynamics: theory and practice, 3rd ed. Baltimore: Williams and Wilkins, 1991: 143–163.
50. Benson JT. Pelvic floor neuropathy: electrodiagnosis. In: Benson JT, ed. Female pelvic floor disorders: investigation and management. New York: Norton Medical Books, 1992:157–165.
51. Anderson RS. A neurogenic element to urinary genuine stress incontinence. Br J Obstet Gynaecol 1984;91:41–45.
52. Ekdstedt J, Stalberg E. Single fiber EMG for the study of microphysiology of the human muscle. In: Desmedt TE, ed. New developments in EMG and clinical neurophysiology. Basel, Switzerland: Karger, 1973:89–102.
53. Neill ME, Swash M. Increased motor unit fiber density in the external sphincter muscle in anorectal incontinence: a single fiber EMG study. J Neurol Neurosurg Psychiatry 1980;43: 343–347.
54. Smith ARB, Hosker GL, Warrell DW. The role of partial denervation of the pelvic floor in the aetiology of genitourinary prolapse and stress incontinence of urine. A neurophysiological study. Br J Obstet Gynaecol 1989;96: 24–28.
55. Gilpin SA, Gosling JA, Smith ARB, Warrell DW. The pathogenesis of genitourinary prolapse and stress incontinence of urine. A histological and histochemical study. Br J Obstet Gynaecol 1989; 96:15–23.
56. Snooks SJ, Swash M. Abnormalities of the urethral striated muscular sphincter in incontinence. Br J Urol 1983;56:401–405.
57. Allen RE, Hosker GL, Smith ARB, Warrell DW. Pelvic floor damage and childbirth: a neurophysiological study. Br J Obstet Gynaecol 1990; 97:770–779.
58. Barnick CGW, Cardozo LD. Denervation and re-innervation of the urethral sphincter in the aetiology of genuine stress incontinence: an electromyographic study. Br J Obstet Gynaecol 1993;100:750–753.
59. Tapp A, Cardozo L, Versi E, Montgomery J, Studd J. The effect of vaginal delivery on the urethral sphincter. Br J Obstet Gynaecol 1988; 95:142–146.
60. Sultan AH, Kamm MA, Hudson CN. Pudendal nerve damage during labour: prospective study before and after childbirth. Br J Obstet Gynaecol 1994;101:22–28.
61. Awad SA, Bryniak SR, Lowe PJ, Bruce AW, Twiddy DAS. Urethral pressure profile in female stress incontinence. J Urol 1978;120: 475–479.
62. Barrington FJF. The nervous mechanism of micturition. Q J Exp Physiol 1914;8:33–71.
63. Asmussen M, Miller ER. Clinical gynaecological urology. London: Blackwell Scientific Publications, 1983.
64. Versi E, Cardozo L, Studd J, Awad D, Cooper D. Urethral vascular pulses in peri- and postmenopausal women. Neurourol Urodyn (in press).
65. Rud T. Urethral pressure profile in continent women from childhood to old age. Acta Obstet Gynecol Scand 1980;59:331–335.
66. Versi E. The bladder in menopause: lower urinary tract dysfunction during the climacteric. Curr Prob Obstet Gynecol Fertil 1994;XVII: 193–232.
67. Raz S, Caine M, Ziegler M. The vascular component in the production of intraurethral pressure. J Urol 1972;108:93–96.
68. Rud T, Asmussen M, Andersson K-E, Hunting A, Ulmsten U. Factors maintaining the intraurethral pressure in women. Invest Urol 1980; 17:343–347.
69. Ek A. Innervation and receptor functions of the human urethra. Scand J Urol Nephrol Suppl 1977;45:1–50.
70. Lapides J, Gray HO, Rawling JC. Function of the striated muscles in the control of urination: effect of pudendal block. Surg Forum 1955;6: 611–615.
71. Katz FH, Kappas A. Influence of oestradiol and oestriol on urinary excretion of hydroxyproline in man. J Lab Clin Med 1968;71:65–71.
72. Grosman NH, Vidberg E, Schou J. The effect of oestrogenic treatment on the acid mucopolysaccaride pattern in skin of mice. Acta Pharmacol Toxicol 1971;30:458–464.
73. Brincat M, Moniz CJ, Studd JWW, et al. The long-term effects of the menopause and sex hormones on skin thickness. Br J Obstet Gynaecol 1985;92:256–259.
74. Versi E, Cardozo L, Brincat M, Cooper D, Montgomery J, Studd J. Correlation of urethral physiology and skin collagen in postmenopausal women. Br J Obstet Gynaecol 1988;97:147–152.
75. Friedman DW, Boyd CD, Norton P, et al. Increases in type III collagen gene expression and protein synthesis in patients with inguinal hernias. Ann Surg 1993;218:754–760.
76. Norton P, Boyd C, Deak S. Collagen synthesis in women with genital prolapse or stress urinary incontinence. Neurourol Urodynam 1992;11: 300–311.
77. Donker PJ, Ivanovici F, Noach EL. Analysis of urethral pressure profile by means of electromyography and administration of drugs. Br J Urol 1972;44:180–193.
78. Nordling J. Alpha blockers and urethral pressure in neurological patients. Urol Int 1978;33: 304–309.

79. Mattiason A, Andersson KE, Sjögren C. Urethral sensitivity to alpha adrenoceptor stimulation and blockade in patients with parasympathetically decentralized lower urinary tract and in healthy volunteers. Neurourol Urodynam 1984; 3:230–234.
80. Krahn HP, Morales PA. The effect of pudendal nerve anesthesia of urinary continence after prostatectomy. J Urol 1965;94:282–285.
81. McGuire EJ, Wagner FC. The effect of complete sacral rhizotomy on bladder and urethral function. Surg Gynecol Obstet 1977;144:343–346.
82. Gosling JA. The structure of the bladder and urethra in relation to function. Urol Clin North Am 1979;6:31–38.
83. Lapides J. Structure and function of the internal vesicle sphincter. J Urol 1958;50:341–353.
84. Versi E, Cardozo L, Studd J, Anand D, Cooper D. Distal urethral compensatory mechanisms in women with an incompetent bladder neck who remain continent, and the effect of the menopause. Neurourol Urodynam 1990;9:579–590.
85. Csapo A. Actinomycin content of the uterus. Nature 1948;162:218–219.
86. Batra S. Oestrogen and smooth muscle function. Trends Pharmacol Soc 1980;1:388–396.
87. Andersen J, Grine E, Eng C, et al. Expression of connexi-43 in human myometrium and leiomyoma. Am J Obstet Gynecol 1993;169:1266–1276.
88. DeLancey JOL. Structural aspects of the extrinsic continence mechanism. Obstet Gynecol 1988;72:296–301.
89. DeLancey JOL. Structural support of the urethra as it relates to stress urinary incontinence: the hammock hypothesis. Am J Obstet Gynecol 1994;170:1713–1723.
90. Klutke C, Golomb J, Barbaric Z, Raz S. The anatomy of stress incontinence: magnetic resonance imaging of the female bladder neck and urethra. J Urol 1990;143:563–566.
91. Enhorning G. Simultaneous recording of intravesical and intraurethral pressure. Acta Chir Scand 1961;267(Suppl):1–6.
92. Constantinou CE, Govan DE. Spatial distribution and timing of transmitted and reflexly generated urethral pressures in healthy women. J Urol 1982;127:964–969.
93. Lapides J, Ajemian EP, Stewart BH, et al. Physiopathology of stress incontinence. Surg Gynecol Obstet 1960;3:224–240.
94. Hilton P, Stanton SL. Urethral pressure measurement by microtransducer: the result in symptom-free women and in those with genuine stress incontinence. Br J Obstet Gynaecol 1983; 90:919–933.
95. Toews HA. Intraurethral and intravesical pressures in normal and stress-incontinent women. Am J Obstet Gynecol 1967;29:613–624.
96. Fasal MH, Constantinou CE, Rother LF, Govan DE. The impact of bladder neck suspension on the resting and stress urethral pressure profile: a prospective study comparing controls with incontinent patients preoperatively and postoperatively. J Urol 1981;125:55–60.
97. Gleason DM, Reilly RJ, Bottaccini R, Pierce MJ. The urethral continence zone and its relation to stress incontinence. J Urol 1974;112:81–88.
98. Hilton P, Stanton SL. A clinical and urodynamic assessment of the Burch colposuspension for genuine stress incontinence. Br J Obstet Gynaecol 1983;90:934–939.
99. Green TH. Development of a plan for the diagnosis and treatment of urinary stress incontinence. Am J Obstet Gynecol 1962;83:632–648.
100. Obrink A, Bunne G, Ulmsten U, Ingelman-Sundberg A. Urethral pressure profile before, during, and after pubococcygeal repair for stress incontinence. Acta Obstet Gynecol Scand 1978; 57:49–61.
101. Henricksson L, Ulmsten U. A urodynamic evaluation of the effects of abdominal urethrocystopexy and vaginal sling urethroplasty in women with stress incontinence. Am J Obstet Gynecol 1978;131:77–82.
102. Hertogs K, Stanton SL. Mechanism of urinary continence after colposuspension: barrier studies. Br J Obstet Gynaecol 1985;92:1184–1188.
103. Jeffcoate TNA, Roberts H. Observations on stress incontinence of urine. Am J Obstet Gynecol 1952;64:721–738.
104. Kitzmiller JL, Manzer GA, Nebel WA, et al. Chain cystourethrogram and stress incontinence. Am J Obstet Gynecol 1972;39:333–340.
105. Fantl JA, Hurt WG, Beachley MC, Bosch HA, Konerding KF, Smith PJ. Bead-chain cystourethrogram: an evaluation. Obstet Gynecol 1981; 58:237–240.
106. Hodgkinson CP. Stress urinary incontinence—1970. Am J Obstet Gynecol 1970;108:1141–1168.
107. Hutch JA. A new theory of the anatomy of the internal urinary sphincter and the physiology of micturition: the base plate and stress incontinence. Am J Obstet Gynecol 1967;30:309–317.
108. Chapple CR, Helm CW, Blease S, Milroy EJ, Richards D, Osborne JL. Asymptomatic bladder neck incompetence in nulliparous females. Br J Urol 1989;64:357–359.
109. Asmussen M. Static and dynamic pressures of the lower urinary tract as measured by simultaneous urethral cystometry. In: Ostergard DR, ed. Gynecologic urology and urodynamics: theory and practice, 2nd ed. Baltimore: Williams and Wilkins, 1985:133–165.
110. Anderson RS. A neurogenic element to urinary genuine stress incontinence. Br J Obstet Gynaecol 1984;91:41–45.
111. Constantinou CE. Resting and stress urethral pressures as a clinical guide to the mechanism of continence in the female patient. Urol Clin North Am 1985;12:247–258.
112. Versi E, Cardozo L, Cooper DJ. Urethral pressures: analysis of transmission pressure ratios. Br J Urol 1991;68:266–270.
113. DeLancey JOL, Starr RA. Histology of the connection between the vagina and levator ani muscles: implications for urinary tract function. J Reprod Med 1990;35:765–771.
114. Richardson AC, Edmonds PB, Williams NL. Treatment of stress urinary incontinence due to paravaginal fascial defect. Obstet Gynecol 1981; 57:357–362.

SECTION II

Epidemiology of
Incontinence

CHAPTER 4

Epidemiology of Incontinence

Julie L. Locher and Kathryn L. Burgio

Introduction

Urinary incontinence is a prevalent condition with significant medical, social, and psychological ramifications. Incontinence is so common in older adults that it is often viewed mistakenly as a natural process of aging. However, incontinence is also a significant problem among middle and younger age groups both in community-dwelling populations and in those individuals with particular medical problems. The epidemiology of incontinence, including prevalence, incidence, type, and severity of incontinence, and factors associated with its occurrence may vary according to a number of variables (most notably age, gender, and illness). Most epidemiological studies of urinary incontinence have been conducted with older adults and are covered in Chapter 5. This chapter focuses on the epidemiology of incontinence in individuals under the age of 65. Compared with the literature on older adults, relatively few studies of incontinence have been performed in these younger age groups. We discuss the prevalence of incontinence, including nocturnal enuresis; its incidence and risk factors; and the epidemiology of treatment for this problem.

Prevalence and Incidence of Urinary Incontinence

STUDIES OF WOMEN

Most studies investigating the epidemiology of incontinence have either included only women in their study samples or re-

ported results separately for women and men. The prevalence of urinary incontinence in healthy nonelderly women residing in the community ranges from 11.3 to 62.7% (1–36). In one well-known study, Yarnell and colleagues (32) interviewed a random sample of 842 women (17–64 years of age) of whom 42% acknowledged incontinence. In the subsample of 348 middle-aged women (aged 45–64 years), 52.6% reported incontinence. In another community-based study of 541 healthy middle-aged women (42–50 years of age), Burgio and colleagues (17) found that 58% of participants had urine loss at some time and 31% reported incontinence on a regular basis at least once per month.

Among women less than 45 years of age, prevalence figures ranged from 24 to 52%. In a study of 4211 healthy nulliparous student nurses (17–25 years old), Wolin (36) found some degree of stress incontinence in 51% and a daily problem with urinary leakage in 16%. Similarly, Nemir and Middleton (14) reported that of 1327 nulliparous female college students, 52% had stress incontinence, although only 5% had urine loss on a regular basis.

Stress incontinence is reported to be the predominant type of incontinence, with prevalence rates of 14.7–52%. Mixed incontinence is also quite common with rates of 3.1–47.9%. Urge incontinence occurs less often with rates of 2.4–13.3%.

The tremendous range of prevalence data reported for incontinence in these studies is probably related to the great diversity between the study populations and sampling procedures, the differences in study methodologies, and the various definitions and methods for measurement of incontinence used by the various investigators. These issues are discussed in greater detail in Chapter 5.

Of particular importance in these studies are the ways in which incontinence is defined. Examining measures of frequency or severity allow one to make a distinction between occasional incontinence and regular or severe incontinence that might be seen as a clinical problem. Thus, although urine loss occurred in approximately half of the women surveyed, a much smaller proportion of these had leakage frequently enough to be considered a problem.

Another issue involved in the definition of urinary incontinence in epidemiological studies is the potential for lack of correspondence between incontinence based on the respondent's self-report and clinical or urodynamic findings. For example, in a community-based study by Sandvik and colleagues (1) comparing survey results with urodynamic findings, the survey found that 51% of incontinent women experienced stress incontinence, 39% mixed incontinence, and 10% urge incontinence. In contrast, urodynamic findings revealed that 77% of incontinent women experienced stress, 11% mixed, and 12% urge incontinence.

Longitudinal studies of the incidence of incontinence are lacking in middle-aged and younger populations. Two studies that coincidentally investigated the 3-year incidence rate of incontinence in women report similar findings of 8% and 4.7% (17, 18). In the former study, the criterion for incontinence was based on a frequency of urine loss at least once per month. This higher incidence rate of 8% was found in a group of healthy perimenopausal women who were slightly older than the women in the study reporting the lower rate.

STUDIES OF MEN

Prevalence rates for incontinence in men range from 2 to 11% (7, 9, 16, 34, 35). The epidemiological literature indicates consistently that men are significantly less likely to experience incontinence than are women. All community-based studies that examined gender differences in younger and middle-

aged adults reported lower prevalence rates for men than women (7, 9, 16, 34, 35). Moreover, the range of reported prevalence rates for men is much smaller than that reported for women. For example, although rates for men range from only 2 to 11%, those for women range from 11.3 to 62.7%. These findings have been attributed to differences in urethral length, anatomical structure of the pelvic floor, and the impact of childbearing on the continence mechanisms in women.

STUDIES OF CHILDREN

Once continence has been achieved in early childhood, it is usually maintained into adulthood. The literature indicates consistently that incontinence occurs less frequently among children compared with other age groups. Depending on the age group studied, prevalence rates range from 2.1 to 7.9% (34, 35, 37–39). In one study of 3556 7-year-old Swedish children, approximately 5% of girls experienced daytime incontinence compared with 3% of boys (38, 39). Girls were significantly more likely to experience daytime incontinence than boys.

NOCTURNAL ENURESIS

Nocturnal enuresis is generally defined as incontinence that occurs during sleep. It may be isolated or may occur concomitantly with other forms of incontinence that occur during waking hours. Several studies of the prevalence of nocturnal enuresis show that it is more common in children than adults. It affects approximately 30% of 5 year olds (40), 10% of 6 year olds (41), and approximately 3% of 7-year-old girls and 4–7% of 7-year-old boys (38, 39). Nocturnal enuresis experienced during childhood most often resolves spontaneously with only 4–5% of 12 year olds continuing to "wet the bed" (40, 42, 43). The prevalence of adulthood nocturnal enuresis is low and ranges from 1–3.7% (41, 44–46). Nocturnal enuresis is more common among boys than girls and among younger than older children. Enuresis is more common among younger boys than either older children or girls (38, 39).

Risk Factors for Incontinence

INCONTINENCE IN WOMEN

Several studies have explored the relationship between urinary incontinence and specific predictor variables, some of which suggest causal links between physiological changes and incontinence.

Incontinence in women is perhaps most often attributed to the effects of childbearing. Certainly incontinence is a common concomitant of pregnancy. Three studies of incontinence during pregnancy have revealed prevalence rates of 30.6, 46.4, and 59.5% (13, 20, 47). Although most women recover urine control spontaneously in the weeks or months after delivery, urine loss persists in some, and the effects of childbearing may predispose these women to develop incontinence in the future.

The role of childbearing in predisposing women to incontinence is supported by several studies that have demonstrated a link between incontinence and parity (6, 19, 25, 31, 34, 47). Thomas and colleagues (34) reported in 1980 that incontinence was more common in parous than nulliparous women at all ages (15–64 years) and that it was most common in women who had four or more children. Holst and Wilson (27) reported that incontinence was less common in nulliparous women than women who had one child but that incontinence changed little with increasing parity. However, Jolleys (25) suggested that the relationship was linear with increasing parity associated with increasing rates of incontinence. In addition, pregnant women with incontinence have been found in one study to have a history of more pregnancies and more births than pregnant women who were continent (47).

Inconsistent with these findings are two studies that found no association between parity and incontinence. Hording and colleagues (30) found that the frequency of urinary incontinence in 45-year-old women did not increase with higher parity. Burgio and colleagues (17) found that healthy perimenopausal women with incontinence did not deliver more children than continent women. Therefore, the nature of the relationship between childbearing and incontinence remains somewhat unclear.

Incontinence is often attributed to aging and associated with age-related changes such as decreased bladder capacity or loss of estrogen. Some studies have shown a relationship between incontinence and age (8, 11, 15, 18, 19, 21, 34).

In women, the relationship between age and incontinence is not always a consistent one. This means that at the aggregate level, it is not necessarily the case that older women are more likely to experience incontinence than younger women. For example, although some studies present a monotonic relationship between increasing age and increasing prevalence of incontinence (3, 8, 21), others have reported no relationship (17) or that incontinence is more prevalent in women in their 30s and 40s than in other age groups, including those over 60 (11, 15).

The literature has not provided support for the role of menopause and estrogen loss as significant contributors to incontinence. One study of menopause status found that among 45-year-old women, the frequency of incontinence was not higher among those who were postmenopausal compared with those who were premenopausal (30). Another study found that postmenopausal women were actually less likely to have incontinence on a regular basis (17). A third study showed a significantly lower prevalence rate among postmenopausal women (35%) than among premenopausal women (47%) (25).

There appears to be epidemiological support for the role of obesity in incontinence. Incontinence in women has been associated with higher body mass index (2, 17) and greater weight (19, 31). In one study, a significant monotonic relationship was found between urinary incontinence and body mass index such that women with regular incontinence had the highest mean body mass index and those who had never been incontinent had the lowest mean body mass index. A link between body mass and incontinence supports the concept that weight gain may increase susceptibility to incontinence and suggests that weight loss may decrease incontinence. Despite anecdotal reports of improved urine control associated with weight loss, the effectiveness of weight loss as an intervention has yet to be tested.

There is also evidence that white women may be more susceptible to incontinence than black women. Data on perimenopausal women indicate that white women were more likely than black women to report regular incontinence at least once per month and also more likely to report even infrequent incontinence (17). Racial differences have also been reported among pregnant women. However, the differences were evident only for stress incontinence and not for urge incontinence or other types of urine leakage (47). In addition, Bump (48), in a clinical study of patients referred for evaluation of incontinence or prolapse, found that a larger proportion of white women reported symptoms of stress incontinence (31% versus 7%), and a larger proportion were diagnosed urodynamically as having genuine stress incontinence (61% versus 27%). These findings among white women may be due to a relative weakness of pelvic support.

Other published articles have reported correlations between incontinence and several other variables including cystitis or urinary tract infection (2, 36), previous hysterectomy (8), other gynecological surgery (6, 25), use of diuretics (19), perineal suturing (25), cystocele (30), uterine prolapse (30) impaired function of the levator muscles (30), childhood bed wetting (5), and current and former cigarette smoking (49).

Urinary Incontinence and Medical Problems

Particularly in younger individuals, incontinence can often be attributed to a medical problem, disease, or injury that disrupts the mechanisms of continence. Three groups that have received particular attention in the epidemiological literature are those who are hospitalized or homebound, those who have undergone prostate surgery, and those who have experienced a spinal cord injury.

INCONTINENCE IN MEDICALLY ILL PATIENTS

Few epidemiological studies of community-dwelling populations have focused specifically on persons who are ill. Mohide

and colleagues (28) in their study of patients receiving home health care reported that 22% of patients experienced incontinence as documented by nurses. Fonda and associates (50) studied patients in an acute care teaching hospital and reported an incontinence rate of 23.4%. In 28% of these cases, the incontinence lasted for longer than 10 days. Persons who experienced incontinence were significantly more likely to be older, to have a greater length of hospital stay, and to experience a higher rate of mortality than the continent general hospital population. In another study reporting on incontinence in two general hospitals, Egan and associates (51) found rates of 5 and 7%, respectively, in patients aged 5–64 years. Data were based on staff recording of incontinent episodes and therefore may underestimate the actual rates of incontinence.

INCONTINENCE SECONDARY TO PROSTATECTOMY

Prostate cancer is the most common form of cancer in men, accounting for approximately 28% of cancer diagnosis in 1993 (52). The most common form of treatment of localized prostate cancer is radiation therapy or radical prostatectomy, with radical prostatectomy becoming increasingly the preferred treatment over the past decade (53). One of the most common complications of prostatectomy is postoperative urinary incontinence (54, 55). After removal of the catheter after surgery, most men experience continual leakage of urine. Studies that have followed men postoperatively indicate that 27–50% of men are incontinent 3 months after surgery, 8–33% are incontinent at 6 months, and 5–23% are incontinent at 1 year (56–63). There is some evidence that younger men are less likely to experience incontinence after radical retropubic prostatectomy than older men (64). Postprostatectomy incontinence is most often attributed to urethral or sphincter damage. However, urodynamic findings of one study indicate that detrusor instability is present in 61% of cases compared with stress incontinence found in 5% of cases and mixed detrusor instability and stress in 34% of cases (65).

INCONTINENCE SECONDARY TO SPINAL CORD INJURY

Morbidity related to urological dysfunction including incontinence as a result of injury to the spinal cord is a commonly experienced problem. Van Kerrebroeck and colleagues (66) report incident rates of 34.4% for persistent severe incontinence requiring absorption or collection devices in individuals who experienced spinal cord injury. Incontinence after spinal cord injury was more common in women (60.8%) than men (25.7%) (66). The most common cause of incontinence related to spinal cord injury reported by these investigators was detrusor hyperreflexia. Mohide and associates (28) studied patients receiving home health care and reported that degenerative disorders, including multiple sclerosis and spinal cord injury, were common in younger patients likely to be incontinent.

Seeking Treatment

Several studies have examined how people respond to incontinence and whether they have told a health care provider about their incontinence or sought treatment for their incontinence. Most studies have reported on women and reveal that most women do not seek treatment for their incontinence (17, 25, 27). In middle-aged women, Burgio and associates (17) found that only 25.5% of respondents sought treatment for their incontinence. Similarly, Holst and Wilson (27) found in their New Zealand sample that only one third of women sought treatment for incontinence and that most of those who did not seek treatment (81%) perceived incontinence as normal. Ten percent of women also believed that there was no benefit to be gained from treatment. Similarly, Jolleys (25) found that 35% of women who had not told their doctor about their incontinence thought that their incontinence was not a serious enough problem. Ten percent thought of their incontinence as typical for women, and 4% were too embarrassed to speak with their doctors about incontinence. Rekers and colleagues (11) reported that 26.1% of their sample aged 35–80 sought treatment and that premeno-

pausal women were even more likely to seek treatment at 38.2%.

Prevalence rates of incontinence may not reflect the need for treatment of incontinence. This chapter highlights the rather high prevalence rates among young and middle-aged persons yet the low rates of seeking treatment. Most epidemiological studies focus on the prevalence and incidence of incontinence, type and severity of incontinence, and the factors associated with incontinence. On their own, these data provide incomplete insight into what factors might account for treatment-seeking behavior. Burgio and collages (67) found that seeking treatment for incontinence was associated not only with severity of incontinence but also with the extent to which the incontinence restricted their activity and affected their mood. Other studies also have indicated that seeking treatment is related to individuals' beliefs and perceptions regarding incontinence (25, 27). Thus, to fully understand the impact of incontinence and needs for clinical services and the barriers to service utilization, future epidemiological studies should address a broad range of factors including psychosocial issues and perceptions.

REFERENCES

1. Sandvik H, Hunskaar S, Vanvik A, Seim A, Hermstad R. Diagnostic classification of female urinary incontinence: an epidemiological survey corrected for validity. J Clin Epidemiol 1995;48: 338–343.
2. Mommsen S, Foldspang A. Body mass index and adult female urinary incontinence. World J Urol 1994;12:319–322.
3. Nielsen AF, Walter S. Epidemiology of infrequent voiding and association symptoms. Scand J Urol Nephrol 1994;157(suppl):49–53.
4. Mommsen S, Foldspang A, Elving L, Lam GW. Association between urinary incontinence in women and a previous history of surgery. Br J Urol 1993;72:30–37.
5. Foldspang A, Mommsen S. Adult female urinary incontinence and childhood bedwetting. J Urol 1994;152:85–88.
6. Harrison GL, Memel DS. Urinary incontinence in women: its prevalence and its management in a health promotion clinic. Br J Gen Pract 1994;44: 149–152.
7. Lagace EA, Hansen W, Hickner JM. Prevalence and severity of urinary incontinence in ambulatory adults: an UPRNet study. J Fam Pract 1993; 36:610–614.

8. Milsom I, Ekelund P, Molander U, Arvidsson L, Areskoug B. The influence of age, parity, oral contraception, hysterectomy and menopause on the prevalence of urinary incontinence in women. J Urol 1993;149:1459–1462.

9. Brocklehurst JC. Urinary incontinence in the community analysis of a MORI poll. BMJ 1993; 306:832–834.

10. Foldspang A, Mommsen S, Lam GW, Elving L. Parity as a correlate of adult female urinary incontinence prevalence. J Epidemiol Commun Health 1992;46:595–600.

11. Rekers H, Drogendijk AC, Valkenburg HA, Riphagen F. The menopause, urinary incontinence and other symptoms of the genito-urinary tract. Maturitas 1992;15:101–111.

12. Minaire P, Jacquetin B. The prevalence of female urinary incontinence in general practice [abstract]. J Gynecol Obstet Biol Reprod 1992;21: 731–738.

13. Metanyi S. Urinary incontinence in pregnancy and puerperium [abstract]. Orvosi Hetilap 1992; 133:2551–2553.

14. Nemir A, Middleton RP. Stress incontinence in young nulliparous women: statistical study. Am J Obstet Gynecol 1954;68:1166–1168.

15. Rekers H, Drogendijk AC, Valkenburg H, Riphagen F. Urinary incontinence in women from 35 to 79 years of age: prevalence and consequences. Eur J Obstet Gynecol Reprod Biol 1992;43: 229–234.

16. O'Brien J, Austin M, Sethi P, O'Boyle P. Urinary incontinence: prevalence, need for treatment, and effectiveness of intervention by nurse. BMJ 1991;303:1308–1312.

17. Burgio KL, Matthews KA, Engel BT. Prevalence, incidence and correlates of urinary incontinence in healthy, middle-aged women. J Urol 1991;146: 1225–1229.

18. Krsnjavi H, Uglesic M. Urinary incontinence in female workers in the area of Zagreb [abstract]. Arch Za Higijenu Reda Toksikol 1991;43: 235–238.

19. Simeonova Z, Bengtsson C. Prevalence of urinary incontinence among women at a Swedish primary health care center. Scand J Private Health Care 1990;8:203–206.

20. Mellier G. Delille MA. Urinary disorders during pregnancy and post-partum [abstract]. Rev Franc Gynecol Obstet 1990;85:525–528.

21. Lam GW, Foldspang A, Elving LB, Mommsen S. Urinary incontinence in women aged 30–59 years. An epidemiological study. Ugeskrift for Laeger 1990;152:3244–3246.

22. Sommer P, Bauer T, Neilsen KK, Kristensen ES, Hermann GG, Steven K, Nordling J. Voiding patterns and prevalence of incontinence in women. A questionnaire survey. Br J Urol 1990; 66;12–15.

23. Elving LB, Foldspang A, Lam GW, Mommsen S. Descriptive epidemiology of urinary incontinence in 3,100 women age 30–59. Scand J Urol Nephrol Suppl 1989;125:37–43.

24. Iosif CS, Bekassy Z, Rydhstrom H. Prevalence of urinary incontinence in middle-aged women. Int J Gynecol Obstet 1988;26:255–259.

25. Jolleys JV. Reported prevalence of urinary incontinence in women in a general practice. Br Med J Clin Res Ed 1988;296:1300–1302.

26. Hagstad A. Gynecology and sexuality in middle-aged women. Women Health 1988;13:57–80.

27. Holst K, Wilson PD. The prevalence of female urinary incontinence and reasons for not seeking treatment. N Z Med J 1988;101: 756–758.

28. Mohide EA, Pringle DM, Robertson D, Chambers LW. Prevalence of urinary incontinence in patients receiving home care services. Can Med Assoc J 1988;139:953–956.

29. Hagstad A, Janson PO. The epidemiology of climacteric symptoms. Acta Obstet Gynecol Scand Suppl 1986;134:59–65.

30. Hording U, Pedersen KH, Sidenius K, Hedegaard L. Urinary incontinence in 45-year-old women. An epidemiological survey. Scand J Urol Nephrol 1986;20:183–186.

31. Yarnell JW, Voyle GJ, Richards CJ, Stephenson TP. Factors associated with urinary incontinence in women. J Epidemiol Commun Health 1982;36: 58–63.

32. Yarnell JW, Voyle GJ, Richards CJ, Stephenson TP. The prevalence and severity of urinary incontinence in women. J Epidemiol Commun Health 1981;35:71–74.

33. Iosif S, Henriksson L, Ulmsten U. The frequency of disorders of the lower urinary tract, urinary incontinence in particular, as evaluated by a questionnaire survey in a gynecological health control population. Acta Obstet Gynecol Scand 1981;60:71–76.

34. Thomas T, Plymat K, Blannin J, et al. Prevalence of urinary incontinence. Br Med J 1980;281: 1243–1245.

35. Feneley R, Shepherd A, Powell P, et al. Urinary incontinence: prevalence and needs. Br J Urol 1979;51:493–496.

36. Wolin L. Stress incontinence in young, healthy nulliparous female subjects. J Urol 1969;101: 545–549.

37. Mattsson S. Urinary incontinence and nocturia in healthy schoolchildren. Acta Paediatr 1994;83: 950–954.

38. Hansson S. Urinary incontinence in children and associated problems. Scand J Urol Nephrol 1992; 141:47–55.

39. Hellstrom AL, Hanson E, Hansson S, Hjalmas K, Jodal U. Mictruition habits and incontinence in 7-year-old Swedish school entrants. Eur J Pediatr 1990;149:434–437.

40. Foxman B, Valdez RB, Brook RH. Child enuresis: prevalence, perceived impact, and prescribed treatment. Pediatrics 1986;77:482–487.

41. De Jonge GA. Bladder control and enuresis. In: Kolvin I, MacKeith RC, Meadow SR, eds. Clinics in developmental medicine. Philadelphia: JB Lippincott, 1973:39–46.

42. Oppel WC, Harber PA, Rider RV. The age of attaining bladder control. Pediatrics 1968;42: 614–626.

43. Rutter M, Yule W, Graham P. Enuresis and behavioral definace: some epidemiological considerations. In: Kolvin I, MacKeith RC, Meadow SR, eds. Bladder control and enuresis. Philadelphia: JB Lippincott, 1973:137–147.

44. Cushing FC, Baller WR. Problem of nocturnal enuresis in adults, with special references to managers and managerial aspirants. J Psychol 1975;89:203–213.
45. Bransby ER, Blomfield JM, Douglas JWB. The prevalence of bedwetting. Med Officer 1955; 94:5–7.
46. McGrother CW, Castleden CM, Duffin H, Clarke M. A profile of disordered micturition in the elderly at home. Age Ageing 1987;16: 105–110.
47. Burgio KL, Locher JL, Zyczynski H, et al. Urinary incontinence during pregnancy in a racially mixed sample: characteristics and predisposing factors. Int Urogynecol J (in press).
48. Bump RC. Racial comparisons and contrasts in urinary incontinence and pelvic organ prolapse. Obstet Gynecol 1993;81:421–425.
49. Bump RC, McClish DK. Cigarette smoking and urinary incontinence in women. Am J Obstet Gynecol 1992;167:1213–1218.
50. Fonda D, Nickless R, Roth R. A prospective study of the incidence of urinary incontinence in an acute care teaching hospital and its implications on future service development. Aust Clin Rev 1988;8:102–107.
51. Egan M, Plymat K, Thomas T, Mead T. Incontinence in patients in two district general hospitals. Nursing Times 1983;79:22–24.
52. Boring CC, Squires TS, Tong T. Cancer statistics, 1993. CA-A Cancer J Clin 1993;43:7–26.
53. Mettlin C, Jones GW, Murphy GP. Trends in prostate cancer care in the United States, 1974–1990. CA-A Cancer J Clin 1993;43:83–91.
54. Diokno AC, Hollander JB. Prostate gland disease. In: Calkins E, Ford AB, Katz PR, eds. Practice of geriatrics, 2nd ed. Philadelphia: WB Saunders, 1992.
55. Doll HA, Black NA, McPherson K, Flood AB, Williams GB, Smith JC. Mortality, morbidity and complications following transurethral resection of the prostate for benign prostatic hypertrophy. J Urol 1992;147:1566–1573.
56. Steiner MS, Morton RA, Walsh PC. Impact of anatomical radical prostatectomy on urinary continence. J Urol 1991;145:512–514.
57. Brendler CB, Walsh PC. The role of radical prostatectomy in the treatment of prostate cancer. CA-A Cancer J Clin 1992;42:212–222.
58. Ishii T, Takamura C, Esa A, Park YC, Mitsubayashi S, Kaneko S, Kurita T. A study of urinary incontinence after prostatectomy. Jpn J Urol 1989;80: 1474–1480.
59. Pedersen KV, Herder A. Radical retropubic prostatectomy for localised prostatic carcinoma: a clinical and pathological study of 201 cases. Scand J Urol Nephrol 1993;27:219–224.
60. Ramon J, Leandri P, Rossingnol F, Gautier JR. Urinary continence following radical retropubic prostatectomy. Br J Urol 1993;71:47–51.
61. Rossignol G, Geandri P, Gautier JR, Quintens H, Gabay-Torbiero L, Tap G. Radical retropubic prostatectomy: complications and quality of life (429 cases, 1983–1989). Eur Urol 1991;19: 186–191.
62. Sole-Balcells F, Villavicencio H, Oritz A. Postsurgical management of the patient undergoing radical prostatectomy. Br J Urol 1992;70(Suppl 1): 43–49.
63. Leandri P, Rossignol G, Gautier JR, Ramon J. Radical retropubic prostatectomy: morbidity and quality of life. Experience with 620 consecutive cases. J Urol 1992;147(3 Pt 2):883–887.
64. Kerr LA, Zincke H. Radical retropubic prostatectomy for prostate cancer in the elderly and the young: complications and prognosis. Eur Urol 1994;25:305–311.
65. Goluboff ET, Chang DT, Olsson CA, Kaplan SA. Urodynamics and the etiology of post-prostatectomy urinary incontinence: the initial Columbia experience. J Urol 1995;153:1034–1037.
66. Van Kerrebroeck PE, Koldewijn EL, Scherpenhuizen S, Debruyne FM. The morbidity due to lower urinary tract function in spinal cord injury patients. Paraplegia 1993;31:320–329.
67. Burgio KL, Ives DG, Locher JL, et al. Treatment seeking for urinary incontinence in older adults. J Am Geriatr Soc 1994;42:208–212.

CHAPTER 5

Epidemiology of Urinary Incontinence in Older Adults

Patrice Artress Cruise and Joseph G. Ouslander

Introduction

Urinary incontinence (UI) is a major clinical problem and a significant cause of disability and dependency in older adults. It is prevalent, disruptive, and complex, affecting approximately 10 million Americans of all ages, particularly older adults. UI can be devastating physically, psychologically, and economically. Physically, UI is associated with symptomatic urinary tract infections when urinary retention with overflow incontinence remains undiagnosed or when UI is inappropriately managed with long-term use of an indwelling catheter (1, 2). UI can predispose persons to skin problems and make pressure ulcers difficult to heal (3, 4). Psychologically, persons with UI often suffer from embarrassment, depression, and isolation (5). Economically, the direct health-care costs related to UI have been conservatively estimated to be over 10 billion annually in 1987 prices. This does not include indirect costs, which would make the total economic impact of UI even more profound (6, 7). One recent study demonstrated that those low-income elderly persons with UI generate significantly greater public costs for home care services (8).

Despite its prevalence and high cost, research indicates that less than 50% of people who suffer from UI seek help for this problem (5, 9–12). The reasons for this are unclear but include embarrassment, denial, and ignorance regarding treatment options. Unfortunately, even when individuals do seek help, evidence exists that older adults with UI are frequently not evaluated and treated appropriately (13–16). They are sometimes told by health care professionals that UI is a normal consequence of aging and that nothing can be done (17). Although normal aging is not a cause of UI, there are age-related and age-associated changes in the lower urinary tract that can predispose the elderly person to this condition (18–22). Finally, additional anatomic and/or physiological problems associated with other medical conditions, including functional problems such as mobility and dexterity, may be predisposing factors for UI (23, 24). However, it is important to remember that UI is always manageable and, in many cases, curable in older adults.

Definitions and Terminology

Urinary incontinence, as defined by the Urinary Incontinence Guideline Panel, is the "involuntary loss of urine which is sufficient to be a problem" (18), which is similar to the International Continence Society's definition (25). These definitions imply that the involuntary loss of urine should meet some criteria to be clinically significant; however, these criteria are not specified, which makes comparisons between studies difficult. Subjective definitions may vary: what is a "problem" for one person may not be for another. If persons are able to "manage" their incontinence satisfactorily, they may not consider themselves incontinent. Definitions of urinary incontinence also vary in terms of severity of incontinence (i.e., volume of urine lost, frequency of urine loss episodes, and over what time period, and so on).

Prevalence refers to all cases of a specific condition at a certain point in time, whereas incidence refers to the risk of developing a disease or condition during a specified time period (26). Estimates of prevalence and incidence are usually obtained by surveying a sample of the population to which generalizations can then be made. Surveys are typically conducted as personal interviews, telephone surveys, self-administered questionnaires, or reports (either verbal or written) from health care professionals. Survey research is especially appropriate for making descriptive studies of large populations and may be used for explanatory purposes as well (27).

However, for survey information to be accurate and generalizable to the population under study, several factors must be addressed, including proper sampling methodology, adequate sample size for generalizing to the population, and appropriate adjustments for any systematic differences between respondents and nonrespondents. Systematic bias, including threats to validity and reliability, may be introduced during the survey process if questions are not asked in an appropriate manner, if response scales are not relevant, or if the definition of incontinence is inaccurate for the questions being asked (27).

A common problem that affects the accuracy of prevalence surveys of UI is underreporting. Often, the incontinent person is embarrassed to report the condition to a health care professional, perhaps because she or he believes that incontinence is a normal part of aging. Incontinent persons often choose to manage the incontinence on their own (e.g., the use of protective pads, undergarments, and/or toileting behaviors) (28, 29). Many health care professionals also underreport incontinence because of lack of knowledge regarding UI and the fact that their patients often do not self-report this problem.

Therefore, the following issues should be kept in mind when reviewing prevalence and incidence studies of UI: (*a*) definition of UI used in the study, including the types and patterns relevant to the population being studied; (*b*) sampling methodology; (*c*) description of the setting; (*d*) description of the sample (demographic information, functional status, and so on); (*e*) reliability and validity of the measurement instrument; (*f*) data collection methods and procedures that minimize biases and underreporting; and (*g*) adequate response rates, description of nonrespondents, and adjustments made for differences between respondents and nonrespondents.

Incontinence in Community Settings

The prevalence of UI in community-dwelling older adults is reported to range from 15 to 36% (30–35). The prevalence of severe UI (where severe is defined as a frequency of "weekly" or more, "regularly," or "most of the time") ranges from 3 to 25%, with prevalence and severity increasing with age and women more often affected than men. Incidence rates among this group are much harder to track, and few efforts have been made. However, a large epidemiological study of UI in community-dwelling older adults found that incidence rates for developing UI over a 1-year period were 10% for elderly men and 20% for elderly women, with remission rates during this same time period of 12% for women and about 30% for men. Those who changed their severity level were most likely to progress from mild to moderate (36).

Most estimates of the prevalence and incidence of UI in community-dwelling persons rely on self-reported continence status. One recent study assessed the reliability of this measure in older adults by telephone interviews administered approximately 2 weeks apart and found that the prevalence of UI was 40% at baseline and 44% on reinterview, revealing the stability of incontinence estimates over this 2-week period (37).

One large population-based cross-sectional study found that 28% of the study participants reported having "difficulty holding urine until they can get to a toilet" at least some of the time, and 8% reported difficulty "most" or "all of the time" (38). Significant age and gender differences in difficulty were found: 44% of women and 34% of men reported some difficulty, and 9% of women and

4% of men reported difficulty most of the time. Difficulty was reported twice as much among those aged 85 and over (12%) compared with those aged 65 to 74 years (6%). Although the question used in this study investigated trouble holding urine and not actual urine loss, the two have been shown to be strongly correlated (39). Trouble holding urine may or may not include actual urine loss but may dominate a person's life by the recurrent and often urgent need to find a toilet. The person may be more susceptible to falls and subsequent fractures in their haste to find a bathroom. Difficulty holding urine was also associated with important functional and health measures, including depression, stroke, chronic cough, night awakening, fecal incontinence, and problems with activities of daily living.

Nocturia is another problem that may or may not result in actual urine loss. However, one study reported that persons who get up several times during the night to use the toilet are often bothered by this and that they experience major disruptions in sleep and fatigue the following day (40). Nocturia episodes are often associated with falls and resulting hip fractures. Furthermore, if nocturia is a problem for a frail older adult with functional impairments, the caregiver, often an elderly spouse, must also get up to help the person to the bathroom, thus disrupting their sleep also.

The effect of UI on caregivers of older adults in the community appears to be profound, both physically and economically (8). In a study of homebound older adults who were cared for at home by family caregivers, the prevalence of UI was 53%. Of those who were incontinent, 40% suffered from isolated UI, whereas 60% had combined incontinence. Both the frequency and severity of UI were greater when the person also suffered from fecal incontinence (41). Many people with UI prematurely use absorbent materials and/or devise other management strategies to conceal and control their incontinence (12, 28, 42). One study of community-dwelling elderly in a large urban setting found that almost all study participants used more than one management strategy to control urine loss and that some strategies were so elaborate they took most of the day to implement (43). For example, one woman constructed a mental map of all the toilets in her shopping area and planned her activities so that a toilet was always within easy access. In general, men in this study used fewer strategies and were less successful than women.

Incontinence in Acute Care Settings

Previous studies report that the prevalence of urinary incontinence ranges from 15 to 21% in acute-care hospital settings (44–47). One study reports that over one third of admissions of elderly persons to the medical and surgical wards of a major teaching hospital had UI at some time during their hospital stay (48). The study also found that UI was more common in women, and that in persons over 75 years old, UI was associated with other functional disabilities, such as mobility problems. Another finding was that the UI persisted and was not just a transient problem associated with the hospitalization.

Incontinence in Long-Term Care Settings

The prevalence of urinary incontinence among residents in nursing homes (NH) varies according to the resident case mix and ranges from 40 to 70% or even higher in facilities with more functionally impaired residents (49, 50). Because incontinence is often a critical factor in the decision to place someone in an NH, a substantial proportion of NH residents are already incontinent at the time of admission (15). In contrast to UI among ambulatory community-dwelling older adults, NH residents suffer from UI that is more severe and more commonly associated with fecal incontinence. Incontinent nursing home residents generally have multiple episodes of UI throughout the day and night, and approximately 50% of these are also incontinent of stool more than one time per week (51).

Urinary incontinence among NH residents is associated with substantial morbidity and cost, including skin irritation and symptomatic urinary tract infection. UI may also lead to falls among residents with mobility limitations (impaired balance or gait) who suffer from frequency, urge incontinence, and/or nocturia. The adverse psychological effects of UI have been difficult to document systematically, but embarrassment and frustration among those residents are common. NH staff generally consider UI to be a very difficult and labor-intensive duty, and they perceive that they spend a disproportionate amount of time caring for incontinent residents. The economic costs of UI in NHs have been estimated to be close to $5 billion annually, including the costs of staff time, laundry, and supplies (7).

Summary

UI is a prevalent, disruptive, and complex problem affecting a large number of older adults and constitutes a major burden on health and economic resources. UI is not a normal consequence of aging and is curable, or at least manageable, in many instances. However, many older adults with this condition are not seriously evaluated and treated by health care professionals. The prevalence and incidence of UI among community-dwelling older adults and in acute and long-term care settings is difficult to measure because of methodological problems with study designs and underreporting. Estimates of UI prevalence in older adults in community settings range from 15 to 36%, from 15 to 25% in acute-care settings, and from 40 to 70% in long-term care settings.

REFERENCES

1. Warren JW, Damron D, Tenney JH, Hoopes JM, Deforge B, Muncie HL Jr. Fever, bacteremia and death as complications of bacteriuria in women with long-term urethral catheters. J Infect Dis 1987;155:1151–1158.
2. Ouslander JG, Greengold BA, Chen S. Complications of chronic indwelling urinary catheters among male nursing home patients: a prospective study. J Urol 1988;138:1191–1195.
3. Panel for the Prediction and Prevention of Pressure Ulcers in Adults. Pressure ulcers in adults. Prediction and prevention. Clinical Practice Guideline, Number 3. Rockville, MD: U.S. Department of Health and Human Services. AHCPR Publication Number 92–0047. May 1992.
4. Bergstrom N, Bennett MA, Carlson CE, et al. Treatment of pressure ulcers. Clinical Practice Guideline, Number 15. Rockville, MD: U.S. Department of Health and Human Services. AHCPR Publication No. 95–0652. December 1994.
5. Wyman JF, Harkins SW, Fantl JA. Psychosocial impact of urinary incontinence in the community-dwelling population. J Am Geriatr Soc 1990;38:282–288.
6. Hu TW. Impact of urinary incontinence on health-care costs. J Am Geriatr Soc 1990;38: 292–295.
7. Hu TW. The cost impact of urinary incontinence on health-care services. Urinary incontinence in adults. Clinical Practice Guideline. Rockville, MD: U.S. Department of Health and Human Services. AHCPR Publication Number 92-0038. March 1992.
8. Baker DI, Bice TW. The influence of urinary incontinence on publicly financed home care services to low-income elderly people. Gerontologist 1995;35:360–369.
9. Branch LG, Walker LA, Wetle TT, DuBeau CE, Resnick NM. Urinary incontinence knowledge among community-dwelling people 65 years of age and older. J Am Geriatr Soc 1994;42:1257–1262.
10. Burgio KL, Ives DG, Locher JL, Arena VC, Kuller LH. Treatment seeking for urinary incontinence in older adults. J Am Geriatr Soc 1994;42: 208–212.
11. Goldstein M, Hawthorne ME, Engeberg S, McDowell BJ, Burgio KL. Urinary incontinence: why people do not seek help. J Gerontol Nurs 1992;18: 15–20.
12. Herzog AR, Fultz NH, Normolle DP, Brock BM, Diokno AC. Methods used to manage urinary incontinence by older adults in the community. J Am Geriatr Soc 1989;37:339–347.
13. McDowell BJ, Silverman M, Martin D, Musa D, Keane C. Identification and intervention for urinary incontinence by community physicians and geriatric assessment teams. J Am Geriatr Soc 1994;42:501–505.
14. Mitteness LS. So what do you expect when you're 85? Urinary incontinence in late life. In: Roth J, Conrad P, eds. Research in the sociology of health care: the experience of illness, vol. 6. Connecticut: JAI Press, 1987:177–219.
15. Ouslander JG, Kane RL, Abrass IB. Urinary incontinence in elderly nursing home patients. JAMA 1982;248:1194–1198.
16. Starer P, Libow LS. Obscuring urinary incontinence: diapering the elderly. J Am Geriatr Soc 1985;12:842–846.
17. Resnick NM, Yalla SV. Management of urinary incontinence in the elderly. N Engl J Med 1985; 313:800–805.
18. Urinary Incontinence Guideline Panel. Urinary incontinence in adults. Clinical Practice Guideline. Rockville, MD: U.S. Department of Health and Human Services. AHCPR Publication Number 92–0038. March 1992.
19. Staskin DR. Age-related physiologic and pathologic changes affecting lower urinary tract function. Clin Geriatr Med 1986;2:701–710.

20. Diokno AC, Brown MB, Brock BM, et al. Clinical and cystometric characteristics of continent and incontinent noninstitutionalized elderly. J Urol 1988;140:567–571.

21. Resnick NM. Initial evaluation of the incontinent patient. J Am Geriatr Soc 1990;38:311–316.

22. Diokno AC. Diagnostic categories of incontinence and the role of urodynamic testing. J Am Geriatr Soc 1990;38:300–305.

23. Diokno AC, Brock BM, Herzog AR, Bromberg J. Medical correlates of urinary incontinence in the elderly. Urology 1990;32:129–138.

24. Williams ME, Gaylord SA. Role of functional assessment in the evaluation of urinary incontinence. J Am Geriatr Soc 1990;38:296–299.

25. Abrams P, Blaivas JG, Stanton SL, Andersen JT. Standardisation of terminology of lower urinary tract function. Neurourol Urodyn 1988;7:403–427.

26. Clayton D, Hills M. Statistical models in epidemiology. New York: Oxford University Press, 1993.

27. Babbie E. The practice of social research, 5th ed. California: Wadsworth Publishing, 1989.

28. Brink CA. Absorbent pads, garments, and management strategies. J Am Geriatr Soc 1990;38:368–373.

29. Fultz NH, Herzog AR. Measuring urinary incontinence in surveys. Gerontologist 1993;33:708–713.

30. Diokno AC, Brock BM, Brown MB, Herzog AR. Prevalence of urinary incontinence and other urological symptoms in the noninstitutionalized elderly. J Urol 1986;136:1022–1025.

31. Harris T. Aging in the eighties, prevalence and impact of urinary problems in individuals age 65 and over. NCHS Adv Data 1986;121:1–7.

32. Herzog AR, Fultz NH. Prevalence and incidence of urinary incontinence in community-dwelling populations. J Am Geriatr Soc 1990;38:273–281.

33. Jeter KF, Wagner DB. Incontinence in the American home: a survey of 36,500 people. J Am Geriatr Soc 1990;38:379–383.

34. Somer P, Bauer T, Neilson KK, et al. Voiding patterns and prevalence of incontinence in women: a questionnaire survey. Br J Urol 1990;66:12–15.

35. Vetter NJ, Jones DA, Victor CR. Urinary incontinence in the elderly at home. Lancet 1981;2:1275–1277.

36. Herzog AR, Diokno AC, Brown MB, Normolle DP, Brock BM. Two-year incidence, remission, and change patterns of urinary incontinence in non-institutionalized older adults. J Gerontol 1990;45:M67–74.

37. Resnick NM, Beckett LA, Branch LG, Scherr PA, Wetle T. Short-term variability of self-report of incontinence in older persons. J Am Geriatr Soc 1994;42:202–207.

38. Wetle T, Scherr P, Branch LG, Resnick NM, Harris T, Evans D, Taylor JO. Difficulty with holding urine among older persons in a geographically defined community: prevalence and correlates. J Am Geriatr Soc 1995;43:349–355.

39. Yarnell JWG, Voyle GJ, Richards CJ, Stephenson TP. The prevalence and severity of urinary incontinence in women. J Epidemiol Commun Health 1981;35:71–74.

40. Barker JC, Mitteness LS. Nocturia in the elderly. Gerontologist 1988;28:99–104.

41. Noelker LS. Incontinence in elderly cared for by family. Gerontologist 1987;27:194–200.

42. Mitteness LS. Knowledge and beliefs about urinary incontinence in adulthood and old age. J Am Geriatr Soc 1990;38:374–378.

43. Mitteness LS. The management of urinary incontinence by community-living elderly. Gerontologist 1987;2:185–192.

44. Paillano M, Resnick NM. Natural history of nosocomial urinary incontinence. Gerontologist 1984;24:212.

45. Sullivan DH, Lindsay RW. Urinary incontinence in the geriatric population of an acute hospital. J Am Geriatr Soc 1984;32:646–650.

46. Warshaw GA, Moore JT, Friedman W, et al. Functional disability in the hospitalized elderly. JAMA 1982;248:847–850.

47. Harris T. Urinary incontinence among hospitalized persons aged 65 years and older—United States, 1984–1987. MMWR 1991;40:433—436.

48. Sier H, Ouslander JG, Orzeck S. Urinary incontinence among geriatric patients in an acute-care hospital. JAMA 1987;257:1767–1771.

49. Ouslander JG. Urinary incontinence in nursing homes. J Am Geriatr Soc 1990;38:289–291.

50. Ouslander JG, Schnelle JF. Incontinence in the nursing home. Ann Intern Med 1995;122:438–449.

51. Ouslander JG, Morishita L, Blaustein J, Orzeck S, Dunn S, Syre J. Clinical, functional and psychosocial characteristics of an incontinent nursing home population. J Gerontol 1987;42:631–637.

SECTION III

Evaluation of the Lower Urinary Tract and Pelvic Floor

CHAPTER 6

Differential Diagnosis of Urinary Incontinence

Michael W. Weinberger

It is estimated that between 10 and 12 million American adults suffer from urinary incontinence. Urinary incontinence affects 15–30% of noninstitutionalized women over age 60 and more than half of nursing home residents (1). Nongynecologists are often surprised to learn that young nulliparous women occasionally experience urinary incontinence. Of nulliparous female varsity athletes, 28% reported urine loss while participating in their sport and 42% reported leakage during their daily activities (2).

The International Continence Society defines urinary incontinence as involuntary urine loss that is severe enough to constitute a social or hygienic problem and that is objectively demonstrable (3). According to this definition, urinary incontinence may be a symptom, sign, or diagnosis. The symptom is the patient's report of urine loss, the sign is objective demonstration of urine loss, and the diagnosis is established with urodynamic testing.

We discuss the varied causes of incontinence in women (Table 6.1). In many instances, the cause for incontinence is multifactorial. Knowledge of the multiple causes of incontinence facilitates diagnosis and treatment.

Genuine Stress Incontinence

Genuine stress incontinence is involuntary urine loss in the absence of a detrusor contraction. Intravesical pressure exceeds the maximum urethral pressure and urine is lost (4). A major cause of genuine stress incontinence is the loss of anatomic support of the urethra, bladder, and urethrovesical junction. When the bladder and proximal urethra are supported in a retropubic position, increases in intraabdominal pressure are transmitted equally to both structures and continence is maintained. Lack of anatomic support displaces the proximal urethra outside the abdominal pressure zone. Intraabdominal pressure increases are then fully transmitted to the bladder but to a lesser extent to the urethra, and urine loss occurs.

Genuine stress incontinence also occurs when the urethra, regardless of support, fails to function as an effective sphincter. Various terms have been used to describe this condition: type III urethra, low pressure urethra, and intrinsic urethral sphincter deficiency (ISD). ISD may result from congenital weakness secondary to myelomeningocele or epispadias. It may be acquired after trauma, radiation, or a sacral cord lesion. In women, ISD is common after multiple antiincontinence surgeries (Table 6.2).

The importance of identifying patients with ISD before surgery is the 33–54% failure rate after conventional urethral suspension procedures (4, 5). By contrast, suburethral sling operations effectively restore long-term continence in 76–96% of these patients (6, 7). Periurethral collagen injection cures ISD in 45% of cases and improves incontinence severity in an additional 34–55% of patients (8, 9).

Many urodynamic and radiographic tests are used to evaluate genuine stress incontinence, but none are considered diagnostic by all investigators. Early research emphasized

Table 6.1. Causes of Urinary Incontinence

Genuine stress incontinence
Detrusor instability
Mixed incontinence
Overflow incontinence
Bypass of anatomic continence mechanism
Functional incontinence
Transient causes of incontinence

Table 6.2. Causes of Genuine Stress Incontinence

Anatomic
    Inadequate support of urethrovesical
        junction
Intrinsic sphincter deficiency
    Congenital
        Meningomyelocele
        Epispadias
    Acquired
        Trauma
        Postradiation
        Spinal cord injury
        Previous antiincontinence surgery

the importance of the posterior urethrovesical angle (PUVA) at maintaining continence. Using lateral cystourethrography, Jeffcoate and Roberts (10) reported 80% of patients with stress incontinence had loss of the PUVA. Green (11) used bead chain cystograms to classify patients with stress incontinence based on the support of the urethrovesical junction. Type I incontinence is characterized by loss of the PUVA and type II, by loss of the PUVA with posterior, inferior, and rotational descent of the bladder base and urethra (11). Green advocated treating type I defects with anterior colporrhaphy and type II defects with retropubic bladder neck suspension. Most authorities have abandoned Green's approach.

Blaivas and Olsson (12) recommend video urodynamics to evaluate the urethral sphincter mechanism. They found in stress incontinent women that the bladder neck is closed at rest but opens with increased intraabdominal pressure. Their modification of Green's classification system includes types 0, I, IIA, and IIB, distinguished by the resting position of the bladder neck relative to the symphysis pubis. The finding that 25–50% of continent women have an incompetent bladder neck during straining has led to considerable controversy about the role of the bladder neck in maintaining continence (13, 14).

In 1981, McGuire (15) reported 75% of women who failed previous antiincontinence operations had an open fibrotic urethra at rest. Resting proximal urethral closure pressure in these individuals was less than 20 cm H_2O. McGuire called this condition the type III urethra, and subtracted urethral pressure profilometry became widely used to evaluate urethral function.

Recently, abdominal leak point pressure has been advocated as a test of urethral sphincteric function (16). Leak point pressure was originally used to determine whether a myelodysplastic child was at risk of developing vesicoureteral reflux and hydronephrosis. It is measured by inserting a pressure catheter into the bladder and infusing water until leakage occurs around the catheter; intravesical pressure at that time is the leak point pressure. McGuire modified this technique to determine the abdominal leak point pressure (16). Urethral and bladder pressure are recorded as contrast is infused into the bladder under fluoroscopic guidance. After filling the bladder to 150 mL, the patient increases abdominal pressure by straining and coughing. The process is videotaped, and the abdominal pressure at the time of urine leakage is noted. McGuire found that 76% of patients with leakage at low abdominal pressures (5–60 cm H_2O) had type III incontinence on video urodynamic testing. In contrast, 90% of patients with leak point pressure greater than 60 cm H_2O had type I or II incontinence. Currently, measurements to determine leak point pressure have not been standardized.

Detrusor Instability

The overactive bladder is one that contracts spontaneously or with provocation when the patient attempts to inhibit micturition (4). When the International Continence Society first standardized urodynamic terminology in 1976, the diagnosis of detrusor instability required a rise in bladder pressure of 15 cm H_2O during filling cystometry. A less restrictive definition was adopted in 1988 when it was recognized that contractions measuring less than 15 cm H_2O often cause symptoms of frequency, urgency, and incontinence (17). Currently, detrusor instability is diagnosed during provocative cystometry when the true detrusor pressure increases by 15 cm H_2O or when smaller increases cause urgency or incontinence. A gradual increase in bladder pressure without subsequent decrease reflects a change of compliance rather than detrusor instability.

The term detrusor hyperreflexia is used when bladder overactivity is due to disturbance of the central nervous mechanism. Neurological disorders commonly associated with detrusor hyperreflexia include stroke, dementia, multiple sclerosis, brain tumor, and Parkinson's disease.

Mixed Incontinence

Detrusor instability and genuine stress incontinence coexist in 4–30% of patients (18, 19). The degree to which each component contributes to the patient's urinary incontinence varies, but one factor often predominates. Patients with mixed incontinence leak larger volumes of urine and tend to have more incontinent episodes per week than patients with either pure stress incontinence or detrusor instability alone (20).

There is controversy whether coexisting detrusor instability decreases the surgical cure rate of genuine stress incontinence. Stanton et al. (21) reported that colposuspension cured stress incontinence in 85% of patients when this was the singular diagnosis but only 43% of patients with mixed incontinence. Lockhart et al. (22) divided patients with mixed incontinence into two groups based on the increase in detrusor pressure during bladder filling. If the pressure increase was less than 25 cm H_2O, the stress incontinence cure rate was 90%; when the pressure increase exceeded 25 cm H_2O, the cure rate was only 50%. Other investigators have reported that detrusor instability does not affect the ability to surgically cure genuine stress incontinence (19, 23). Differing patient selection criteria, definitions of detrusor instability, diagnostic techniques, and outcome analysis may account for the discrepancies.

Overflow Incontinence

The International Continence Society defines overflow incontinence as the involun-

tary loss of urine associated with overdistension of the bladder (4). In most cases, overdistension is caused by outflow tract obstruction or detrusor underactivity.

Outflow tract obstruction is uncommon in women. Pelvic prolapse, uterine leiomyomata, ovarian neoplasms, acutely retroverted gravid and nongravid uteri, and large vaginal wall mesonephric and paramesonephric cysts are reported as causes of urethral obstruction (24).

Detrusor function may be compromised by neurogenic or myogenic factors (Table 6.3). Herniated intervertebral disks, peripheral neuropathy (caused by diabetes mellitus, hypothyroidism, vitamin B_{12} deficiency, or tabes dorsalis), spinal cord injury, and central nervous system lesions may produce a hypotonic or acontractile bladder. Medications that induce overflow incontinence include anticholinergics, calcium channel blockers, alpha- and beta-adrenergic agonists, and diuretics.

The bladder wall may be damaged by radiation therapy, interstitial cystitis, or recurrent urinary tract infection. Overflow incontinence can develop if bladder fibrosis produces a small-volume, noncompliant, functionally inadequate urine reservoir.

Patients with overflow incontinence commonly complain of unconscious urine loss throughout the day and night. Many experience hesitancy, intermittent flow with diminished stream, having to lean or bend to a

Table 6.3.   Causes of Overflow Incontinence

Bladder atony
  Neurological causes
    Autonomic neuropathy
    Peripheral neuropathy
    Central nervous system pathology
  Pharmacological
    Anticholinergic agents
    Calcium channel blockers
    Alpha-adrenergic agonists
    Beta-adrenergic agonists
  Endocrine disease
    Diabetes mellitus
    Hypothyroidism
Decreased bladder wall compliance
  Radiation fibrosis
  Intrinsic bladder disease
    Interstitial cystitis
    Recurrent urinary tract infection
Outflow tract obstruction

certain position, or using suprapubic pressure to empty their bladders. Increased residual urine volumes predispose these individuals to recurrent urinary tract infections. During physical examination, the bladder may be palpable above the pubic symphysis.

Overflow incontinence is always included in the differential diagnosis of urinary incontinence. In practice, overflow incontinence is rarely diagnosed unless one is dealing with a special patient population, such as the elderly or the neurologically impaired. Measurement of postvoid residual urine identifies patients at risk for overflow incontinence.

Bypass of Anatomic Continence Mechanism

An uncommon cause of incontinence is the bypass of the normal continence mechanism (Table 6.4) by nonphysiological conduits for urine such as epispadias, ectopic ureters, and fistulae (ureterovaginal, vesicovaginal, urethrovaginal, or vesicouterine). These patients usually experience continuous urine loss, and the diagnosis is relatively easy.

In some cases, diagnosis may be more difficult. For example, patients with epispadias may occasionally reach adulthood before an association is made between the incomplete midline fusion of their genitalia, the absence of pubic hair at the center of the mons pubis, and lifelong urinary incontinence. An ectopic ureter can cause incontinence if it empties distal to the urethral sphincter mechanism. One third of ectopic ureters empty at the level of the bladder neck; these women are usually continent. When

Table 6.4.   Bypass of Anatomic Continence Mechanism

Ectopic ureter
Epispadias
Fistula
Ureterovaginal
Urethrovaginal
Vesicouterine
Vesicovaginal
Urethral diverticulum

the ureter opens the mid or distal urethra (33% of cases), the vagina (25%), or the cervix or uterus (5%), urine loss may be continuous or infrequent.

Patients with urethral diverticula present with dysuria, dyspareunia, and postmicturition dribbling. Urine accumulates within the diverticulum and empties when the patient stands. Urethroscopy, urethral pressure profilometry, or radiographic techniques may be used to confirm the diagnosis.

Functional Incontinence

Functional incontinence occurs when a patient with an intact lower urinary tract is unable or unwilling to reach the toilet to urinate. Visual impairment, limited manual dexterity, and multiple layers of undergarments or pads may prevent undressing before urine loss occurs. Patients should be encouraged to wear comfortable loose-fitting clothing that is easy to remove.

Environmental factors may impair the elderly patient's ability to reach the bathroom before incontinence occurs. These factors may include inaccessible facilities, unfamiliar surroundings, inattentive staff, and physical restraints. Correcting environmental factors may restore continence.

Effects of Aging

The prevalence and type of urinary incontinence vary with the age and health of the population being evaluated. Several investigators have reported that the prevalence of genuine stress incontinence decreases with advancing age, with commensurate increases in detrusor instability and mixed incontinence (25, 26). Among ambulatory adult incontinent women, genuine stress incontinence is diagnosed in 50–70% of cases. In this population, detrusor instability and mixed incontinence each account for 20–40% of cases. Among elderly community-dwelling incontinent women undergoing urodynamic testing, genuine stress incontinence is diagnosed less frequently (36–46% of cases); detrusor instability and mixed incontinence are more common, accounting for 27–46% and 19% of diagnoses, respectively (27, 28). Urodynamic evaluation of incontinent institutionalized elderly women diagnosed detrusor instability in 61%, genuine stress incontinence in 21%, and mixed incontinence in 4% (29).

The effect of aging on urinary tract function has not been studied longitudinally. Cross-sectional observations suggest that bladder capacity, the ability to postpone voiding, maximal urethral closure pressure, and urinary flow rate decrease with age. Postvoid residual urine volume and the prevalence of uninhibited detrusor contractions are probably increased (30). Even in the absence of congestive heart failure, peripheral venous insufficiency, or renal disease, an age-related decline in glomerular filtration rate causes the elderly to excrete the bulk of their daily ingested fluid at night. As a result, the healthy 80 year old may experience one to two episodes of nocturia.

None of these age-related changes cause incontinence, but they reduce the capacity of the lower urinary tract to withstand further insult. Factors outside the urinary tract often precipitate or exacerbate incontinence. Reversal of the precipitating factor will restore continence even if underlying urogynecological abnormalities are not corrected.

Transient Causes of Incontinence

Recognizing that physiological changes in lower urinary tract function make the elderly more susceptible to incontinence, Resnick devised the mnemonic "DIAPPERS" to categorize the causes of transient incontinence (Table 6.5) (31).

DELIRIUM

Delirium is a confusional state characterized by acute or subacute onset. Its insidious onset and slow progression distinguish it from dementia. Delirium may result from any drug or medical illness, including pneumonia, deep venous thrombosis, congestive heart failure, or the pain associated with a fracture. These underlying causes may present atypically and, if unrecognized, may

Table 6.5.   Reversible Causes of Urinary Incontinence

Delirium
Infection
Atrophic vaginitis
Pharmacological
Psychological
Endocrine
Restricted mobility
Stool impaction

be associated with significant morbidity and mortality. Incontinence is a symptom that will abate when the cause of the patient's confusion is identified and treated.

INFECTION

Increased postvoid residual urine and postmenopausal urogenital atrophy predispose elderly women to develop urinary tract infections. Symptoms of urinary tract infection in the elderly may differ from those in younger patients. Dysuria is often absent and incontinence may be the patient's only symptom.

Bacteriuria can cause mucosal irritation leading to unsuppressible detrusor contractions and urge incontinence. Bacterial endotoxins inhibiting alpha-adrenergic receptors may cause urethral relaxation and stress incontinence (32). Among patients with undiagnosed urinary tract infections at the time of urodynamic evaluation, 30% of those with stress incontinence and 60% of those with detrusor instability became continent after treatment of bacteriuria (33).

ATROPHIC URETHRITIS

Postmenopausal estrogen deficiency causes increased genitourinary tract sensitivity and irritative symptoms. Patients may complain of urethral burning, dysuria, dyspareunia, urinary urgency, or urge incontinence.

PHARMACOLOGICAL CAUSES

Virtually any medication that affects the autonomic nervous system also influences lower urinary tract function. Commonly prescribed antihypertensives, antidepressants, and sedative hypnotics may exacerbate incontinence. Many over-the-counter multi-component cold medications, decongestants, and antihistamines can affect the lower urinary tract. Incontinent patients should be asked about nonprescription medication use.

PSYCHOLOGICAL CAUSES

Incontinence may occasionally be used to gain attention or to manipulate others. Patients may be so profoundly depressed that they do not care about continence.

ENDOCRINE CAUSES

Diabetes mellitus and hypercalcemia may induce an osmotic diuresis that exacerbates other causes of incontinence.

RESTRICTED MOBILITY

Arthritis, hip deformity, or gait instability may impair the elderly patient's ability to reach the bathroom. If mobility cannot be improved, a nearby commode may improve the incontinence.

STOOL IMPACTION

Fecal impaction is a common cause of urinary incontinence in bedridden or immobile patients. It should be suspected in the patient who develops fecal oozing and urinary incontinence with a palpable bladder.

Summary

The etiologies of urinary incontinence are many. The pathophysiology may be multifactorial. History alone is inadequate to establish the etiology of incontinence. It is incumbent on the clinician to perform a thorough evaluation of all incontinent patients before any therapy. Many patients will benefit from comprehensive urodynamic evaluation before treatment.

REFERENCES

1. Urinary Incontinence Guideline Panel. Urinary incontinence in adults. Clinical Practice Guideline. Rockville, MD: U.S. Department of Health and Human Services. AHCPR Publication No. 92–0038. 1992.
2. Nygaard IE, Thompson FL, Svengalis SL, Albright JP. Urinary incontinence in elite nulliparous athletes. Obstet Gynecol 1994;84:183–187.
3. Abrams P, Blaivas JG, Stanton SL, et al. The standardization of terminology of lower urinary tract function. Scand J Urol Nephrol 1988; 114(Suppl):5–19.
4. Koonings PP, Bergman A, Ballard CA. Low urethral pressure and stress urinary incontinence in women: risk factor for failed retropubic urethropexy. Urology 1990;36:245–248.
5. Sand PK, Bowen LW, Pangamiban R, Ostergard DR. The low pressure urethra as a factor in failed retropubic urethropexy. Obstet Gynecol 1987;69:399–402.
6. Weinberger MW, Ostergard DR. Long-term clinical and urodynamic evaluation of the polytetrafluoroethylene suburethral sling for treatment of genuine stress incontinence. Obstet Gynecol 1995;86:92–96.
7. McGuire EJ, Lytton B. Pubovaginal sling procedure for stress incontinence. J Urol 1978;119:82–84.
8. McGuire EJ, Appell RA. Transurethral collagen injection for urinary incontinence. Urology 1994;43:413–415.
9. Herschorn S, Radomski SB, Steele DJ. Early experience with intraurethral collagen injections for urinary incontinence. J Urol 1992;148:1797–1800.
10. Jeffcoate TNA, Roberts H. Observations on stress incontinence of urine. Am J Obstet Gynecol 1952;64:712–738.
11. Green TH. Development of a plan for the diagnosis and treatment of urinary stress incontinence. Am J Obstet Gynecol 1962;83:632–648.
12. Blaivas JG, Olsson CA. Stress incontinence: classification and surgical approach. J Urol 1988;139:727–731.
13. Versi E, Cardozo LD, Studd, JWW, Brincat M, O'Dowd TM, Cooper DJ. Internal urinary sphincter in maintenance of female continence. BMJ 1986;292:166–167.
14. Hilton P, Stanton SL. Urethral pressure measurement by microtransducer: the results in symptom-free women and in those with genuine stress incontinence. Br J Obstet Gynecol 1983;90:919–933.
15. McGuire EJ. Urodynamic findings in patients after failure of stress incontinence operations. Prog Clin Biol Res 1981;78:351–360.
16. McGuire EJ, Fitzpatrick CC, Wan J, et al. Clinical assessment of urethral sphincter function. J Urol 1993;150:1452–1454.
17. Coolsaet BLRA, Blok C, van Venrouijj GEFM, Tan B. Subthreshold detrusor instability. Neurourol Urodyn 1985;4:309–311.
18. McGuire EJ, Savastano JA. Stress incontinence and detrusor instability/urge incontinence. Neurourol Urodyn 1985;4:313–316.
19. Herzog AR, Fultz NH. Prevalence and incidence of urinary incontinence in community-dwelling populations. J Am Geriatr Soc 1990;38:273–280.

20. Fantl JA, Bump RC, McClish DK. Mixed urinary incontinence. Urology 1990;36(Suppl):21–24.
21. Stanton SL, Cardozo L, Williams J, Allen V. Clinical and urodynamic features of failed incontinence surgery in the female. Am J Obstet Gynecol 1978;15:515–520.
22. Lockhart J, Vorstman B, Politano VA. Anti-incontinence surgery in females with detrusor instability. Neurourol Urodyn 1984;3:201–207.
23. Bowen LW, Sand PK, Ostergard DR, Franti CE. Unsuccessful Burch urethropexy: a case-controlled urodynamic study. Am J Obstet Gynecol 1989;160:452–458.
24. Polsky MS, Agee RE, Berg SR, Weber CH. Acute urinary retention in women: brief discussion and unusual case report. J Urol 1973;110:541–543.
25. Yarnell JWG, Voyle GJ, Richards CJ, Stephenson TP. The prevalence and severity of urinary incontinence in women. J Epidemiol Community Health 1981;35:71–74.
26. Brocklehurst JC, Fry J, Griffith LL, Kalton G. Urinary infection and dysuria in women aged 45–64 years: their relevance to similar findings in the elderly. Age Ageing 1972;1:41–47.
27. Ouslander J, Staskin D, Raz S, Hong-Lin S, Hepps K. Clinical versus urodynamic diagnosis in an incontinent female population. J Urol 1987;137:68–71.
28. Bent AE, Richardson DA, Ostergard DR. Diagnosis of lower urinary tract disorders in postmenopausal patients. Am J Obstet Gynecol 1883;145:218–222.
29. Resnick NM, Yalla, SV, Laurino E. The pathophysiology of urinary incontinence among institutionalized elderly persons. N Engl J Med 1989;320:1–7.
30. Resnick NM, Yalla SV. Aging and its effect on the bladder. Semin Urol 1987;5:82–86.
31. Resnick NM, Yalla SV. Management of urinary incontinence in the elderly. N Engl J Med 1985;313:800–805.
32. Nergardh A, Boreus LO, Holme T. The inhibitory effect of coli-endotoxin on alpha-adrenergic receptor functions in the lower urinary tract. An in vitro study in cats. Scand J Urol Nephrol 1977;11:219–224.
33. Bergman A, Bhatia NN. Urodynamics: effect of urinary tract infection on urethral and bladder function. Obstet Gynecol 1985;66:366–371.

CHAPTER 7

Guide to Investigation of the Incontinent Patient

John J. Klutke and Arieh Bergman

Introduction

Incontinence is a symptom and not a diagnosis. The symptom of urinary incontinence results from several distinct defects in lower urinary tract function: an incompetent outlet (stress urinary incontinence [SUI]), inappropriate contraction of the bladder (detrusor instability), or bypass of the bladder outlet (fistula, diverticulum, or ectopic ureter). Each condition has a different treatment, making the diagnostic distinction crucial.

Investigation of the incontinent patient should start with simple and noninvasive tests and, if necessary, proceed in a logical sequence to more complex ones. Often, simple diagnostic tests will suffice to establish the diagnosis. The diagnostic approach has four general components:

1. Urinalysis and urine culture;
2. History;
3. Physical examination;
4. Urodynamic testing.

This formula aims to establish the cause of the incontinence, its effect on the individual, and the presence of related urinary tract pathology. The history and physical examination will provide the framework for diagnosis. A careful history can establish transient causes of incontinence like stool impaction, restricted mobility, etc., which simple, practical therapeutic steps will alleviate. The physical examination should confirm the history and exclude related pathology.

Urodynamic testing is an adjunct to the history and physical examination. The bladder is an "unreliable witness" because the symptoms and signs elicited in the incontinent patient are not specific to any one diagnosis (1). Cardozo and Stanton (2) demonstrated that 55% of patients proven to have SUI had symptoms suggesting a diagnosis of detrusor instability. Conversely, 49% of patients with detrusor instability had the symptom of stress incontinence. Other investigators have documented similar findings in incontinent patients (3, 4). Symptoms of the lower urinary tract are thus overlapping and nonspecific. Simple urodynamic tests include uroflow, measurement of residual urine volume after voiding, and simplified cystometry. These tests should be accessible to and understood by all clinicians providing primary care to women and will suffice to adequately evaluate 80% of incontinent patients. The other patients will require more complex testing.

Urinalysis and Urine Culture

Urinary tract infection can mimic any lower urinary tract condition, including detrusor instability or SUI. Urinalysis and culture, therefore, is an essential screening test for the patient with urinary tract symptoms. Failure to culture the urine of the incontinent patient before performing more complex and invasive tests is akin to working up the amenorrheic patient without checking a pregnancy test (5).

History

Incontinence is defined as the involuntary loss of urine that is a social or hygienic problem and that can be objectively demonstrated (6). The history should note the onset of the problem, its duration, severity, associated symptoms, and precipitating conditions. The character of the incontinence should be elicited: is the leakage continuous or intermittent? Many patients will hesitate to talk about their problem. The interviewer should anticipate this and make every effort to allay embarrassment.

RELATED SYMPTOMS

Symptoms reflect alteration of the normal physiology. The bladder is a compliant organ, storing urine at low pressure throughout its filling phase until its capacity of 350–500 mL is reached. The detrusor muscle does not normally contract during filling. A patient will generally first sense filling with 100–200 mL of urine in the bladder, but a strong desire to void occurs only at capacity. Women normally void about six times per day, with an average volume of 250 mL at each void.

Related symptoms are defined by convention:

1. Urgency—a strong desire to void accompanied by a fear of leakage or pain;
2. Frequency—voiding more than seven times per day;
3. Nocturia—arousal from sleep to void twice or more times per night;
4. Nocturnal enuresis—incontinence during sleep.

Despite general "normal" voiding patterns, symptoms have very little meaning without a context of information in which to interpret them. Voiding twice or more per night, for example, may not be pathological in the patient who drinks gallons of water during the daytime. Before her interview, the patient should complete a voiding record or urolog to provide this context. This urolog is a 24-hour record of the patient's fluid intake and output, in which the patient notes incontinent episodes, associated symptoms, and activities.

A past medical and surgical history is important. Nonurological disease processes commonly cause urological symptoms. Is there an associated systemic disease or is the patient on a medication that affects the kidneys and urinary tract? Previous attempts at correction, surgical or nonsurgical, should be described.

Examination of the Incontinent Woman

General reference is made to the patient's mental status, mobility, and body habits. Many incontinent women will prove to be best managed with surgery. Knowledge of the patient's general status of health should precede any consideration of elective surgery. A general physical examination is performed in this light. Examination of the incontinent woman should specifically focus on

1. Reproducing the incontinence;
2. Excluding related neurological disorders;
3. Assessing pelvic support;
4. Excluding pelvic pathology.

Additional components of the examination therefore focus on neurologic screening and the pelvic examination.

Reproducing the problem is important, particularly if the history seems unreliable. Patients may, alternatively, mistake sweating or vaginal discharge for urinary incontinence. The patient who complains of stress incontinence initially stands with a full bladder and coughs. The examiner observes the external urethral meatus by separating the labia. This is repeated in the seated position if loss of urine is not demonstrated. When the patient implicates a particular activity in the incontinence (e.g., heavy lifting, step aerobics, and so on), exactly recreating the activity may help to demonstrate the leakage. If urine accumulates in the vagina but does not visibly escape from the urethra, a fistula is likely. Instilling the bladder with methylene blue dye before a careful speculum examination can diagnose this condition. Patients who do not demonstrate incontinence despite a diligent search can be given pyridium

30 minutes before ambulating with an absorbent pad in the vagina. Such a "pad test," of course, does not differentiate the cause of the incontinence nor does it rule out a voluntary condition.

PELVIC EXAMINATION

The examination should emphasize several key features. The vaginal mucosa should be examined closely for fistulae. Excoriation is sometimes seen and provides a clue to the severity of the problem. Signs of hypoestrogenic atrophy include a thin friable mucosa, urethral caruncle, and obliteration of the vaginal fornices and rugae. The capacity and mobility of the vagina are noted. The paravaginal tissues normally allow mobilization of the vagina to the iliopectineal ligament. The examiner's two fingers should be easily allowed on digital examination, and the strength of a voluntary contraction of the pelvic floor muscles should be assessed. Digital rectal examination will rule out the presence of stool impaction and make possible assessment of rectal sphincter tone.

Stress incontinence is commonly associated with pelvic organ prolapse. Given the association, the vagina and cervix should be inspected carefully for signs of this surgically correctable problem. It should be remembered that the presence or absence of genitourinary prolapse reveals nothing about the cause of the incontinence. A large cystocele, for example, can exist independently or concurrently with detrusor instability, SUI, or both. A Sims speculum or the disarticulated blade of a Graves speculum will facilitate the identification of prolapse by isolating the anterior vaginal wall from the posterior wall. The type of prolapse (i.e., uterine, cystocele in anterior wall defects, rectocele, and/or enterocele in posterior wall defects) is described as well as its grade. Because a large cystocele or vault prolapse can obstruct the urethra, the stress test should be performed after reduction of the prolapsed segment with a pessary (7, 8).

COTTON SWAB TEST

Descent of the bladder neck and proximal urethra out of the realm of intraabdominal pressure appears to be a primary factor in the development of stress incontinence (9). The examiner evaluates the degree of this descent with a simple and painless test (10). The test is performed in the following manner. With the patient in the supine position, the urethral meatus is cleaned with povidone-iodine and a cotton swab is introduced into the bladder. The cotton tip should be well lubricated with anesthetic cream so that discomfort is avoided. The cotton swab is then gently pulled back out of the bladder until some resistance is encountered. At this point, the cotton tip is at the level of the urethrovesical junction. The accurate placement of the cotton is important because placement too deep in the bladder or too far into the urethra may alter the test's result (11). A change in the angle of the cotton swab of more than 30 degrees from the horizontal indicates poor anatomic support to the bladder base and urethrovesical junction (10, 11).

Normal continent women commonly have a positive cotton swab test (12). The test is therefore nonspecific, and a positive test does not necessarily imply a diagnosis of stress incontinence (13). The test is, however, quite sensitive, and most patients with stress incontinence have a positive test (11, 12). A negative cotton swab test, that is, the absence of bladder neck hypermobility in a woman with SUI, serves as a red flag in the diagnosis. Women with stress incontinence and a negative cotton swab test before a bladder neck suspension had failure rates of up to 50% (14).

NEUROLOGICAL SCREENING

Significant and relatively common neurological diseases frequently manifest initially as a loss of bladder control. It is known that 20–30% of patients with multiple sclerosis or Parkinson's disease have primary complaints of urinary incontinence (15, 16). Although the neurology of continence is complex and poorly understood, the clinician providing primary care can and should effectively screen the incontinent patient for major neurological disease. The notion of a neurourological axis of bladder control simplifies this screening. The general aim in screening is to establish an intact axis from the cortex to the brainstem and pons and through spinal cord to the peripheral nerves that innervate the bladder.

Mental status, gait, and balance will have been noted in the general examination. Because of the importance of the sacral cord in the continence mechanism, the neurological examination concentrates on the innervation of the lower extremities and sacral reflexes. The lower back should be inspected for dimpling over the lumbosacral cord that could indicate a fusion defect (17). Assessment of the strength in the lower extremities as well as the deep tendon reflexes are important, particularly in a patient with low back pain or sciatica. The sharp and dull sensation in the perineum, buttocks, and inner thigh are randomly tested in the distribution of the pudendal nerve (S2-S4). If a patient can discriminate sharp from dull in these areas, the examiner can conclude that the sensory part of S2-S4 (lower micturition center) is intact.

Three simple tests of the sacral reflex arc demonstrate an intact motor component of the pudendal nerve: tapping the clitoris causes a visible contraction of the bulbocavernosus muscle (bulbocavernosus reflex), coughing causes contraction of the pelvic floor musculature (cough reflex), and, finally, stroking the skin adjacent to the anus elicits a reflex contraction of the anal sphincter muscle ("anal wink"). Inability to elicit the sacral reflex arc may not be pathological because it will be encountered in 20% of neurologically intact women (18). However, if these screening tests of S2-S4 are normal, any pathology found in the bladder is a local problem of the lower urinary tract and not secondary to central nervous system neuropathy.

Neurological testing in this manner will be easily and quickly performed. Such testing is for screening purposes and significant abnormal findings will merit referral to a neurologist.

URETHROSCOPY

Urethroscopy using a 0-degree urethroscope is a simple and quick office procedure (19). The test is performed with a small instrument (18 or 22F in diameter) without local anesthesia. The test is performed after voiding, with the patient in the supine position. The assessable bladder is then carefully inspected for foreign bodies, urethritis (red and shaggy proximal urethral mucosa and urethrovesical junction with or without mucosal polyps), or urethral diverticula. Urethritis can simulate clinical symptoms and urodynamic findings of detrusor instability, whereas urethral diverticula can simulate SUI (20). The only way to diagnose these conditions is by urethroscopy.

The urethrovesical junction is inspected with the urethroscope 1 cm distal to the junction. The patient is then asked to hold her urine. In the presence of an intact internal pudendal nerve and a pliable urethra, she should be able to close the urethrovesical junction. Inability to close the urethrovesical junction on command may indicate peripheral neuropathy or a fibrotic urethra, conditions that are contraindications to a suspending antiincontinence operation and indicate referral for further evaluation. The patient is then asked to cough or strain, during which the urethrovesical junction is expected to close with a well-supported and competent urethra or open if the urethral sphincter is incompetent (19).

Uroflow

This noninvasive test screens for disturbances in the emptying phase of the micturition cycle. Normal flow rates should exceed 15 mL/s. If the voided volume is less than 100 mL, the test is unreliable and may be repeated after instillation of 200 mL of saline in the bladder. Residual urine after spontaneous voiding is then measured. More than 50 mL of residual urine also raises the suspicion of a problem in the emptying phase. Such an emptying disorder may result from detrusor dysfunction or obstruction, and further testing is required for the differentiation.

Cystometry

Cystometry is a test of the bladder's filling and storage function. It allows differentiation of incontinence due to a problem primarily related to the detrusor (detrusor instability) from incontinence due to a defective outlet

(SUI) (21). One of the main reasons for recurrent symptoms after an antiincontinence operation is detrusor instability not diagnosed preoperatively (22). Cystometry should be performed with the patient in the standing position and with periodic cough provocations. The same test performed in the supine position without provocation may miss more than 30% of women with detrusor instability (23).

Single-channel cystometry can be easily performed in the office. In the absence of a cystometry machine, a fetal cardiotocographic monitor can be used with instillation of saline into the bladder with a pediatric feeding tube to measure bladder pressure with filling (24). The interpretation of a single-channel technique is reliable provided the detrusor is stable. Apparent bladder contractions suggest either combined stress incontinence and detrusor instability or detrusor contractions stimulated by Valsalva maneuver.

Guide to Triage

Recent advances in diagnosis of urinary tract disorders have resulted in the development of highly complex testing procedures. The clinician should bear in mind the principle of performing the simplest, least invasive, and most informative test first. Incontinence should be approached as a puzzle, and each piece of diagnostic information should point to a definite clinical impression. A simple workup consisting of tests accessible to the primary care clinician will establish a clear clinical impression in most incontinent patients. Approximately 20% of patients in unselected populations will require more sophisticated urodynamic testing.

Urinalysis and culture is performed before the first visit, and antibiotic treatment is initiated if necessary. The patient can complete a urolog and urinary questionnaire at home before the first visit. The initial evaluation consists of a detailed history and physical examination. Uroflow and measurement of postvoid residual can subsequently be performed. Urethroscopic findings of urethritis indicate that the inflammatory condition should be treated first, before the cysto-

metric examination. Simple cystometry may then be performed. Patients who undergo instrumentation of the urethra and bladder should receive 2 days of antibiotic prophylaxis.

If a patient gives a history of loss of urine on stress, has a normal urine test, normal screening neurologic test of S2-S4, positive cotton swab test, and stable bladder on simple cystometry, one can conclude that the loss of urine is from stress incontinence and anatomic defect. Such an evaluation can be done at the physician's office at relatively low cost, with no need for sophisticated urodynamic testing.

Indications for Referral

Complex urodynamic testing includes multichannel cystometry, pressure-flow voiding studies, measurement of Valsalva leak point pressure, urethral profilometry, and/or videourodynamic studies. Such testing is done at a referral center by specialists who primarily treat incontinent women.

The following are suggested criteria for referral for further testing.

UROLOG OF HIGH URINE OUTPUT

Total 24-hour urinary output that exceeds 2000 mL suggests possible diabetes mellitus or diabetes insipidus. These two conditions should be ruled out before final diagnosis is established.

NEUROPATHY

Any S2–S4 abnormality should result in referral of the patient to a neurologist to rule out central neuropathy as a possible cause of the urinary incontinence. Many patients with multiple sclerosis or Parkinson's disease (up to 25%) have urinary incontinence as their first symptom of the disease. The neurological disease should be treated first, before any further treatment for urinary incontinence is considered.

HEMATURIA

Gross or microscopic hematuria will frequently be related to a significant urological lesion, including carcinoma (25). Such findings should be explained before further treatment.

ABNORMAL URETHROCYSTOSCOPY

Urethral diverticula can simulate stress incontinence by lowering urethral closure pressure. Urethroscopic findings of urethral diverticula necessitate urodynamic testing, mainly a static urethral pressure profile to indicate which kind of surgical procedure should be selected (26). Inability to close the urethrovesical junction on command while performing the urethroscopic dynamic evaluation of this junction indicates that the patient may have a peripheral neuropathy as the cause for her incontinence, and a neurological consultation should be obtained (27). Mucosal lesions of the bladder noted on cystoscopy should be properly evaluated to rule out malignancy.

NEGATIVE COTTON SWAB TEST

Women with genuine stress incontinence not previously operated on almost always have hypermobility of the urethrovesical junction, resulting in a positive cotton swab test (12). A well-supported urethrovesical junction and a negative cotton swab test should serve as a red flag for the diagnosis of genuine stress incontinence, and further in-depth urodynamic studies should be ordered. If urodynamic testing confirms the diagnosis of SUI, an obstructive surgical procedure (such as the sling operation) should be considered, because procedures to suspend the bladder base in women with stress incontinence and negative cotton swab test are accompanied by an unacceptably high failure rate (14).

ABNORMAL UROFLOW OR POSTVOID RESIDUAL

Screening tests that suggest an emptying disorder should result in pressure-flow voiding tests to establish its cause.

DETRUSOR INSTABILITY ON SIMPLIFIED CYSTOMETRY

Findings of bladder contractions during cystometry in a woman with SUI necessitate multichannel urodynamic evaluation. It is very helpful to have simultaneous abdominal pressure readings in these patients to rule out periodic Valsalva maneuvers simulating detrusor contractions (28). It is important to assess the contribution of uninhibited bladder contractions versus the urethral factor to the patient's urinary incontinence. It is similarly helpful to determine whether there was an uninhibited urethral relaxation before the detrusor contraction before establishing a treatment plan (29, 30). All the foregoing information can be obtained only by a multichannel urodynamic testing.

PRIOR SURGICAL FAILURES

Women who were previously operated on for SUI and in whom the operation failed should have multichannel urodynamic evaluation before another operative procedure is planned. Such women may have unrecognized lower urinary tract pathology causing their incontinence other than simple "technical failure" of the surgeon. They may have peripheral neuropathy or periurethral scarring resulting in intrinsic urethral damage that requires a different operation than bladder neck suspension.

REFERENCES

1. Stanton SL. Principles of investigation. In: Stanton SL, ed. Clinical gynecologic urology. St. Louis: CV Mosby Company, 1984:45.
2. Cardozo L, Stanton SL. Genuine stress incontinence and detrusor instability: a review of 200 patients. Br J Obstet Gynaecol 1980;87:184–190.
3. Jarvis GJ, Hall S, Millar DR, et al. An assessment of urodynamic examination in incontinent women. Br J Obstet Gynaecol 1980;87:893–896.
4. Stanton SL, Ozsoy C, Hilton P. Voiding difficulties in the female: prevalence, clinical and urodynamic review. Obstet Gynecol 1983;61: 144–147.
5. Thompson JD, Wall LL, Growdon WA, Ridley JH. Urinary stress incontinence. In: Thompson JD, Rock JA, eds. TeLinde's operative gynecology. 7th ed. Philadelphia: JB Lippincott Company, 1992: 887–940.
6. Abrams P, Blaivas JG, Stanton SL, et al. Standardization of terminology of lower urinary tract function. Intern Urogyn J 1990;1:45–48.
7. Richardson DA, Bent AE, Ostergard DR. The effect of uterovaginal prolapse on urethrovesical pressure dynamics. Am J Obstet Gynecol 1983; 146:901–905.
8. Wall LL, Hewitt JK. Urodynamic characteristics

of women with complete posthysterectomy vaginal vault prolapse. Urology 1994;44:336–341.

9. Enhörning G. Simultaneous recording of intra vesical and intra urethral pressure: a study on urethral closure in normal and stress incontinent women. Acta Chir Scand Suppl 1971;276:1–68.

10. Crystle CD, Charme LS, Copeland WE. Q-tip test in stress urinary incontinence. Obstet Gynecol 1971;38:313–315.

11. Karram MM, Bhatia NN. The Q-tip test: standardization of the technique and its interpretation in women with urinary incontinence. Obstet Gynecol 1988;71:807–811.

12. Bergman A, McCarthy TA, Ballard CA, et al. Role of the Q-tip test in evaluating stress urinary incontinence. J Reprod Med 1987;32:273–275.

13. Montz FJ, Stanton SL. Q-tip test in female urinary incontinence. Obstet Gynecol 1986;67:258–260.

14. Bergman A, Koonings PP, Ballard CA. Negative Q-tip test as a risk factor for failed anti-incontinence surgery. J Reprod Med 1989;34:157–160.

15. Beck RP, Warren KG, Whitman P. Urodynamic studies in female patients with multiple sclerosis. Am J Obstet Gynecol 1981;139:273–276.

16. Galloway NTM. Urethral sphincter abnormalities in parkinsonism. Br J Urol 1983;55:691–693.

17. Stanton SL. History and examination. In: Stanton SL, ed. Clinical gynecologic urology. St. Louis: CV Mosby Company, 1984:46–58.

18. Wein AJ. Neuromuscular dysfunction of the lower urinary tract. In: Walsh PC, Retik AB, Stamey TA, Vaughan ED, eds. Campbell's urology. 6th ed. Philadelphia: WB Saunders, 1992:573–642.

19. Robertson JR. Gynecologic urethroscopy. Am J Obstet Gynecol 1973;115:986–990.

20. Scotti RJ, Ostergard DR. The urethral syndrome. Clin Obstet Gynecol 1984;27:515–529.

21. Reid RE, Owens LF, et al. Unstable bladder: urodynamic diagnosis and observations in evaluating urinary incontinence in the female. Urology 1987;29:107–110.

22. Hodgkinson CP. Recurrent stress urinary incontinence. Am J Obstet Gynecol 1978;132:844–854.

23. Godec CJ, Cass AS. Cystometric variations during postural changes. J Urol 1980;123:722–725.

24. Bergman A, Nguyen H, Koonings PP, et al. Use of fetal cardiotocographic monitor in the evaluation of urinary incontinence. Isr J Med Sci 1988;24:291–294.

25. Carson CC III, Segura JW, Greene LF. Clinical importance of microhematuria. J Am Med Assoc 1979;241:149–150.

26. Bhatia NN, McCarthy TA, Ostergard DR. Urethral pressure profiles of women with urethral diverticulae. Am J Obstet Gynecol 1981;58:375–378.

27. Bhatia NN, Bradley WE. Neuroanatomy and physiology: innervation of the lower urinary tract. In: Raz S, ed. Female urology. Philadelphia: WB Saunders, 1983:12–32.

28. Fantl JA, Hurt WG, Dunn LJ. Urinary incontinence due to unconscious abdominal contractions. Am J Obstet Gynecol 1983;147:137–140.

29. Koonings PP, Bergman A, Ballard CA. Urodynamics: combined detrusor instability and stress urinary incontinence: where is the primary pathology? Gynecol Obstet Invest 1989;26:250–256.

30. Sand PK, Bowen LW, Ostergard DR. Uninhibited urethral relaxation: an unusual cause of incontinence. Obstet Gynecol 1986;68:645–648.

CHAPTER 8

Urologically Oriented Neurological Examination

Lawrence R. Lind, Bruce A. Rosenzweig, and Narender N. Bhatia

A comprehensive neurological examination and its interpretation form an integral part of the history and physical examination of female patients with lower urinary tract symptomatology. Electrophysiological studies over the past 10 years have demonstrated an increasing role of neurological evaluation for patients with voiding dysfunction (1–6). The urogynecologist must understand the neurophysiology of normal voiding (see Chapter 3), must be familiar with the physical findings that may suggest a neurological explanation for voiding dysfunction, and must know which urodynamic and electrophysiological tests are required as they relate to neurological causes of voiding dysfunction (see Chapter 17). This chapter describes the details of the neurologically oriented physical examination followed by a clinical overview of the most common neurological disorders that have urological sequelae. Guidelines are provided for selecting patients who require formal neurological consultation or advanced electrophysiological testing. It is emphasized that to perform a meaningful neurological examination for a patient with lower urinary complaints, the combined understanding of neuroanatomy and neurophysiology is essential.

Neurological Evaluation

The neurological history and examination should immediately follow the general physical examination. To perform an effective general screening neurological examina-

tion, a basic understanding of neuroanatomy is necessary (see Chapter 3). The localization of a lesion to the cerebrum, brainstem, cerebellum, spinal cord, or peripheral nervous system is accomplished by the systematic examination of the cranial nerves, neck, and trunk; motor, reflex, and sensory function of the upper and lower extremities; and an assessment of sphincteric and autonomic nervous system functions, gait, and station. Each component of the neurological examination is presented with emphasis on the clinical correlations between findings on the neurological examination and concomitant voiding abnormalities.

History

The neurological examination always begins with a detailed and focused history. Attention is necessary not only to the presented facts but to the speech and manner of patient responses to questions. The mode of onset, evolution, and course of each symptom are of paramount importance. It is tempting to shorten the time spent on history taking when the patient is a poor historian. The presence of poor speech or disorganized thoughts may be the first clue to a central nervous system lesion also related to the urological complaints. Differentiating between the various etiologies of mental deficits may assist in understanding the nature of the urinary complaints.

Because historical events may be the most important consideration, extensive details of voiding difficulties, as well as information regarding bowel and sexual function, are essential to the proper interpretation of neurological findings. History should include sequentially the same categories to be explored in the neurological examination: mental status, strength and sensory changes of the upper and lower extremities, and gait and station.

General Screening Neurological Examination

MENTAL STATUS

Mental status testing is performed by determining the accuracy of recent and past memory, orientation, calculations, comprehension, and fund of general knowledge. More precise information can be obtained by psychometric testing. Disorders associated with mental status aberrations that may also produce urological abnormalities include senile and presenile dementia, Parkinson's disease, brain tumors, and normal pressure hydrocephalus. Patients with these disorders may present with either detrusor instability (when the frontal lobe is primarily affected) or overflow incontinence (when the paracentral gyrus is primarily affected). It is important to define the severity of the dementia because the patient's ability to understand and subsequently to comply with various tasks such as intermittent self-catheterization and pharmacological management will to a large degree determine whether these treatment plans will be successful. Further details regarding cerebral injuries, neurological evaluation, and urinary function may be found in the clinical correlations section.

CRANIAL NERVES

A detailed review of each cranial nerve is beyond the scope of this chapter. Most of the nerves can be evaluated in a series of maneuvers that takes less than 1 minute. A reasonably thorough examination includes assessment of smell; eye movements; fundoscopic examination; facial symmetry; use of eye, facial, and tongue muscles; jaw strength; head movement; and shoulder shrug.

MUSCLE STRENGTH

Muscle strength, sensory examination, reflexes, and tests for sacral integrity must be interpreted as a group because they all add information to spinal and peripheral nerve function. Skeletal muscles should be inspected for muscle atrophy and fasciculations, spasticity, rigidity, and strength. Muscle strength is assessed by having the patient either resist movement or by actively moving against resistance. Strength is graded on a scale of 0 to 5: 0, no movement; 1, trace of contraction; 2, active movement when gravity eliminated; 3, active movement against gravity only; 4, active movement against resistance but less than normal; and 5, normal strength.

Evaluation of the motor function reflecting the sacral spinal cord involves testing the patient's ability to perform specific movements of the lower extremities. The basic maneuvers are extension and flexion of the hip, knee, and ankle and inversion or eversion of the foot. Figure 8.1 illustrates the maneuvers and the segments of the spinal cord involved.

DEEP TENDON REFLEXES

Evaluation of the deep tendon reflexes provides information regarding segmental and suprasegmental spinal cord function. The important reflexes to be evaluated in each patient are the jaw jerk, the biceps, triceps, knee, ankle, and plantar responses. Any asymmetry of the reflexes may closely reflect the nature of bladder dysfunction. In supranuclear lesions, there is hyperreflexia of the deep tendon reflexes. This is often associated with uninhibited detrusor contractions as demonstrated by cystometry.

An upper motor neuron lesion may also be detected with the plantar toe reflex. The plantar toe reflex is elicited by stroking the handle of a reflex hammer along the lateral aspect of the foot from the heel to the ball of the foot and then curving medially. A normal response produces plantar flexion of the toes. An abnormal (Babinski) response produces fanning of the toes and dorsiflexion of the big toe and indicates interruption of the corticospinal tracts, an upper motor neuron lesion.

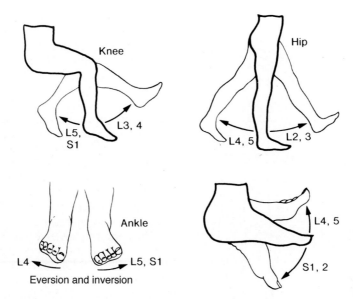

Figure 8.1. Testing of motor strength. Lower extremity movements and the corresponding spinal cord segments are indicated.

In patients with cauda equina lesions or with peripheral neuropathy (lower motor neurons), the deep tendon reflexes may be diminished or absent. Urologically, these findings are most commonly associated with detrusor areflexia or varying degrees of decreased bladder contractility. The presence of peripheral nerve impairment, autonomic neuropathy, or spinal cord disease below T12 may be suggested by absent or diminished reflexes and clinically correlated with symptoms of urinary retention or voiding difficulties.

SENSORY FUNCTION

Accurate assessment of sensory function is difficult because of the subjective nature of the response and the need for patient cooperation. Despite these limitations, the examiner can usually determine whether the patient can perceive the stimulus and whether the response is symmetrical. The spinal pathways of importance are the lateral spinothalamic tract (pain and temperature), the posterior columns (position, vibration, and light touch), and the anterior spinothalamic tract (crude touch). Only the distal extremities need to be evaluated for position sense and vibration; however, both proximal and distal extremities should be evaluated for pain, touch, and temperature.

A dermatome is an area of skin innervated by a sensory nerve from a single nerve root. Dermatome charts (Fig. 8.2) may be referred to if a deficit is noted on examination. Dermatomes overlap and levels can vary considerably.

SACRAL CORD INTEGRITY

Spinal cord segments S2 to S4 contain important neurons involved with micturition. Therefore, the screening neurological examination related to the lower urinary tract encompasses the sensory and motor functions represented in this area. Detailed neuroanatomy of this region is described in Chapter 3. In the context of the physical examination, parasympathetic detrusor muscle fibers arise from the intermediolateral cell column of the spinal cord at levels S2 and S3 with minor contributions from S1 and S2. The principal action of these fibers, traveling as the pelvic nerve, is contraction of the detrusor muscle. Sympathetic motor neurons, traveling with the hypogastric nerve, regulate bladder storage. Alpha adrenergic stimulation primarily affects the proximal urethra, causing constriction. Beta adrenergic stimulation has minor detrusor effect causing relaxation, whereas the predominant regulator of detrusor activity is the parasympathetic system as described above.

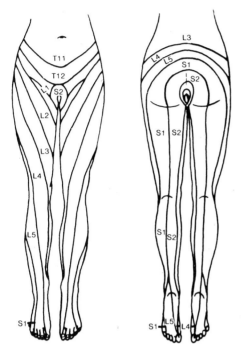

Figure 8.2. An exemplary dermatome map for use with sensory testing.

Separate from the autonomic innervation, the periurethral striated muscle is also innervated by the pudendal nerve, originating in the S2–4 segments. Stimulation of this nerve causes contraction of the distal periurethral striated muscle.

The external voluntary anal sphincter is representative of the pelvic floor musculature. Anal sphincter testing involves a determination of resistance to the entry of the examining finger and the ability of the patient to voluntarily contract the anal sphincter. A full bladder or rectal ampulla may interfere with anal sphincter reflex activity but will not change muscle tone. The presence of a voluntary contraction indicates integrity of the pelvic floor innervation, both segmental and suprasacral. Preservation of tone in the absence of a voluntary contraction indicates a suprasacral lesion; diminished tone implies a sacral or peripheral nerve abnormality.

Reflexes, including the anal sphincter, bulbocavernosus, and cough reflexes, can produce contraction of the pelvic floor. Stroking the skin lateral to the anus elicits the anal reflex. Contraction of the anus should be observed. When the contraction is not visible, often a contraction can be palpated with an examining finger (Fig. 8.3). The bulbocavernosus reflex involves contraction of the bulbocavernosus and ischiocavernosus muscles in response to tapping or squeezing of the clitoris (Fig. 8.3). Pulling on a suprapubic or intraurethral Foley catheter or touching the urethral or vesical mucosa also stimulates this reflex. Because the external anal sphincter is part of this same pelvic floor musculature, it also responds in most patients. Intactness of these reflexes indicates functional normality of the fifth lumbar to the fifth sacral segments.

The cough reflex involves the same spinal cord efferents and also the volitional innervation of the abdominal muscles (T6 to L1). Both coughing and deep inspiration cause a contraction of the periurethral striated sphincter (Fig. 8.4). Unfortunately, these reflexes are sometimes difficult to evaluate clinically because of the rapidity of response. The ability to detect the responses of all three reflexes is improved by placing a pressure-sensitive catheter in either the urethra or the anal sphincter and recording pressure changes. In approximately 10% of normal adults, the reflex response may not be strong enough to be appreciated on physical examination (7). In these patients, EMG and latency studies may be helpful in distinguishing diminished responses from absence of reflex activity (8).

CEREBELLUM

Truncal ataxia and the ataxic gait characteristic of midline cerebellar dysfunction are frequently observed in patients with multiple sclerosis. Additional cerebellar testing consists of evaluation of finger–nose and heel–shin coordination and examination of the patient's gait, including tandem gait. The cerebellum has four major functions in the control of micturition: maintenance of the tone of the periurethral striated muscle and the pelvic floor, suppression of the detrusor reflex by modulation of the brainstem detrusor centers, coordination of bladder contraction with urethral relaxation, and regulating the strength of detrusor and periurethral muscle contractions.

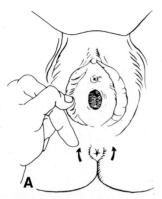 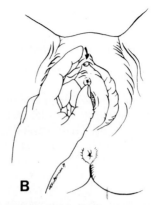

Figure 8.3.   Tests of sacral cord integrity. **A,** The anal reflex. The skin lateral to the anus is stroked. Contraction of the anus is observed or palpated with an examining figure. **B,** The bulbocavernosus reflex.

Contraction of the bulbocavernosus and ischiocavernosus muscles is observed in response to tapping or squeezing the clitoris.

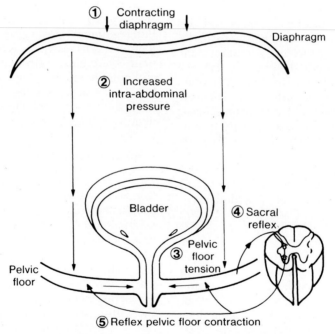

Figure 8.4.   Tests of sacral cord integrity. The cough reflex. Contraction of the diaphragm during cough generates increased abdominal pressure that places tension on the pelvic floor. Tension on the pelvic floor initiates a sacral reflex, resulting in contraction of the pelvic floor and periurethral striated muscles.

Cerebellar disease characteristically produces spontaneous high-amplitude detrusor reflex contractions as observed during cystometry. Poor hand coordination in these patients can impede the use of intermittent self-catheterization.

The sequential steps of the general screening neurological examination have been presented above. To present the examination in sequence, details of clinical entities related to each aspect of the examination were briefly described. Detailed clinical correlations between several neurological disorders and their urological sequelae are presented below.

Clinical Correlations

DISEASES AT OR ABOVE THE BRAINSTEM

Cerebrovascular Disease

Disorders affecting the cerebrum include dementia, atrophy, cerebral vascular accident, tumor, trauma, and hydrocephalus. Neurological examination may reveal abnormal mental status, speech impairment, and asymmetry in strength and reflexes. At the time of the acute episode, urinary retention may occur. After a variable recovery period, the most common expression of lower urinary tract dysfunction is detrusor hyperreflexia because there is release of the detrusor reflex response from voluntary control. Sensation is variable but usually intact, and thus the patient complains of urgency. When sensation is intact and the cerebral insult has not affected the patient's awareness of the problem, voluntary contraction of the urethral sphincter mechanism may maintain continence. This compensation makes the difference between urgency and urgency with incontinence. Smooth and striated muscle activity is usually synergic. Urodynamic findings suggesting detrusor sphincter dyssynergia may truly represent appropriate sphincter activity in a patient who is attempting not to soil herself, a syndrome named "pseudodyssynergia" (9, 10).

Brain Tumor

Voiding dysfunction secondary to a solid mass is dependent on the localized region involved. The most frequent area that affects voiding function is the frontal lobe with resultant detrusor hyperreflexia. Mass lesions in this area often result in decreased awareness of all voiding events. The patient thus has no thoughts concerning voluntary suppression of the reflex and may not care to wait for a socially acceptable time before soiling herself. Mental status abnormalities in this situation are easily elicited on examination. When the cerebral insult is in the midline affecting the paracentral gyrus, volitional control of urethral sphincteric relaxation is lost, resulting in urinary retention.

Parkinson's Disease

This disease is characterized by a relative dopamine deficiency with a predominance of cholinergic activity in the corpus striatum. Neurological findings include bradykinesia, tremor, and skeletal rigidity. Voiding dysfunction occurs in 25–75% of patients and is usually characterized by urgency, frequency, nocturia, and urge incontinence (10). Urodynamically, detrusor hyperreflexia is the most common finding. Smooth and striated muscle activity is synergic, but it is less clear whether these patients retain striated sphincter control (11).

Shy-Drager Syndrome

Shy-Drager syndrome is a rare degenerative disorder affecting the cerebellum, brainstem, peripheral autonomic ganglia, and thoracolumbar preganglionic sympathetic neurons (11). Patients present with parkinsonian symptoms, orthostatic hypotension, and anhidrosis. Voiding dysfunction varies but most often includes detrusor hyperreflexia and an open bladder neck at rest with denervation of the striated sphincter.

Cranial Nerve Abnormalities

Cranial nerve involvement is usually relevant to urinary dysfunction when it suggests a brainstem lesion or a generalized neurological disorder. A history of optic neuritis, the detection of pallor of the optic disks, or the presence of nystagmus suggest the diagnosis of multiple sclerosis. Although brainstem plaques related to the systemic disorder may not be responsible for the urinary symptoms, the finding of cranial nerve dysfunction promotes the search for similar plaques elsewhere in the nervous system. Because the lesions of multiple sclerosis may be in the upper spinal cord, lower spinal cord, or in both locations, urinary derangements may include detrusor instability, detrusor areflexia, or a combination of detrusor overactivity with incomplete emptying.

DISEASES AFFECTING THE SPINAL CORD

Spinal cord injury may be the result of trauma, vascular disease, arteriovenous mal-

formation, myelopathy, arachnoiditis, or myelitis. The location of insult dictates the
motor and urological sequelae of spinal cord
injury. It is important to recognize that the
vertebral level does not correspond to the
neural cord level. The sacral spinal cord
begins about the level of T12 to L1. The spinal
cord terminates in the cauda equina at about
the level of the second lumbar vertebra.

Suprasacral Injury

Bladder contractility and reflex bladder
contractions require an intact conus medullaris (sacral spinal cord segments) and its
afferent and efferent connections. Complete
lesions above this level but below the level of
sympathetic outflow usually result in detrusor hyperreflexia, absent sensation below the
level of the lesion, smooth sphincter synergia, and striated sphincter dyssynergia (10). If
the insult is above the spinal column level of
T6 (spinal cord level T7–8), there may also be
dyssynergia of the smooth muscle sphincter.

General neurological and urological findings vary depending on the amount of time
that has passed before the physical evaluation. Immediately after a major spinal injury,
"spinal shock" occurs. There is a global
decrease in nerve excitability below the level
of the lesion. There are decreased or absent
somatic reflexes and flaccid muscle paralysis
below the level of the injury (12, 13). The
exception to this rule is that the peripheral
somatic reflexes (anal and bulbocavernosus
reflexes) may never disappear. If they do,
they may return in hours or minutes (13).
Autonomic activity is depressed, resulting in
an acontractile and areflexic bladder. The
smooth component of the sphincter usually
is intact, and EMG recordings can usually be
obtained from the striated sphincter (14).
Continence is usually preserved secondary to
the sphincter tone, and urinary retention is
the usual clinical problem requiring intermittent or continuous catheterization. If the
distal cord is intact but isolated (via the
insult) from the upper cord, detrusor contractility will eventually return, causing involuntary voiding usually with incomplete
emptying secondary to weak involuntary detrusor contractions. Bladder reflex activity
should parallel return of lower extremity
reflex activity. In these patients, preserving

low pressure bladder storage is a priority.
After a period of spinal shock, the long-
standing dysfunction that follows a complete
lesion above the sacral spinal cord includes
detrusor hyperreflexia, smooth sphincter
synergia (unless the lesion is above T6), and
striated sphincter dyssynergia (10). Neurological examination demonstrates skeletal
muscle spasticity below the level of the insult, hyperreflexic deep tendon reflexes, extensor plantar reflexes (Babinski), and decreased sensation. Bladder emptying is
usually incomplete as a result of striated
sphincter dyssynergia.

There are patients with upper spinal lesions in which reflex activity of the spinal
cord does not follow the areflexic stage and
the bladder remains hypotonic. In these patients, referral for electrophysiological testing is indicated. Abnormalities in evoked
potential from the perineal region may be
demonstrated.

The pontine-mesencephalic formation is
responsible for coordinating bladder and striated sphincter activity. Any lesion between
this center and the sacral spinal cord may
interfere with this coordination, resulting
in true detrusor-sphincter dyssynergia. Although management of the incontinence is
often of great concern to the patient, clinical
priority lies with protecting the upper urinary tracts from the sequelae of high intravesical pressure. Cystometry is essential to
determine the bladder pressure before detrusor contractions occur, the bladder capacity
at a safe intravesical pressure, and to detect
the pressure at which leakage occurs. To
avoid upper tract injury, bladder pressures at
vesical volumes obtained during the intermittent catheterization schedule must be less
than 40 cm H_2O. Alternatively, the pressure
at which the bladder involuntarily empties
must be below 40 cm H_2O.

Lesions Above T6

Many of the findings with lesions above T6
are the same as those below T6 but above the
sacral cord. As mentioned previously, there
may be smooth sphincter dyssynergia in addition to the dysfunctions described above
for lower lesions. Autonomic dysreflexia is a
syndrome of exaggerated sympathetic activity below the level of the spinal lesion (12, 13,

15). It occurs most often in patients with cervical spine injuries but can occur with any lesion above T6. The syndrome includes hypertension, headache, profuse sweating, and reflex bradycardia. The stimulus for this response usually comes from the rectum or bladder. Hemodynamic effects of the syndrome can be managed acutely with parenteral ganglionic alpha adrenergic blockade or parenteral chlorpromazine (Thorazine). Stimuli that initiate this reflex must be identified on an individual case basis. Catheter management protocols often must be altered to decrease bladder overactivity that is often the stimulus for acute exacerbations. Alternatively, surgical measures may be required to decrease outlet resistance so that leakage occurs at lower bladder volumes and pressures.

Lesions of the Sacral Spinal Cord

After sacral spinal injury and spinal shock, there is depression of the deep tendon reflexes, varying degrees of flaccid paralysis, and absent sensation below the level of the lesion. This is in contrast to upper spinal lesions in which hyperreflexia and muscle spasticity are the rule. Detrusor areflexia is the most common urological result. The smooth sphincter is competent but fails to relax. The striated sphincter retains some tone (diminished EMG activity) but is usually no longer under voluntary control. The classic description of urological findings includes a reasonable bladder capacity with high compliance; however, depending on the obstructive abilities of the nonrelaxing sphincter, decreased compliance is a possible clinical outcome. When bladder pressure becomes greater than urethral pressure, leakage occurs. If this leak point is high enough, the upper tracts are affected.

Multiple Sclerosis

Multiple sclerosis is one of the most common neurological causes for voiding dysfunction (16). The pathophysiology involves impaired nerve conduction secondary to focal neural demyelination. Neurological abnormalities are subject to exacerbation and remission over time. Symptoms are dependent on the extent and locations of the demyelinating plaques. Cranial nerve findings are

common, but all levels of the spinal cord are vulnerable.

Voiding abnormalities are common because the process commonly involves the posterior and lateral columns of the spinal cord, which are of import for bladder and outlet function. Fifty to 80% of patients with this disease have voiding complaints, and in 10%, a voiding complaint will be a part of the initial symptom complex. Patients may present with acute urinary retention, but detrusor hyperreflexia is the most common abnormality. In addition, 30–65% of patients with detrusor hyperreflexia secondary to multiple sclerosis will also have striated sphincter dyssynergia (15–17). Bladder areflexia may occur but is less common. Voiding function in the presence of detrusor sphincter dyssynergia is variable, and physician priority lies with protecting the upper tracts from the potential consequences of elevated bladder pressures.

DISEASES OF THE PERIPHERAL NERVOUS SYSTEM

Diabetes Mellitus

Diabetes is the most common cause for peripheral and autonomic neuropathies. The pathophysiology involves segmental demyelination and impaired nerve conduction secondary to metabolic abnormalities of the Schwann cell (16, 17). Physical examination may reveal decreased sensation in the lower extremities secondary to vascular and nerve compromise. Urinary symptoms are insidious in onset as bladder sensation gradually diminishes. Typically, with impaired sensation, voiding intervals increase and may progress to only once or twice daily with no real sensation or urgency. Stretch of the detrusor muscle and neural impairment eventually result in decreased contractility. Recruitment of abdominal muscles or use of mechanical maneuvers is common to initiate and maintain a weak stream of urine. Urodynamic testing demonstrates decreased sensation to bladder filling, large bladder capacity, poor contractility, prolonged voiding time with low peak flows, and high residual volumes. Early diagnosis and institution of timed voiding with periodic evaluation of residual volumes is the best treatment. Tabes dorsalis and pernicious anemia may result in similar sensory neurogenic voiding abnormalities (12).

Herpes Zoster

Invasion of the sacral spinal ganglia with the herpes virus results in typical vesicular skin eruptions, reflecting the affected dermatomes. Urgency and frequency followed by urinary retention are the typical urological sequelae (12). This disease usually resolves within weeks to months depending on host factors and treatment.

Spinal Disk Disease

Patients with spinal disk disease usually present with low back pain radiating down the back of the thigh (12). When spinal root compression in the L4–5 or L5 to S1 disk interspace causes voiding dysfunction, the most common urodynamic finding is detrusor hyperreflexia. The striated sphincter may be normal or show signs of decreased function. The status of the striated sphincter will dictate whether the patient experiences incontinence secondary to involuntary detrusor contractions versus retention or straining secondary to the failure of relaxation of the striated sphincter. Laminectomy may not restore bladder function. It is thus important to identify the problem preoperatively to separate disk protrusion from the surgical intervention as the causative agent.

Radical Pelvic Surgery

Voiding dysfunction after surgery is most common after abdominoperineal resection and radical hysterectomy (10). The frequency varies with reports of up to 60% of patients having voiding difficulties with 15–20% experiencing permanent dysfunction (15). Neurological examination in these patients may be normal. Urinary retention with varying degrees of sensory awareness are usually the first abnormal urological findings. In the long term, there is absent or diminished bladder contractility with distal obstruction secondary to preserved striated sphincter tone that is no longer under voluntary control. Decreased compliance is common. Depending on the degree of distal obstruction, the patient may manifest both storage and emptying dysfunction. Urodynamic studies are essential in such complex patients. Risks to the upper urinary tracts depend on the filling leak point. Therapy is directed to establish low pressure storage and periodic emptying.

Neurological Consultation and Electrophysiological Testing

In certain patients, urinary bladder dysfunction could be the initial manifestation of an underlying neurological disease. On the other hand, many patients with multiple urinary symptoms have no symptoms or signs suggestive of overt neurological disease. In these patients, detailed electrophysiological and urodynamic testing of the lower urinary tract may suggest neuropathy as the underlying cause of the symptomatology. In patients with known neurological disease and associated bladder symptoms, the urodynamic and related testing could be used to define the nature, location, and extent of end organ involvement. The question of when and to whom to refer is often a difficult one. Any patient with a neurological deficit and voiding complaints should undergo multichannel urodynamics, including uroflowmetry, cystometry, and pressure-voiding studies. Patients with established neurological diagnoses whose urinary complaints, physical examination, and urodynamics are in agreement regarding the mechanism of the voiding disorder do not require advanced electrophysiological testing. However, if a treatment plan fails or when history, physical, and urodynamics do not lead to a clear etiology of the voiding dysfunction, electrophysiological testing is indicated by a qualified specialist. This may be a neurologist, urologist, or urogynecologist, depending on specialized training. In addition, patients presenting with incontinence or pelvic organ prolapse despite having no risk factors may also be good candidates for electrophysiological testing. In this scenario, evoked responses may localize an atypical explanation for the voiding dysfunction such as a paraspinal mass. In this case, imaging studies can be selected more specifically, and perhaps inappropriate surgical intervention may be avoided for the elective problem of incontinence.

Similar reasoning applies to patients with intrinsic sphincter deficiency. In the absence of established risk factors (age greater than 50, previous incontinence surgery, radiation, known neurological impairment [18]), patients with urodynamic evidence of intrinsic sphincter deficiency may also benefit from electrophysiological testing. The association of intrinsic sphincter deficiency with myelomeningocele is well established (19, 20), and thus in the absence of historical or examination evidence to explain the sphincter incompetence, electrophysiological testing to investigate spinal cord integrity is indicated. The specific tests available and their applications are discussed in Chapter 17.

There should be a low threshold for referral to a neurologist. Although the mechanism of correcting a voiding dysfunction may be clear after history, physical, and urodynamics, the presence of any underlying neurological disorder necessitates ongoing care by a neurologist. Any patient with a new neurological finding or a change in character of existing deficits requires neurological consultation.

Conclusion

A variety of diseases cause urethral and bladder disturbances and associated neurological signs and symptoms. Although the urologic neuroanatomy is complex, some patterns of neurological deficits and their urological manifestations are well established. Familiarity with these patterns combined with appropriate neurology history and physical examination are essential for evaluation of women with lower urinary complaints. Gynecologists and urologists need to be familiar with the clinical correlations between general neurological findings and urological dysfunction to properly treat and triage patients with lower urinary tract complaints.

REFERENCES

1. Kiff ES, Swash M. Slowed conduction in the pudendal nerves in idiopathic (neurogenic) fecal incontinence. Br J Surg 1984;71:614–616.

2. Bradley WE, Timm GW, Rockswold GL, Scott FB. Detrusor and urethral electromyelography. J Urol 1975;114:69–71.
3. Swash M, Henrey MM, Snooks SJ. Unifying concept of pelvic floor disorders and incontinence. J R Soc Med 1985;78:906–911.
4. Benson JT, editor. Female pelvic floor disorders: investigation and management. New York: Norton Medical Books, 1992:142–166.
5. Benson JT. Neurophysiologic control of lower urinary tract. Obstet Gynecol Clin North Am 1989;16:733–740.
6. Benson JT, McClellen E. The effect of vaginal dissection on the pudendal nerve. Obstet Gynecol 1993;82:387–389.
7. Bruskewitz R. Female incontinence: signs and symptoms. In: Raz S, ed. Female urology. Philadelphia: WB Saunders, 1983:45–50.
8. Ortiz OC, Bertitti AC, Nunez JD. Female pelvic floor responses. Int J Urogynecol 1994;5:278–282.
9. Wein AJ, Barrett DM. Etiologic possibilities for increased pelvic floor electromyography activity during bladder filling. J Urol 1982;127:949–952.
10. Barrett DM, Wein AJ. Voiding dysfunction: diagnosis, classification, and management. In: Gillenwater JY, Grayhack JT, Howards SS, Duckett JW, eds. Adult and pediatric urology, 2nd ed. St. Louis: Mosby Year Book, 1991:1001–1099.
11. Blaivas JG. Non traumatic neurogenic voiding dysfunction in the adult. I. Physiology and approach to therapy. AUA Update Series; 1985 lesson 11, vol 4.
12. Hald T, Bradley WE. The urinary bladder-neurology and dynamics. Baltimore: Williams and Wilkins, 1982:160–165.
13. Thomas DG. Spinal cord injury. In: Mundy AR, Stephenson TP, Wein AJ, eds. Urodynamics: principles, practice, and application. Great Britain: Churchill Livingstone, 1984:260–272.
14. Awad S, Bryniak SR, Downie JN, et al. Urethral pressure profile during spinal shock stage in man: a preliminary report. J Urol 1777;117:91–94.
15. McGuire EJ. Clinical evaluation and treatment of neurogenic vesical dysfunction. In: Libertino J, ed. International perspectives in urology. Baltimore: Williams and Wilkins, 1984:303–312.
16. Blaivas JG. Non traumatic neurogenic voiding dysfunction in the adult. II. Multiple sclerosis and diabetes melitus. AUA Update Series; 1985b lesson 12, vol 4.
17. Mundy AR, Blaivas JG. Non-traumatic neurologic disorders. In: Mundy AR, Stephenson TP, Wein AJ, eds. Urodynamics: principles, practice and application. New York: Churchill Livingstone, 1984:278–287.
18. Horbach NS, Ostergard DR. Predicting intrinsic sphincter deficiency in women with stress incontinence. Obstet Gynecol 1994;84:188–192.
19. McGuire EJ, Woodside JR, Borden TA, Weiss RM. Prognostic value of urodynamic testing in myelodysplastic children. J Urol 1980;126:205–208.
20. Wan J, McGuire EJ, Bloom DA, Ritchey ML. Stress leak point pressure: a diagnostic tool for incontinent children. J Urol 1993;150:700–702.

CHAPTER 9

Standardization of the Description of Pelvic Organ Prolapse

Kimberly W. Coates and Bob L. Shull

Introduction

Lack of a standardized system for the objective description of pelvic organ prolapse is a significant problem in gynecology. Although multiple systems have been tried, no consensus has been reached. Consequently, gynecologists have been unable to document physical findings objectively and follow them longitudinally and to compare preoperative and postoperative pelvic support in series reported by different investigators. These handicaps have adversely affected the advancement of knowledge of the natural history of pelvic organ prolapse and refinement of surgical techniques for treatment of pelvic organ prolapse. A standardized system that allows reproducible and reliable descriptions of pelvic organ support is imperative.

History

Dr. Norman Miller, one of the early American gynecologic surgeons to note the importance of observing "end results" of surgical therapy, reported a creative system for quantifying the size of cystoceles (1). "Enormous" was used to describe a cystocele the size of an "average orange," "large" for the size of a "lemon," "moderate" for the size of a "hen's egg," and "small" for the size of a "bantam's egg or plum." Although he aspired to quantify the amount of prolapse observed, his system was fraught with limitations because descriptions such as these are subjective and vary greatly between observers. The use of multiple classification methods for pelvic organ prolapse has lead some investigators to become frustrated about the lack of a standardized description for grading prolapse. In 1961, Friedman and Little (2) concisely summarized the state of disarray: "Specious and misleading discrepancies exist with reference to classification of the extent of descent of the uterus in disorders involving fascial relaxation."

In 1980, Dr. C. T. Beecham (3) proposed a grading system "in the interests of standardization" that included three degrees of severity to describe "rectocele," "cystocele," "uterine prolapse" or "vaginal apex prolapse," and "enterocele." His classification system strictly prohibited straining by the patient or the examiner's use of traction on pelvic structures. Digital depression of the perineum was an integral part of this method. Each site of prolapse was graded by degree, from first to third, based on visual inspection. When the site of evaluation was seen with depression of the perineum, a first-degree grade of severity was assigned to that site. For example, when the perineum was depressed and the cervix was visible, first-degree uterine prolapse was diagnosed. For second- and third-degree prolapse, the examiner would note progressively more descent of the prolapsing site with the patient at rest. Specific definitions were assigned for each site of prolapse. A major fallacy of this classification is the requirement that the patient is not allowed to strain during the examination. Consider how much could be learned from auscultation of the lungs if the patient was asked *not* to breathe. We know patients must be examined with a maximum increase in intraabdominal pressure to reproduce prolapse findings at their worst. All recently proposed grading systems recommend the use of straining efforts or standing to elicit the maximum amount of prolapse.

Brubaker and Norton (personal communication, 1994) reviewed a sample of 157 manuscripts published in the English language from 1966 to 1990 and found the state of affairs described by Little and Friedman has not improved in the subsequent three decades (Tables 9.1 and 9.2). While pelvic reconstructive surgeons saddled themselves with the lack of any precise classification

Table 9.1. Overall Category of Disorder

Prolapse	53 (34%)
Genital prolapse	37 (24%)
Pelvic relaxation	14 (9%)
Procidentia	4 (3%)
Other	

Descensus	Pelvic floor lesion
Descent	Pelvic prolapse
Eversion	Perineal hernia
Genital relaxation	Perineal relaxation
Genital tract prolapse	Urogenital prolapse
Genitourinary prolapse	Uterovaginal prolapse
Pelvic floor defect	Vaginal inversion
Pelvic floor dysfunction	Vaginal prolapse

From Brubaker L, Norton P, personal communication, 1994.

Table 9.2. Grading Systems Used in 157 Prolapse Papers

	N
Mild/moderate/severe	19
Grade 0–3/1–3	12
Grade 0–4/1–4	8
Incomplete/complete	3
Alternative grading system	37
No grading system	78

From Brubaker L, Norton P, personal communication, 1994.

system, oncologists developed clinical and surgical staging systems and infertility surgeons introduced staging for endometriosis. Now all scientific reports regarding outcome of cancer therapy can be understood by gynecologists worldwide, results from different treatment modalities can be critically compared, and patients can be given information about treatment options and prognosis for cure. Pelvic reconstructive surgeons and their patients, on the other hand, have not been able to enjoy these advantages.

The Halfway System

From the late 1960s to the 1990s, Drs. Baden and Walker (4) developed and refined a site-specific classification for pelvic organ prolapse that addresses all potential sites of support loss. Initially published in 1968 and known as the "vaginal profile," their original classification was perceived to be too difficult for general use. After review of their original classification by a committee of the American College of Obstetricians and Gynecologists, Baden and Walker created a simplified version known as the Halfway System (Table 9.3).

For almost two decades, we have used the halfway system for describing pelvic organ prolapse. Consequently, we have been able to follow patients longitudinally to determine whether their pelvic support changes and to document long-term responses to surgical intervention. This site-specific analysis of pelvic organ prolapse has led to significant refinement in our diagnostic skills and to modifications in surgical techniques (5–8). Although this system provides a means to quantify the amount of prolapse at six vaginal sites, it provides only an estimate and not an exact measurement of descent of the prolapsing structure proximal and distal to the hymen (9).

Standardization of Terminology

In September 1993, a subcommittee of the International Continence Society met in

Table 9.3. Halfway System for Grading Relaxations

Urethrocele, cystocele, uterine prolapse, culdocele, or rectocele: patient strains firmly. Grade descent of desired sites
Grade posterior urethral descent, lowest part other sites
    Grade 0: normal position *for each* respective site
    Grade 1: descent *halfway* to the hymen
    Grade 2: descent to the hymen
    Grade 3: descent *halfway past* the hymen
    Grade 4: maximum possible descent for each site
Anterior perineal laceration: grade with patient holding
    Grade 0: normal; superficial epithelial laceration
    Grade 1: laceration *halfway* to the anal sphincter
    Grade 2: laceration to the anal sphincter
    Grade 3: laceration involves anal sphincter
    Grade 4: laceration involves rectal mucosa

When choosing between two grades, use the greater grade (i.e., if there is a question as to grade 2 or 3 cystocele, use cystocele, grade 3). Grade still in doubt? = Regrade with patient standing. Grade worst site, worst segment, or vaginal canal PRN. Grades are interchanged with mild to severe and degrees methods.
From Baden W, Walker T. Surgical repair of vaginal defects. Philadelphia, PA: JB Lippincott Company, 1992.

Rome to draft a system to enable accurate quantitative description of pelvic support findings (10). The subcommittee completed a final draft of their recommendations that was distributed to members of the International Continence Society, the American UroGynecologic Society, and the Society of Gynecologic Surgeons in late 1994 and early 1995. The system is an adaptation of Baden and Walker's site-specific system that requires measuring eight sites to create a tandem vaginal profile before assigning site-specific stages.

Observation and description of the maximum amount of pelvic organ prolapse are critical and must be consistent with the amount of prolapse experienced by the patient. Criteria for demonstration of maximum prolapse may include use of Valsalva's maneuver, traction, standing and straining, or patient use of a mirror to observe and confirm the prolapse. Other variations of examination technique should be described, including detailed descriptions of patient position, type of examination table or chair, type of speculum, type of strain, and fullness of bladder and rectum.

Keys to this classification scheme are the use of a defined anatomic landmark as a fixed point of reference and specifically defined points of measurement. The hymen is the fixed point by which measurements of six vaginal points are referenced. The report discourages the use of imprecise terms such as "introitus." Points of measurement within the vaginal canal are defined for the anterior and posterior vaginal wall and vaginal apex. Anteriorly, the two points of reference include a point 3 cm proximal to the external urethral meatus and a point that represents the most distal or dependent portion of the anterior vaginal wall. Posteriorly, the points of reference are similar by use of a midline posterior point 3 cm proximal to the hymen and a point representing the most distal or dependent position of the posterior vaginal wall. The vaginal apex is defined by two points: the most distal edge of the cervix or vaginal cuff and the location of the posterior fornix or pouch of Douglas. This last point is omitted in patients who have no cervix. Measurements of the genital hiatus, perineal body, and the total vaginal length are also included in this classification scheme.

All measurements are made in centimeters and expressed as above (proximal) or below (distal) the hymen and designated negative or positive, respectively. The numbers may then be listed as a simple line of numbers (tandem profile) or as a three by three grid (Table 9.4). In addition, the report establishes an ordinal staging system to be used after the quantitative description is completed (Table 9.5). The committee acknowledges the arbitrary nature of such a staging system but concludes that it is necessary. Staging allows for description and comparison of populations of patients, correlation of symptoms with severity of prolapse, and assessment of treatment outcomes.

Table 9.4. A Three-by-Three Grid for Recording the Quantitative Description of Pelvic Organ Prolapse

Point Aa Anterior Wall	Point Ba Anterior Wall	Point C Cervix or Cuff
Genital Hiatus	Perineal Body	Total Vaginal Length
Point Ap Posterior Wall	Point Bp Posterior Wall	Point D Posterior Fornix

From Bump R, Bo K, Brubaker L, et al. The International Continence Society Committee on Standardization of Terminology, Subcommittee on Pelvic Organ Prolapse and Pelvic Floor Dysfunction. The standardization of terminology of female pelvic organ prolapse and pelvic floor dysfunction. Am J Obstet Gynecol (in press).

Table 9.5. International Continence Society Pelvic Organ Prolapse Ordinal Staging System

Stage 0	Points Aa, Ap, Ba, and Bp are all at −3 cm and either point C or D is at no more than $-(X-2)$ cm
Stage I	The criteria for stage 0 are not met and the leading edge of prolapse is less than −1 cm
Stage II	Leading edge of prolapse is at least −1 cm but no more than +1 cm
Stage III	Leading edge of prolapse is greater than +1 cm but less than $+(X-2)$ cm
Stage IV	Leading edge of prolapse is at least $+(X-2)$ cm

X, total vaginal length in centimeters in stages 0, III, and IV. Stages I through IV can be subgrouped according to which portion of the lower reproductive tract is the leading edge of the prolapse using the following qualifiers: a, anterior vaginal wall; p, posterior vaginal wall; C, vaginal cuff; Cx, cervix; and Aa, Ba, Ap, Bp, and D for the defined points of measurement (e.g., IV-Cx, II-a, or III-Bp).
From Bump R, Bo K, Brubaker L, et al. The International Continence Society Committee on Standardization of Terminology, Subcommittee on Pelvic Organ Prolapse and Pelvic Floor Dysfunction. The standardization of terminology of female pelvic organ prolapse and pelvic floor dysfunction. Am J Obstet Gynecol (in press).

The subcommittee report also addresses the use of ancillary techniques for describing pelvic organ prolapse. These ancillary techniques may be used to characterize further the observed prolapse; however, careful description by investigators of the technique and the methods used is essential. Ancillary techniques may include digital rectal-vaginal examination, cotton swab testing for mobility of the urethral axis, and endoscopic or imaging studies.

The subcommittee report addresses the presence of functional symptoms related to the presence of pelvic organ prolapse. Although the functional deficits are not well established, there is a great need to characterize the occurrence of these symptoms with prolapse. The report acknowledges four functional symptom groups including urinary, bowel, sexual, and other local symptoms. They recommend that investigators attempt to standardize and validate symptom scales when possible. Specifically, investigators should ask precisely the same questions before and after the treatment has been implemented.

The subcommittee's efforts in creating this classification scheme and incorporating objective criteria for the description of pelvic organ prolapse are a first step toward establishing a standard, reliable, and validated description of pelvic anatomy and function. They acknowledge the need for studies designed to evaluate and validate the descriptions and definitions they propose.

REFERENCES

1. Miller NF. End-results from correction of cystocele by the simple fascia pleating method. Surg Gynecol Obstet 1928;46:403–410.
2. Friedman EA, Little WA. The conflict in nomenclature for descensus uteri. Am J Obstet Gynecol 1961;81:817–820.
3. Beecham CT. Classification of vaginal relaxation. Am J Obstet Gynecol 1980;136:957–958.
4. Baden W, Walker T. Surgical repair of vaginal defects. Philadelphia, PA: JB Lippincott Company, 1992.
5. Shull BL, Baden WF. Paravaginal defect repair for urinary incontinence: a six year experience. Am J Obstet Gynecol 1989;160:1432–1440.
6. Shull BL, Capen CV, Riggs M, Kuehl T. Pre- and postoperative analysis of site-specific pelvic support defects in 81 women treated by sacrospinous ligament suspension and pelvic reconstruction. Am J Obstet Gynecol 1992;166:1764–1768.
7. Shull BL, Capen CV, Riggs M, Kuehl T. Bilateral attachment of the vaginal cuff to iliococcygeus fascia: an effective method of cuff suspension. Am J Obstet Gynecol 1993;168:1669–1677.
8. Shull BL, Benn SJ, Kuehl TJ. Surgical management of prolapse of the anterior vaginal segment: an analysis of support defects, operative morbidity, and anatomic outcome. Am J Obstet Gynecol 1994;171:1429–1439.

9. Coates KW, Galan HL, Shull BL, Kuehl TJ. The squirrel monkey: an animal model of pelvic relaxation. Am J Obstet Gynecol 1995;172:588–593.
10. Bump R, Bo K, Brubaker L, et al. The International Continence Society Committee on Standardization of Terminology, Subcommittee on Pelvic Organ Prolapse and Pelvic Floor Dysfunction. The standardization of terminology of female pelvic organ prolapse and pelvic floor dysfunction. Am J Obstet Gynecol (in press).

CHAPTER 10

Urodynamic Evaluation

Janine K. Jensen

Urodynamic tests measure and record physiological parameters related to lower urinary tract function. The goal of urodynamic testing is to determine the cause of the patient's symptoms, whether the problem be urinary incontinence, voiding dysfunction, or lower urinary tract irritative symptoms. For any test to be valuable to the clinician, the patient's symptom complex must be reenacted during testing and the appropriate parameters must be monitored during the reenactment. Correlation of the objective data obtained by urodynamic evaluation with the patient's clinical history allows accurate diagnosis and appropriate therapy. This chapter covers the urodynamic tests currently available to evaluate lower urinary tract symptomatology in the female patient.

Cystometry

Cystometry measures bladder filling and storage functions, specifically addressing the pressure-volume relationship (compliance) of the bladder. Cystometry also measures bladder capacity, sensation to filling, and contractility.

NORMAL VERSUS ABNORMAL

The normal bladder relies on the inherent accommodative properties of the smooth muscle bladder wall to store an increasing volume of fluid at a near constant pressure. The normal cystometric curve is divided into three phases: an initial phase of pressure elevation to reach a resting bladder pressure of 2–8 cm H_2O (determined by the viscoelas-

tic properties of the bladder wall), a second tonic phase with minimal pressure increase during accommodation of a large volume of fluid, and a final evacuation phase during which intravesical pressure increases to empty the bladder of fluid. During the second phase of "tonic" bladder filling, bladder pressure should not rise more than 15 cm H_2O (Fig. 10.1). An elevation in bladder pressure greater than 15 cm H_2O or less than 15 cm H_2O in the presence of urgency is considered to reflect detrusor activity.

Normal bladder capacity is typically 350–500 mL in the average female. Decreased bladder capacity is found in association with infection, upper motor neuron lesions, a contracted bladder wall, and incontinence. Increased bladder capacity can also result from a variety of causes, including sensory neuropathy, lower motor neuron lesions, outflow obstruction, megalocystitis, and social inhibition. By itself, capacity has little meaning without the simultaneous measurement of intravesical pressure; an increased or decreased bladder capacity with normal intravesical pressures typically has little significance. However, a reduced capacity associated with elevated pressure (hypertonic bladder) or an increased capacity combined with diminished intravesical pressure (hypotonic bladder) usually signifies an underlying pathological process. Low intravesical pressure and increased bladder capacity may result from sensory neurological dysfunction, lower motor neuron injury, outflow obstruction, or chronic infrequent voiding habits (Fig. 10.2). Two cystometric tracing patterns have been associated with high intravesical pressure. A rapidly rising pressure during bladder filling is seen in the presence of conditions that cause decreased bladder wall compliance (Fig. 10.3). A pattern composed of a series of progressively increasing intravesical pressure spikes, with intravesi-

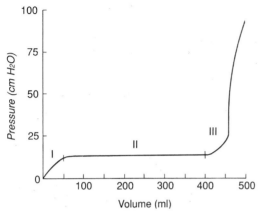

Figure 10.1. Triphasic cystometric curve.

cal pressure never returning to baseline, has also been identified and usually occurs in conjunction with decreased bladder capacity and compliance with associated detrusor overactivity (Fig. 10.4).

Individuals normally sense bladder filling and are able to determine the need to urinate based on this sensation of bladder fullness (1). Females typically report first sensation of bladder filling at 150 mL, fullness at 200–300 mL, and maximum bladder capacity at 400–700 mL. Variation from these normative values can be classified as either hyposensitive or hypersensitive conditions. The patient's position during measurement will effect these volumes, with increased sensation at lower volumes in the standing position than in the sitting or supine positions. Finally, it is important to realize that maximum cystometric capacity is not equivalent to bladder

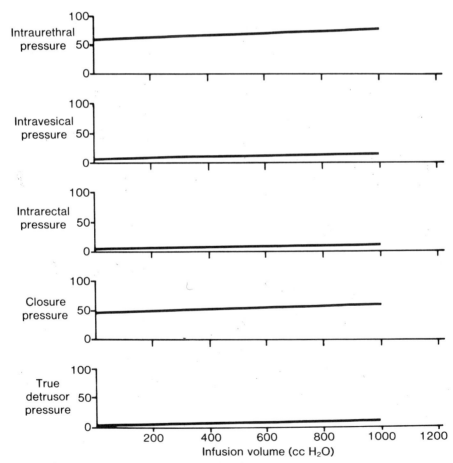

Figure 10.2. The cystometrogram of a hypotonic bladder. Minimal intravesical pressure increase occurs despite a large intravesical volume. No terminal contraction occurs.

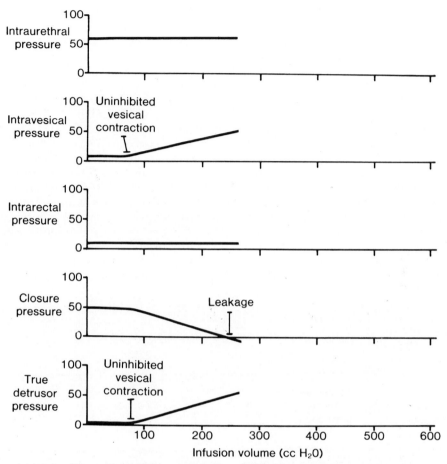

Figure 10.3. The cystometrogram of a hypertonic bladder. Characteristically, a gradual increase of uninhibitable bladder pressure occurs at low bladder volumes.

capacity, the former being approximately 60% of maximum functional bladder capacity (2).

One of the most important features of the bladder is its ability to contract. The bladder is unique in that it is an involuntary smooth muscle organ that is partially under voluntary control. During bladder filling and normal daily activity, the detrusor muscle is relatively quiet; voluntary cortical activity suppresses bladder contractions. However, once the bladder contracts on its own, it normally sustains the contraction until completely empty. It is important on cystometry to determine whether detrusor contractions occur and whether they are of sufficient strength and duration to completely evacuate intravesical contents.

Uninhibited detrusor contractions signify a decrease or lack of accommodative prop-erties during bladder filling. The other part of the equation is to assess the patient's voluntary control over the bladder, an involuntary organ. This voluntary control has two aspects: the ability to initiate a bladder contraction and the ability to inhibit the contraction. A neurologically intact individual should have the volition to both initiate and inhibit bladder detrusor activity despite the bladder's smooth muscle composition.

TECHNIQUE

Cystometry involves the instillation of a filling media into the bladder with simultaneous measurement of intravesical pressure as the bladder fills, producing a curve of intravesical pressure plotted against volume. Cystometry can be performed by several different methods using simple to complex recording techniques.

Regardless of the method used, many factors can influence the results of the test, including patient position, method of bladder filling, filling media used, medium temperature, rate of filling, and the inclusion or exclusion of provocative maneuvers. It is well recognized that patient position influences sensation to bladder filling, with the erect position being the most sensitive. In general, cystometry is best performed in the sitting or standing position. Supine cystometry has been shown to be a less sensitive test, missing up to 50% of women with detrusor instability or hyperreflexia (3).

The bladder can be filled either antegrade or retrograde. The latter is used more commonly in the office setting because of the time factor of fluid processing by the body. Bladder filling may be physiological, incremental, or continuous by catheter either under gravity or using a calibrated electronic pump. The rate of bladder filling also influences test results because rate of filling challenges the bladder's ability to accommodate an increasing volume over a variable amount of time (4). The International Continence Society defines slow fill as less than 10 mL/min, medium fill as 10–100 mL/min, and fast fill as greater than 100 mL/min (5). Fast-fill methods appear more effective in provoking detrusor overactivity, which may or may not be erroneous. For this reason, medium-fill rates are typically used.

The type of filling media will also influence testing. Current choices for media in-

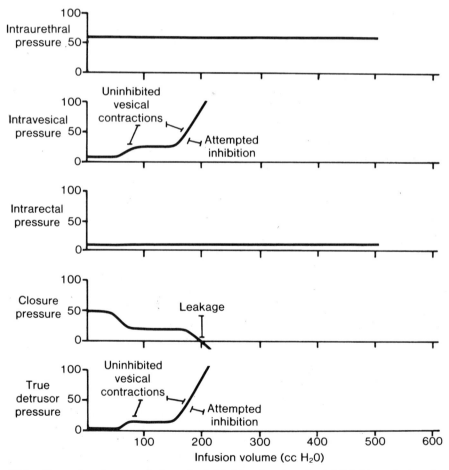

Figure 10.4. The cystometrogram of a hypertonic bladder. A series of uninhibitable vesical contractions occur with a stair-step increase in intravesical pressure.

clude carbon dioxide, saline, or radiographic dye. Multiple investigators evaluated the use of these media (2, 6–9). Carbon dioxide offers the advantages of being neat, simple, and speedy because it can be infused at rates up to 300 mL/min. However, the use of carbon dioxide can result in a false-positive test for detrusor overactivity for several reasons. Fast filling of the bladder with CO_2 tests bladder compliance because bladder pressure and wall tension rise rapidly and a contraction is difficult to inhibit. Carbon dioxide has also been found to be a bladder mucosal irritant due to its reaction with urine to produce carbonic acid. Irritation of the urothelium acts to decrease bladder capacity, increase sensitivity to bladder filling, and provoke increased bladder wall activity, resulting in a false-positive test for detrusor overactivity. Wein et al. (9) found considerable variation in all parameters measured on CO_2 cystometry performed on two different occasions and questioned the reproducibility of gas cystometry.

Saline, although somewhat "messy," is more physiological than carbon dioxide and does not cause bladder wall irritability if warmed to room temperature. If unwarmed saline is used, an increased incidence of detrusor activity may occur. Another advantage to the use of saline includes clear visibility of leakage from the urethral meatus during testing to determine when the patient experiences incontinence with different maneuvers (stress test, other provocative tests, or leak point pressure).

Radiographic contrast is used only when combining cystometric evaluation with simultaneous radiographic techniques such as fluoroscopy or ultrasonography. It is important to avoid the use of these agents in patients with a history of allergy to iodine or in those with previous allergic or anaphylactic reaction specifically related to radiographic contrast.

Just as it is important to avoid factors that falsely increase the production of uncontrolled bladder activity and lead to misdiagnosis, it is equally important to have the patient perform activity during cystometry that typically elicits her symptoms. This inclusion of provocative maneuvers is a critical part of urodynamic testing. The patient should be asked to cough, heel bounce, walk, squat, and hear or feel running water as necessary to provoke her symptoms during urodynamic monitoring. Failure to include such provocative maneuvers can result in false-negative test results.

Single-Channel Cystometry

Simple single-channel cystometry can be performed manually. The "poor man's" cystometric evaluation consists of a Foley catheter in the bladder attached to a wide-mouthed syringe (without the plunger) and held at the level of the superior edge of the symphysis pubis. Saline is incrementally poured into the syringe and, thus, retrograde into the bladder. The height of the column of water in the syringe indicates the pressure of the tonic segment of the cystometric curve; a detrusor contraction during any part of bladder filling results in a rapid sustained rise in the column of water.

Single-channel cystometry can also be performed electronically using a pressure transducer held at the level of the superior edge of the symphysis pubis and attached to a printer that generates the pressure versus volume curve. With any single-channel technique, the intravesical pressure recording reflects the cumulative effects of all sources of pressure on the bladder, namely the intraabdominal pressure and the true detrusor pressure (pressure derived from bladder smooth muscle activity). With single-channel recording systems, it can be difficult to ascertain the exact cause of the rise in intravesical pressure, as it may be secondary to an increase in detrusor pressure (a bladder contraction) or the result of increased abdominal pressure (Valsalva, patient movement). One method to distinguish the source of the increased intravesical pressure during single-channel cystometry is to ask the patient to hold her breath. This action will result in a decrease in intraabdominal pressure and can be used to differentiate between the possible sources of increased intravesical pressure.

Multichannel Cystometry

Multichannel cystometry involves the placement of microtip pressure transducer catheters to allow the concurrent measurement of total intravesical pressure, intraab-

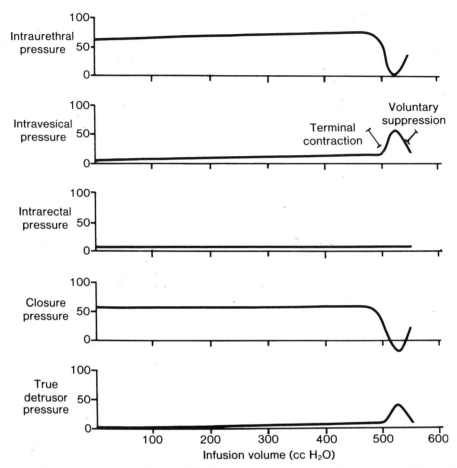

Figure 10.5. The cystometrogram of a normal bladder with an inhibitable terminal contraction. This diagrammatic representation of a urodynamic tracing shows the simultaneous measurement of intraurethral, intravesical, and intrarectal pressures. The intrarectal pressure, when subtracted from the intravesical pressure, gives the true detrusor pressure. The closure pressure results from subtraction of the intravesical pressure from the intraurethral pressure. All measurements of pressure are in cm H_2O.

dominal pressure, urethral pressure, and the digitally subtracted true detrusor pressure (Fig. 10.5). True detrusor pressure equals the intravesical pressure minus the intraabdominal pressure. True detrusor pressure recordings are necessary to make deductions regarding the authentic muscle activity of the detrusor muscle. A real bladder contraction will be depicted on multichannel cystometrogram by a rise in both intravesical and true detrusor pressure, whereas intraabdominal pressure remains constant. Other events associated with this change in true detrusor pressure with a real bladder contraction include a fall in urethral pressure, indicating urethral relaxation, and either a momentary increase in electromyographic

(EMG) activity if the bladder contraction is involuntary or a sustained decrease in EMG activity if the act is voluntary (voiding).

To perform multichannel cystometry, the patient's bladder is drained to ensure a starting zero volume and surface electrodes are placed adjacent to the anus to detect pelvic floor striated muscle activity. A double microtip pressure transducer catheter is placed such that the distal pressure transducer is located in the bladder (to measure total intravesical pressure) and the proximal pressure transducer is positioned in the urethra at the point of maximal urethral pressure (to measure urethral pressure). Another microtip pressure transducer is placed in either the vagina or the rectum to measure intraabdominal pressure. Both the vagina and rectum have been shown to accurately measure and reflect changes in intraabdominal pressure (10, 11). The choice of site to measure intraabdominal pressure often depends on the presence of severe vaginal prolapse or rectal conditions that dictate the placement of the catheter. If the patient has severe vaginal prolapse, the catheter may not be retained in the vagina over the duration of the test. If the catheter is placed rectally, the presence of feces and colonic movement may produce some degree of artifact. To avoid this, some investigators have the patient perform a bowel preparation before multichannel urodynamic testing.

During the test, the bladder is filled retrograde with filling media. The patient is asked to report the volume of first sensation of bladder filling, sensation of fullness, and the point of maximum bladder capacity. During bladder filling the patient performs directed provocative maneuvers (cough, specific activity, hear or feel running water). Valsalva leak point pressures may be obtained (with at least 150 mL bladder fullness) by having the patient Valsalva, and the lowest intravesical pressure that results in urine leakage is recorded as the stress leak point pressure (12–14) (see Fig. 11.4). The stop test may also be performed, testing voluntary control of micturition. The patient is asked to void and then requested to inhibit the voiding act.

The addition of electromyography is an important adjunct to multichannel cystometry. Surface or needle electrodes measure the change in electrical potential produced by striated muscle activity and are used to monitor activity of the pelvic floor and striated urethral sphincter. Direct measurement of these potentials requires the insertion of needle electrodes into the muscle of interest, which may be uncomfortable for the patient. Surface electrodes placed superficially on the perineum adjacent to the anus or in the form of an inserted anal plug record mass local contractions. Although easy to use and more comfortable for the patient, surface electrodes measuring anal sphincter activity may not be representative of urethral sphincter activity.

Normally during bladder filling on cystometry, the EMG signal will increase, re-flecting heightened activity in the urethral voluntary sphincter and increased pelvic floor tone. In contrast, the EMG signal ceases with voluntary micturition and remains silent until voiding is completed (Fig. 10.6). The EMG recording may also assist in distinguishing involuntary from voluntary bladder contractions during cystometry, based on the timing of bladder contraction in relation to decreased or increased EMG activity (Fig. 10.7).

Ambulatory Cystometry

Most urodynamic testing is conducted in the laboratory under artificial conditions and for a brief duration of time. As such, urodynamic studies can fail to reveal the underlying pathophysiology resulting in incontinence, not unlike the limitations of capturing a cardiac arrhythmia during a twelve-lead echocardiogram. Over the past 15 years, improved telemetric techniques to monitor pressure changes in the lower urinary tract have allowed the development of continuous ambulatory monitoring to record static and reflex changes in urethral and bladder pressure during daily activities (15–19).

Comparative studies of conventional office and ambulatory urodynamic techniques have indicated that continuous monitoring during daily activity significantly increases the diagnosis of detrusor instability. Webb et al. (20) diagnosed detrusor instability among 60% of patients with symptoms of urge incontinence but a negative office cystometrogram. van Waalwijk van Doorn et al. (21) performed conventional and ambulatory urodynamics on 100 patients. Conventional urodynamic evaluation produced a diagnosis in 68% of patients compared with a 97% diagnostic rate when ambulatory urodynamic monitoring was used. Although ambulatory urodynamic evaluation remains a research tool at present, the merits of the technique are fully apparent. For further in-depth discussion of this emerging technique, please refer to Chapter 14.

CLINICAL APPLICATION

Sutherst and Brown (22) compared single-channel standing cystometry to multichan-

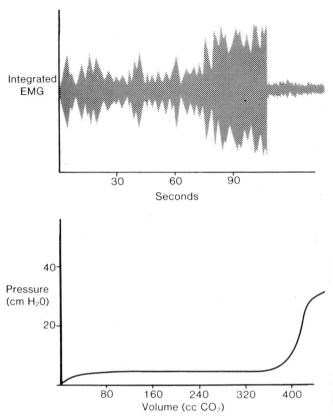

Figure 10.6. Normal combined tracing of EMG activity during the cystometrogram. There is a gradual increase in EMG activity. The patient successfully suppresses all detrusor activity until the end of the evaluation when a detrusor contraction occurs and EMG activity of the pelvic floor ceases.

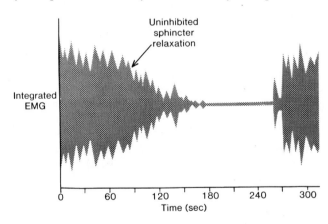

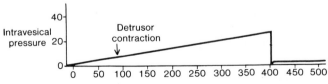

Figure 10.7. Uninhibited or reflex urethral sphincter relaxation. The detrusor contraction occurs at a very low volume of CO_2 and precedes the decrease of EMG activity in the urethral sphincter. The patient cannot inhibit this event. Bottom figure: x axis, mL CO_2; y axis, cm H_2O.

nel cystometry and found the former to be 100% sensitive and 83.3% specific in the diagnosis of detrusor instability. Sand et al. (3) tested the utility of single-channel cystometry as a screening method to detect detrusor instability and found it to be relatively specific (82.4%) with a negative predictive value of 82.4% but a low sensitivity (59.3%) that marred its use as a screening test. Single-channel cystometry has also been used clinically to assess patients with symptoms of stress incontinence. Studies have shown that when combined with other screening tests in a low-risk population, single-channel cystometry can be used effectively to rule out the presence of detrusor instability (23–25).

However, if readily available, most investigators prefer to use multichannel technique to evaluate patients with symptoms of urge incontinence and, specifically, in patients with mixed symptoms of urge and stress loss to clearly document the etiology of the patient's incontinence. Clearly, multichannel cystometry gives the most definitive diagnosis, as it is able to distinguish the source of increased intravesical pressure and the cause of urine leakage (26, 27). The other advantage to multichannel cystometry with electromyography is the detection of other causes of urinary incontinence and lower urinary tract symptomatology, including overflow incontinence, uninhibited urethral relaxation, sensory urgency, and urethral instability (28–31). The use of multichannel cystometry is clearly indicated in patients with recurrent urinary incontinence after incontinence surgery, patients with a history of radical pelvic surgery or radiation therapy, and those with suspected neurological conditions. However, this type of evaluation is not available uniformly and for many practitioners the method used to perform cystometry depends on the availability of equipment and trained personnel.

Urethral Pressure Profilometry

Continence depends on the relationship between urethral and bladder pressure, re-

quiring that urethral pressure exceed intravesical pressure at all times other than during micturition (32). Urethral pressure profilometry, the measurement of urethral pressure, has developed over the last 75 years as a means to investigate normal urethral function and abnormalities that result in incontinence. Over time, several different techniques to record urethral pressure have been described and perfected.

In 1923, Bonney (33) was the first to attempt measurement of urethral pressure via the method of retrograde sphincterometry. Lapides in 1957 used a whistletip catheter in the urethra to discharge fluid into the urethra from a water manometer filled with fluid. Flow of fluid ceased when the height of the water column equaled urethral wall pressure and the pressure in the manometer was recorded. Repetition of measurement at several points along the urethra produced a crude urethral pressure curve (34). The balloon catheter technique, as first described by Barnes in 1940 (35) and later used by Enhorning (32), consisted of a fluid-filled balloon positioned at the tip of a catheter that was connected to a pressure transducer to record urethral resistance to distension. This technique does not produce a true depiction of urethral pressure but rather measures pressure over a finite length of the urethra equal to the length of the balloon.

In 1967, Toews (36) described fluid perfusion through a catheter combined with the use of strain gauges to continuously measure urethral pressure at consecutive points along the length of urethra. The fluid perfusion technique was perfected by Brown and Wickham in 1969 (37) with the addition of a special catheter, with multiple side holes to diminish rotational error, connected to a pressure transducer; a mechanical pump to provide a constant fluid flow rate of 1–2 mL/min and a mechanical device to withdraw the catheter along the length of the urethra at a constant rate of 1–2 mm/s.

The perfusion technique measures resistance of the urethral wall to the inflow of fluid, averaging the pressure around the catheter at any given point along the length of the urethra. The result is a continuous pressure curve depicting the effective pressure exerted by the urethral wall at every point along the length of the urethra (Fig.

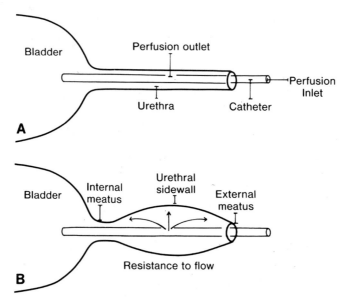

Figure 10.8. The perfusion urethral closure pressure profile. **A.** The catheter in the urethra before infusion. **B.** During perfusion, resistance to flow at the internal and external urethral meatus occurs as well as from the urethral sidewall.

10.8). In studies designed to test accuracy and reproducibility, the fluid perfusion technique was found to be consistent regardless of catheter size, infusion rate (subject to specific limits), or patient position and is considered to be an accurate and reproducible method for obtaining resting urethral pressure profiles (38–40).

The perfusion of gas instead of water, specifically carbon dioxide, has also been widely used by clinicians because of simplicity and availability (41–44). However, when compared with fluid perfusion, gas perfusion methods have been found to be less reliable, less reproducible, and less accurate (6, 45). Gleason et al. (6), in a comparison of water and gas urethral pressure profile data, found little similarity between urethral pressure profile curve configuration, peak pressure, or continence zone areas; overall it was impossible to extrapolate water and gas data or to interpret one in terms of the other. Much of the discrepancies between gas and fluid perfusion are secondary to the compressibility of gas that results in a lag in registering pressure changes along the urethra. Other drawbacks to the use of gas include the irritation of urethral and bladder mucosa that may alter test results and the inability to detect leakage of gas from the urethra. Using a mechanical

model, Gilmour et al. (46) found that both gas and water profilometry had limitations and set specific guidelines for the use of each media to optimize results. Regardless of the media perfused, the perfusion technique has limits due to the lack of responsiveness and inability to measure the pressure at a particular level of the urethra as a pressure profile implies.

Membrane catheters, introduced in the 1970s, give an added level of sensitivity and accuracy, with reproducible results that measure localized intraurethral pressure along the length of the urethra (45–48). The membrane catheter is a four-channel silicone 6F catheter with two membranes about 1.5 cm apart, with the first membrane located approximately 7 cm from the tip (Fig. 10.9). Each membrane measured pressure of the immediate opposing urethral wall. Drawbacks to the use of this methodology include the difficulty of obtaining specially constructed catheters and the need to constantly calibrate and adjust the catheters with each use.

Each method described above involves the transmission of pressure from the urethra to a distant transducer, a setup that may be adequate for recording resting urethral pressure profiles but is inadequate for dynamic or stress urethral profilometry. Detailed studies of the urethral musculature response to cough indicate that any system designed to measure urethral pressure changes produced by coughing should be capable of a rise time of 16 ms or have a frequency response of at least 30 Hz (49, 50). None of the systems described above have such a capability.

Karlson (51) was the first to directly measure urethral pressure with a measuring device within the urethral lumen. Millar and Baker (52) miniaturized the technique by mounting pressure-sensitive piezoelectric units onto a small catheter, producing microtip pressure transducer catheters for simultaneous urethrocystometry and urethral pressure measurement. The piezoelectric units are located at the catheter tip and 6 cm proximally to measure bladder pressure and urethral pressure, respectively (Fig. 10.10).

These units measure the pressure exerted relative to atmospheric pressure and are highly sensitive to rapid changes in pressure, with a frequency response rate of 2000 Hz. Although expensive and delicate, requiring special care to ensure longevity of use, these catheters are currently the technique of choice.

TECHNIQUE

The patient is placed in the dorsal lithotomy position, the urethral meatus cleaned with antiseptic, and the bladder drained of urine. Surface electrodes to measure EMG activity of the pelvic floor are placed close to the anal opening and on the inner thigh. The microtip pressure transducer catheters are calibrated at the level of the bladder. The catheter to measure intraabdominal pressure

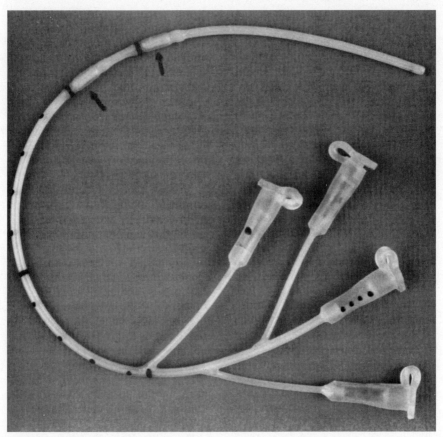

Figure 10.9. The membrane catheter. This catheter has four channels. Two open at the end of the catheter for intravesical pressure measurements and for intra- vesical perfusion during the cystometrogram. The two balloons *(arrows)* measure intraurethral pressures.

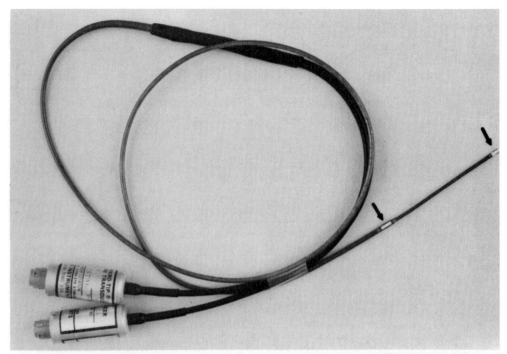

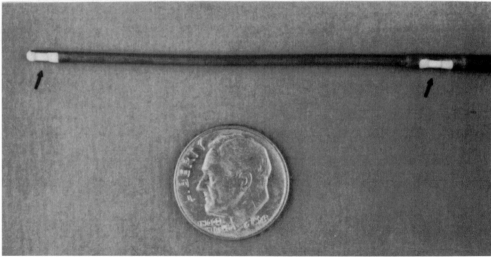

Figure 10.10. The microtransducer catheter. The two microtransducers *(arrows)* measure intravesical and intraurethral pressures.

is placed either vaginally or rectally, depending on the presence or absence of significant pelvic prolapse (53). The microtip catheter is then placed in the bladder and attached to the mechanical arm that will withdraw the catheter through the urethra at a set speed, typically 1 mm/s. At this point, pressures recorded on the urethral channel and intravesical channel should be identical, as both microtip transducers are located in the bladder. Care is taken to position the microtip transducer laterally because of documented impact of transducer orientation on accurate urethral pressure measurement (54, 55).

The patient is moved to the sitting position and the bladder filled with warmed saline to the patient's level of bladder fullness. Position of the patient and bladder fullness at the time of urethral pressure profilometry have been found to significantly alter test results; a sitting or standing position with a full bladder is required to maximize the sensitivity of the test (56).

By activating the mechanical arm, the catheter is withdrawn through the urethra at a set rate and a resting urethral profile produced. Two to three resting profiles are obtained to ensure reproducibility. A cough or stress urethral pressure profile is then obtained by having the patient cough intermittently as the catheter is withdrawn through the urethra. During each urethral profile, five concurrent pressure curves are recorded: intravesical pressure, intraabdominal pressure, detrusor pressure, urethral pressure, and urethral closure pressure (Fig. 10.11). The urethral clo-

sure pressure, like detrusor pressure, is a derived product calculated by subtracting intravesical pressure from urethral pressure (Fig. 10.12). The urethral pressure curve represents the absolute pressure required to overcome urethral resistance to the flow of fluid.

PARAMETERS

The static or resting urethral pressure profile measures intraluminal pressure along the length of the urethra with the bladder at rest (5). Parameters measured and recorded during the urethral pressure profile include the maximum urethral pressure, the maximum urethral closure pressure, the functional urethral length, and the total urethral length. Maximum urethral pressure is the maximum pressure of the measured profile, whereas

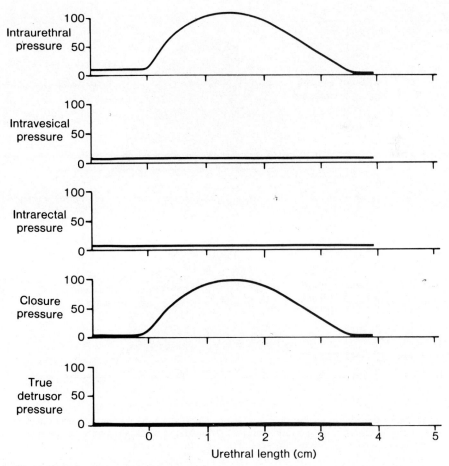

Figure 10.11. The urethral closure pressure profile in the normal female. Subtraction of intravesical pressure from simultaneously measured intraurethral pressure provides a recording of the urethral closure pressure.

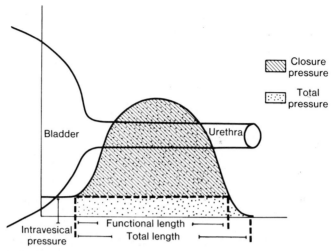

Figure 10.12.   The urethral closure pressure profile of a normal patient. The hatch lines outline the area of closure pressure and the dotted area represents the area of total urethral pressure.

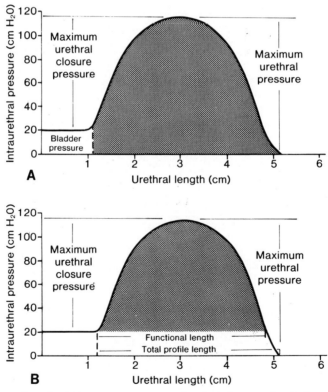

Figure 10.13.   Integrated urethral closure pressure profile. **A.** The shaded area under the upper curve constitutes the integrated *total* urethral pressure. **B.** The shaded area under the lower curve indicates the integrated urethral *closure* pressure (also called the *continence* area).

maximum urethral closure pressure is the difference between the maximum urethral pressure and the bladder pressure. The functional urethral length is the length of the urethra along which the urethral pressure exceeds bladder pressure. The total urethral length equals the functional urethral length plus the additional length to reach atmospheric pressure; it is not considered to be a clinically useful parameter. The continence area (mm^2) or integrated urethral closure pressure is the area encompassed by the urethral closure pressure profile at rest and at baseline (57) (Fig. 10.13).

Normative values for these parameters have been described by several different investigators using different measurement techniques (32, 58–61). Urethral closure pressure has been noted to decrease with age with a mean urethral closure pressure of 90 cm H$_2$O at age 25 compared with a mean urethral closure pressure of 65 cm H$_2$O at age 64 (58, 61). The functional urethral length

averages 2–5 cm and has been noted to decrease after menopause (32, 62, 63). In the continent patient, both functional urethral length and maximal urethral closure pressure increase with the assumption of an increasingly upright position (Fig. 10.14). In contradistinction, these parameters decrease in the incontinent patient (Fig. 10.15).

The resting urethral closure pressure profile also gives information regarding the distribution of the closure pressure along the anatomic length of the urethra, tending to be symmetric. Urethral closure pressure increases to a maximum level located in the midsegment of the urethra corresponding to the anatomic position of the urethral sphincter musculature. The urethral closure pressure profile clearly indicates the relationship of the maximum point of closure pressure to the bladder neck and, likewise, the location of lowest closure pressure along the urethral length. Alteration in the normal distribution of the closure pressure along the urethral

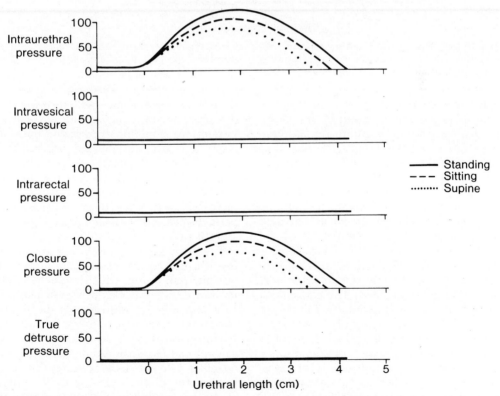

Figure 10.14. Superimposed urethral closure pressure profiles in the supine, sitting, and standing positions in the normal patient. Characteristically, closure pressure and/or functional length increases with assumption of a more upright position.

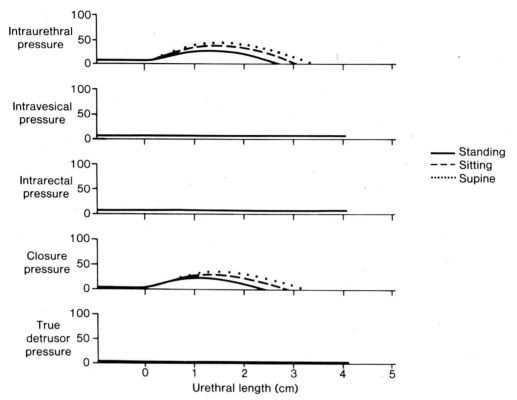

Figure 10.15. Superimposed urethral closure pressure profiles in the supine, sitting, and standing positions in the patient with genuine stress incontinence. Characteristically, there is a decrease of closure pressure and/or functional length.

length has been noted to be important in the diagnosis of incontinence and in the detection of areas of stricture, kinking, or urethral muscle attenuation or absence. These abnormalities should not be confused with the common finding of rapid changes in urethral pressure at the peak of the urethral pressure profile that reflect pulsation in the urethral submucosal vasculature and can fluctuate by as much as 25 cm H_2O (32, 63).

The cough or stress urethral closure pressure profile measures urethral intraluminal closure pressure along the length of the urethra during physical stress. The cough urethral closure pressure profile is defined as positive when equalization of pressure occurs with each cough along the length of the urethra and negative when positive pressure transmission is present at any point along the urethral length. In the continent patient, the pressure rises significantly higher in the urethra than the bladder with each cough, due to transmission of abdominal pressure to both the urethra and bladder. However, in the stress incontinent patient, equal transmission of abdominal pressure does not occur and urethral closure pressure will drop to zero or "equalize" (Fig. 10.16). The degree of bladder fullness does not effect the ability of the stress continent patient to remain dry but does test the stress incontinent patient's protective mechanisms (Figs. 10.17 and 10.18).

The dynamic cough urethral pressure profile allows objective assessment of pressure transmission from the abdomen to the urethra under episodes of stress. The pressure transmission ratio equals the ratio of change in intraurethral pressure to change in intravesical pressure during a cough. The pressure transmission ratio for each cough is calculated by dividing the amplitude of the urethral rise by the amplitude of the corresponding bladder pressure rise and multiplying the quotient by 100 (Fig. 10.19).

CLINICAL APPLICATION

Over the last 70 years, urethral closure pressure profilometry has greatly increased our understanding of urethral function and urinary incontinence. Specific changes in the parameters measured have been found to occur with age, hormonal status, presence or absence of incontinence, and as the result of successful or unsuccessful incontinence surgery (32, 58, 61, 64, 65). Clinically, the technique has been specifically applied to the diagnosis of genuine stress incontinence, defined by The International Continence Society as "the involuntary loss of urine when the

intravesical pressure exceeds maximum urethral pressure in the absence of vesical contractions" (5). This definition tacitly implies the use of multichannel urodynamic testing to make the diagnosis. However, to date, investigators and clinicians are split as to the clinical usefulness of urethral profilometry in the evaluation of urinary incontinence and genuine stress incontinence specifically. The basis for this lack of consensus is presented below.

Studies have shown a statistically significant difference in the maximum resting urethral closure pressure and functional urethral length between incontinent patients

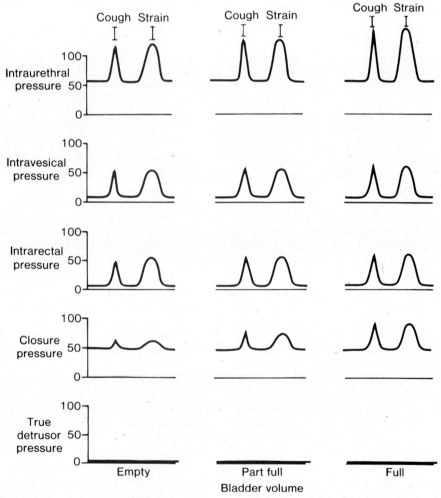

Figure 10.16. Urethral pressures with empty, partially filled, and full bladder during stress in the normal patient. There is a positive transmission of the intraabdominal pressure to the urethra that exceeds the actual pressure increase measured in the bladder and rectum. Closure pressure remains positive throughout.

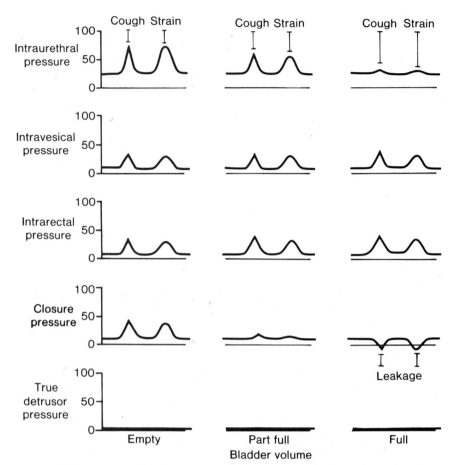

Figure 10.17. Urethral pressures with empty, partially filled, and full bladder during stress in the patient with genuine stress incontinence. Actual pressure transmission to the urethra decreases as the bladder fills, leading to negative closure pressures and urine loss through the urethra.

and continent control subjects, with a lower resting closure pressure and functional urethral length of the former (32, 60, 61). Despite these differences, other investigators have pointed to the wide overlap in values between continent and incontinent patients, making a "cutoff" value for either parameter impossible to define (66–68). Furthermore, in comparing urethral closure pressure profilometry before and after incontinence surgery, significant change in resting closure pressure has not been consistently found, despite restored continence (65, 69–72).

The resting urethral closure pressure has been linked to the severity of incontinence symptoms (61). The presence of low postoperative urethral pressure as a possible cause of surgery failure was first suggested by McGuire (73), who noted that patients with recurrent genuine stress incontinence were more likely to have a maximum urethral closure pressure less than 20 cm H_2O than patients who were continent after urethropexy. In both retrospective and prospective studies, patients with genuine stress incontinence and low urethral closure pressure (<20 cm H_2O in the sitting position and with a full bladder) have been shown to be at significantly higher risk for surgical failure after standard retropubic urethropexy (54% objective failure rate) (74–76). Horbach and Ostergard (77) found that patients over age 50 were more likely to have low urethral pressures and suggested that such patients undergo urethral pressure profilometry for detection of poor urethral sphincter function. More recently, Versi (67), using sophisticated statistical analysis, identified the continence area (area under the urethral closure pressure curve) to be the most discriminatory parameter to separate continent and incontinent subjects. Other investigators suggested residual continence area (the area between the baseline and a line connecting each cough spike on the urethral closure pressure cough profile) as a predictor of the severity of incon-

tinence, finding that patients with a decreased residual continence area leak more (68). These results point to the continued importance of both resting and stress urethral pressure profilometry as methods by which to evaluate urinary incontinence; the results

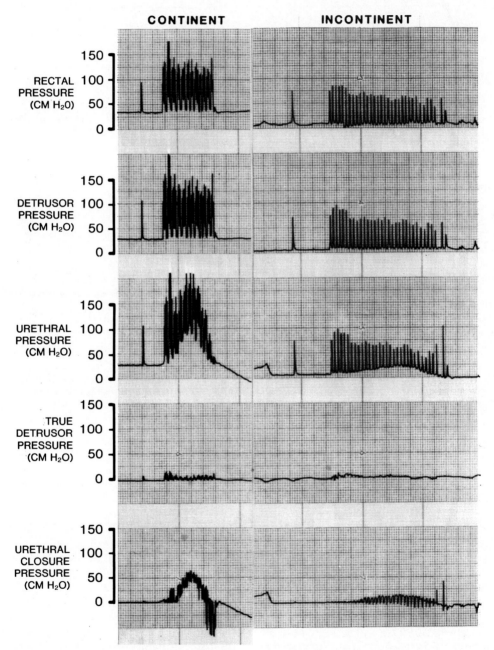

Figure 10.18. Cough urethral pressure profile. As the recording catheter is gradually withdrawn through the urethra, the patient coughs continuously. The continent patient *(left)* has an area of positive pressure under the curve that prevents urine leakage.

The incontinent patient *(right)* lacks any areas of positive pressure. The change in closure pressure during coughing directly indicates the pressure transmission capacity ratio.

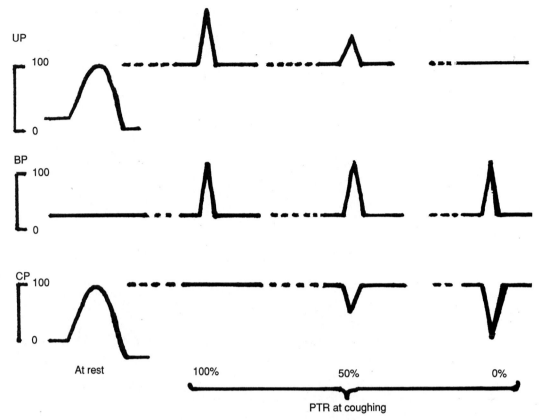

Figure 10.19. The PTR is calculated from the formula

$$\frac{\Delta \text{ MUP}}{\Delta \text{ BP}} \times 100\% = \text{PTR}$$

(MUP = Maximum Urethral Pressure
BP = Bladder Pressure)

The above shown examples provide a pressure transmission of 100% from the intraabdominal cavity to the bladder. If the real transmission to the bladder is only 50%, the PTR is 200%. If the transmission to the urethra is only 50%, the PTR is 100%. If the defect in pressure transmission to the bladder is compensated (e.g., through pelvic floor muscle contraction), the real PTR is 50%.

of resting urethral pressure measurements do have an impact on diagnosis and treatment.

The cough or stress urethral pressure profile has performed better as a diagnostic test for genuine stress incontinence but is also not perfect. Originally defined as an "all or none" phenomenon of equalization along the entire length of the urethra under stress, many investigators found limitations in application of the cough profile (61, 78–80). These studies showed that pressure equalization on cough urethral profile (performed in the sitting position with a full bladder) has a high specificity (92–100%) and a high positive predictive value (86–100%) but suffers from low sensitivity (41–50%) and a low negative predictive value (52–58%). In conclusion, these authors cautioned against the use of the cough urethral profile as the sole criterion for the diagnosis of genuine stress incontinence; patients with genuine stress incontinence do not always have pressure equalization along the entire urethra.

To address these issues, Bump et al. (81) suggested a quantitative method of analysis using the pressure transmission ratio to replace the qualitative all or none approach of pressure equalization on cough profile. Hilton and Stanton (61) and Bump et al. (81) found the pressure transmission ratio to discriminate well between patients with genuine stress incontinence and those without; the discriminatory cutoff value defining an abnormal continence mechanism has consistently been reported to be a ratio less than or equal to 90–95%. These authors and others also consistently reported a statistically significant difference in the pressure transmission ratio between continent women and those with genuine stress incontinence (61, 81, 82). Farghaly et al. (83) and Shephard et al. (84) both support the view that the pressure transmission ratio is a reliable clinical test to distinguish stress incontinent from continent women. However, others believe that the marked overlap in pressure transmission ratios between continent and incontinent subjects, like the parameters measured on static profilometry, leaves the test with limited clinical usefulness (82, 85–87).

Pressure transmission ratio measurement may be a means by which to determine surgical success. In a retrospective study, Bump et al. (88) found that patients with unsuccessful incontinence surgery had pressure transmission ratios much less than 100%, similar to incontinent patients before surgery. Multiple investigators found increased pressure transmission ratios after incontinence surgery, even on long-term follow-up at 5 and 10 years (67, 69, 70, 89–91). Rosenzweig et al. (82) reported that a greater change in pressure transmission ratio measured preoperatively and postoperatively correlated highly with surgical success.

The problems encountered in the use of stress urethral profiles and pressure transmission ratios to detect genuine stress incontinence involve multiple factors. The degree of bladder filling and patient position both influence the cough profile and pressure transmission ratio (60, 86). The difficulty in eliciting adequate cough intensity to challenge the urethral continence mechanism is recognized by clinicians on a day-to-day basis and is compounded by the fact that no consistent relationship between cough strength and pressure transmission ratio has been found (87). With some subjects, increased cough intensity produces an augmentation in pressure transmission ratio, whereas in others, the opposite occurs (86). This variable effect of cough strength on urethral sphincteric function directly influences any test that measures urethral response to dynamic activities.

In addition to its clinical use in the evaluation of urinary incontinence, urethral closure pressure profilometry has been found to assist in the detection of urethral stricture, kinking, diverticulum, and, potentially, urethrovesical fistula (92–95). Urethral stricture presents itself as a high rapid elevation in urethral pressure on profilometry. On the other hand, the presence of a urethral diverticulum is represented on urethral profilometry by a loss of urethral pressure at the point of urethral wall disruption from the diverticular ostia. The result is a double-peaked urethral closure pressure profile. Although urethral diverticula are usually diagnosed by radiographic means, urethral pressure profilometry may be helpful in determining the surgical procedure of choice for correction. Bhatia et al. (93) used the urethral pressure profile to ascertain the position of the diverticulum in relation to the point of maximum urethral pressure and used this information to select the surgical corrective procedure. Like a urethral diverticulum, a urethrovesical fistula would be expected to cause a decrease in urethral pressure at the area of the breach in the urethral wall.

At this time, the clinical use of urethral closure pressure profilometry remains controversial. Many investigators view the technique purely as a research tool with limited clinical applications, whereas others find the test easy to perform in conjunction with other multichannel tests and clinically useful in the diagnosis and management of incontinence and other urethral conditions. Urethral function, specifically the generation of urethral closure pressure, is the result of multiple contributing factors. It may be unrealistic to believe that one test or parameter alone will be able to separate patients with stress incontinence from other causes of incontinence or from those who are continent.

Uroflowmetry and Pressure Voiding Studies

Normal voiding requires neurological coordination of both the urethral and bladder musculature. Simultaneous urethral smooth and striated muscle relaxation occurs first, followed in 2–3 seconds by a detrusor contraction of adequate magnitude, which is sustained until bladder emptying is accomplished. During this concomitant urethral

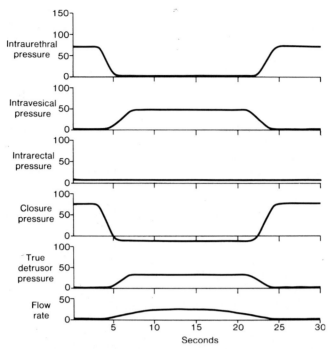

Figure 10.20. Diagrammatic representation of the normal female voiding act. Urethral relaxation precedes the vesical contraction, which continues for about 20 seconds and is associated with a normal flow rate of greater than 20 mL/s. All pressures on the graphs in this chapter are in cm H_2O.

relaxation and detrusor contraction, the normally high urethral sphincteric pressure drops significantly, remaining at a low pressure until voiding is complete, after which it resumes its high prevoiding pressure. The initial detrusor contraction produces a rise in detrusor pressure of no more than 30–40 cm H_2O, exceeding the urethral pressure to result in urine flow, and then levels off over time as the bladder is emptied (Fig. 10.20). Beyond this coordinated interplay between urethra and bladder musculature, successful micturition also requires the absence of anatomic outflow obstruction.

The normal female voids via a variety of mechanisms, all of which include urethral relaxation as the major component. Abnormal voiding mechanisms, on the other hand, occur without urethral relaxation or as an actual increase in urethral sphincteric contraction (Tables 10.1 and 10.2).

Evacuation of the bladder may be evaluated by simple uroflowmetry or by multichannel pressure voiding studies. These methods and their clinical utility are described below. The Second Report on the Standardization of Terminology of Lower

Table 10.1. Normal Female Voiding Mechanisms

	Pressure Changes	
Urethra	Bladder	Abdomen
Complete relaxation	Mild increase	Absent
Complete relaxation	None	Absent
Complete relaxation	None	Present

Table 10.2. Abnormal Female Voiding Mechanisms

	Pressure Changes	
Urethra	Bladder	Abdomen
No change	Increase	Absent
Increase	Increase	Absent

Urinary Tract Function presents the recommendations of the International Continence Society regarding the flow rate and pressure measurement during micturition (96).

UROFLOWMETRY

Assessment of a patient's urine flow is a good gauge of the integrity of the voiding mechanism and outflow tract. The simplest assessment can be done by sound alone, in addition to timing the duration of flow and measuring the total voided volume. Basic mathematics allow the calculation of the average urine flow rate (total volume voided divided by total time).

Uroflowmetry, on the other hand, is performed by having the patient void on a special commode that funnels the urine onto a device that measures the volume voided over time. Various measurement techniques have been used, such as the analysis of the change of fluid weight, air displacement, capacitance, intensity of sound, and force on a rotating disc (97–100). Fluid weight uroflowmetry has become the most common method used to assess female micturition. The data include the total volume voided, total voiding time, maximum flow rate, and time to maximum flow. The pattern of urine flow may also be identified.

When performing and reporting uroflowmetry, the patient's position, the mechanism of bladder filling (spontaneous or forced diuresis, or by catheter), and the type of fluid used needs to be recorded. Bergman and Bhatia (101) found equivalent uroflowmetric results when filling by catheter or by normal diuresis. Two more recent studies indicated that uroflowmetry performed after urethral instrumentation results in reduced peak and mean urine flow rates when the data are corrected for the relative voided volume (102, 103). The amount of urine voided during the study also bears importance to the results. Drach et al. (104) studied 364 female patients with uroflowmetry and reported that a minimum of 100 mL was satisfactory for adequate test interpretation, noting also that the peak flow increased by a rate of 5.6 mL/s with each increase of 100 mL voided volume. Other authors have set the required volume for adequate test interpretation at 200 mL (105–107).

The results of any voiding study depend on the recorded micturition being representative of the patient's normal urine flow. To obtain this goal, the patient should void in private, where she is more likely to be uninhibited and relaxed. It is also important she understand what is being asked of her and should be able to state, after the test, whether the void was "normal" for her. If not, the test should be repeated.

Uroflowmetric parameters to be recorded and reported include total volume voided, total voiding time, peak flow rate, mean flow rate, and time to maximum flow. Urine flow rate, in general, is defined as the volume of urine (mL) expelled through the urethra per unit time (s). The uroflowmetric curve is a graphic representation of the flow rate and depicts the ratio between the change in urine volume and the change in time. The voided volume represents the total volume voided during a single micturition event. The flow time is the time over which measurable urine flow occurs. Flow rate is measured from a point of initiation (a) to a point of termination (b) and is considered unmeasurable when equal to or less than 2 mL/s. Any further flow after the drop to less than or equal to 2 mL/s is noted but not included in the flow time and is considered to represent terminal events. The peak flow rate equals the maximum flow rate measured during a single void that is sustained for a minimum duration of 1 second. The average flow is calculated by dividing the total voided volume by the total flow time. The time to peak flow rate measures the time required to reach the peak flow rate. Many authors suggested values for the minimum voided volume required for an adequate study, normal peak flow rate, and time to peak flow (104, 105, 107, 108) (Table 10.3). Although investigators have not reached a consensus as to the normative values for the parameters described above, consistent relationships between certain parameters have been described. Fantl et al. (100) and Meunier (108) both found that flow time, peak flow rate, peak time, and average flow rate increased with larger voided volumes. Similarly, Karl et al. (109) described an increase in peak flow rate with increased voided volume but only up to a voided volume of 200 mL.

Nomograms are available to assess normal urine flow rates relative to the volume voided and patient age, although not all studies showed a change in uroflow parameters with increasing age (110–112). Parity, weight, height, and menstrual phase do not influence uroflowmetric parameters. Most clinicians would agree that a "normal" uroflow study would consist of a total volume of over 200 mL, voided over 15–20 seconds, with a maximum flow rate of greater than 20 mL/s and with a smooth continuous

Table 10.3. Published "Normal" Uroflowmetry Parameters

Author	Minimum Voided Volume (mL)	Peak Flow Rate (mL/s)	Residual Volume (mL)
Stanton	200	≥15	<200
Barrett	—	>10	<50
Drach	100	Varies with volume voided	—
Meunier	All volumes acceptable	Varies with volume voided	—
Bhatia and Bergman	200	≥20 ≥10[a]	≤50

[a]Mean flow.

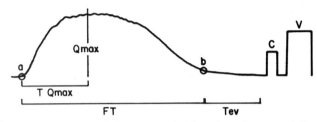

Figure 10.21. Uroflowmetric curve, continuous flow pattern. *a*, point of initiation; *b*, point of termination; *C*, calibration signal; *V*, total volume voided; *FT*, flow time; *Qmax*, peak flow rate; *T Qmax*, time to peak flow rate; *Tev*, terminal events. (From Fantl JA, et al. Am J Obstet Gynecol 1983;145:1017.)

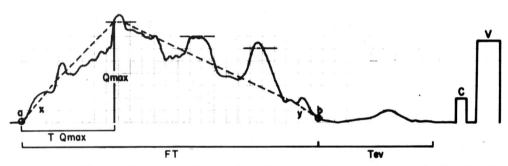

Figure 10.22. Uroflowmetric curve, multiple peak pattern. *a*, point of initiation; *b*, point of termination; *x*, ascending segment; *y*, descending segment; *Qmax*, peak flow rate; *T Qmax*, time to peak flow rate; *FT*, flow time; *Tev*, terminal events; *C*, calibration signal; *V*, total volume voided. (From Fantl JA, et al. Am J Obstet Gynecol 1983;145:1017.)

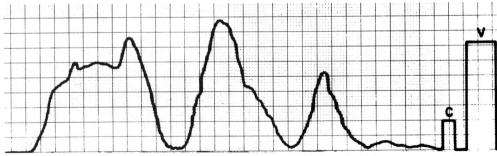

Figure 10.23. Uroflowmetric curve, interrupted pattern. *C*, calibration signal; *V*, total volume voided. (From Fantl JA, et al. Am J Obstet Gynecol 1983;145:1017.)

crescendo-decrescendo curve (113). On the other hand, voiding dysfunction is suggested when uroflow parameters are not within normative values for a given volume and require further evaluation.

Beyond absolute uroflow values, the other, possibly better, indicator of voiding dysfunction is the urine curve pattern (97, 100). Uroflowmetric curve patterns reflect the graphic representation of urine flow over time. Several distinguishable curve patterns have been described and can be said to be normal or abnormal. Normal urine flow is usually continuous with a crescendo-decrescendo curve, minimal fluctuations, and with the peak flow rate reached within one third of the total voiding time (Fig. 10.21). Intermittent urine flow is defined by one or more decreases in flow rate with subsequent increases. Intermittent flow rate can be divided into either a multiple peak pattern, where the downward deflection of the flow rate never descends below 2 mL/s (Fig. 10.22), or an interrupted pattern, where the downward deflection of the urine flow becomes unmeasurable at less than or equal to 2 mL/s (Fig. 10.23). Intermittent flow rate patterns occur

in approximately 17% of asymptomatic women and therefore are not considered necessarily to be pathological (100).

The uroflowmetric parameters of a multiple peak pattern can be assessed by reconstructing the flow curve (Fig. 10.22). This is performed by drawing a line (X) from the point of initiation of micturition to a point 2 seconds after the point of initiation and a line (Y) from the point of termination to a point 2 seconds before the point of termination, determining the peak flow rate that equals the highest flow rate with a duration of at least 1 second, and drawing lines connecting the point of peak flow to both line X and Y (100). Uroflowmetric parameters of interrupted flow patterns are usually not estimated, as it is difficult to determine the volume of each aliquot. Flow time of the interrupted pattern can be roughly assessed by ignoring the time during which no measurable urine flow occurred (114).

On uroflowmetry, obstructive urine flow patterns in the female are suggested by a slow urine flow rate and a prolonged voiding time (Fig. 10.24). In 1983, Meunier (108) suggested that the percent difference be-

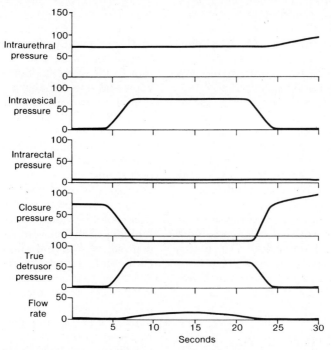

Figure 10.24. An obstructive voiding pattern. No decrease in intraurethral pressure occurs with voiding, and closure pressure approaches zero due to an abnormally high intravesical pressure. A low flow rate occurs due to this abnormal voiding pattern.

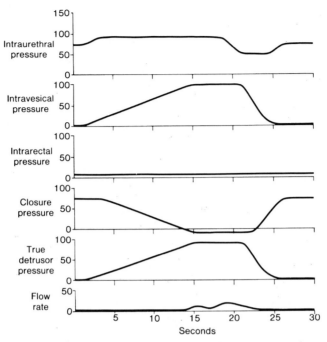

Figure 10.25. Obstructive voiding with detrusor sphincter dyssynergia. The detrusor pressure increases during a series of voiding attempts, but micturition does not occur due to a positive closing pressure. Finally, poor urethral relaxation allows an intermittent pattern of flow.

tween the peak flow and the average flow might better identify obstructive flow patterns, with a decreased percent difference specific for an obstructive flow (108). Obstructive voiding patterns in females can result from mechanical factors such as a urethral stricture, kinking secondary to pelvic prolapse, or direct compression due to periurethral masses. Overall, outlet resistance secondary to mechanical factors is rare in women. Difficulty in initiation of the urinary stream can also be psychogenic in origin or may be the result of infectious or inflammatory processes in the urethra (115–117). The more important factor determining urine flow rate rests with the voluntary urethral sphincter mechanism. Patients who void without urethral relaxation (i.e., detrusor sphincter dyssynergia) must rely on a strong detrusor contraction to overcome urethral pressure and as a result have a slow urinary flow rate (Fig. 10.25).

MULTICHANNEL PRESSURE VOID

Multichannel pressure voiding studies allow further assessment of abnormal uroflow-metry parameters and curve patterns. Pressure flow study requires the same setup and equipment as for multichannel cystometry or urethral pressure profilometry: a microtip transducer catheter in the bladder and urethra to measure bladder and urethral pressures and one catheter in the vagina or rectum to measure abdominal pressure. Surface electrodes are placed adjacent to the anus to record pudendal nerve activity reflecting urethral striated muscle activity. The pressure voiding study reports the same parameters as uroflowmetry: total volume voided, total voiding time, peak flow rate, mean flow rate, and time to maximum flow. Added information gained from the pressure void study includes direct measurement of the detrusor contraction, urethral relaxation, and any intraabdominal pressure elevation (Valsalva). A normal detrusor contraction measures up to 40 cm H_2O; a contraction greater than 50 cm H_2O suggests increased outflow resistance. Likewise, the presence of detrusor hypocontractility or atony can be diagnosed. Unfortunately, there is no clear cutoff between normal and abnormally high or low detrusor pressures during voiding.

The multichannel pressure voiding study also allows assessment of the patient's mechanism of voiding, which can then be classified as normal or abnormal (Tables 10.1 and 10.2). Although classic normal micturition results from urethral relaxation followed by detrusor contraction, other mechanisms of voiding are also considered normal. Voiding can occur in the absence of a bladder contraction, resulting from total rapid urethral sphincteric relaxation alone (Fig. 10.26) or coupled with increased intraabdominal pressure from Valsalva straining (Fig. 10.27). The common factor to all normal voiding mechanisms in the female is urethral relaxation. Voiding in the absence of urethral sphincteric relaxation is considered abnormal but can occur if the detrusor contraction is strong enough to overcome urethral pressure. Simultaneous urethral and detrusor contraction during micturition is called detrusor sphincter dyssynergia and results when a detrusor contraction stimulates a concomitant contraction of the urethral sphincter. No voiding or a very low urine flow occurs because the urethral closure pressure never becomes negative (Fig. 10.25). In detecting this pathological entity, the EMG recording during the act of micturition is essential; an increase in sphincteric activity is diagnostic when occurring in conjunction with a rise in urethral pressure and at the same time as voluntary detrusor contraction.

Unfortunately, the technique involved in multichannel pressure void studies is invasive, complicated by artifact, and may be practically difficult to interpret. Furthermore, although the methodology is theoretically sound, it is unknown whether instrumented micturition truly reflects typical urinary flow that occurs in the absence of recording instruments. It has been noted that 20–30% of patients are unable to void with such catheters in place (114).

CLINICAL APPLICATION

The major application of uroflowmetry in clinical urology to date has been in the assessment of obstructive voiding in males; the utility of uroflow studies in the assessment of female urinary tract complaints remains controversial. However, female patients do present with a multitude of "abnormal" voiding complaints that require evaluation. Such abnormal micturition may reflect a local in-

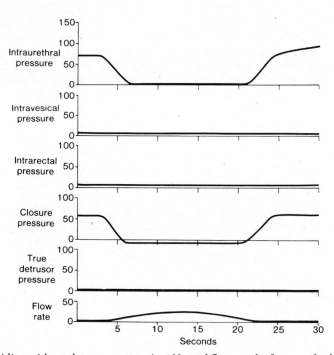

Figure 10.26. Voiding without detrusor contraction. Normal flow results from urethral relaxation alone.

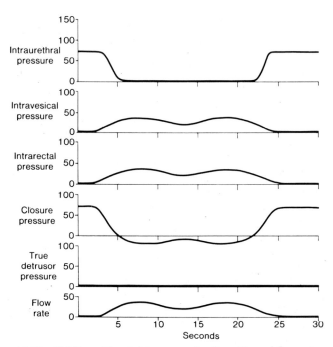

Figure 10.27.   Voiding without detrusor contraction. Normal flow rate results from urethral relaxation with pressure augmentation from Valsalva.

fectious inflammatory or obstructive process, a neurologic problem at the peripheral or central level, a psychogenic origin, or a variety of systemic disease processes. Fantl et al. (100) reviewed the fluid weight uroflowmetric parameters in 60 normal women, with each woman voiding six different times. No significant statistical difference was noted based on patient age, weight, height, parity, phase of menstrual cycle, or menopausal status. A wide range of normal values was observed, with variation in peak flow rate and flow time recorded in the same patient with varying voided volumes (Fig. 10.28). The configuration of flow rate patterns was more consistent over multiple voids by the same patient. The authors concluded that uroflowmetry is an indirect method by which to evaluate micturition and is best used as a screening method to identify voiding dysfunction. If abnormal uroflow parameters or curve patterns are noted, further urodynamic evaluation with multichannel pressure void studies are indicated (100).

More recently clinical studies investigated the role of uroflowmetry and pressure voiding studies to identify patients at risk for postoperative voiding dysfunction (105–

107). Bhatia and Bergman (106) found that neither elevated postvoid residuals nor abnormal peak flow rates, defined as less than 20 mL/s, in the presence of a voided volume greater than 200 mL, were predictive of prolonged postoperative voiding difficulties. The same investigative team then assessed the utility of combined uroflowmetry with pressure-voiding studies and found that the preoperative group with an inadequate detrusor contraction (less than 15 cm H_2O) had a 36% incidence of prolonged postoperative catheterization (greater than 7 days). In addition, all patients with an inadequate detrusor contraction in conjunction with an abnormal uroflow (peak flow less than 20 mL/s, mean flow less than 10 mL/s) also required prolonged postoperative catheterization (107). Some authors recommended that all patients who undergo incontinence surgery should be evaluated to adequately inform the patient of postoperative voiding difficulties (105). The clinical utility of uroflowmetry and pressure voiding studies in the female patient requires further investigation. At this point, simple uroflowmetry has been suggested to be beneficial in the following areas: as a screening test for voiding abnormalities before incontinence surgery; assessment of urinary frequency, urgency, nocturia, and urge incontinence, otherwise known as the frequency-urgency syndrome; voiding dysfunction; and neurological disease. Pressure void studies have the major ability to document the patient's voiding mechanism. This type of evaluation is most helpful to determine voiding abnormalities before incontinence surgery and to evaluate voiding dysfunction that has developed after incontinence surgery, radical pelvic surgery, pelvic radiation, or serious lower urinary tract or nervous system injury.

Postvoid Residual

Residual urine is defined as the volume of fluid remaining in the bladder immediately after a voluntary void (118). The postvoid residual measures the patient's ability to empty the bladder and is an indirect reflection of bladder contractility. As such, the postvoid residual is an essential adjunct to any assessment of voiding ability. The absence of residual urine is clinically relevant, whereas the significance of an elevated postvoid residual is unclear, requiring confirmation on several occasions to be considered important. An elevated residual urine can be caused by many acute and chronic conditions.

There is no real consensus regarding what amount of residual urine is normal. Most physicians consider a residual less than 50 mL to be adequate bladder emptying and that greater than 200 mL to be inadequate bladder emptying (119). Many factors need to be considered when interpreting the significance of a postvoid residual volume, including the environmental setting, the voided volume before postvoid residual measurement, and the patient's readiness to void. In many instances, more than one postvoid residual measurement may be necessary to fully assess the patient's ability to void, in terms of adequacy of emptying.

There are several ways by which the postvoid residual can be measured. Simple palpation of the suprapubic area either abdominally or on bimanual pelvic examination after a patient has voided will detect gross retention of urine. Radiographic means of assessing residual urine within the bladder include intravenous urography and micturition urography, both of which require the use of radiographic contrast. Radioisotopes have also been used to determine the adequacy of micturition. Although invasive and associated with a small risk of infection (less than 3%), the most common method used clinically is transurethral catheterization immediately after a voluntary void. This technique should result in an accurate measure of the amount of urine remaining in the bladder, unless the measurement is complicated by presence of bladder diverticula or vesicoureteric reflux.

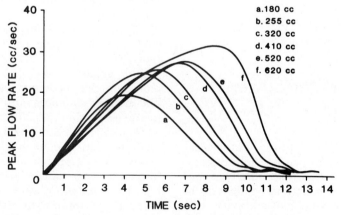

Figure 10.28. Six consecutive voidings in one volunteer subject. Note variations in the uroflowmetric parameters.

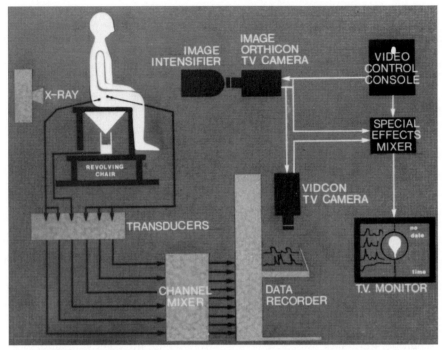

Figure 10.29. The urodynamic recording method. The urodynamic data and the video image are mixed and displayed on the television monitor.

A newer method being used with greater frequency is that of ultrasound measurement. Multiple studies, initially using large stationary ultrasound units and more recently small portable scanners, indicate that ultrasound measurement of postvoid residual is simple, accurate, reproducible, and noninvasive (120–125). Ultrasound assessment of the bladder volume is particularly useful in institutional care of chronic urinary retentive states as a means to decrease the frequency of catheterization.

Endoscopy of the Lower Urinary Tract

Visualization of the urethra, urethrovesical junction, and bladder can provide information of lower urinary tract structure and function and is an important counterpart to urodynamic testing for lower urinary tract function. Cystourethroscopy is presented in Chapters 12 and 13.

Combined Studies

Investigative techniques that allow visualization of lower urinary tract anatomy and function and measurement of urodynamic parameters of bladder and urethral function during urine storage and voiding have been developed over the last 30 years (126–132). To this end, videourodynamic studies of the lower urinary tract combine videocystourethrography and the standard techniques of multichannel urodynamic evaluation. Highly technical and expensive equipment is required to simultaneously project the radiographic image of the bladder and urethra alongside the recorded pressure channels obtained by standard multichannel urodynamic evaluation (Fig. 10.29). Radiographic opaque dye is used for bladder filling for easy visibility. This combined radiographic and urodynamic approach allows visualization of bladder neck descent with activity, bladder neck funneling, and leakage of urine through the urethra and the corresponding changes in bladder, intraabdominal, detrusor, and urethral pressures.

Considered by some to be the ultimate evaluation of the lower urinary tract, others see no additional benefit over nonimaged multichannel studies. Detractors find the videourodynamic evaluation prohibitive on the basis of cost, limited availability, and radiation exposure. In an effort to overcome some of the disadvantages of videourodynamics yet retain the advantages of concurrent imaging and pressure measurement of lower urinary tract function, investigators combined ultrasound and urodynamic assessment. First described by Kohorn et al. (133) and confirmed by Koelbl et al. (134) to be possible, further advances in ultrasound imaging continue to improve visualization of the periurethral structures. Recently, Schaer et al. (135) presented the simultaneous recording of urodynamic tracings during real-time transperineal ultrasonagraphy of the bladder neck, bladder, and urethra, with both modalities projected onto the same screen for easy visualization and comparison. This use of ultrasound has the distinct advantage of avoiding exposure to radiation or radiographic dye and, furthermore, should reduce costs. Only further study will tell how this new combination of radiographic imaging and urodynamic evaluation adds to the current understanding and clinical evaluation of lower urinary tract dysfunction.

Conclusions

Urodynamics may be defined as the medical science concerned with the physiology and pathophysiology of the transport of urine from the kidneys to the bladder and its storage and drainage (34). The urodynamic techniques of cystometry, urethral pressure profilometry, and uroflowmetry are invaluable methods by which to understand normal urinary tract function and pathophysiology that results in incontinence and voiding dysfunction. The same methods of evaluation have been applied clinically and found to be instrumental in the diagnosis and treatment of lower urinary tract symptoms.

Many have questioned the need for urodynamic evaluation on all patients with incontinence, although it is well established that the patient's symptoms do not necessarily reflect the etiology of urinary leakage (136, 137). A recent metaanalysis of 19 articles comparing patients' symptoms to urodynamic diagnosis indicated that approximately one quarter of all patients presenting with urine loss associated with cough, sneeze, or physical activity were not found to actually have genuine stress incontinence on evaluation. Worse yet, basing treatment on a history of urge loss of urine results in a misdiagnosis in 45% of patients (138). Furthermore, other causes of urinary incontinence exist, including retention and overflow incontinence, fistula, intrinsic sphincter deficiency, urinary tract infection, and uninhibited urethral relaxation. The evaluation of female incontinence requires a thorough systematic approach using an appropriate combination of available urodynamic tests to make the distinction between possible diagnoses and to ensure appropriate management.

REFERENCES

1. Rose DK. Cystometric bladder pressure determinations. J Urol 1927;17:487–494.
2. Torrens M, Abrams P. Cystometry: symposium on clinical urodynamics. Urol Clin North Am 1979;6:71–88.
3. Sand PK, Hill RC, Ostergard DR. Supine urethroscopic and standing cystometry as screening methods for the detection of detrusor instability. Obstet Gynecol 1987;70:57–60.
4. Cass AS, Ward BD, Markland C. Comparison of slow and rapid fill cystometry using liquid and air. J Urol 1970;104:104–108.
5. Bates P, Bradley WE, Glen E, et al. First report on the standardization of terminology of lower urinary tract function. Urinary incontinence. Procedures related to the evaluation of urine storage-cystometry, urethral pressure profile, units of measurement. Scand J Urol Nephrol 1976;11:193–196.
6. Gleason DM, Bottaccini MR, Reilly RJ. Comparison of cystometrograms and urethral profiles with gas and water media. Urology 1977;6:155–160.
7. Gleason DM, Reilly RJ. Gas cystometry in cystometry: symposium on clinical urodynamics. Urol Clin North Am 1979;6:85–88.
8. Jorgensen L, Lose G, Andersen JT. Cystometry: water or carbon dioxide as filling medium? A literature survey of the influence of the filling medium on the qualitative and quantitative cystometric parameters. Neurourol Urodyn 1988;7:343–350.
9. Wein AJ, Hanno PM, Dixon DO, Raezer D, Benson GS. The reproducibility and interpretation of carbon dioxide cystometry. J Urol 1978;120:205–206.

10. McCarthy TA. Validity of rectal pressure measurements as indication of intra-abdominal pressure changes during urodynamic evaluation. Urology 1982;10:657–660.

11. Al-Taher H, Sutherst JR, Richmond DH, Brown MC. Vaginal pressure as an index of intra-abdominal pressure during urodynamic evaluation. Br J Urol 1987;59:529–532.

12. McGuire EJ, Fitzpatrick CC, Wan J, et al. Clinical assessment of urethral function. J Urol 1993; 150:1452–1454.

13. Swift SE, Ostergard DR. A comparison of stress-leak-point pressure and maximal urethral closure pressure in patients with genuine stress incontinence. Obstet Gynecol 1995;85:704–708.

14. Montella JM. Valsalva leak point pressure. AUGS Quarterly Report 1994;12:3.

15. James D. Continuous monitoring. Urol Clin North Am 1979;6:125–135.

16. Bhatia NN, Bradley WE, Haldeman S, Johnson BK. Continuous monitoring of bladder and urethral pressures: new technique. Urology 1981; 18:207–210.

17. Bhatia NN, Bradley WE, Haldeman S, Johnson BK. Continuous ambulatory urodynamic monitoring. Br J Urol 1982;54:357–359.

18. Bhatia NN, Bradley WE, Haldeman S. Urodynamics: continuous monitoring. J Urol 1982; 128:963–968.

19. Griffiths CJ, Assi MS, Ramsden PD, Neal DE. Ambulatory monitoring of bladder and detrusor pressure during natural filling. J Urol 1989;142: 780–783.

20. Webb RJ, Ramsden PD, Neal DE. Ambulatory monitoring and electronic measurement of urinary leakage in the diagnosis of detrusor instability and incontinence. Br J Urol 1991;68: 148–152.

21. van Waalwijk van Doorn ESC, Remmers A, Janknegt RA. Extramural ambulatory urodynamic monitoring during natural filling and normal daily activities: evaluation of 100 patients. J Urol 1991;146:124–131.

22. Sutherst JR, Brown MC. Comparison of single and multichannel cystometry in diagnosing bladder instability. Br Med J 1984;288:1720–1722.

23. Fonda D, Brimage PJ, D'Astoli. Simple screening for urinary incontinence in the elderly: comparison of simple and multi-channel cystometry. Urology 1984;42:536–540.

24. Scotti RJ, Myers D. A comparison of the cough stress test and single-channel cystometry with multichannel urodynamic evaluation in genuine stress incontinence. Obstet Gynecol 1994; 81:430–433.

25. Wall LL, Wiskind AK, Taylor PA. Simple bladder filling with cough stress test compared with subtracted cystometry for the diagnosis of urinary incontinence. Am J Obstet Gynecol 1994; 171:1472–1479.

26. Webster GD, Older RA. Value of subtracted bladder pressure measurement in routine urodynamics. Urology 1980;16:656–661.

27. Blaivas J. Multichannel urodynamic studies. Urology 1984;23:421–438.

28. Sand PK, Bowen LW, Ostergard DR. Uninhibited urethral relaxation: an unusual cause of incontinence. Obstet Gynecol 1986;68:645–649.

29. Ulmsten U, Hendricksson L, Iosif S. The unstable female urethra. Am J Obstet Gynecol 1992;144:93–97.

30. Versi E, Cardozo L. Urethral instability: diagnosis based on variations of the maximum urethral pressure in normal climacteric women. Neurourol Urodyn 1986;5:535–540.

31. Fossberg E, Beisland HO, Sander S. Sensory urgency in females. Treatment with phenylpropanolamine. Eur Urol 1981;7:157–159.

32. Enhorning G. Simultaneous recording of the intravesical and intraurethral pressure. Acta Chir Scand Suppl 1961;276:1–68.

33. Bonney V. On diurnal incontinence of urine in women. J Obstet Gynaecol Br Emp 1923;30: 358–365.

34. Perez LM, Webster GD. The history of urodynamics. Neurourol Urodyn 1992;11:1–21.

35. Barnes AC. A method for evaluating the stress of urinary incontinence. Am J Obstet Gynecol 1940;40:381–390.

36. Toews H. Intraurethral and intravesical pressure in normal and stress incontinent women. Obstet Gynecol 1967;29:613–624.

37. Brown M, Wickham JEA. The urethral pressure profile. Br J Urol 1969;41:211–217.

38. Edwards L, Malvern J. The urethral pressure profile: theoretical considerations and clinical applications. Br J Urol 1976;46:325–342.

39. Abrams PH, Martin S, Griffith DJ. The measurement and interpretation of urethral pressures obtained by the method of Brown and Wickham. Br J Urol 1978;50:33–40.

40. Ghoniem MA, Rottembourg JL, Fretin J, Susset JG. Urethral pressure profile: standardization of technique and study of reproducibility. Urology 1975;5:632–637.

41. Robertson JR. Gas cystometrogram with urethral pressure profile. Obstet Gynecol 1974;44:72–76.

42. Tscholl R, Tettamanti F, Worsdorfer O. The urethral pressure profile recorded as a means of CO_2-perfusion at high flow rates. Br J Urol 1976;48:337–339.

43. Raz S, Kaufman JJ. Carbon dioxide urethral pressure profile. J Urol 1976;115:439–442.

44. Merrill DC. Determination of peak urethral pressure by retrograde gas studies. Urology 1977;10: 236–238.

45. Schmidt RA, Witherow R, Tanagho EA. Recording the urethral pressure profile. Urology 1977; 10:390–396.

46. Gilmour RF, James DF, Toguri AG, Churchill BM. Analysis of the urethral pressure profile using a mechanical model. Invest Urol 1980;18: 54–60.

47. Drouin G, McCurry EH. Catheters for studies of urinary tract pressure. Invest Urol 1970;8: 195–201.

48. Tanagho EA, Jones U. Membrane catheter: effective for recording pressure in the lower urinary tract. Urology 1977;10:173–178.

49. Lindstrom K, Ulmsten U. Some methodological aspects of the measurement of intra-luminal

pressures of the female urogenital tract in vivo. Acta Obstet Gynecol Scand 1978;57:63–66.

50. Asmussen M, Ulmsten U. Simultaneous urethrocystometry and urethral pressure profile measurement with a new technique. Acta Obstet Gynecol Scand 1975;54:385–386.

51. Karlson S. Experimental functioning of the female urinary bladder and urethra. Acta Obstet Gynecol Scand 1953;32:285–286.

52. Millar HD, Baker LE. Stable ultraminiature catheter-tip pressure transducer. Med Biol Eng 1973;11:86–91.

53. Richardson DA. Use of vaginal pressure measurements in urodynamic testing. Obstet Gynecol 1985;66:581–584.

54. Bunne G, Obrink A. Urethral closure pressure with stress. A comparison between stress incontinent and continent women. Urol Res 1978;6:127–134.

55. Hilton P, Stanton SL. Urethral pressure measurement by microtransducer. I. An analysis of variance. Presented at the 11th annual meeting of the International Continence Society, Lund, 1981.

56. Awad SA, Bryniak SR, Lowe PJ, Bruce AW, Twiddy AS. Urethral pressure profile in female stress incontinence. J Urol 1978;120:475–479.

57. Abrams P, Blaivas JG, Stanton SL, Andersen JT. The standardization of terminology of the lower urinary tract function by the International Continence Society Committee on Standardization of Terminology. Scand J Urol Nephrol 1978;114(Suppl):5–19.

58. Rud T. Urethral pressure profile in continent women from childhood to old age. Acta Obstet Gynecol Scand 1980;59:331–335.

59. Beck RP, Maughan GB. Simultaneous intraurethral and intravesical pressure studies in normal women and those with stress incontinence. Am J Obstet Gynecol 1964;89:746–756.

60. Tanagho AE. Urodynamics of female urinary incontinence with emphasis on stress incontinence. J Urol 1979;122:200–203.

61. Hilton P, Stanton SL. Urethral pressure measurements by microtransducer: the results in symptom-free women and in those with genuine stress incontinence. Br J Obstet Gynaecol 1983;90:919–933.

62. Tanagho AE, Miller ER. Functional considerations of urethral sphincteric dynamics. J Urol 1973;109:273–278.

63. Asmussen M. Intraurethral pressure recordings. Scand J Urol Nephrol 1976;10:1–6.

64. Rud T. The effects of estrogen and gestagens on the urethral pressure profile in urinary continent and stress incontinent women. Acta Obstet Gynecol Scand 1980;59:265–270.

65. Hilton P, Stanton SL. A clinical and urodynamic assessment of the Burch colposuspension for genuine stress incontinence. Br J Obstet Gynaecol 1983;90:934–939.

66. Cadogan M, Awad S, Field C, Acker K, Middleton S. A comparison of the cough and standing urethral pressure profile in the diagnosis of stress incontinence. Neurourol Urodyn 1988;7:327–341.

67. Versi E. Discriminant analysis of urethral pressure profilometry data for diagnosis of genuine stress incontinence. Br J Obstet Gynaecol 1990;97:251–259.

68. Meyer S, De Grandi P, Schmidt N, Sanzeni W, Spinosa JP. Urodynamic parameters in patients with slight and severe genuine stress incontinence: is the stress profile useful? Neurourol Urodyn 1994;13:21–28.

69. Faysal MH, Constantinou CE, Rother LF, Govan DE. The impact of bladder neck suspension on the resting and stress urethral pressure profile: a prospective study comparing controls with incontinent patients preoperatively and postoperatively. J Urol 1981;125:55–60.

70. Bhatia NN, Ostergard DR. Urodynamics in women with stress urinary incontinence. Obstet Gynecol 1982;60:552–559.

71. Beisland HO, Fossberg E, Sander S, Moer A. Urodynamic studies before and after retropubic urethropexy for stress incontinence in females. Surg Gynecol Obstet 1982;155:333–336.

72. Weil A, Reyes H, Bischoff P, et al. Modification of urethral rest and stress profiles after different types of surgery for urinary stress incontinence. Br J Obstet Gynaecol 1984;91:46–55.

73. McGuire EJ. Urodynamic findings in patients after failure of stress incontinence operations. Prog Clin Biol Res 1981;78:351–356.

74. Sand PK, Bowen LW, Panganiban R, Ostergard DR. The low pressure urethra as a factor in failed retropubic urethropexy. Obstet Gynecol 1987;69:399–402.

75. Bowen LW, Sand PK, Ostergard DR. Unsuccessful Burch retropubic urethropexy: a case controlled urodynamic study. Am J Obstet Gynecol 1989;160:451–458.

76. Koonings PP, Bergman A, Ballard CA. Low urethral pressure and stress urinary incontinence in women: risk factor for failed retropubic surgical procedure. Urology 1990;16:245–248.

77. Horbach NS, Ostergard DR. Predicting intrinsic urethral sphincter dysfunction in women with stress urinary incontinence. Obstet Gynecol 1994;84:188–192.

78. Richardson DA. Value of the cough pressure profile in the evaluation of patients with stress incontinence. Am J Obstet Gynecol 1986;155:808–811.

79. Fantl JA, Hurt WG, Bump RC, Dunn L, Choi SC. Urethral axis and sphincteric function. Am J Obstet Gynecol 1986;155:554–556.

80. Hanzal E, Berger E, Koelbl H. Reliability of the urethral closure pressure profile during stress in the diagnosis of genuine stress incontinence. Br J Urol 1991;68:369–371.

81. Bump RC, Copeland WE, Hurt WG, et al. Dynamic urethral pressure profilometry pressure transmission ratio determinations in stress-incontinent and stress-continent subjects. Am J Obstet Gynecol 1988;159:749–755.

82. Rosenzweig BA, Bhatia NN, Nelson AL. Dynamic urethral pressure profilometry pressure transmission ratios: what do the numbers really mean? Obstet Gynecol 1991;77:586–590.

83. Farghaly SA, Shah J, Worth P. The value of

transmission pressure ratios in the assessment of female stress incontinence [abstract 14.42.01]. Arch Gynecol 1991;237(Suppl):366.

84. Shephard A, Lewis P, Howell SC, Abrams PH. Video screening and stress profiles—unnecessary investigations in the diagnosis of genuine stress incontinence. Proc Int Cont Soc 1985;15:262–264.

85. Lose G, Thind P, Colstrup H. The value of pressure transmission ratio in the diagnosis of stress incontinence. Neurourol Urodyn 1990;9: 323–324.

86. Versi E, Cardozo L, Cooper DJ. Urethral pressures: analysis of transmission pressure ratios. Br J Urol 1991;68:266–270.

87. Richardson DA, Ramahi A. Reproducibility of pressure transmission ratios in stress incontinent women. Neurourol Urodyn 1993;12: 123–130.

88. Bump RC, Fantl JA, Hurt WG. Dynamic urethral pressure profilometry pressure transmission ratio determinations after continence surgery: understanding the mechanism of success, failure, and complications. Obstet Gynecol 1988;72: 870–874.

89. Eriksen BC, Hagen B, Eik-Nes SH, Molne K, Mjølnerød OK, Romslo I. Long-term effectiveness of the Burch colposuspension in female urinary stress incontinence. Acta Obstet Gynecol Scand 1990;69:45–50.

90. Herbertsson G, Iosif CS. Surgical results and urodynamic studies 10 years after colpourethrocystopexy. Acta Obstet Gynecol Scand 1993; 72:298–301.

91. Baker KR, Drutz HP. Retropubic colpourethropexy: clinical and urodynamic evaluation in 289 cases. Int Urogynecol J 1991;2:196–200.

92. Højsgaard A. The urethral pressure profile in female patients with meatal stenosis. Scand J Urol Nephrol 1976;10:97–99.

93. Bhatia NN, McCarthy TA, Ostergard DR. Urethral pressure profiles of women with diverticula. Obstet Gynecol 1981;58:375–378.

94. Asmussen M, Ulmsten U. The role of urethral pressure profile measurement in female patients with urethral carcinoma. Ann Chir Gynecol 1982;71:122–126.

95. Richardson DA, Bent AE, Ostergard DR. The effect of uterovaginal prolapse on urethrovesical pressure dynamics. Am J Obstet Gynecol 1982; 146:901–905.

96. Bates P, Glenn E, Griffiths D, et al. Second report on the standardization of terminology of lower urinary tract function. Procedures related to the evaluation of micturition—flow rate, pressure measurement, symbols. Scand J Urol Nephrol 1977;11:197–199.

97. Von Garretts B. Analysis of micturition: a new method of uroflowmetry of recording the voiding of the bladder. Acta Chir Scan 1956;112: 326–330.

98. Susset JG, Picker P, Kretz M, et al. Critical evaluation of uroflowmetry and analysis of normal curves. J Urol 1973;109:874–878.

99. Abrams P, Torrens M. Urine flow studies. Urol Clin North Am 1979;6:71–82.

100. Fantl JA, Smith PJ, Schneider V, Hurt WG, Dunn IJ. Fluid weight uroflowmetry in women. Am J Obstet Gynecol 1983;145:1017–1023.

101. Bergman A, Bhatia NN. Uroflowmetry: spontaneous versus instrumental. Am J Obstet Gynecol 1983;150:788–790.

102. Tessier J, Schick E. Does urethral instrumentation affect uroflowmetry measurements? Br J Urol 1990;65:261–263.

103. Wall LL, Hewitt JK. A statistical study of the effects of urethral instrumentation on urine flow in women. Int Urogynecol J 1994;5:341–344.

104. Drach GW, Ignatoff J, Layton T. Peak urinary flow rate: observations in female subjects and comparison to male subjects. J Urol 1979;122: 215–219.

105. Stanton SL, Ozsoy C, Hilton P. Voiding difficulties in the female: prevalence, clinical and urodynamic review. Obstet Gynecol 1983;61: 144–147.

106. Bhatia NN, Bergman A. Uroflowmetry and simultaneous for predicting post-operative voiding difficulties in women with stress urinary incontinence. Br J Obstet Gynaecol 1985;92: 835–838.

107. Bhatia NN, Bergman A. Use of preoperative uroflowmetry and simultaneous urethrocystometry for predicting risk of prolonged postoperative bladder drainage. Urology 1986;28: 440–445.

108. Meunier P. Study of micturition parameters in healthy young adults using a uroflowmetric method. Eur J Clin Invest 1983;13:25–32.

109. Karl C, Gerlach R, Hannappel J, Lehnen H. Uroflow measurements: their information yield in a long-term investigation of pre- and postoperative measurements. Urol Int 1986;41: 270–275.

110. Backman KA. Urinary flow during micturition in normal women. Acta Chir Scand 1965;130: 357–361.

111. Frimodt-Moller C. A urodynamic study of micturition in healthy men and women. Dan Med Bull 1973;21:41–45.

112. Bottaccini MR, Gleason DM. Urodynamic norms in women. I. Normal versus stress incontinent. J Urol 1980;124:659–682.

113. Karram MM. Urodynamics: voiding studies. In: Walters MD, Karram MM, eds. Clinical urogynecology. St. Louis, MO: Mosby-Year Book, 1993:77–88.

114. Fantl JA, Farrel SA. Clinical Uroflowmetry. In: Ostergard DR, Bent AE, eds. Urogynecology and urodynamics: theory and practice. 3rd ed. Baltimore, MD: Williams and Wilkins, 1991: 108–114.

115. Larson JW, Swenson WA, Utz DC, et al. Psychogenic urinary retention in women. JAMA 1993; 184:697–700.

116. van Gool J, Tanagho EA. External sphincter activity and recurrent urinary tract infection in girls. Urology 1977;10:348–351.

117. Bergman A, Karram M, Bhatia NN. Urethral syndrome: a comparison of different treatment modalities. J Reprod Med 1989;34:157–161.

118. Bates P, Bradley WE, Glen E et al. Third report on

the standardization of terminology of lower urinary tract function. Procedures related to the evaluation of micturition: pressure flow, relationships residual urine. Scand J Urol Nephrol 1980;12:191–193.

119. Urinary Incontinence Guideline Panel. Urinary Incontinence in adults: clinical practice guideline. Rockville, MD: Department of Health and Human Services. AHCPR Publication No. 92-0038. March 1992.

120. McLean GK, Edell SL. Determination of bladder volumes by gray scale ultrasonagraphy. Radiology 1978;128:181–184.

121. Ravichandran G, Fellows GJ. The accuracy of a hand-held real time ultrasound scanner for estimating bladder volume. Br J Urol 1983;55:25–27.

122. Griffiths CJ, Murray A, Ramsden PD. Accuracy and repeatability of bladder volume measurement using ultrasonic imaging. J Urol 1986;136:808–812.

123. Roehrborn CG, Peters PC. Can transabdominal ultrasound estimation of postvoid residual (PVR) replace catheterization? Urology 1988;31:445–449.

124. Haylen BT. Residual urine volumes in a normal female population: application of transvaginal ultrasound. Br J Urol 1989;64:353–356.

125. Ireton RC, Krieger JN, Cardenas DD, et al. Bladder volume determination using a dedicated, portable ultrasound scanner. J Urol 1990;143:909–911.

126. Enhorning G, Miller ER, Hinman F. Urethral closure studies with cine roentgenography and bladder urethral recording. Surg Gynecol Obstet 1964;118:507–513.

127. Whiteside CG. Videocystographic studies with simultaneous pressure and flow recordings. Br Med Bull 1972;28:214–219.

128. McGuire EJ. Combined radiographic and manometric assessment of urethral sphincter function. J Urol 1977;118:632–635.

129. Webster GD, Older RA. Videourodynamics. Urology 1980;16:106–114.

130. McGuire EJ, Woodside JR. Diagnostic advantages of fluoroscopic monitoring during urodynamic evaluation. J Urol 1981;125:830–834.

131. DeSai P. Bladder pressure studies combined with micturating cystourethrography. Radiography 1985;51:2–7.

132. Benness C, Barnick CG, Cardozo LD. Use of routine videocystourethrography in the evaluation of female lower urinary tract dysfunction. Neurourol Urodyn 1989;8:447–451.

133. Kohorn E, Scioscia AL, Jeanty P, Hobbins JC. Ultrasound cystourethrography by perineal scanning for the assessment in patients with genuine stress incontinence. Obstet Gynecol 1986;68:289–372.

134. Koelbl E, Bernaschek G, Wolf G. A comparative study of perineal ultrasound scanning and urethrocystography in patients with genuine stress incontinence. Arch Gynecol Obstet 1988;244:39–45.

135. Schaer GN, Koechli OR, Schuessler B, Haller U. Simultaneous perineal ultrasound and urodynamic assessment of female urinary incontinence: initial observations. Int Urogynecol J 1995;6:168–174.

136. Haylen BT, Sutherst JR, Frazer MI. Is the investigation of most stress incontinence really necessary? Br J Urol 1989;64:147–149.

137. Evans AT, Felker JR, Shank RA, Sugarman SR. Pitfalls of urodynamics. J Urol 1979;122:220–222.

138. Jensen JK, Nielsen FR, Ostergard DR. The role of patient history in the diagnosis of urinary incontinence. Obstet Gynecol 1994;83:904–910.

CHAPTER 11

Intrinsic Urethral Sphincteric Deficiency

Steven E. Swift

The term "intrinsic urethral sphincteric deficiency" (ISD) was first coined by a panel formed to set down clinical practice guidelines for the care and management of the incontinent adult by the Agency for Health Care Policy and Research (AHCPR). In this document, ISD was defined as a cause of genuine stress urinary incontinence:

...which may be due to congenital sphincter weakness such as myelomeningocele or epispadias or may be acquired after prostatectomy, trauma, radiation, or sacral cord lesion. In this condition, the urethral sphincter is unable to coapt and generate enough resistance to retain urine in the bladder, especially during stress maneuvers. In women, ISD is commonly associated with multiple anti-incontinence procedures. Patients with ISD often leak continuously or with minimal exertion (1).

This description defines patients who have a deficient or severely defective urethral sphincter mechanism. They are set apart as a subgroup of genuine stress incontinence (GSI) patients who are believed to be at high risk to fail standard antiincontinence procedures and conservative nonsurgical therapy. Therefore, it is imperative that they are identified before embarking on any therapeutic measures.

The definition of ISD as set down by the AHCPR mentions some testing procedures that can suggest the diagnosis but does not establish a set of specific or objective criteria that can be used to make the diagnosis. However, the testing procedures and findings that are described correlate with two clinical entities known as the low pressure urethra

and type III incontinence. Therefore, because no agreed upon criteria to establish the diagnosis of ISD exists, most investigators equate ISD with a low pressure urethra and/or type III incontinence.

Because ISD remains a somewhat elusive diagnosis, we present a discussion on the clinical significance and management of the low pressure urethra and type III urinary incontinence. Throughout this chapter, we focus on these two entities and present them as if they represent ISD, but it should be kept in mind that the terms are not necessarily interchangeable. Also, in the only study comparing type III incontinence and low pressure urethra, a poor correlation was demonstrated (2).

Background

Since the introduction of surgery to correct GSI, investigators have been searching for ways to improve success rates and avoid failures. There are several ways to accomplish this: improve the surgical procedure and identify preoperatively those patients at high risk of failure. There are over 100 surgical procedures to correct GSI. New procedures and modifications of existing techniques are constantly being introduced and advocated. Currently, the retropubic urethropexies (Marshall-Marchetti-Krantz and Burch) remain, for many, as the procedure of choice in the uncomplicated patient. However, even in the best of hands, there remains a 10–20% long-term failure rate with these procedures (3, 4).

Almost since the introduction of the retropubic urethropexies, investigators have been searching for a commonality among those patients who fail surgical correction to screen them preoperatively. It was noted early on that failure of a previous antiincontinence procedure put one at risk for subsequent failure, but the reason for this was largely unknown (5, 6). McGuire et al. (7) were the first to note that patients who failed surgical correction of incontinence had a low urethral closure pressure (less than 20 cm H_2O). McGuire (8) later defined type III incontinence as a low maximal urethral closure pressure (less than 20 cm H_2O) in the proximal one half of the urethra and noted that type III incontinence was found in 75% of patients who had failed multiple procedures and in only 13% of those with no previous antiincontinence surgery. However, he could not determine whether this was the cause or the effect of these failed procedures. Sand et al. (9) were the first to report that those patients who demonstrated preoperatively a low pressure urethra (maximal urethral closure pressure of less than or equal to 20 cm H_2O throughout its entire length) were at a higher risk of failure when undergoing a Burch retropubic urethropexy than those patients with "normal" closure pressures (maximal urethral closure pressure of greater than 20 cm H_2O). At a 3-month follow-up, the failure rate in the low pressure urethra group was 54% versus 18% in the normal pressure urethra group. Thus, the concepts of type III incontinence and the low pressure urethra were born. Now patients could be screened for the presence of these entities preoperatively and appropriate measures could be taken to ensure surgical success. However, this prompted a new controversy: which surgery is most effective in patients with type III incontinence or a low pressure urethra?

Urethral Sphincter Mechanism

A full discussion of the urethral sphincter mechanism is presented in Chapters 1 and 4 and is only briefly reviewed here.

The intact urethral sphincter mechanism is made up of both active and passive components that maintain apposition of the urethral mucosa or closure at all times except during the voluntary act of voiding. The active mechanism is comprised of the striated muscle of the voluntary urethral sphincter and the pelvic floor or levator ani muscles. The passive mechanism is composed of the inherent elasticity of the periurethral tissue, the smooth muscle of the urethra, the high retropubic position of the proximal urethra, the urethral mucosa, and the submucosal vascular plexus (10, 11).

The active mechanism, also referred to as the extrinsic urethral sphincter, has two roles: to maintain a constant tone, which it accomplishes through the action of slow twitch muscle fibers, and to actively contract during periods of stress through fast twitch fibers (10, 12, 13). This active contraction of the external urethral sphincter occurs milliseconds before the intraabdominal pressure generated by the cough or Valsalva reaching the bladder and probably represents a reflex that is centrally mediated (14).

The passive mechanism, also referred to as the intrinsic urethral sphincter, maintains adequate resting closure pressure and provides a mucosal seal. There are several factors that make up this sphincter and act through a variety of mechanisms. The urethral mucosa and elasticity of the periurethral tissue maintain coaptation of the mucosa and a water-tight seal. The vascular submucosal cavernous plexus acts as a cylindrical bladder or cushion applying external compression to the urethra, whereas the smooth muscle exerts a constant tone and may play a role modulating blood flow into the vascular plexus (15, 16). All of these components contribute to the resting urethral closure pressure. The high retropubic position of the bladder neck and proximal urethra give it a mechanical advantage, such that rises in intraabdominal pressure are transmitted equally to the bladder and proximal urethra (17). Although this is an element of the passive continence mechanism, it helps maintain urethral closure under stress.

From this discussion, it is apparent that the mechanism responsible for maintaining coaptation and compression of the urethra under periods of rest and stress is a complicated interplay of several components, any one of which might fail and lead to incontinence. Where the defect occurs in patients with ISD is not known, and it may be a different combination of factors in each patient.

Development of ISD

As mentioned in the introduction, ISD is roughly equated with two recognized entities: the low pressure urethra and type III incontinence. The data regarding the prevalence and development of these entities are presented as if they are equated with ISD.

The defects in the urethral sphincter that lead to ISD are largely unknown. The term suggests that there is a deficiency or defect in the "intrinsic urethral sphincter" as defined above. However, this is not necessarily the case, and it may be that a host of factors play a role in its development. As noted in the AHCPR definition, ISD can occur as a result of surgical trauma, pelvic irradiation, sacral cord lesion, or myelomeningocele (1). Women over the age of 50 are another group noted to be at risk (18). It is apparent that this entity can result from a variety of insults and probably represents the end point of multiple different processes that damage some or all of the components of the urethral sphincter.

The earliest reports on surgical failures noted that previous failure of an antiincontinence procedure put one at risk for subsequent failure (5–8, 19, 20). Subjects with ISD are also noted to have a high incidence of previous failed surgical correction. It has been documented that between 58 and 98% of patients diagnosed with either type III incontinence or a low pressure urethra had undergone previous antiincontinence surgery (21, 22). It has also been shown that the maximal urethral closure pressure and number of previous procedures are inversely related (Fig. 11.1) (23). The reason for this may be related to scarring of the periurethral tissue and possibly to damage of the nerves innervating the muscular component of the sphincter mechanism that occurs as a result of the periurethral dissection at the time of surgery. This is particularly true when the procedure involves extensive vaginal dissection (24). An alternative explanation for this apparent association is that subjects with ISD

are at risk to fail antiincontinence procedures and therefore are more likely to undergo repeated procedures. Not all reports identify previous antiincontinence surgery as a predisposing factor for ISD (9, 25, 26), and the data on the effect of antiincontinence surgery on the maximal urethral closure pressure do not confirm this apparent association. The few studies that measure maximal urethral closure pressures pre- and postoperatively show little difference and generally note a slight overall increase in values after surgery (3, 27). In one study with a 10-year follow-up, the mean maximal urethral closure pressure increased from 41 cm H_2O preoperatively to 53 cm H_2O postoperatively in 72 subjects who underwent a Burch retropubic urethropexy. In only 15 of 72 (21%) was there a postoperative decrease in the maximal urethral closure pressure, but none of these patients were incontinent postoperatively (27). The association between previous failed antiincontinence surgery and intrinsic urethral sphincter deficiency exists, but whether it is a cause or effect is unclear.

Surgical trauma during a radical hysterectomy for cervical cancer is a recognized cause of genuine stress urinary incontinence and can occur in up to 50% of patients postoperatively (28, 29). Resection of the posterior aspect of the cardinal ligament (pars nervosa) that contains the sympathetic and parasympathetic fibers results in a significant fall in the maximal urethral closure pressure (Fig. 11.2) (29). This is believed to be responsible for weakening the urethral sphincter mechanism resulting in incontinence. The number of patients experiencing ISD after radical hysterectomy is unknown, but as noted in Figure 11.2, the standard deviation for the maximal urethral closure pressure at 12 months follow-up falls below 20 cm H_2O, demonstrating that several subjects in this study developed a low pressure urethra postoperatively.

One area where the cause of ISD is well recognized is in the patient with a meningomyelocele. These patients tend to have two urologic disorders: incontinence and upper tract deterioration. The upper tract deterioration stems from outlet obstruction with a hypertonic urethral sphincter mechanism, whereas the incontinence can occur from either detrusor hyperreflexia or GSI

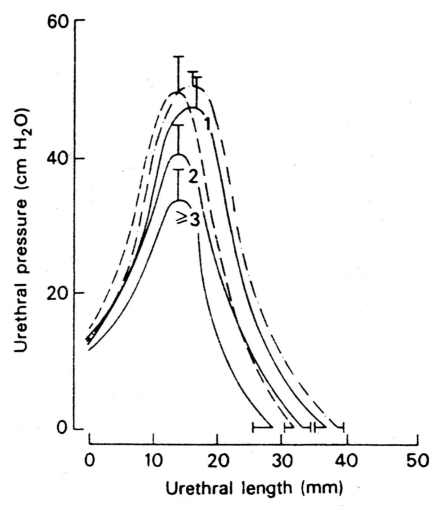

Figure 11.1. Average resting urethral pressure for stress incontinent patients subdivided according to previous surgery: -.-.-, no previous surgery, ---, previous pelvic surgery other than for incontinence, —, one, two, or three or more previous antiincontinence procedures. (From Hilton P, Stanton SL. Urethral pressure measurement by microtransducer: results in symptom-free women and in those with genuine stress incontinence. Br J Obstet Gynaecol 1983;90: 919–933.)

(30, 31). If stress incontinence is present, patients tend to have an open bladder neck and low urethral closure pressure (type III incontinence). This can be seen in up to 86% of these patients, particularly if the lesion involves the lumbosacral segment of the spinal cord (31).

Other types of spinal cord lesions are not necessarily associated with ISD. Nordling et al. (32) studied 57 patients with a variety of spinal cord lesions, from the cervical cord to the cauda equina, and found no association between incontinence with an open patulous bladder neck and the level of cord injury. McGuire and Wagner (33) also noted that

interruption of the sacral nerve roots S2–S4, to control detrusor hyperreflexia in paraplegics, did not alter urethral pressures but that high spinal anesthesia (involving the thoracic cord) did result in complete loss of resting urethral pressure. This suggests that a large part of urethral sphincter function is maintained by the sympathetic nervous system (which originates in the thorax and sacral cord segments) and that simple disruption of the sacral cord segments alone (where a portion of the pelvic sympathetic nerves and the motor fibers of the striated urethral sphincter originate) does not uniformly result in ISD.

The effect of radiation therapy on urethral sphincter function has been poorly studied. There are no studies comparing pre- and postradiation changes in the continence mechanism to determine what effect radiation therapy has on the development of ISD. In one study, it was demonstrated that subjects who were treated with intracavitary and external beam radiotherapy for cervical cancer had a lower maximum urethral closure than matched control subjects who were awaiting therapy for their cervical cancer (34). However, the mean postradiotherapy closure pressure was still 56.7 ± 4.5 cm H_2O, well above the 20 cm H_2O used as a cutoff to diagnose a low pressure urethra. Also, the posttreatment group in this study was older, which probably contributed to the difference

noted. In another study that evaluated 11 patients presenting to a referral center for postirradiation bladder complications, they noted that 5 had an open nonfunctional bladder neck, suggesting that in patients with urinary tract complaints after radiotherapy, there is a significant number with ISD (35).

Other historical factors believed to aid in identifying patients at risk for ISD are age, parity, and menopausal status. It has been demonstrated that the maximal urethral closure pressure falls with advancing age (Fig. 11.3) but not with increasing parity. Only increasing age has been consistently correlated with ISD (9, 18, 23, 25). In a recent multivariate analysis, only age greater than 50 was found to be an independent predictor for the presence of a low pressure urethra,

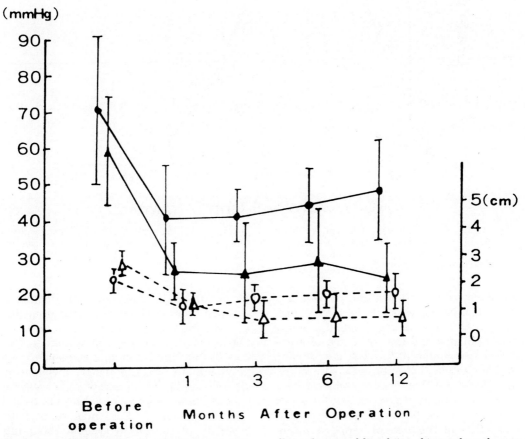

Figure 11.2. Mean maximal urethral closure pressure and mean functional urethral length with a full bladder for subjects before and 3, 6, and 12 months after a radical hysterectomy. •, pressure in subjects in whom the pars nervosa was spared; ▲, pressure in subjects where the pars nervosa was resected bilater-ally; ○, functional length in subjects where the pars nervosa was spared; △, functional length in subjects where the pars nervosa was resected bilaterally. (From Sasaki H, Yoshida T, Noda K, et al. Urethral pressure profiles following radical hysterectomy. Obstet Gynecol 1982;59:101–104.)

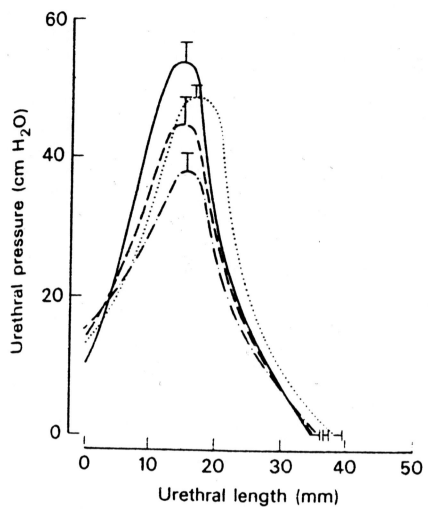

Figure 11.3. Average resting urethral pressure for stress incontinent subjects subdivided by age: —, 31–40 years; ···, 41–50 years; ---, 51–60 years; -·-·-, ≥61 years. (From Hilton P, Stanton SL. Urethral pressure measurement by microtransducer: results in symptom-free women and in those with genuine stress incontinence. Br J Obstet Gynaecol 1983;90: 919–933.)

whereas parity was not found to have any effect (18). In the same article, menopausal status and hormone replacement therapy were evaluated and the incidence of estrogen use was similar in both the low pressure urethra group and the normal pressure urethra group (18). Menopausal subjects have been shown to be at greater risk for a low pressure urethra; however, whether this is a function of the loss of estrogen or increased age has not been conclusively demonstrated (36).

The variety of insults described in this section demonstrate the various etiologies of ISD. Surgical trauma may promote scarring of the periurethral tissue, adversely affecting its elastic properties and may directly injure the striated urethral sphincter muscle or its innervation. Central nervous system lesions may damage the autonomic and somatic innervation to the sphincter mechanism, whereas radiation therapy and age-associated changes may damage the suburethral vascular plexus, urethral mucosa, and the elasticity of the entire system. From this discussion, it is apparent that no one defect results in ISD but rather it represents an end point of a variety of insults to the various components of the urethral continence mechanism.

After close scrutiny of the data, only age greater than 50, failure of a previous antiincontinence procedure, and the presence of stress incontinence in a patient with a meningomyelocele (particularly one involving the lumbosacral region) place the individual at risk for ISD. Whether radical pelvic surgery and radiation therapy lead to the development of ISD have yet to be fully determined. If these are a part of the subject's past medical history, then a thorough evaluation of the urethral sphincter mechanism should be done before any antiincontinence procedures.

Evaluation of ISD

The diagnostic criteria of a low pressure urethra or type III incontinence is well recognized (Table 11.1) (37). However, the question arises, do all subjects with GSI require sophisticated urodynamic studies to exclude ISD? This question is currently open to debate because there is no good data on the prevalence of ISD in the general population. In a study by Bergman et al. (3), they noted that 17 of 127 patients (13%) presenting to the USC Medical Center with a diagnosis of

GSI and no previous antiincontinence surgery had a low pressure urethra. Rates as high as 50% have been reported in other referral populations. However, the rates of previous failed incontinence surgery in these populations were also in the 50% range (18, 30). In a referral practice, routine sophisticated urodynamic studies seem indicated, but in a general practice population, the debate remains as to which subjects should be extensively evaluated for ISD.

From the above discussion, there are certain historical findings that suggest the presence of ISD in the patient with GSI (Table 11.2). The patient with meningomyelocele or previous failed antiincontinence surgery deserves the benefit of a thorough evaluation before recommending surgical correction. In the individual who is over age 50 or postmenopausal, the presence of ISD should always be considered, but routine use of sophisticated studies in these women may not be indicated. Other historical clues to the presence of ISD are the severity of the patient's incontinence symptoms. An inverse relationship has been shown between the subjective severity of the patient's incontinence and the maximal urethral pressures (38, 39). However, a specific association between the grade of severity of a subject's

Table 11.1. Diagnostic Techniques for Identifying a Deficient or Severely Defective Urethral Sphincter Mechanism

Entity	Diagnostic Technique	Diagnostic Criteria
Low pressure urethra (9)	Urethral pressure profile (multichannel urodynamics)	Maximal urethral closure pressure throughout the entire functional urethral length of less than or equal to 20 cm H$_2$O in the sitting position with a subjectively full bladder.
Type III incontinence (8)	Videocystourethrography (multichannel urodynamics with simultaneous fluoroscopy)	Urethral closure pressure of less than 20 cm H$_2$O in the proximal 1.5 cm of the urethra. Open patulous urethra at rest.
Type III incontinence (37)	Videocystourethrography	Vesical neck and proximal urethra are open at rest and obvious urinary leakage that may be gravitational or associated with minimal increases in abdominal pressure.
Intrinsic sphincter deficiency (2, 41)	Stress leak point pressure (multichannel urodynamics or videocystourethrography)	Gross or fluoroscopically visualized urine loss during Valsalva at a vesical pressure of less than 60 cm H$_2$O with a bladder volume of 150 mL or less than 45 cm H$_2$O in a symptomatically full bladder.

Table 11.2. Historical and Physical Findings Suggestive of ISD

Finding	Comment
Historical	
Failed previous incontinence surgery	Found in up to 95% of subjects with ISD
Meningomyelocele	If it involves the lumbosacral vertebrae, up to 86% will have ISD
Age greater than 50	The incidence of ISD in this population is unknown, but it is the most consistent historical finding
Prior pelvic irradiation	Presumed cause of ISD, little data in this area
Postoperative from a radical hysterectomy	Destruction of the autonomic components of the cardinal ligament results in weak urethral sphincter
Severe incontinence complaints (i.e., continuous loss or loss with minimal exertion such as rising to a standing position)	Some correlation with the presence of ISD
Physical[a]	
Gross loss of urine with cough or Valsalva and normal urethrovesical support	Some consider this diagnostic of ISD
Gross loss with cough or Valsalva with a small bladder volume	For example, gross urine loss is seen during the pelvic examination with cough or Valsalva immediately after the patient has voided and a normal voiding mechanism is present

[a]There are no studies correlating physical findings and ISD; however, these findings are believed by many to be suggestive.

incontinence and the presence of ISD has not been consistently demonstrated. McGuire et al. (2) noted that 81% of patients with grade 3 incontinence (defined as incontinent without regard to effort, position or activity) had ISD. Horbach and Ostergard (18) found no relationship between grade of incontinence and the presence or absence of a low pressure urethra. Therefore, there are no clearcut recommendations regarding which patients require extensive evaluation based on subjective symptoms. However, complaints of continuous urine loss should be considered and arouse suspicion in the evaluation process. A thorough history and physical examination should be carried out in all patients with complaints of incontinence to look for any physical evidence of ISD, and particular attention should be paid when evaluating those patients over the age of 50.

Certain findings during a physical examination may allow the physician to suspect the presence of ISD (Table 11.2). It has been suggested that if the patient has gross urine loss with cough in the supine or upright position with a moderately full bladder and no hypermobility of the urethrovesical junction (as demonstrated by a negative Q-tip test or normal position by ultrasound or cystoure-

thrography), then this is suspicious for, and possibly diagnostic of, ISD (1, 40). Another suspicious finding is gross urine loss with cough or Valsalva in the supine position with a scant amount of urine in the bladder. Clinically, if the patient has voided immediately before the examination, has a normal voiding mechanism, and gross urine loss with cough or Valsalva is noted with the subject in the dorsal lithotomy position, then ISD should be suspected.

Sophisticated urodynamic studies are still the mainstay of diagnosing ISD: either urethral pressure profilometry, to diagnose a low pressure urethra, or videocystourethrography to diagnose type III incontinence. Urethroscopy can aid in the diagnosis by visualizing a fixed, scarred, open urethra. However, the presence of an open bladder neck by itself is not diagnostic of ISD or even GSI (41). Therefore, a urethroscopic examination or a voiding cystogram by itself is not sufficient and must be accompanied by pressure studies of the urethra for a proper diagnosis. The drainpipe urethra is an older description of a fixed, scarred, open urethra that is diagnosed by urethroscopic examination. There is little data in the literature regarding this finding or its treatment, but it probably represents the worst form of ISD where the urethra has no ability to coapt and urine flows freely as if through a drainpipe. Even in this setting, a sophisticated urodynamic evaluation to confirm these findings would be appropriate, although not absolutely necessary.

There is a new technique, the leak point pressure, that has been introduced to diagnose ISD (Table 11.1). As with most of the current discussion surrounding this entity, there is controversy here regarding the ability of this test to diagnose a disease that is not well defined. It is being used and advocated as the best technique to diagnose ISD, despite a lack of outcome data regarding therapeutic measures in patients diagnosed with ISD. There is one study in the literature that shows an apparent correlation between leak point pressure data and type III incontinence; however, only 76% of the subjects diagnosed with ISD by leak point pressures had type III incontinence (2). In another study comparing leak point pressure with maximal urethral closure pressure, there was noted to be a statistically significant, but weak, clinical correlation (42).

The leak point pressure is performed by inserting a small-caliber (7–8F) catheter with microtransducers into the bladder. The blad-

der is filled to a given volume (suggested as 150 mL by some) and then the subject is asked to Valsalva. The lowest intravesical pressure that causes gross urine leakage is recorded as the stress leak point pressure (Fig. 11.4) (2, 42, 43). A stress leak point pressure of less than 60 cm H_2O in the standing position with 150 mL in the bladder has been correlated with type III incontinence (2), and a stress leak point pressure of less than 45 cm H_2O in the sitting position with a subjectively full bladder has been correlated with a low pressure urethra (41). Before further evaluation of this test and its ability to diagnose ISD, a standard technique for performing it must be established and adhered to.

There does appear to be some correlation between leak point pressures and the diagnostic techniques that are currently used to evaluate subjects with ISD. However, it is not strong enough to recommend leak point pressures as the definitive diagnostic test at this time, particularly because there is no surgical outcome data on patients diagnosed with ISD by this technique. This does not mean that this test is without merit but that before advising its use as the technique of choice for diagnosing ISD, it should be fully evaluated with respect to treatment outcomes.

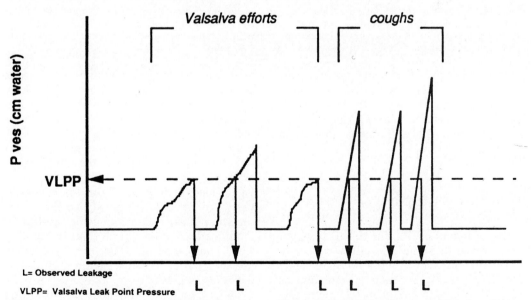

Figure 11.4. Performance of a Valsalva leak point pressure (also known as stress or abdominal leak point pressure). The patient is asked to Valsalva and the intravesical pressure at the moment of leakage, noted either grossly or fluoroscopically, is recorded. This is then checked with repeated Valsalva efforts or coughs for reproducibility and accuracy. (From Montella JM. Valsalva leak point pressure. AUGS Q Rep 1994;12:3.)

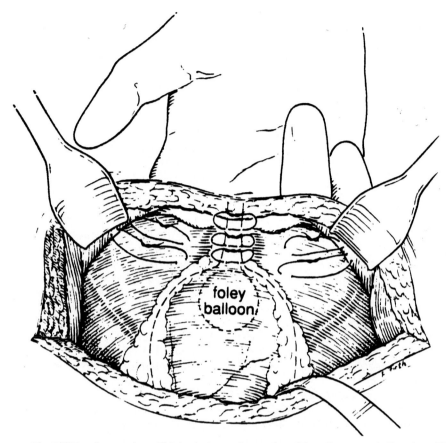

Figure 11.5. The Ball-Burch procedure. This is similar to the standard Burch retropubic urethropexy except for the addition of three pairs of imbrication sutures placed along the dorsal or superior aspect of the urethra. (From Bergman A, Koonings PP, Ballard CA. The Ball-Burch procedure for stress incontinence with low pressure urethra. J Reprod Med 1991;36: 137–140.)

One other area of controversy regarding this examination is the name of the leak point pressure study. Some prefer the term "stress leak point pressure," others "Valsalva leak point pressure." and still others "abdominal leak point pressure."

Treatment of ISD

The treatment of GSI due to ISD is generally surgical in nature. Certainly conservative treatments can provide relief in many patients with GSI, but their role in subjects with ISD is largely unknown. There are several surgical procedures that have been recommended for the correction of ISD. Generally, they are based on retrospective data, and to date, no prospective randomized study has been done to determine which procedure is best for patients with ISD. Most data show that simple elevation of the bladder neck to a high retropubic position will be ineffective in restoring continence in these patients. Currently, most authors recommend more obstructive procedures (i.e, suburethral slings, artificial sphincters, and periurethral collagen injections) (3, 9, 22, 40, 44). However, there are several reports of excellent cure rates in subjects with ISD using the Burch, modifications of the Burch (Ball-Burch, Fig. 11.5), and modifications of the Stamey needle (Stamey-Martius, Figure 11.6) procedures (21, 45, 46).

The current recommendations regarding selection of a surgical procedure to restore continence in subjects with ISD that are generally, but not universally, accepted are as follows (1). If the urethrovesical junction is well supported (as determined by a negative Q-tip test, normal positioning on ultrasound, no descent on lateral straining cystourethrography, or an open bladder neck with minimal mobility on urethroscopic examination), then either an artificial urethral sphincter, obstructive suburethral sling, or periurethral collagen injections are indicated (1, 40, 47). The role of a suburethral sling placed under excessive tension, intended to obstruct the urethra at rest resulting in intermittent self-catheterization for voiding, has not been fully evaluated. There is one study, involving small numbers, that suggests a suburethral

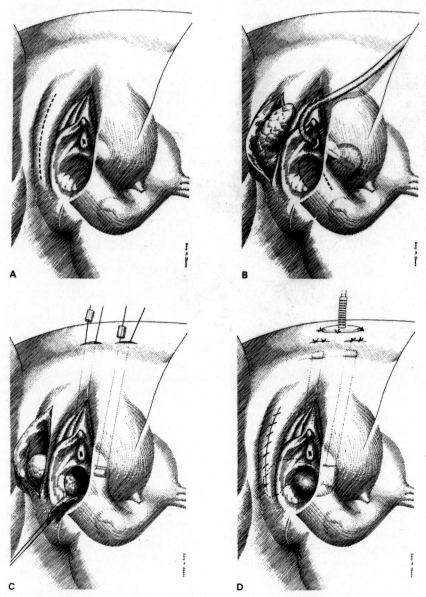

Figure 11.6. Stamey-Martius procedure. **A.** Vertical incision in the labia majora to dissect free the Martius fat pad. **B.** Inverted U-shaped incision in the anterior vaginal wall with its apex at the mid urethra. **C.** After performing the Stamey procedure, the Martius fat pad is tunneled under the labia minora into the anterior vaginal wall defect and fixed with sutures under the urethrovesical junction. **D.** A suprapubic catheter is placed, the Stamey sutures are tied down, and the anterior vaginal wall defect is closed. (From Ganabathi K, Abrams P, Mundy AR, Dwyer PL, Glenning PP. Stamey-Martius procedure for severe genuine stress incontinence. Br J Urol 1992;69:34–37.)

sling placed under normal tension is ineffective in this setting (48). They demonstrated a 20% success rate in subjects with a low pressure urethra and normal urethrovesical junction support versus a 93% success rate in subjects with a low pressure urethra and urethrovesical junction hypermobility. Currently, most authors are recommending either periurethral collagen injections or artificial sphincters as the treatment of choice in this setting (2). If urethrovesical junction hypermobility is present, then many authors believe that a suburethral sling is the procedure of choice (49, 50). Periurethral collagen injections play a role in this setting as well, but they are probably most effective in the patient without hypermobility. However, as stated above, there have been no prospective randomized trials to determine which surgical procedure is the most effective in treating ISD. Until this is done, no recommendations can be universally accepted.

Summary

ISD appears to be a severe form of GSI that puts one at risk to fail standard antiincontinence procedures. There is no one cause for its development, and any insult that severely damages the urethral sphincter mechanism can result in ISD. Although there are several techniques for evaluation of the individual at risk for ISD, there is not a definitive universally accepted test for its diagnosis. Therapy is generally surgical in nature, and obstructive procedures appear to offer the best results, but again, there are no absolute recommendations on which procedure is best. The biggest problem with ISD, at present, is that no agreed upon definition exists that uses specific objective criteria. Until this is done, individual investigators will use various definitions of ISD. This will make it difficult, if not impossible, to pool data from various centers to make any recommendation regarding diagnosis and therapy.

REFERENCES

1. Urinary Incontinence Guidelines Panel. Urinary incontinence in adults. Clinical practice guidelines AHCPR publication 9-2-0038. Rockville, MD: Agency for Health Care Policy and Research, PHS,HHS, March 1992.
2. McGuire EJ, Fitzpatrick CC, Wan J, et al. Clinical assessment of urethral function. J Urol 1993;150: 1452–1454.
3. Bergman A, Ballard CA, Koonings PP. Comparison of three surgical procedures for genuine stress incontinence: prospective randomized study. Am J Obstet Gynecol 1989;160:1102–1106.
4. Herbertsson G, Iosif CS. Surgical results and urodynamic studies 10 years after retropubic colpourethropexy. Acta Obstet Gynecol Scand 1993;72:298–301.
5. Stanton SL, Cardozo L, Williams JE, Ritchie D, Allan V. Clinical and urodynamic features of failed incontinence surgery in the female. Obstet Gynecol 1978;51:515–520.
6. Arnold EP, Webster JR, Loose H, et al. Urodynamics of female incontinence: factors influencing the results of surgery. Am J Obstet Gynecol 1973; 117:805–813.
7. McGuire EJ, Lytton B, Pepe V, Kohorn EI. Stress urinary incontinence. Obstet Gynecol 1976;47: 255–264.
8. McGuire EJ. Urodynamic findings in patients after failure of stress incontinence operations. Prog Clin Biol Res 1981;78:351–360.
9. Sand PK, Bowen LW, Panganiban R, Ostergard DR. The low pressure urethra as a factor in failed retropubic urethropexy. Obstet Gynecol 1987;68: 399–402.
10. Staskin DR, Zimmern PE, Hadley HR, Raz S. The pathophysiology of stress incontinence. Urol Clin North Am 1985;12:271–278.
11. DeLancey JOL. Structural aspects of the extrinsic continence mechanism. Obstet Gynecol 1988;72: 296–301.
12. Shafik A. Stress urinary incontinence: an alternative concept of pathogenesis. Int Urogynecol J 1994;5:3–11.
13. Constantinou CE, Govan DE. Spatial distribution and timing of transmitted and reflexively generated urethral pressures in healthy women. J Urol 1982;127:964–969.
14. Shafik A. Straining urethral reflex: description of a reflex and its clinical significance. Acta Anat 1991;140:104–107.
15. Rud T, Andersson KE, Asmussen M, Hunting A, Ulmsten U. Factors maintaining the intraurethral pressure in women. Invest Urol 1980;17: 343–347.
16. Huisman AB. Aspects on the anatomy of the female urethra with special relation to urinary incontinence. Contrib Gynecol Obstet 1993; 10:1–31.
17. Summit RL, Bent AE, Ostergard DR. The pathophysiology of genuine stress incontinence. Int Urogynecol J 1990;1:12–18.
18. Horbach NS, Ostergard DR. Predicting intrinsic urethral sphincter dysfunction in women with stress urinary incontinence. Obstet Gynecol 1994;84:188–192.
19. Sundin T, Petterssen S. Anterior urethropexy according to Lapides in stress urinary incontinence. Scand J Urol Nephrol 1975;9:28–31.
20. Jeffcoate TNA. The principles governing the

treatment of stress incontinence of urine in the female. Br J Urol 1965;37:633–643.

21. Bergman A, Koonings PP, Ballard CA. The Ball-Burch procedure for stress incontinence with low pressure urethra. J Reprod Med 1991;36:137–140.

22. Blavis JG, Salinas J. Type III urinary incontinence: importance of proper diagnosis and treatment. Surg Forum 1984;35:473–475.

23. Hilton P, Stanton SL. Urethral pressure measurement by microtransducer: results in symptom-free women and in those with genuine stress incontinence. Br J Obstet Gynaecol 1983;90:919–933.

24. Benson JT, McClellan E. The effect of vaginal dissection on the pudendal nerve. Obstet Gynecol 1993;82:387–389.

25. Summitt RL, Sipes DR, Bent AE, Ostergard DR. Evaluation of pressure transmission ratios in women with genuine stress incontinence and low urethral pressure: a comparative study. Obstet Gynecol 1994;83:984–988.

26. Sand PK, Bowen LW, Ostergard DR, Nakanishi AM. Hysterectomy and prior incontinence surgery as risk factors for failed retropubic cystourethropexy. J Reprod Med 1988;33:171–174.

27. Herbertsson G, Iosif CS. Surgical results and urodynamic studies 10 years after retropubic colpourethrocystopexy. Acta Obstet Gynecol Scand 1993;72:298–301.

28. Scotti RJ, Bergman A, Bhatia NN, Ostergard DR. Urodynamic changes in urethrovesical function after radical hysterectomy. Obstet Gynecol 1986;68:111–120.

29. Sasaki H, Yoshida T, Noda K, et al. Urethral pressure profiles following radical hysterectomy. Obstet Gynecol 1982;59:101–104.

30. McGuire EJ, Woodside JR, Borden TA, Weiss RM. Prognostic value of urodynamic testing in myelodysplastic patients. J Urol 1981;126:205–209.

31. Barbalias GA, Blavis JG. Neurologic implications of the pathologically open bladder neck. J Urol 1983;129:780–782.

32. Nordling J, Meyhoff HH, Olesen KP. Cysto-urethrographic appearance of the bladder and posterior urethra in neuromuscular disorders of the lower urinary tract. Scand J Urol Nephrol 1982;16:115–124.

33. McGuire EJ, Wagner FC. The effects of sacral denervation on bladder and urethral function. Surg Obstet Gynecol 1977;164:343–346.

34. Parkin DE, Davis JA, Symonds RP. Urodynamic findings following radiotherapy for cervical carcinoma. Br J Urol 1988;61:213–217.

35. Zoubek J, McGuire EJ, Noll F, DeLancey JOL. The late occurrence of urinary tract damage in patients successfully treated by radiotherapy for cervical carcinoma. J Urol 1989;141:1347–1349.

36. Meschia M, Bruschi F, Barbancini P, Amicarelli F, Crosignani PG. Recurrent incontinence after retropubic surgery. J Gynecol Surg 1993;9:25–28.

37. Blavis JG, Olsson CA. Stress incontinence: classification and surgical approach. J Urol 1988;139:727–731.

38. Toews HA. Intraurethral and intravesical pressures in normal and stress-incontinent women. J Obstet Gynecol 1967;29:613–623.

39. Low JA, Kao MS. Patterns of urethral resistance in deficient sphincter function. Obstet Gynecol 1972;40:634–637.

40. McGuire EJ, Appell RA. Transurethral collagen injection for urinary incontinence. Urology 1994;43:413–415.

41. Versi E. The significance of an open bladder neck in women. Br J Urol 1991;68:42–43.

42. Swift SE, Ostergard DR. A comparison of stress-leak-point pressure and maximal urethral closure pressure in patients with genuine stress incontinence. Obstet Gynecol 1995;85:704–708.

43. Montella JM. Valsalva leak point pressure. AUGS Q Rep 1994;12:3.

44. Bowen LW, Sand PK, Ostergard DR, Franti CE. Unsuccessful Burch retropubic urethropexy: a case controlled study. Am J Obstet Gynecol 1989;160:452–458.

45. Richardson DA, Ramahi A, Chalas C. Surgical management of stress incontinence in patients with low urethral pressure. Gynecol Obstet Invest 1991;31:106–110.

46. Ganabathi K, Abrams P, Mundy AR, Dwyer PL, Glenning PP. Stamey-Martius procedure for severe genuine stress incontinence. Br J Urol 1992;69:34–37.

47. Scotti RJ, Mendelovici R. Periurethral bulking agents. AUGS Q Rep 1994;12:1–2.

48. Summitt RL, Bent AE, Ostergard DR, Harris TA. Stress incontinence and low urethral closure pressure: correlation of preoperative urethral hypermobility with successful suburethral sling procedures. J Reprod Med 1990;35:877–890.

49. Horbach NS, Blanco JS, Ostergard DR, Bent AE, Cornella JLA. Suburethral sling procedure with polytetrafluoroethylene for the treatment of genuine stress incontinence in patients with a low urethral closure pressure. Obstet Gynecol 1988;71:648–652.

50. McGuire EJ, Lytton B, Kohorn EI, Pepe V. The value of urodynamic testing in stress urinary incontinence. J Urol 1980;124:256–258.

CHAPTER 12

Dynamic Urethroscopy

Jack R. Robertson

The female urethra is a neglected structure. Physicians seldom recognize its importance in the genesis of pelvic or lower urinary tract symptoms. Today, urogynecologists realize the true role of the urethra in pelvic pathology and view its interior with the 0° urethroscope. All physicians who deal with the symptomatic lower urinary tract should develop facility in the use of the urethroscope.

Modern urethroscopic technique is dynamic in its approach. It stresses not only visualization of the interior of the urethra and the base of the bladder but also the response of the urethral sphincteric mechanism to bladder filling and to various commands and stressful maneuvers. With this emphasis on dynamic urethral function, a new and important dimension is added to the evaluation of the functional integrity of the lower urinary tract.

Historical Perspective

Bozzini developed the first endoscope about 1805 (1). A candle provided a sufficient light source to allow visualization of the interior of the bladder. His pioneering efforts led to his expulsion from the local medical society.

At Johns Hopkins Hospital, Kelly (2) established the first residency training program in gynecology in which gynecologists became genitourinary surgeons for women. Kelly developed a cystoscope consisting of a tube with a handle and used a head mirror for the light source. He discovered that the bladder ballooned with air when the patient assumed the knee-chest position (Fig. 12.1). With the patient in this position, Kelly examined the interior of the bladder and became the first person to pass ureteral catheters under direct vision.

About this time, Nitzke (3) developed the new indirect water endoscope, and urologists recognized the advantages of lower urinary tract endoscopy. They built a medical specialty around this instrument. This male-oriented panendoscope is inadequate for female urethroscopy due to its 30° view, which limits urethral visualization.

The Robertson TM urethroscope is about 8 inches long with a sleeve that locks over the outside (Fig. 12.2). There is an inlet for gas, which is essential for urethroscopic examination.

Technique of Urethroscopy

The technique for female urethroscopy uses a single channel gas cystometer as the source of carbon dioxide. The tip of the urethroscope is 24F in diameter and tapered. Table 12.1 outlines the procedure for the clinical evaluation of patients who have genuine stress incontinence or other genitourinary problems.

Under direct endoscopic view and with the carbon dioxide flowing at 150 mL/min, the physician obtains an opening urethral pressure (see Fig. 12.5). This is not a urethral closure pressure profile but simply the pres-

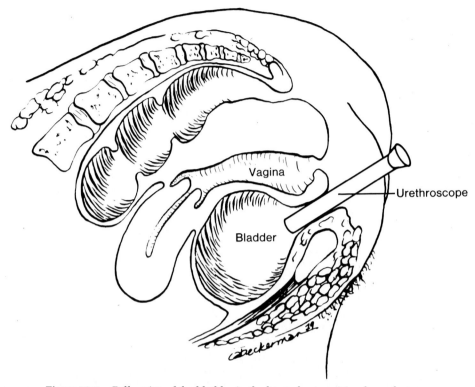

Figure 12.1. Ballooning of the bladder in the knee-chest position for endoscopy.

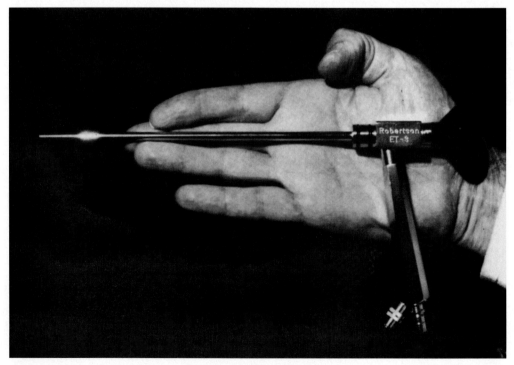

Figure 12.2. The urethroscope.

Table 12.1.   Sequence of Endoscopic Evaluation of the Urethra and Trigone

Urethral opening pressure
Urethral visualization from external meatus
  to urethrovesical junction
Trigonal and ureteral orifice visualization
With observation of the urethrovesical
  junction
  During bladder filling
  With hold command
  With Valsalva and cough
Observation of urethra for exudate and
  abnormal orifices
  Posterior urethral glandular exudate
  Diverticula
  Fistula
  Ectopic ureter
Continued urethral observation
  Occlusion of urethrovesical junction
  Urethral palpation for expression of exudate

sure necessary to open the urethra. The gas is the obturator and provides a less traumatic entry.

Because the manipulation of the urethroscope in the urethra causes erythema, it is important to visualize the interior of the urethra during the initial introduction of the instrument. After visualization of the urethra, the urethroscope enters the bladder through the urethrovesical junction. Evaluation of the trigone follows with visualization of the ureteral orifices.

The endoscopist withdraws the instrument to the urethrovesical junction and views this area during bladder filling and during other superimposed dynamic activities. An evaluation of the responsiveness of the urethrovesical junction to the command of "hold urine" and to the stress of Valsalva and cough when the bladder is nearly full follows.

A search for the orifices of diverticula, an ectopic ureter, or fistulae and exudate from the posterior urethral glands or diverticula completes the urethral visualization sequence. A continuous flow of CO_2 and the occlusion of the urethrovesical junction aid in the search for abnormal orifices within the urethra, enabling better visualization of the area. Simultaneous urethral palpation and massage frequently express exudate under direct visualization.

Endoscopy of Normal Urethra

Endoscopically, the normal urethra has a lush pink epithelium (Fig. 12.3, *top left*). The urethrovesical junction is round and symmetrical (Fig. 12.3, *top right*), and the trigone is pale pink with smooth epithelium and slit-like ureteral orifices (Fig. 12.3, *middle left*).

Dynamic Urethroscopy in the Normal Patient

During carbon dioxide cystometrography with endoscopic control, various changes occur in the urethrovesical junction. As the bladder fills, the inverted U-shaped urethrovesical junction closes (Fig. 12.4). With further bladder filling, there is further urethral tightening ahead of the endoscope. This represents the increased tone of the periurethral striated muscle that develops as the bladder fills.

During bladder filling, the endoscopist uses various challenge maneuvers to test the integrity of the urethrovesical junction. These challenges include asking the patient to hold urine, to bear down, and to cough. In the normal patient, these challenges cause further tightening of the vesical neck, which remains stationary. It is not possible to stimulate a vesical contraction without the volitional agreement of the patient. If a vesical contraction does occur, the normal patient always suppresses it.

In a retrospective chart review of 204 patients who underwent dynamic urethroscopy, Scotti et al. (4) found 99 patients with a diagnosis of genuine stress incontinence. These patients were evaluated urodynamically and urethroscopically to determine the predictive accuracy of the sensitivity and specificity of each of these diagnostic methods. The urodynamic cough profile was both highly reactive and specific for genuine stress incontinence, with sensitivity and specificity of 90 and 100%, respectively. Dynamic urethroscopy yielded sensitivity and specificity of 68.2 and 79.1%, respec-

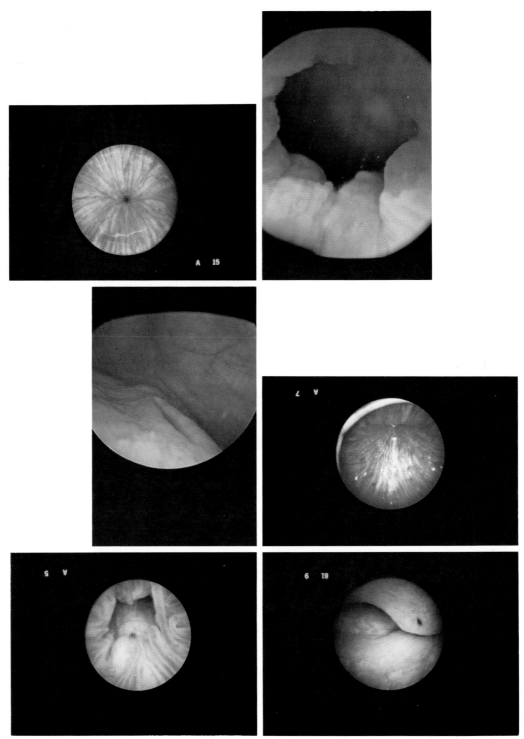

Figure 12.3. Urethroscopic views of the female urethra: the normal urethra (*top left*); the normal urethrovesical junction (*top right*); the normal trigone with one of the ureteral orifices (*middle left*); the red urethra in a patient with urethritis (*middle right*); urethral inflammatory polyps and fronds at the urethrovesical junction (*lower left*); and a urethral diverticular orifice (*lower right*).

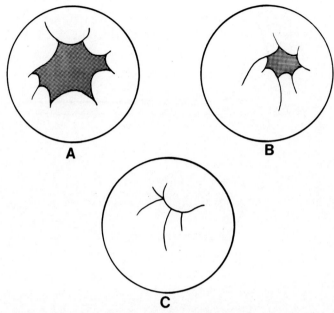

Figure 12.4. Diagram of the normal urethrovesical junction and its changes with bladder filling: (**A**) empty bladder; (**B**) partially filled bladder; (**C**) full bladder.

tively. The researchers concluded that the urodynamic cough urethral pressure profile is recommended for diagnosing this condition.

Women are usually continent when lying down. If there is any question about the findings with dynamic urethroscopy, the patient must be examined in the standing position for confirmation. A Teflon sheath, which keeps the sheath from falling out, is used instead of the conventional stainless steel sheath. With this method, the patient is examined in the standing position with ease by attaching a video camera to the endoscope. Urethral tone is markedly increased when the patient stands. The increased tone in the pelvic floor greatly enhances the endoscopic view over that seen in a supine patient.

The investigators failed to examine the patients in the standing position in their comparison of the two methods. Urodynamics may be the superior of the two methods; however, it requires time-consuming procedures and expensive equipment not available to most clinicians.

Cornella (5), in a recent report, states that the diagnosis of intrinsic sphincteric deficiency is made by clinical opinion. It is his view that this diagnosis is not made by any one urodynamic measurement. He notes that

urethroscopy is an essential part of making the clinical diagnosis of intrinsic sphincteric deficiency.

Urethroscopy for diagnosis must be used in conjunction with history-taking, physical and neurological examination, measurement of postvoiding residual, and especially a voiding diary. This is a clinical diagnosis.

If the diagnosis is genuine stress incontinence or bladder instability, the patient receives behavioral therapy such as bladder drill and Kegel's exercises. There is no risk or side effect from this kind of treatment. Medication is used if indicated. As with most medications, there may be side effects. It is extremely important to review for possible bladder side effects from the medications the patient may already be taking. Some medications may be the cause for incontinence.

If there is no improvement after 6 weeks, surgery is discussed with the patient. Surgery has risks and possible complications. The patient should be offered formal urodynamics at this time.

Recently, Ulmsten (6), one of the founders of urodynamics, stated the belief that the diagnosis of urinary stress incontinence is a clinical diagnosis. He argued that pressure studies are only a part of making this diagnosis.

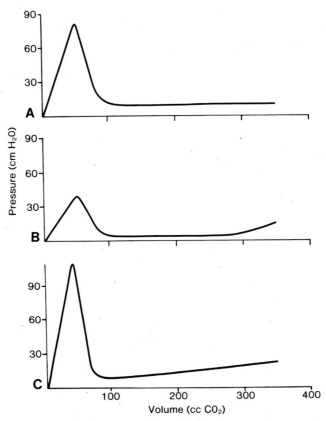

Figure 12.5. Urethral opening pressures (**A**) in the normal patient, (**B**) in the patient with genuine stress incontinence, and (**C**) in the patient with detrusor instability.

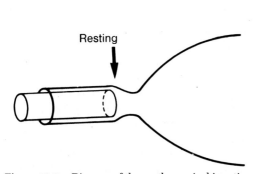

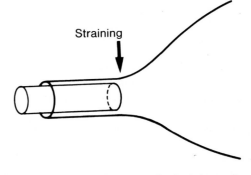

Figure 12.6. Diagram of the urethrovesical junction in the patient with genuine stress incontinence. The end of the urethroscope is located at the junction of the midurethra and the upper third of the urethra (*arrows*). With straining, funneling is characteristic.

Opening Pressures in Normal and Incontinent Patients

The urethral opening pressure in the normal patient registers between 70 and 90 cm H_2O, and the urethroscope easily enters the urethra at an angle from 0° to 45° horizontally (Fig. 12.5). Figure 12.6 diagrammatically demonstrates the urethrovesical junction in patients with genuine stress incontinence. These patients have vesical necks with minimal anatomic support. During stress, the vesical neck behaves like an inelastic rubber band. After three or four vigorous coughs, the vesical neck opens (funnels) and descends. It is very slow to reform and to return to its normal position. Similarly, the vesical neck reacts sluggishly, if at all, to the "hold" command.

Urethroscopy and Unstable Bladder

With a cough, the patient with an unstable bladder will demonstrate an increase in intravesical pressure; several seconds later, the vesical neck will open, and urine will escape from the external meatus (Fig. 12.5). In some patients, bladder filling will stimulate this reaction; in others, one of the detrusor activating procedures will cause vesical contraction. These patients cannot suppress these detrusor contractions.

Urethroscopy in Urethral Syndrome

Those patients whose incontinence results from the urethral syndrome characteristically have a red urethra with exudate from the posterior periurethral glands, particularly with visualization during urethral massage (Fig. 12.3, *middle right*). Commonly, the

inflamed urethra contains polyps and fronds, particularly at the urethrovesical junction (Fig. 12.3, *lower left*). The physician must be careful to distinguish inflammatory polyps from condyloma acuminata. The latter usually appears as a small "forest" of villi and occupies a larger area of the proximal urethra and also the trigone. Condyloma acuminata is best visualized with the CO_2 off while the urine is allowed to bathe the trigone and proximal urethra. Condyloma may also occur at the urethral meatus.

Urethroscopy and Diverticula

The endoscopist attempts to visualize urethral diverticula during urethral distention (Fig. 12.3, *lower right*). Urethral palpation frequently reveals puffs of exudate that aid in the localization of diverticular orifices.

Urethroscopy of Ectopic Ureter, Fistula, and Frozen Urethra

Although the ectopic ureter is rare, the characteristic spurts of urine reveal its identity. Urethrovaginal fistulae also have a characteristic appearance.

Table 12.2. Urethroscopy of Normal and Abnormal Patients

Dynamic Function of the Urethrovesical Junction During	Normal	Genuine Stress Incontinence	Unstable Bladder
Empty bladder		Closed	Closed
Partially filled bladder	Closed	Slowly opens	Closed if no vesical contraction
Full bladder			
Holding	Closes	Sluggish closure	Closes
Straining	Remains closed	Opens	Remains closed if no vesical contraction
Coughing			
Vesical contraction	Opens and then closes, with suppression		Opens and remains open due to inability to suppress
Ability to suppress a vesical contraction	Present	Present	Absent

Urethroscopy of the frozen urethra in a patient who has had multiple surgical procedures in or about the urethra not uncommonly demonstrates a rigid fibrotic functionless urethra with no response to any functional command. These patients require an obstructive surgical procedure using suburethral slings or an artificial sphincter to cure their genuine stress incontinence. This is a major triage junction in the selection of an appropriate surgical procedure for a given patient.

Summary

The direct visualization of urethral-trigonal anatomy with the 0° urethroscope reveals the existence of previously unrecognized pathological entities. This dynamic technique also provides a method for evaluation of the functional integrity of the urethral sphincteric mechanism during bladder filling and with superimposition of varying commands and stressful situations (Table 12.2). The localization of diverticular orifices, ectopic ureters, and fistulae is also possible. Finally, when coordinated with urodynamic techniques, urethroscopy completes the essential composite evaluation of normal and abnormal urethrovesical function.

REFERENCES

1. Bozzini P. Lichteiter, eine Erfindung zur Anschung Innerer Theile, und Krankheiten nebst Abbildung. J Pract Arzeykunde 1805;24:107.
2. Kelly HA. Bull Johns Hopkins Hosp 1893.
3. Nitzke M. Eine Neue Balbachtungs- und Untersuchunigsmethods fur Harnrohre, Harnblase and Rectum. Wein Med Wochenschr 1879;24:659.
4. Scotti R, Ostergard D, Guillaume A, Kohatsu K. Predictive value of urethroscopy as compared to urodynamics in the diagnosis of genuine stress incontinence. J Reprod Med 1990;35:772–776.
5. Cornella J. Intrinsic sphincteric deficiency: a clinical opinion. AUGS Q Rep 1995;XIII:1–3.
6. Ulmsten U. Female urinary incontinence-a symptom, not a urodynamic disease. Some theoretical and practical aspects on the diagnosis and treatment of female urinary incontinence. Int Urol J 1995;6:2–3.

SUGGESTED READINGS

Robertson JR. Gynecologic urethroscopy. Am J Obstet Gynecol 1973;115:986.
Robertson JR. Ambulatory gynecologic urology. Clin Obstet Gynecol 1974;17:255.
Robertson JR. Gas cystometrogram with urethral pressure profile. Obstet Gynecol 1974;44:72.
Robertson JR. Genitourinary problems in women. Springfield, IL: Charles C Thomas, 1978.

CHAPTER 13

Cystoscopy for the Urogynecologist

Geoffrey W. Cundiff and Alfred E. Bent

Cystoscopy provides a noninvasive method of visually evaluating the lower urinary tract. It has broad diagnostic and therapeutic applications in urogynecology. Once one has a basic understanding of the equipment and the ability to recognize normal and pathological findings, the techniques of cystoscopy are easily mastered. Its simplicity and utility make it indispensable in the practice of urogynecology.

Historical Perspective

Although Kelly is often credited with developing the female cystoscope, endoscopy of the female bladder preceded his report by half a century. Bozzini (1) described an endoscopic technique for evaluating the female bladder in the early 19th century. His invention consisted of a stand that supported different-sized hollow funnels, a candle for illumination, and a reflector to direct the light into the funnel when it was placed into the urethra. Visibility with this device was limited by both poor illumination and the tendency of the operator to burn himself if the stand was tilted for a better view. His invention was not favorably received.

Desmormeaux (2) introduced a more practical endoscope in 1853 that used different-sized angulated tubes. The angulated tubes increased the surface area of the bladder that could be inspected and use of an alcohol lamp significantly improved illumination. By 1877 Grünfeld's (3) modification of the endoscope still used a hollow tube but added

an obliquely placed glass lens at the vesical end. His endoscope was vastly improved by the adaptation of an electrical light source reflected by mirrors. Even with this improvement, visualization was poor without bladder distention, and endoscopy was considered to be an adjunct to the established method of urethral dilation followed by bimanual palpation. Nitze (4) developed a compound lens system that increased the field of vision and used an incandescent light source to provide illumination, but this cystoscope was considered to be too complicated for all but the specialist.

Kelly's contribution was in overcoming the deficiencies of both Grünfeld's and Nitze's instruments and techniques. The Kelly cystoscope was a hollow tube, without glass, that used an obturator for placement (5). By placing the patient in the knee-chest position, introduction of the cystoscope allowed air to distend the bladder. A head mirror was used to reflect an electric light into the bladder for illumination (Fig. 13.1). The technique was simple yet provided an excellent view. Its simplicity made cystoscopy available to all physicians for the first time.

Modern endoscopy started with the development of the Hopkins fiber-optic telescope in 1954 (6). The use of glass fibers in place of an air chamber dramatically improved light transmission and resolution and also provided a wider viewing angle. The viewing angle could also be changed, which improved the extent of visualization and facilitated more invasive procedures. Later modi-

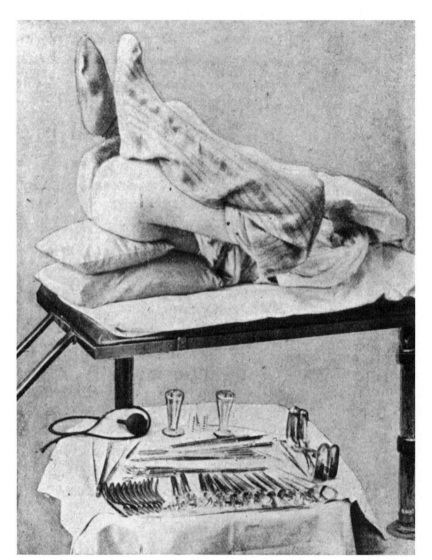

Figure 13.1. Cystoscopy as described by Kelly used a supine position with the hips elevated. The instruments used by Kelly are arranged in the foreground. (From Kelly HA. The direct examination of the female bladder with elevated pelvis—the catheterization of the ureters under direct inspection, with and without elevation of the pelvis. Am J Obstet Dis Wom Child 1894;25:7.)

fications of the Hopkins system incorporated a series of glass rods with optically finished ends separated by intervening spaces.

The improved view of the bladder provided by the Hopkins cystoscope came at the price of a compromised view of the urethra. Not only is the angled telescope not effective for evaluating the urethral mucosa, but most cystoscope sheaths have a terminal fenestra for use with a catheter deflector mechanism that allows the irrigant to escape during urethroscopy. Robertson (7) addressed the com-

promised view of the urethra by applying the fiber-optic technology of the Hopkins cystoscope to a shorter straight-on telescope designed specifically for viewing the urethra. Subsequently, he outlined the use of this urethroscope for evaluating women with incontinence, and his technique came to be known as dynamic urethroscopy. Many gynecological surgeons treating incontinence at that time relied solely on the findings from the history and physical examination. Dynamic urethroscopy offered a simple office procedure that considerably improved the diagnostic evaluation of the lower urinary tract.

The most recent development in cystoscopy is the flexible cystoscope. A flexible endoscope takes advantage of the flexibility of the fiber-optic lens system to create an endoscope that bends, thereby increasing the range of the field of view. Tsuchida and Sugawara (8) reported that using a flexible fiber cystoscope provided an improved view of the bladder neck. Others have advocated flexible cystoscopy as a means to limit the necessary instrumentation and improve patient tolerance (9). The flexible endoscope, although providing flexibility, sacrifices some of the resolution; however, several recent comparisons of flexible cystoscopes with rigid cystoscopes have reported the two techniques to be diagnostically equivalent (10, 11).

Modern cystoscopy is an easily mastered skill with many applications in urogynecology. It should be part of the armamentarium of all pelvic surgeons.

Equipment

RIGID CYSTOSCOPY

Three parts make up the rigid cystoscope: the telescope, the bridge, and the sheath (Fig. 13.2). Each component serves a different function and is available with various options to facilitate this role.

The telescope transmits light to the bladder cavity and an image to the viewer. Today

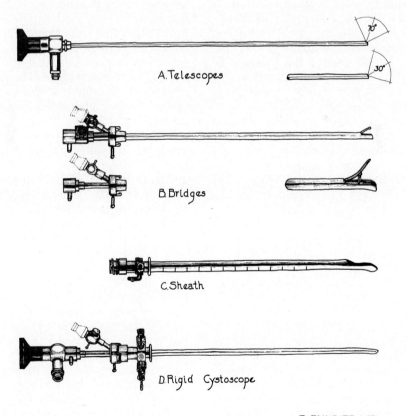

Figure 13.2. The rigid cystoscope. **A,** Telescopes. The 70° lateral angled-view telescope (*above*) and the 30° forward-oblique telescope (*below*). **B,** Bridges. Single-port bridge (*below*) and dual-port bridge with an Albarran deflecting mechanism (*above*). The position of the deflecting mechanism within the fenestra of the operating sheath is shown. **C,** Sheath. 22F operating sheath. **D,** Assembled cystoscope with a diagnostic 17F sheath.

virtually all rigid telescopes use a modification of the fiber-optics developed by Hopkins. Telescopes designed for cystoscopy are available with several viewing angles, including 0° (straight), 3° (forward-oblique), 70° (lateral), and 120° (retro view). The angled telescopes have a field marker that maintains orientation. It is visible as a blackened notch at the outside of the visual field and opposite the angle of deflection.

The different angles facilitate the inspection of the entire bladder wall. Although the 0° lens is essential to adequate urethroscopy, it is insufficient for cystoscopy. The 30° lens provides the best view of the bladder base and posterior wall, whereas the 70° lens permits inspection of the anterolateral walls. The retro view of the 120° lens is not usually necessary for cystoscopy of the female bladder but can be useful for evaluating the urethral opening into the bladder. For many applications, a single telescope is preferable. In diagnostic cystoscopy, the 30° telescope is usually sufficient, although a 70° telescope may be required in the presence of fixation of the urethrovesical junction. For operative cystoscopy, the 70° telescope is preferable.

The cystoscope sheath provides a vehicle for introducing the telescope and distending media into the vesical cavity. They are available in various calibers ranging from 17 to 28F. When placed within the sheath, the telescope, which is 15F, only partially fills the lumen, leaving an irrigation-working channel. The smallest diameter sheath is useful for diagnostic procedures, whereas the larger calibers provide space for the placement of instruments into the irrigation-working channel. The proximal end of the sheath has two irrigating ports, one for introduction of the distending medium and another for removal. The distal end of the cystoscope sheath is fenestrated to permit the use of instrumentation in the angled field of view. It is also beveled, opposite the fenestrae, to increase the comfort of introduction of the cystoscope into the urethra. Bevels increase with the diameter of the cystoscope, and larger diameter sheaths may require an obturator for placement.

The bridge serves as a connector between the telescope and sheath and forms a water-tight seal with both. It may also have one or two ports for the introduction of instruments into the irrigation-working channel. The Albarran bridge is a variation of the bridge that has a deflector mechanism at the end of an inner sheath. When placed within the cystoscope sheath, the deflector mechanism is located at the distal end of the inner sheath within the fenestra of the outer sheath. In this location, elevation of the deflector mechanism assists the manipulation of instruments within the field of view.

FLEXIBLE CYSTOSCOPY

Unlike the rigid cystoscope, the flexible cystoscope combines the optical systems and irrigation-working channel in a single unit. The optical system consists of a single image-bearing fiber-optic bundle and two light-bearing fiber-optic bundles. The fibers of these bundles are coated parallel coherent optical fibers that transmit light even when bent. This permits incorporation of a distal-tip deflecting mechanism that will deflect the tip 290° in a single plane. The deflection is controlled by a lever at the eyepiece. The optical fibers are fitted to a lens system that magnifies and focuses the image. A focusing knob is located just distal to the eyepiece. The irrigation-working port enters the instrument at the eyepiece opposite the deflecting mechanism. The coated tip is 15–18F in diameter and 6–7 cm in length, with the working unit constituting half the length.

Because of the individual coating of the fibers, there is a small space between each fiber in the image guide. Consequently, the image appears somewhat granular. The delicate 5- to 10-μm diameter of the fibers makes them susceptible to damage, which can further compromise the transmission of image or light. Gentle handling is therefore essential to good visualization and to longevity of the instrument. The flow rate of the irrigation-working channel is approximately one fourth that of a rigid cystoscope of similar size and is further curtailed by the passage of instruments down this channel. Some tip deflection is also lost with use of the instrument channel.

Despite these restrictions, several studies comparing flexible to rigid cystoscopy have found no compromise of diagnostic capabilities (10, 11). Many urologists prefer the flexible cystoscope because of improved patient comfort, but the improvement in patient comfort primarily applies to male patients, who often require general anesthesia for diagnostic cystoscopy with a rigid instrument. The absence of a prostate and the short length of the female urethra make rigid cystoscopy well tolerated by women. This may offset any perceived advantage of flexible cystoscopy in female patients.

LIGHT SOURCES AND VIDEO MONITORS

Any light source that provides adequate illumination via a fiber-optic cable is sufficient, although a high-intensity (xenon) light source is recommended for the use of video monitoring or photography. The fiber-optic cable attaches to the telescope at the eyepiece. It uses flexible optic fibers comparable with those of the flexible cystoscope and is similarly prone to damage.

Although all cystoscopic procedures can be performed with direct visualization through the eyepiece, video monitoring eliminates the awkward positioning required for direct visualization. It also permits video documentation, which facilitates teaching, and often improves patient toleration by providing distraction during the procedure. The video camera attaches directly to the eyepiece and should be maintained in an upright orientation. Changing the direction of view is accomplished by rotating the cystoscope without moving the camera itself.

DISTENDING MEDIA

Urethrocystoscopy was originally described with carbon dioxide used as a distending medium, but many practitioners prefer to use water or saline to distend the bladder and urethra. A liquid medium prevents the bubbling associated with carbon dioxide, which can limit visualization; furthermore, the bladder volumes achieved using a liquid medium more accurately approximate physiological volumes. If a liquid medium is used, the water is instilled by gravity through a standard intravenous infusion set. The bag should be at a height of at least 100 cm above the patient's pubic symphysis to provide adequate flow.

INSTRUMENTATION

A wide range of instrumentation is available for use through a cystoscope. Those most pertinent to urogynecology are grasping forceps with either rat-tooth or alligator jaws, biopsy forceps, and scissors. They can be obtained in semirigid or flexible varieties and come in various diameters. A flexible monopolar ball electrode (Karl Storz, Culver City, CA) is useful for electrocautery during operative cystoscopy.

Cystoscopic Techniques

DIAGNOSTIC CYSTOSCOPY

Diagnostic cystoscopy in women is easily performed as an office procedure and is well tolerated without anesthesia. Indications for the procedure are a source of some debate. There is general agreement that cystoscopy is indicated for patients complaining of irritative symptoms or hematuria. Most urogynecologists would also use cystoscopy to evaluate persistent incontinence or voiding dysfunction after incontinence surgery. There is less agreement about the role of cystoscopy in the baseline evaluation of the incontinent patient.

The refinement of urodynamic techniques over the last 3 decades has fostered the uncertain role of cystoscopy. There have been several comparisons of urethrocystoscopy to multichannel urodynamics that have shown the former to be less sensitive and less specific in diagnosing genuine stress incontinence and detrusor instability (12, 13). These comparisons fail to recognize the unique information that urethrocystoscopy provides when combined with urodynamics. Urethrocystoscopy provides an anatomic assessment of the urethra and bladder that permits the discovery of benign and malignant mucosal lesions missed by urodynamics alone. A recent study of 84 women evaluated for lower urinary tract dysfunction with combined urodynamics and urethrocystoscopy reported that 7% of the women had findings at urethrocystoscopy that were not suspected after urodynamics. These included two cases of papillary transitional cell carcinoma, two cases of cystitis glandularis, an intravesical suture, and a urethral diverticulum. All patients presented for urinary incontinence and none had a history of pain or hematuria. Moreover, there were no significant predictors of these critical urethrocystoscopic findings in an analysis that included age over 60, symptoms of urgency, or a urodynamic diagnosis of detrusor instability (14).

Urethrocystoscopy may also have a role in diagnosing conditions for which the urodynamic criteria are inaccurate or ill-defined, such as intrinsic sphincter deficiency. Although many diagnostic parameters have been recommended based on retrospective data, the clinical criteria and therapeutic implications of intrinsic sphincter deficiency are uncertain. Although fluoroscopic demonstration of urethrovesical funneling has been purported to represent so-called type III incontinence, this finding has been demonstrated in up to half of asymptomatic continent women (15). More recently, efforts have been made to generate functional criteria, including low leak point pressures and low urethral closure pressure (16, 17). Unfortunately, the sensitivity and specificity of both leak point pressures and urethral closure pressures are poor (18, 19). In the absence of proven criteria for diagnosing intrinsic sphincter deficiency, a combined clinical approach to making the diagnosis seems logical. In such an approach, the historical risk factors for intrinsic sphincter deficiency and urodynamic evidence of stress incontinence with functional compromise of the urethral sphincter are supplemented by an anatomic assessment using urethrocystoscopy.

Another function of diagnostic cystoscopy is ensuring normal ureteral function preoperatively. This provides a baseline for intraoperative and postoperative evaluation of ureteral integrity.

Most indications for diagnostic cystoscopy warrant evaluation of both the bladder and urethra. Urethroscopy is easily performed in conjunction with cystoscopy and usually precedes the cystoscopic examination. Because urethroscopy is well covered in Chapter 12, this discussion only addresses cystoscopy.

The technique described uses room-temperature sterile water as a distending medium. Instillation is by gravity through a standard intravenous infusion set with the bag at a height of 100 cm above the patient's pubic symphysis. Cystoscopy is performed using a 30° or 70° rigid telescope in a 17F sheath. Topical anesthetics are typically avoided during urethroscopy, because they can affect the color of the urethral mucosa. After urethroscopy, however, 2% lidocaine jelly may be used as a lubricant and topical anesthetic, although the procedure is usually well tolerated without topical anesthesia. The cystoscope is placed into the urethral meatus with the bevel directed posteriorly and is advanced to the bladder under direct visualization. An obturator is not necessary, because downward pressure on the posterior lumen of the urethra with the blunt bevel of a 17F sheath fully opens the urethral lumen and is well tolerated by most patients. The infusion of water is maintained at a slow rate until a volume of 300–400 mL is reached or until the patient reports fullness. At this volume, the flow may be stopped unless it is required to improve the endoscopic view, in which case a small volume can be removed for patient comfort. Orientation is easily established by identifying an air bubble at the anterior dome of the bladder. This serves as a landmark during the remainder of the examination of the bladder mucosa. Beginning at the superior dome to the urethrovesical junction, the survey progresses in 12 sweeps, mimicking the points of a clock. Orientation is maintained by placing the field marker directly opposite the portion of the bladder to be inspected. Visualization of the bladder base can be difficult in patients with a large cystocele, although reduction of the prolapse with a vaginal finger easily circumvents this problem. The mucosa is examined for color, vascularity, trabeculation, and abnormal lesions such as plaques or masses. Once the survey is complete, the telescope is removed while leaving the sheath in place. This allows the bladder to drain and permits measurement of the drained fluid, giving an estimate of the bladder volume. The approach to diagnostic cystoscopy using a flexible cystoscope follows an approach similar to that described for rigid cystoscopy.

ANTIMICROBIAL PROPHYLAXIS

Infection is one of the leading causes of morbidity associated with cystourethroscopy, yet the actual rate of procedure-related bacteriuria is not well defined. In the literature, the rate of bacteriuria after cystoscopy ranges from 2.8–16.6% (20–22). The upper limits of these ranges represent significant factors of potential morbidity that have prompted many clinicians to use prophylactic antibiotics. Approaches vary considerably, in terms of both choice of antimicrobial agents and route of administration. The most common prophylactic regimen used for cystoscopy is probably oral nitrofurantoin. Some practitioners use antibiotic bladder irrigation in lieu of oral antibiotics.

Operative Cystoscopy

Urogynecologists generally leave most operative cystoscopies to urologists. There are, however, several minor procedures that are easily performed in the office during diagnostic cystoscopy. These include biopsy of mucosal lesions and removal of small foreign bodies or intravesical sutures. Because these procedures require a larger cystoscope sheath (22F) and may cause some patient discomfort, anesthesia is recommended. Intravesical instillation of anesthetic is often sufficient but can be augmented by a bladder pillar block. For bladder instillation, the bladder is catheterized and drained. Fifty milliliters of 4% lidocaine solution is instilled and left in place for 5 minutes. The bladder pillar block can be placed before the lidocaine is drained from the bladder. The block is performed by injecting 5 mL of 1% lidocaine solution submucosally at the bladder pillars. After placement of a bivalve speculum, the bladder pillars are located in the lateral fornices at 2 and 10 o'clock with respect to the cervix. If the uterus is absent, placement of a Sims speculum reveals the location of the bladder pillars on the anterior vaginal wall just superior and lateral to the urethrovesical junction (23).

Because of the focal length of the optics, the best view is immediately in front of the telescope; this is where operative procedures should take place. After introduction of the cystoscope into the bladder and instillation of a sufficient volume to view the entire vesical wall, the instrument is introduced into the operative port and advanced until it is visible just at the end of the cystoscope. Gross movements should be made by moving the cystoscope, whereas minor adjustments are made by moving the instrument itself. This approach keeps the operation in the optimal field of view. Irrigation at a brisk rate prevents the field from being obscured by hemorrhage. The bleeding that occurs with biopsy will usually stop by itself, although the patient should be apprised of potential minor hematuria immediately after the procedure. If excessive hemorrhage occurs, this can be controlled by electrocautery using the ball electrode.

Intraoperative Cystoscopy

Cystoscopy is an important adjuvant to surgery of the female genitourinary system. It is commonly used to judge coaptation during periurethral injections, to assess the elevation of the urethrovesical junction during needle urethropexies, to facilitate the safe placement of suprapubic catheters, and to evaluate the ureters and bladder mucosa for inadvertent damage.

Cystoscopy is essential to both the periurethral and the transurethral approach to periurethral injections. Visualization of the urethral lumen with the urethroscope allows the surgeon to advance the needle to the proper position just lateral to the urethrovesical junction. It also permits injection of sufficient material to achieve coaptation without breaching the urethral mucosa.

For placement of a suprapubic catheter, cystoscopy increases the safety of the suprapubic stab technique. It facilitates intelligent insertion by confirming proper orientation and providing visualization of the entry. It also guarantees accurate final positioning of the catheter (24).

As part of his modification of the needle urethropexy, Stamey (25) advocated use of a cystoscope to ensure correct suture placement and to avoid bladder injuries. Cystoscopy is now commonly used during needle urethropexies to assess the elevation of the urethrovesical junction and to ensure that the needle has not breached the integrity of bladder mucosa. A recent report suggests that the intraoperative endoscopic view of the bladder neck is neither reproducible nor predictive of postoperative success (RC Bump, WG Hurt, DM Elser, JP Theofrastous, JA Fantl, DK McClish, unpublished data, 1995). This does not, however, detract from the value of cystoscopy in the intraoperative evaluation for damage to the ureters and bladder mucosa.

The approach to assessment of the integrity of the bladder mucosa after pelvic surgery is similar to the approach described for diagnostic cystoscopy. A thorough survey of the bladder is made with special attention to the portions of the bladder potentially jeopardized by the given procedure. Inspection of the anterolateral aspects of the mucosa is important after a retropubic urethropexy, whereas inspection of the trigone is warranted after a difficult vaginal hysterectomy or dissection of an anterior enterocele sac from the bladder. An assessment of ureteral integrity is warranted after any retropubic suspension or culdoplasty but is also warranted in any case in which there is a suspicion of ureteral injury. Visualization of the ureteral orifice during efflux is sufficient and is facilitated by intravenous administration of indigo carmine approximately 5 minutes before initiating cystoscopy. The absence of efflux is an indication for the passage of ureteral catheters to evaluate for potential obstruction.

URETERAL CATHETERIZATION

Catheterizing the ureteral orifices has been a goal of the endoscopist since the early use of cystoscopes in the 19th century. With today's technology, catheterization is accomplished with ease and safety. In gynecology, the primary indications for ureteral catheterization are to evaluate potential ureteral obstruction and to place ureteral markers. Ureteral markers are useful for any surgery with a high potential for ureteral injury, including radical surgery and surgery with abnormal pelvic anatomy.

Ureteral catheters are available in various sizes and with a number of specialized tips. Although available from 3 to 12F, the most useful calibers are from 4 to 7F. The most common catheters are the general-purpose and the whistle-tip catheters. Specialized tips include the spiral filiform for negotiating strictures and curves and the acorn tip for obtaining retrograde pyelograms. Catheters are fabricated from plastic or Dacron and are generally radiopaque. They also have graduated centimeter markings for judging the depth of insertion.

Once the ureteral orifice is located, the ureteral catheter is advanced into the field of view. Although the deflecting mechanism of the Albarran bridge facilitates ureteral catheterization, it is usually not essential. The catheter is placed just outside the fenestrated end of the cystoscope with the catheter tip oriented in the axis of the ureteral lumen. The tip is threaded into the ureteral orifice by advancing the entire cystoscope. Once the tip passes the ureteral orifice, the catheter is gently advanced until it meets resistance as it passes into the renal pelvis, which is generally at 25–30 cm.

Difficulty in passing the catheter may be due to an anatomic variation such as a stenotic orifice, mucosal fold, or ureteral tortuosity. A stenotic orifice is suspected in the presence of immediate resistance to the catheter tip. Using a smaller caliber catheter and withdrawing the catheter tip slightly into the sheath to minimize its bending will often overcome the stenosis. A mucosal fold can be conquered by repositioning the patient, bladder, or cystoscope. Placing the patient in the Trendelenburg position helps to alter the position of the intramural ureter, as does further filling or emptying the bladder. A filiform tip catheter is also valuable for negotiating strictures or tortuosities.

If the catheter is to be left in place, it should be secured to a transurethral catheter and connected to a drainage device. Gentle technique is essential to prevent hematuria and resulting colic. Other potential complications include perforation and ureteral spasm, but with proper methods the risk of complication is minimal.

SUPRAPUBIC TELESCOPY

Transurethral cystoscopy is well suited to evaluating vesical and ureteral integrity when pelvic surgery is performed from a vaginal approach, but it is inconvenient in conjunction with an abdominal approach.

Valuable operative time is lost by closing the abdominal wound to permit repositioning and preparing for transurethral cystoscopy. Moreover, any significant cystoscopic findings mandate reopening the abdomen for surgical correction. Despite these inconveniences, most ureteral injuries occur during abdominal pelvic surgery (26). Suprapubic telescopy addresses this dilemma by providing a method to perform endoscopy from an abdominal approach (27). Because of the simplicity of the technique, suprapubic telescopy compares favorably with the alternatives of open cystotomy or dissection of ureters in terms of required operating time and morbidity. Moreover, it is an easy transition for an endoscopist experienced in transurethral cystoscopy.

Suprapubic telescopy is an extraperitoneal technique that begins with closure of the anterior peritoneum to prevent vesicoperitoneal fistulas and contamination of the peritoneal cavity with spilled urine. If indigo carmine is to be used to help identify the ureteral orifices, it should be administered at this juncture to permit time for renal excretion. Efflux of indigo carmine is usually visible in 5–10 minutes but sometimes takes up to 20 minutes. The bladder cavity is filled through a transurethral Foley catheter to at least 400 mL. This is simplified by placing a triple-lumen Foley catheter before beginning surgery. A 1- to 2-cm purse-string suture is placed into the muscularis layer of the dome of the bladder, using a 2-0 absorbable suture. Two stay sutures are placed within the purse-string suture using similar suture material but with a full-thickness purchase to facilitate introduction of the telescope. A stab incision made between the stay sutures provides an opening for insertion of the telescope. Because distention of the bladder is achieved through the transurethral catheter, the sheath and bridge are not necessary, and only the telescope is inserted. The purse-string suture is tightened sufficiently to prevent leakage without limiting the movement of the telescope. A 30° telescope provides the best view of the trigone and ureteral orifices whereas also permitting a thorough bladder survey. Orientation can be achieved by identifying the transurethral Foley catheter bulb. The trigone is beneath the bulb, with the urethral and ureteral orifices at its apices.

In the event that ureteral catheterization is planned, a sheath with a sufficient irrigation-working channel can be used with the telescope. If suprapubic catheterization is planned, the catheter can be placed through the same stab incision when telescopy is completed.

Cystoscopic Findings

NORMAL CYSTOSCOPIC FINDINGS

In its normal state, the bladder mucosa has a smooth surface with a pale pink to glistening white hue. The translucent mucosa affords easy visualization of the branched submucosal vasculature. As the mucosa of the dome gives way to the trigone, it thickens and develops a granular texture. The reddened granular surface of the trigone is commonly covered by a thickened white membrane with a villous contour. Histological evaluation of the layer reveals squamous metaplasia, but it is usually referred to simply as metaplasia (Fig. 13.3). Metaplasia outside of the trigone warrants biopsy and pathologic evaluation.

The trigone is triangular, with the inferior apex directed toward the urethrovesical junction and the ureteral orifices forming the superior apices. As the cystoscope is advanced past the urethrovesical junction, the trigone is apparent at the bottom of the field. The interureteric ridge is a visible elevation that forms the superior boundary of the trigone and runs between the ureteral orifices. The intramural portion of the ureters can often be seen as they course from the lateral aspect of the bladder toward the trigone and ureteral orifices. There is marked variation in the ureteral orifices, but they are generally circular or slit-like openings at the apex of a small mound. With efflux of urine, the slit opens and the mound retracts in the direction of the intramural ureter.

When distended, the bladder is roughly spherical, but numerous folds of mucosa are evident in the empty or partially filled bladder. The uterus and cervix can usually be seen indenting the posterior wall of the bladder, which creates posterolateral pouches where the bladder drapes over the uterus into the paravaginal spaces. At times, visualiza-

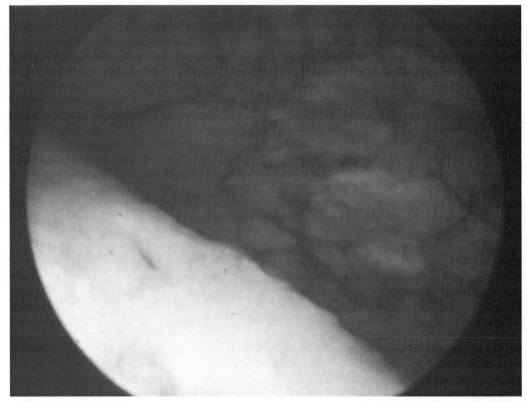

Figure 13.3. Trigonal metaplasia.

tion of the bowel peristalsis is possible through the vesical wall.

PATHOLOGICAL CYSTOSCOPIC FINDINGS

Pathology affecting the bladder can be categorized as mucosal lesions or structural variations. Mucosal lesions are either inflammatory or neoplastic, although coexistence of the two types is not uncommon.

Despite common use of the term to describe infection of the bladder, cystitis in its broadest definition refers to inflammation of the bladder mucosa, of which there are several varieties. Cystoscopy should not be performed in the presence of active infectious cystitis, but if it is done inadvertently it may provide variable findings. In its mildest form, bacterial cystitis can be rather inconspicuous, manifesting little more than pink or peach-colored macules or papules. With increasing severity, mucosal edema and hypervascularity are evident with the loss of the submucosal vascular pattern and marked vascular dilation. In hemorrhagic cystitis,

this can progress to individual or confluent mucosal hemorrhages and may be associated with hematuria in addition to irritative voiding symptoms.

The symptoms of hematuria and irritative voiding are typical to several other less common inflammatory conditions, which can often be distinguished by cystoscopy. The hemorrhagic cystitis that follows bladder infusion with toxins such as cyclophosphamide is characterized by diffuse mucosal hemorrhage. In radiation cystitis, areas of hemorrhage are surrounded by pale mucosa, which may be fibrotic and hypovascular. An indwelling urethral or suprapubic catheter produces an inflammatory reaction of the mucosa that is directly in contact with the catheter. This reaction can range from pseudopapillary edema and submucosal hemorrhages to vesical fibrosis.

Interstitial cystitis, another form of chronic inflammation, is often associated with hematuria and fibrosis. Although interstitial cystitis may be suspected in patients with frequency and urgency, cystoscopy with biopsy is essential to its accurate diagnosis. The pathognomonic lesions appear on refilling the bladder, after initially filling to maximum cystometric capacity. General anesthesia is usually required to fill to maximum cystometric capacity, because the associated fibrosis often makes filling intolerable. Glomerulations are the primary finding in very mild cases. These petechial hemorrhages are small red dots, which may coalesce to form larger hemorrhagic areas. Petechiae are sometimes seen in normal patients, especially on the posterior wall and trigone due to cystoscope trauma. In contrast, patients with interstitial cystitis will have at least 10–20 glomerulations per field of vision. The classic Hunner ulcer is seen in more severe cases of interstitial cystitis. These appear as velvety red patches or linear cracks with a granulating base and surrounding vascular congestion.

Recurrent or chronic inflammation can produce characteristic lesions as well. Inflammatory polyps are often identified at the urethrovesical junction if the cystoscope is retracted into the proximal urethra and the infusion is interrupted to allow them to float into the field of view. They are usually translucent with a villous appearance but can become large enough to partially fill the urethral lumen. Cystitis cystica consists of clear mucosal cysts, which are usually found on the bladder base and are often found in multiples. The cysts are formed by single layers of subepithelial transitional cells, which degenerate with central liquefaction. Cystitis glandularis has an appearance similar to cystitis cystica, but the cysts are not clear and have a less uniform contour. As in cystitis glandularis, the mechanism of formation is a glandular metaplasia. In cystitis glandularis, however, there is involvement of multiple layers, including the mucus-producing glandular epithelium. Both lesions are associated with chronic irritation of the bladder mucosa and are commonly surrounded by marked inflammation. The frequent association of cystitis glandularis with adenovillous carcinoma of the bladder has led to the belief that cystitis glandularis may be a precursor of adenocarcinoma (28). A proposed metaplastic transformation from epithelial hyperplasia through cystitis glandularis and finally to adenocarcinoma is based on a case presented by Shaw et al. (29)

of a gradual transition of cystitis glandularis to adenocarcinoma over a 5-year period. There have been two subsequent reports of transformation of cystitis glandularis to adenocarcinoma (30, 31).

Although it is twice as common in men, bladder cancer is the most common genitourinary neoplasm in women. Most cases occur past the fifth decade. Transitional cell carcinoma is the most common histological type, followed by adenocarcinoma and squamous cell carcinoma. Transitional cell carcinoma is usually carcinogen induced. Tobacco, dyes, and organic chemicals are known carcinogens for the transitional epithelium. Adenocarcinoma is relatively more common with bladder exstrophy. Squamous cell carcinoma has been reported with chronic indwelling catheters. Cystoscopic appearance is variable depending on histological type and grade, but it usually reveals a raised lesion with a villous feathery or papillary appearance. Circumferential inflammation is ubiquitous. Superficial transitional cell carcinoma may be multicentric or may have associated carcinoma in situ. Carcinoma in situ can be disturbingly inconspicuous, often mimicking the macules or plaques of infectious cystitis.

Vesical and ureteral structural variations may be anatomic or functional anomalies. Auxiliary ureteral orifices are examples of rare anatomic anomalies, which are indicative of renal collecting anomalies. When present, they often enter the vesical wall slightly superior to the trigone in near proximity to the other ureteral orifice. Ureteroceles are caused by laxity of the distal ureteral lumen with herniation into the vesical cavity during efflux (Fig. 13.4).

Trabeculations are considerably more common than auxiliary ureteral orifices or ureteroceles. These smooth ridges become evident with distention of the bladder to volumes approaching maximum cystometric capacity. They appear as interlaced cords of different diameters with intervening sacculations (Fig. 13.5). They represent hypertrophied detrusor musculature associated with detrusor instability and functional or anatomic bladder obstruction. A bladder diverticulum can occur when high intravesical pressure produces an enlargement of the intervening sacculations. The thick muscular band that creates the neck varies in diameter and gives way to an outpouching of bladder mucosa. The interior of the diverticulum has been reported as the site of neoplasm in approximately 7% of cases (32).

Fistulas may also be encountered at cystoscopy. Although approximately 75% of vesicovaginal fistulas result from abdominal hysterectomies, they may also occur after vaginal hysterectomies, urological procedures, radiation exposure, presence of foreign bodies, cancer, and obstetrical trauma (33). Posthysterectomy fistulas are usually located in the bladder base superior to the interureteric ridge, corresponding to the level of the vaginal cuff (34). The fistulous openings range from small to several centimeters in diameter. In the immediate postoperative state, the surrounding mucosa is edematous and hyperemic, whereas in later stages the mucosa has a typical smooth appearance. In contrast, vesicoenteric fistulas uniformly have a sur-

rounding inflammatory reaction often with bulbous edema, and the fistulous tract is not discernible in two thirds of cases (35).

Bladder calculi may result from urinary stasis or the presence of a foreign body, or an inflammatory exudate may coalesce and serve as a nidus for stone formation. Stones have extremely variable cystoscopic appearance in terms of color, size, and shape but generally have an irregular surface. Foreign bodies and stones are usually accompanied by varying degrees of general or localized inflammatory reaction.

Summary

With the technological advances of the last century, cystoscopes have evolved into high-resolution instruments that permit excellent visualization of the entire lower urinary tract.

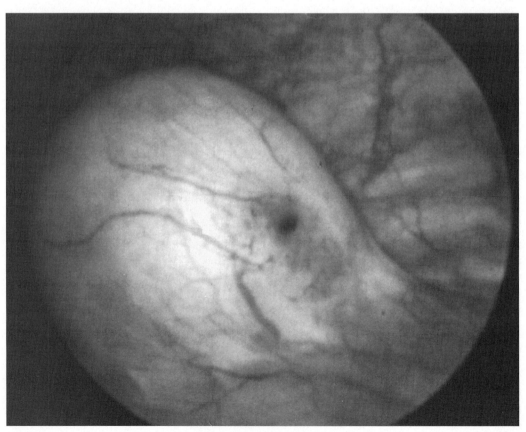

Figure 13.4. Ureterocele.

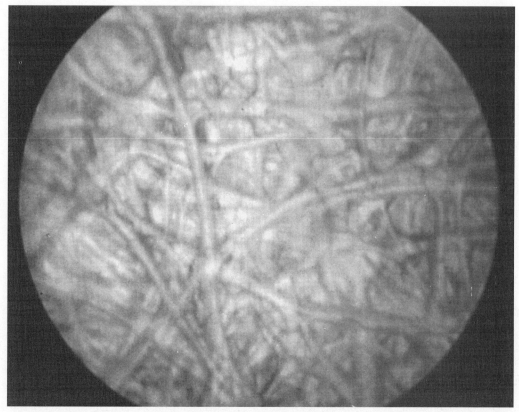

Figure 13.5. Trabeculations.

The instrumentation is available with many modifications that increase the applications of the technique. Within urogynecology, cystoscopy is valuable for diagnosing anatomic lesions of the lower urinary tract that are commonly overlooked by other diagnostic modalities. Cystoscopy is also valuable to assess ureteral function and vesical integrity during pelvic surgery. The simplicity of the techniques and breadth of applications make it invaluable to the pelvic surgeon.

REFERENCES

1. Bozzini P. Lichteiter, eine erfindung zur anschung innerer theile, und krukheiten nebst abbildung. J Pract Arzeykunde 1805;24:107.
2. Desmormeaux AJ. Transactions of the Socíeté Chirurgie, Paris. Gazette des Hop, 1865.
3. Grünfeld I. Der harnröhrenspiegel (das endoscop), seine diagnostische und therapeutische anwendung. Vienna: Deutsch Chirugie, 1881.
4. Nitze M. Eine neue balbachtungs-und untersuchunigsmethods fur harnrohre, harnbiase und rectum. Wien Med Wochenschr 1879;24:649.
5. Kelly HA. The direct examination of the female bladder with elevated pelvis—the catheterization of the ureters under direct inspection, with and without elevation of the pelvis. Am J Obstet Dis Wom Child 1894;25:1–19.
6. Hopkins HH, Kopany NS. A flexible fiberscope, using static scanning. Nature 1954;179:39–41.
7. Robertson JR. Air cystoscopy. Obstet Gynecol 1968;32:328–330.
8. Tushida S, Sugawara H. A new flexible fibercystoscope for visualization of the bladder neck. J Urol 1970;91:830–831.
9. Kavoussi LR, Clayman RV. Office flexible cystoscopy. Urol Clin North Am 1988;15:601–608.
10. Figueroa TE, Thomas R, Moon TD. Taking the pain out of cystoscopy: a comparison of rigid with flexible instruments. J Louisiana St Med Soc 1987;139:26–28.
11. Clayman RV, Reddy P, Lange PH. Flexible fiber optic and rigid-rod lens endoscopy of the lower urinary tract: a prospective controlled comparison. J Urol 1984;131:715–716.
12. Sand PK, Hill RC, Ostergard DR. Supine urethroscopic and standing cystometry as screening methods for detection of detrusor instability. Obstet Gynecol 1987;70:57–60.
13. Scotti RJ, Ostergard DR, Guillaume AA, Kohatsu KE. Predictive value of urethroscopy as com-

pared to urodynamics in the diagnosis of genuine stress incontinence. J Reprod Med 1990;35: 772–776.

14. Cundiff GW, Bent AE. The contribution of urethrocystoscopy added to urodynamics in the evaluation of lower urinary tract dysfunction in women. Am J Obstet Gynecol (in press).

15. Versi E, Cardoza LD, Studd JWW, Brincat M, O'Dowd TM, Cooper DJ. Internal urinary sphincter in maintenance of female continence. Br Med J 1986;292:166–167.

16. McGuire EJ, Fitzpatrick CC, Wan J, Bloom D, Sanaordenker J, Ritchey M, Gormley EA. Clinical assessment of urethral sphincter function. J Urol 1993;150:1452–1454.

17. Sand PK, Bowen LW, Panganiban R, Ostergard DR. The low pressure urethra as a factor in failed retropubic urethropexy. Obstet Gynecol 1987;69: 399–402.

18. Decter RM, Harpster L. Pitfalls in determination of leak point pressure. J Urol 1992;148:588–591.

19. Richardson DA, Ramahi A, Chalas E. Surgical management of stress incontinence in patients with low urethral pressure. Gynecol Obstet Invest 1991;31:106–109.

20. Manson AL. Is antibiotic prophylaxis indicated after outpatient cystoscopy? J Urol 1988;140: 316–317.

21. Richards B, Bastable JRG. Bacteriuria after outpatient cystoscopy. Br J Urol 1977;49:561–564.

22. Hares MM. A double-blinded trial of half-strength Polybactrin soluble GU bladder irrigation in cystoscopy. Br J Urol 1981;53:62–67.

23. Ostergard DR. Bladder pillar block anesthesia for urethral dilation in women. Am J Obstet Gynecol 1980;136:187–188.

24. Cundiff G, Bent AE. Suprapubic catheterization complicated by bowel injury. Int J Urogynecol 1995;6:110–113.

25. Stamey TA. Endoscopic suspension of the vesical neck for urinary incontinence. Surg Gynecol Obstet 1973;6:547–554.

26. Freda VC, Tacchi D. Ureteral injury discovered after pelvic surgery. Am J Obstet Gynecol 1962; 85:406–409.

27. Timmons MC, Addison WA. Suprapubic teloscopy: extraperitoneal intraoperative technique to demonstrate ureteral patency. Obstet Gynecol 1990;75:137–139.

28. Daroca PJ, McKenzie F, Reed RJ, Keane JM. Primary adenovillous carcinoma of the bladder. J Urol 1976;115:41–45.

29. Shaw JL, Gislason GJ, Imbriglia JE. Transition of cystitis glandularis to primary adenocarcinoma of the bladder. J Urol 1958;79:815.

30. Edwards PD, Hurm RA, Jaeesehke WH. Conversion of cystitis glandularis to adenocarcinoma. J Urol 1972;108:568–570.

31. Susmano D, Rubenstein AB, Dakin AR, Loyd FA. Cystitis glandularis and adenocarcinoma of the bladder. J Urol 1971;105:671–674.

32. Kelalis PP, McLean P. The treatment of diverticulum of the bladder. J Urol 1967;98:349–352.

33. Lee RA, Symmonds RE, Williams TJ. Current status of genitourinary fistula. Obstet Gynecol 1988;72:313–319.

34. Jonas U, Petri E. Genitourinary fistulas. In: Stanton SL, ed. Clinical gynecologic urology. St Louis: CV Mosby, 1984:238.

35. Farringer JL, Hrabovsky E, Marsh J, Virajslip P, Pickens DR. Vesicocolic fistula. South Med J 1974;67:1043–1046.

CHAPTER 14

Ambulatory Urodynamic Monitoring

Vik Khullar and Linda Cardozo

Introduction

Laboratory urodynamics is unphysiological and is carried out over a short period of time. The urinary symptoms and the test result may not concur; thus, women with troublesome urinary symptoms may not have an abnormality diagnosed on conventional urodynamic assessment. Ambulatory urodynamics was developed to measure lower urinary tract function under more physiological conditions and improve the sensitivity and accuracy of the urodynamic diagnosis. During laboratory urodynamics, the woman does not void during bladder filling, and this may lead to cortical suppression of abnormal detrusor activity. Ambulatory urodynamics facilitates the observation of bladder function under more "normal" conditions and for longer periods of time and leads to a better understanding of bladder pathophysiology. Increased mobility is facilitated by using either telemetry, long cables, or portable recording units.

Development

Initial attempts involved the use of a pressure-sensitive radio pill (1) in which pressure information was transmitted by telemetry from within the bladder. This method allowed the measurement of intravesical pressure without a foreign body within the urethra, but the cost of the radio pill, the limited range of transmission (30 cm), and occasional difficulty in retrieval

prevented its wider use. The use of fluid-filled lines for ambulatory urodynamics is not recommended because they are prone to movement artefact and the pressures measured are dependent on the relative position of the pressure transducer to the tip of the fluid-filled line, altering the baseline measurement as the woman changes posture. Despite these problems, Tsuji et al. (2) used natural filling and described increased detrusor phasic activity in spinal injury patients.

James (3) described air probes in which a small diameter air-filled tube was inserted into the bladder. The end of the tube was sealed by a meniscus of urine. Air is not prone to movement artifacts, but if fluid traveled down the tube, then artefacts associated with fluid-filled lines appeared. This problem was prevented by covering the tube end with a compliant balloon. The position of the catheter relative to the transducer is unimportant, but changes occur with temperature that can cause drift in the pressure measured. These catheters are also difficult to calibrate.

Initially radio telemetry (4, 5) was used, but at distances greater than 50 m, interference was marked. Thuroff et al. (6) used telemetry to perform urodynamic measurements, allowing the patient to void and exercise without disturbance under closed-circuit television. This method was thorough but prohibitively expensive and time consuming. Thus, a tape-recording system (7) using the analog output of microtip pressure transducers was developed. Because the recorders had a limited capacity, pressures

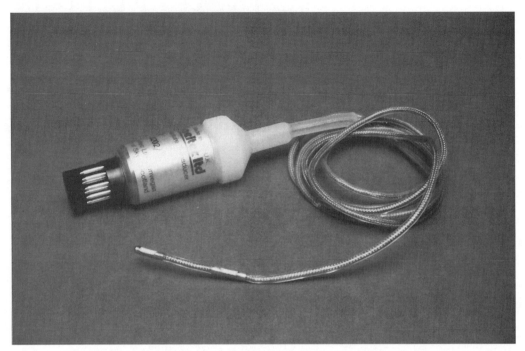

Figure 14.1. Microtip transducer (Gaeltec Dunevegan, Isle of Skye, Scotland). Note the recessed transducer sensing plate.

were only recorded if they went above a threshold value. Unfortunately, if a patient was symptomatic during the test but without recorded pressure at the time, this left a diagnostic quandary about interpretation; also the level of the threshold was difficult to set.

Griffiths et al. (8) developed an ambulatory system that used microtip pressure transducers with a recorder using a digital solid-state memory. This meant that pressures would be recorded digitally and then transferred and reviewed at the end of the test, allowing the trace to be expanded or compressed easily without loss of information.

Equipment

Ambulatory systems have three main components: transducers, recording unit (including patient markers), and the analyzing system. Solid-state transducers (Fig. 14.1) measure the pressure impinging on them and are less likely to have movement artefact. There are problems of drift during the test,

but in most systems this is less than 3 cm H_2O over 5 hours (9). As most transducers have the pressure-sensitive membrane inset a few millimeters from the catheter exterior, artefactual pressure rises may be recorded by the intravesical transducer touching the bladder wall. To detect this, we routinely insert two pressure transducers within the bladder. An intravesical pressure change is only considered significant if it is recorded on both intravesical transducers.

The recording system (Fig. 14.2) should be portable and, ideally, battery powered. Sampling rate of the pressures should be greater than 4 Hz, and the memory should be digital, which enables the trace to be compressed. Some recorders only register pressures if the detrusor pressure is above a threshold value (10) that produces the problems already outlined, so they are not recommended.

The patient's own symptoms are important in the interpretation of the trace, and therefore a diary should be used to record them. The recording system should have a method of marking events onto the trace. This allows accurate interpretation of traces in conjunction with the diary. The diary used in our unit

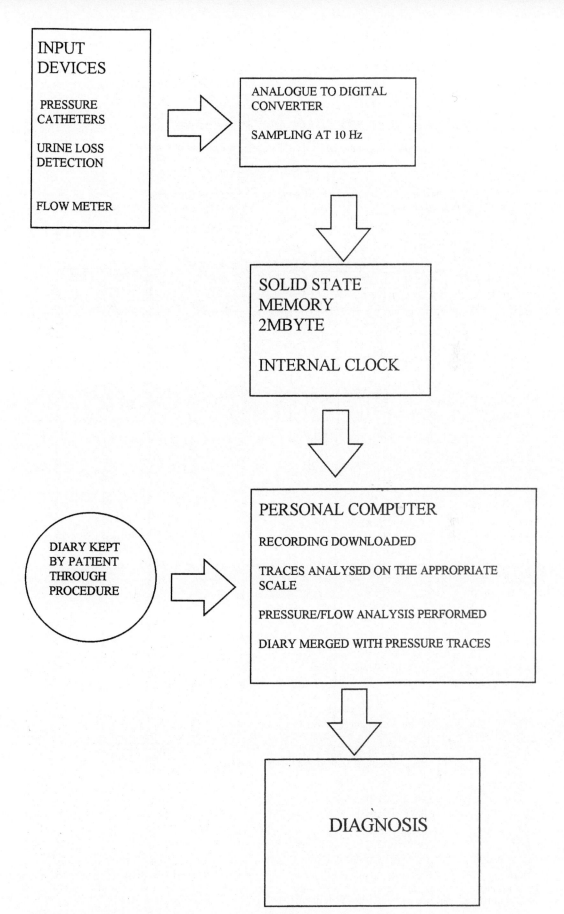

Figure 14.2. Diagrammatic representation of an ambulatory urodynamic system and reviewing system.

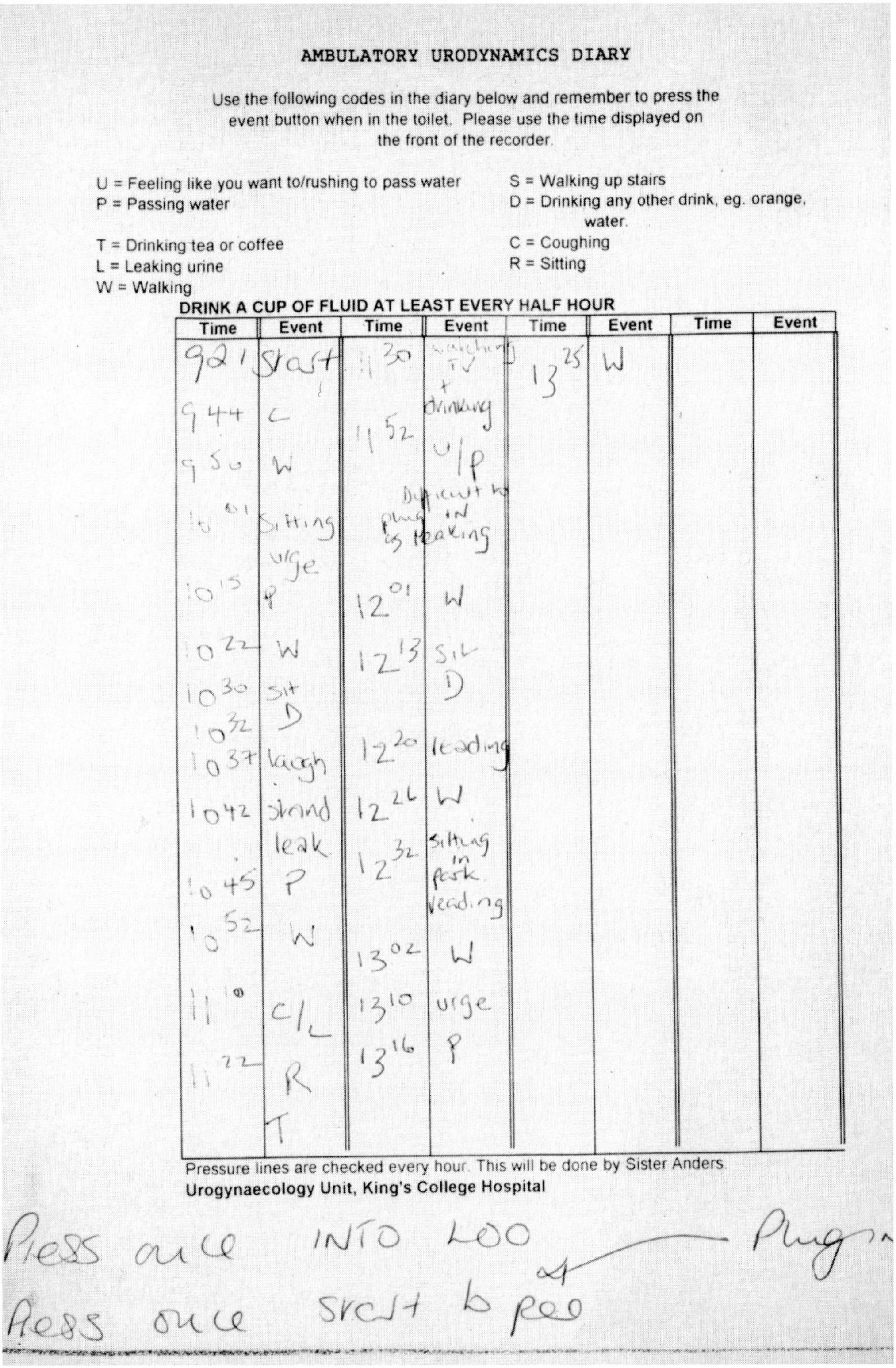

AMBULATORY URODYNAMICS DIARY

Use the following codes in the diary below and remember to press the event button when in the toilet. Please use the time displayed on the front of the recorder.

U = Feeling like you want to/rushing to pass water
P = Passing water
T = Drinking tea or coffee
L = Leaking urine
W = Walking
S = Walking up stairs
D = Drinking any other drink, eg. orange, water.
C = Coughing
R = Sitting

DRINK A CUP OF FLUID AT LEAST EVERY HALF HOUR

Time	Event	Time	Event	Time	Event	Time	Event
921	Start	11 30	watching TV + drinking	13 25	W		
944	C	11 52	U/P				
950	W		Difficult to plug in as leaking				
10 01	Sitting urge	12 01	W				
10 15	P	12 13	Sit D				
10 22	W	12 20	leading				
10 30	sit	12 26	W				
10 32	D	12 32	Sitting in park reading				
10 37	laugh	13 02	W				
10 42	stand leak	13 10	urge				
10 45	P	13 16	P				
10 52	W						
11 10	C/L						
11 22	R T						

Pressure lines are checked every hour. This will be done by Sister Anders.
Urogynaecology Unit, King's College Hospital

Press once INTO LOO —— Plug in
Press once start to pee

Figure 14.3. Ambulatory urodynamic diary filled in by a woman. The commonly used comments have been abbreviated. The diary can also have comments not listed at the top of the diary written in. The timing must relate to the ambulatory unit's internal clock.

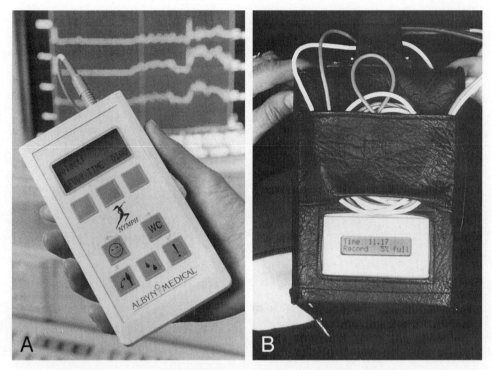

Figure 14.4.   Multiple marker button (**A**) and single button (**B**) ambulatory system (Albyn Medical and Gaeltec systems).

is shown (Fig. 14.3). Many systems have multiple marker buttons on the recorder (Fig. 14.4). Because some patients have difficulty pressing two buttons correctly, the use of multiple buttons may be more confusing for the woman and the physician. If the wrong button is pressed, this does not allow easy interpretation of the trace without the diary. For the diary to be meaningful, times should also be noted. The recorder itself may display the time (Fig. 14.5), or the woman's own watch can be synchronized with the recorder. The recorder should have the option to connect an electronic nappy; this is important to gain information on urine loss. The recorder used in our unit connects to a gravimetric flowmeter (Fig. 14.6). This is useful in calculating pressure/flow curves and checking when detrusor instability has occurred in relation to voiding. Often detrusor instability is seen before a patient voids.

The pressure traces are downloaded onto a computer in various formats. It is important that diary events are displayed once entered with the pressure recordings and that in analyzing the recording, the appropriate

scales are chosen for pressure measurement and time (Fig. 14.7). The trace must be interpreted with the patient present to obtain information not written in the diary at the crucial event on the trace and to obtain further details from the patient while her memory is still fresh.

To evaluate incontinence, it is essential to detect urine loss during the urodynamic test. This allows the interpretation of the pressure changes leading to the urinary loss and is the only method by which urinary incontinence without an increase of intravesical pressure can be detected. This phenomenon is presumably due to urethral relaxation. Using a weighed perineal pad for the length of the test gives an indication of the severity of the incontinence; however, this method does not indicate when the loss occurred. The timing and quantification of urinary loss and pressure change in the bladder are helpful in determining the cause of urinary leakage. Three methods have been described. First, the Urilos (Exeter) electronic nappy (11) uses elongated electrodes arranged in an interleaved fashion embedded in an absorbent

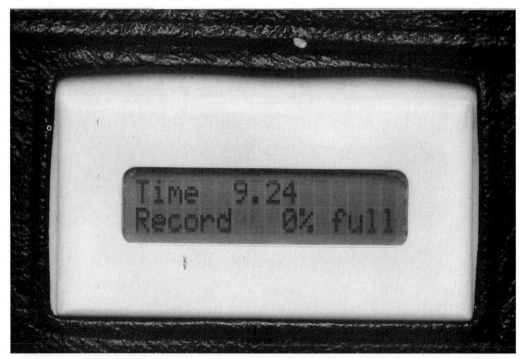

Figure 14.5. Clock on the ambulatory recording unit (MPR2) (Gaeltec).

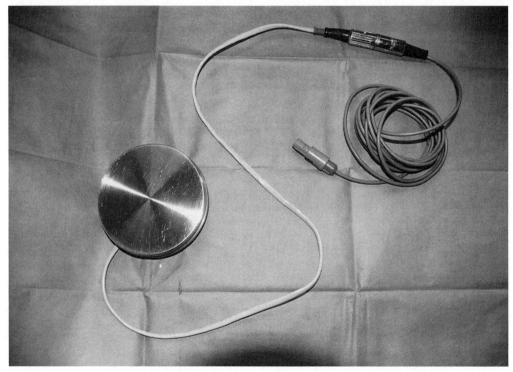

Figure 14.6. Gravimetric flowmeter used with ambulatory urodynamics.

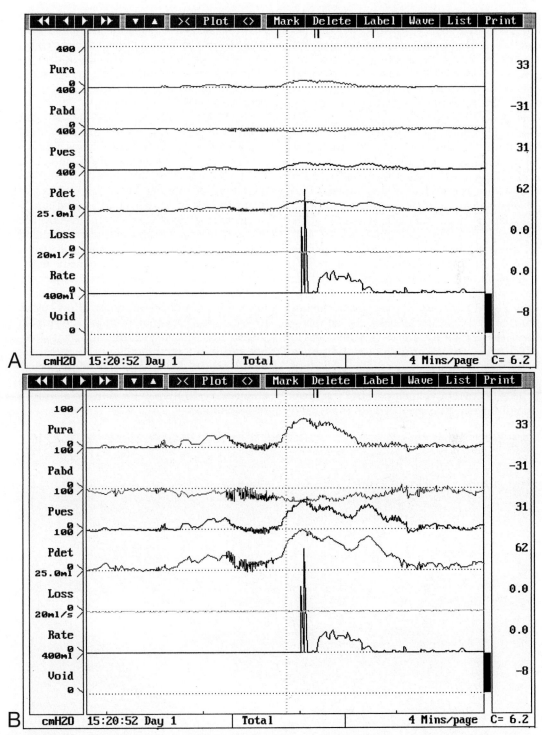

Figure 14.7. **A.** Y axis scale too large to allow meaningful examination of the ambulatory urodynamic trace. **B.** Same trace as **A** appropriately scaled to show the detrusor contraction that could not be seen on the first trace.

material (Fig. 14.8). A low-voltage (50 mV) alternating current is passed between the two electrodes. The current crossing between the electrodes increases as the urine loss increases. Unfortunately, this method depends on the electrolytes within the urine. Because this is not constant, the pad has to be preloaded with a measured volume of a known electrolyte solution. This method is useful for volumes between 1 and 100 mL and is reproducible within 20%. The nappy is bulky but can be cut into a smaller size for ambulatory use and has been found to be adequate in detecting incontinence during ambulatory urodynamic tests (12). This method is quantitative, but losses less than 1 mL may not be detected. Once the pad is soaked, it does not register further loss.

An alternative method has been to measure the perineal temperature. The temperature of urine (37° C) is warmer than the perineum (30–34° C). When urine leaks, the temperature rises transiently. The detection of loss is effective because the urine cools rapidly once it has leaked, allowing detection of further leakage. Using a single temperature detector is not effective in women because the position of the detector in relation to the leaked urine changes; thus, a parallel array of diodes has been used with a separate reference diode (13). The rate of rise in temperature correlates well with the quantity of leaked urine. Problems of interpretation may occur if the patient has her legs together while sitting, as the perineal temperature may rise.

The third technique uses the catheter within the urethra. Distal urethral electrical conductivity can be used to detect urinary leakage (14, 15). Two electrodes are mounted on a catheter, and an electric current is passed between them. Leakage or voiding of urine causes increased conductance and a larger current passes across the electrodes. The positioning of the electrodes is crucial; in the proximal urethra, changes in electrical current indicates the presence of urine in the proximal urethra but not necessarily urinary leakage. This can occur with urethral instability where urethral relaxation allows urine to enter the proximal urethra, interpreted incorrectly as leakage. If the electrodes were not within the urethra, then urinary leakage would not be detected. Distal urethral electrical conductance is not used clinically in ambulatory urodynamics and is mainly a research tool.

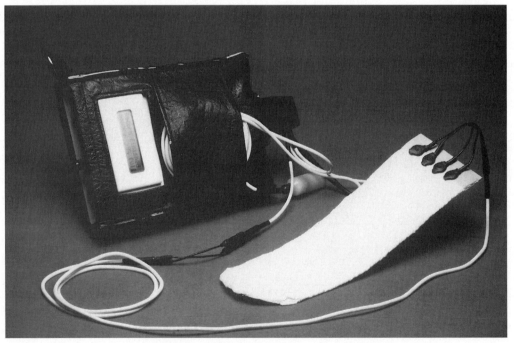

Figure 14.8. Urilos (Exeter) nappy modified for use with an ambulatory system (Lectromed, Ltd., Welwyn Garden City, England).

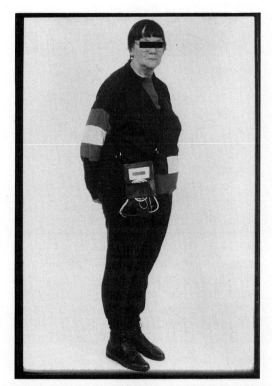

Figure 14.9. Appropriately dressed with ambulatory urodynamic equipment.

Ambulatory Urodynamics Method

At present, the regimen we use is as follows:

1. The urine should be infection free on urinalysis.
2. The woman is requested to wear clothing with a separate top and bottom before the test (Fig. 14.9).
3. If she wishes to evacuate bowels, she should do this before the pressure transducers are inserted.
4. A urethral silastic covered catheter 6F with two pressure transducers (Gaeltec) is inserted with *both* transducers within the bladder. The rectal transducer is on a 6-cm silicone rubber cylinder 7 mm in diameter (Fig. 14.10) covered with a condom. This allows for comfortable insertion and better retention. Both catheters are strapped firmly with plenty of wide tape to the skin close to the site of inser-

tion. This determines how often the lines will need to be resited (Fig. 14.11). The lines are then looped up and fixed onto the abdomen.
5. The woman is asked to void and the lines are rechecked.
6. She is requested to drink 180 mL every hour based on a total daily fluid intake of 2 L/d. Those women who do not drink this amount of fluid during the test often have normal urodynamic tests where no abnormality is detected.
7. When she wishes to void, she must press the event marker button *before* entering the room to void on the flowmeter. Where a urodynamic system does not have a flowmeter, the event marker should be pushed at the initiation of the void.
8. Any other events are noted in the diary (Fig. 14.3) and the event marker is also depressed.
9. After each void, the lines are checked for their position and, if necessary, replaced.
10. Provocative maneuvers are carried out with a "full" bladder for the last half hour of the test. These are listed in Table 14.1.
11. The trace and diary are analyzed with the woman present.

The test length is usually 4 hours. Close supervision is important because patient compliance is essential for a successful test. The diagnosis of detrusor instability is made when the symptom of urgency coincides with a detrusor pressure rise (Fig. 14.12). It is important that this symptom is usually felt by the woman under "normal" circumstances; otherwise, the symptom during the test may be due to the presence of catheters. Prophylactic antibiotics are used in women with a high risk of urinary tract infection such as diabetics, those suffering recurrent urinary tract infections and voiding difficulties, and those with bladder lines repeatedly replaced.

Clinical Applications

At present, in our unit the following groups of women undergo ambulatory urodynamics, a test we found to be useful:

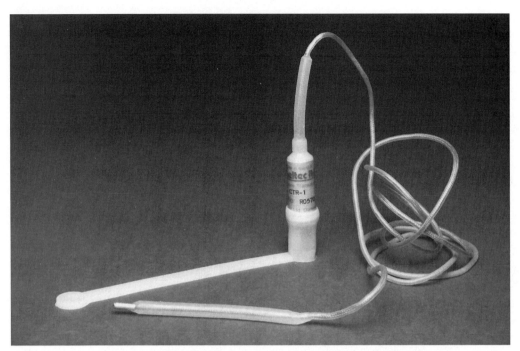

Figure 14.10. Rectal pressure catheter.

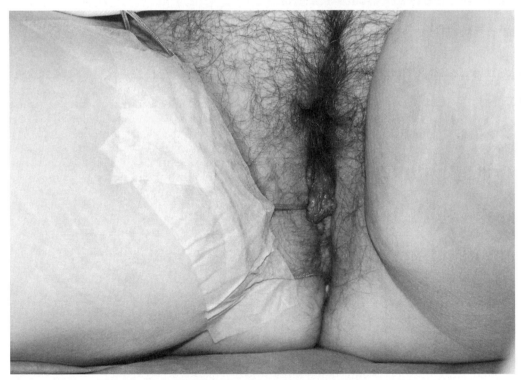

Figure 14.11. Urethral and rectal pressure lines taped into position.

1. No abnormality detected during laboratory urodynamics in symptomatic women;
2. Genuine stress incontinence diagnosed on laboratory urodynamics without complaint of stress incontinence as a symptom;
3. Clarifying the balance between detrusor instability and urethral sphincter incontinence of women with mixed urinary incontinence;
4. Women with voiding difficulties who are unable to void with pressure lines during laboratory urodynamics. Ambulatory urodynamics allows pressure flow studies to be carried out, thus determining the cause of voiding difficulties;

Table 14.1. Provocative Maneuvers Carried Out During the Ambulatory Test

Coughing 10 times
Ten star jumps
Listening to running water
Anything that causes urinary incontinence

5. Women with sensory urgency on laboratory urodynamics but normal cystourethroscopy and bladder histology;
6. Women with suprapubic pain after voiding. This has been found to be detrusor contractions once the bladder is empty (Fig. 14.13) and can be treated as detrusor instability, but cystourethroscopy and bladder biopsy are required.

Clinical Studies

UNEXPLAINED URINARY INCONTINENCE

One hundred symptomatic patients (86 male and 14 female) (16) who underwent standard urodynamic investigations and had a urodynamic result that did not correlate with symptoms or who had previous failed incontinence surgery underwent ambulatory urodynamics. The results were compared with their symptoms and the laboratory urodynamic results. Ambulatory urodynamics diagnosed detrusor instability twice as fre-

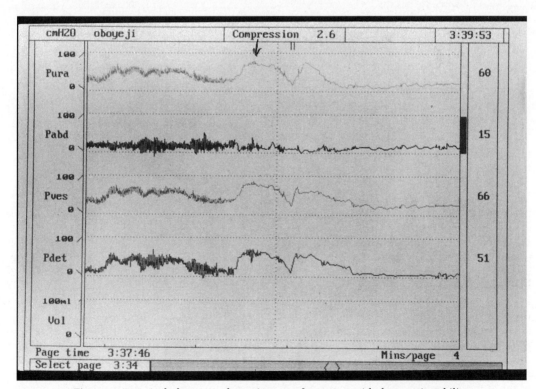

Figure 14.12. Ambulatory urodynamic trace of a woman with detrusor instability. Detrusor contraction marked by an *arrow*.

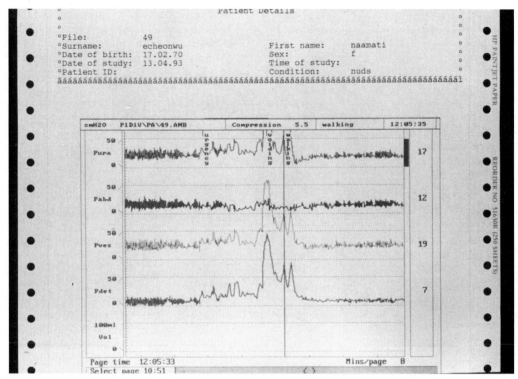

Figure 14.13. Ambulatory urodynamic trace of a woman with pain after voiding. There are large detrusor pressure rises even though the bladder is empty.

quently as laboratory urodynamics. Interestingly, 32 patients were diagnosed as normal on laboratory urodynamics, but on ambulatory testing only 5 patients were considered normal. This result rather begs the question of what is normal. The test could be either very sensitive or, alternatively, have a high false-positive rate for diagnosing detrusor instability. Ambulatory urodynamics only diagnosed eight patients as having urethral sphincter incompetence compared with 13 patients with laboratory urodynamics. Webb et al. (12) studied 52 patients who underwent laboratory urodynamics and then ambulatory urodynamics. Laboratory urodynamics did not provide a diagnosis that correlated well with the patients' symptoms. Detrusor instability was found on ambulatory monitoring in 31 patients whose bladders had not been unstable during laboratory urodynamics, and 11 of these patients were found to have detrusor instability on provocation only, emphasizing the importance of this part of the ambulatory test. Urinary incontinence was detected using the Urilos nappy in 23 women, 13 of whom had detrusor instability and 3 women who had coexisting urethral sphincter incompetence. In this study, detrusor instability and urinary incontinence were detected more frequently on ambulatory monitoring than with laboratory urodynamics.

NORMAL VOLUNTEERS

Ambulatory urodynamics performed on 36 female volunteers (17) without lower urinary tract symptoms found 25 to have "detrusor instability." Unfortunately, only 17 women also underwent standard cystometry and 3 had detrusor instability. In both the above studies, the women were asked to drink more than normal, some drinking up to 530 mL/h. This alters the rate of orthograde bladder filling and changes the behavior of the detrusor muscle. The urinary symptoms the volunteers felt during the ambulatory urodynamic test are not felt during their normal daily activities and thus would be discounted as artefact when analyzed in our unit. The authors suggested the use of the detrusor activity index to determine "normal" limits of bladder activity. This incorporates the number of contractions per hour multiplied by 10 added to the mean amplitude and mean duration of uninhibited detrusor contractions. Unfortunately, this index does not take into account leakage or voiding associated with detrusor instability, which may curtail the pressure rise during the detrusor contraction. "Normal" bladder function in women without urinary symptoms needs to be properly established.

LOW COMPLIANCE AND DETRUSOR INSTABILITY

During laboratory urodynamics, in the filling phase, a tonic detrusor pressure rise (low compliance) may be seen. There are questions about the significance of this finding.

Some authorities assert that the pressure rise is a passive phenomenon related to the reduced elasticity of the bladder wall. In this case the pressure rise should not decrease at the end of filling. The other theory is that the increase in pressure is associated with a tonic detrusor contraction. If this is the case at the end of filling, the detrusor pressure should decay exponentially as the contracting detrusor relaxes. Webb et al. (9) studied patients with neuropathic bladders who developed a detrusor pressure rise greater than 25 cm H_2O at a filling rate of 100 mL/min. When these patients had cystometry at faster filling rates, there was a greater tonic detrusor pressure rise (Fig. 14.14). During the ambulatory test, there was a much smaller detrusor pressure rise on orthograde filling, but the frequency of phasic detrusor instability during the test correlated with the size of the pressure rise during the conventional cystometry. The greater number of phasic detrusor contrac-

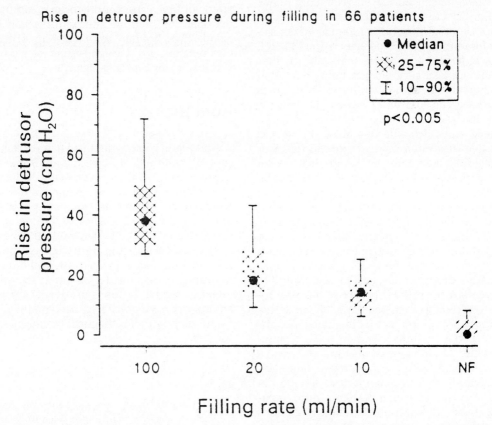

Figure 14.14. Plot showing pressure rise during artificial filling rates of 100, 20, and 10 mL/min and during natural filling. (From Prof. D.E. Neale, Department of Surgery, University of Newcastle, U.K.)

tions during ambulatory monitoring did correlate with dilated upper renal tracts. Unfortunately, the low compliance on filling during laboratory urodynamics did not correlate with the development of upper tract dilatation. Phasic detrusor contractions during ambulatory urodynamics quantified as the area under the detrusor pressure curve 20 minutes before voiding has been found to correlate with upper tract dilatation (18). Ambulatory urodynamic studies have also been used to investigate detrusor activity after "clam" ileocystoplasty (19), showing reduced pressure rises with detrusor instability after the procedure.

Predicting Failure in Women After Continence Surgery

Detrusor instability has to be distinguished from genuine stress incontinence before selecting a woman for continence surgery. Detrusor instability is a major risk factor for failure after colposuspension (20, 21). The appearance of detrusor instability after continence surgery despite being excluded preoperatively with laboratory urodynamics is also associated with failure (22, 23). No specific cause has been found but may be either a result of the operation due to excessive dissection or undiagnosed detrusor instability before surgery. Ambulatory urodynamics is more sensitive at detecting detrusor instability, but can it predict the development of detrusor instability after surgery? We studied 35 women, all of whom were diagnosed as having moderate to severe genuine stress incontinence on laboratory urodynamics (24). All underwent ambulatory urodynamics, and 11 were found to have detrusor instability. Six weeks postoperatively, six women developed the irritative symptoms of urgency and urge incontinence, but all other women were asymptomatic. Nine months postoperatively, 13 women had irritative symptoms. These included all women diagnosed as having detrusor instability on ambulatory urodynamics. On videocystourethrography, after 9 months seven women were diagnosed as having detrusor instability; these were all

women diagnosed as having detrusor instability on ambulatory urodynamics preoperatively. The use of the detrusor activity index (17) or the area under the detrusor curve for 20 minutes before voiding (18) may enable more accurate identification of those women who will develop detrusor instability postoperatively.

Urogynecological Practice

In our unit, 278 women were investigated with "normal urodynamics"(25). Sixty-five percent (180) of these women were found to have detrusor instability on ambulatory urodynamics. Neither the urinary symptoms nor the laboratory urodynamic results predicted detrusor instability on ambulatory urodynamics other than the isometric detrusor pressure generated on interrupting micturition being greater than 50 cmH$_2$O. Three women who complained of suprapubic pain after voiding were found to have multiple detrusor contractions after voiding had finished. Five women with voiding difficulties had successful diagnostic pressure/flow studies during ambulatory tests.

Conclusions

Ambulatory urodynamics is an extremely sensitive method of detecting abnormal detrusor activity and can give useful information where laboratory urodynamics has not. Ambulatory urodynamics enables greater understanding of detrusor instability and its relationship with patient symptoms. The detection of detrusor instability in asymptomatic women leads to questions about the relevance of the results obtained in symptomatic women. If this is resolved, then ambulatory urodynamics may become the most useful technique for diagnosing detrusor instability.

REFERENCES

1. Warrell DW, Watson BW, Shelley T. Intravesical pressure measurements in women during movement using a radio-pill and an air-probe. J Obstet Gynaecol Br Commonw 1963;70:959–967.

2. Tsuji I, Kuroda K, Nakajima F. Excretory cystometry in paraplegic patients. J Urol 1960;83: 839–844.
3. James ED. The behaviour of the bladder during physical activity. Br J Urol 1978;50:387–394.
4. Miyagawa I, Nakamura I, Ueda M, Nishida H, Nakashita E, Goto H. Telemetric cystometry. Urol Int 1993;41:263–265.
5. Vereecken RL, Puers B, Das J. Continuous telemetric monitoring of bladder function. Urol Res 1983;11:15–18.
6. Thuroff JW, Jonas V, Frohneberg D, Petri E, Hohenfellner R. Telemetric urodynamic investigations in normal males. Urol Int 1980;35:427–434.
7. Bhatia NN, Bradley WE, Haldeman S, Johnson BK. Continuous monitoring of bladder and urethral pressures: new technique. Urology 1981;18: 207–210.
8. Griffiths CJ, Assi MS, Styles RA, Ramsden PD, Neal DE. Ambulatory monitoring of bladder and detrusor pressure during natural filling. J Urol 1989;142:780–784.
9. Webb RJ, Styles RA, Griffiths CJ, Ramsden PD, Neal DE. Ambulatory monitoring of bladder pressures in patients with low compliance as a result of neurogenic bladder dysfunction. Br J Urol 1989;64:150–154.
10. McInerney PD, Harris AB, Pritchard A, Stephenson TP. Night studies for primary diurnal and nocturnal enuresis and preliminary results of the "clam" ileocystoplasty. Br J Urol 1991;67:42–43.
11. James ED, Flack FC, Caldwell KPS, Martin MR. Continuous measurement of urine loss and frequency in incontinent patients. Br J Urol 1971; 43:233–237.
12. Webb RJ, Ramsden PD, Neal DE. Ambulatory monitoring and electronic measurement of urinary leakage in the diagnosis of detrusor instability and incontinence. Br J Urol 1991;68:148–152.
13. Eckford SC, Abrams PH. A new temperature sensitive device to detect incontinent episodes during ambulatory monitoring. Neurourol Urodyn 1992;11:448–450.
14. Janez J, Rodi Z, Mihelic M, Vrtacnik P, Vodusek DB, Plevnik S. Ambulatory distal urethral electric conductance testing coupled to a modified pad test. Neurourol Urodyn 1993;12:324–326.
15. Plevnik S, Vrtacnik P, Janez P. Detection of fluid entry into the urethra by electrical impedance measurement: fluid bridge test. Clin Phys Physiol Meas 1983;4:309–313.
16. van Waalwijk van Doorn ESC, Remmers A, Janknegt RA. Extramural ambulatory urodynamic monitoring during natural filling and normal daily activities: evaluation of 100 patients. J Urol 1991;146:124–131.
17. van Waalwijk van Doorn ESC, Remmers A, Janknegt RA. Conventional and extramural ambulatory urodynamic testing of the lower urinary tract in female volunteers. J Urol 1992;47:1319–1326.
18. Webb RJ, Griffiths CJ, Ramsden PD, Neal DE. Ambulatory monitoring in low compliance neuropathic bladder function. J Urol 1992;148:1477–1481.
19. Sethia KK, Webb RJ, Neal DE. Urodynamic study of ileocystoplasty in the treatment of idiopathic detrusor instability. Br J Urol 1991;67:286–290.
20. Arnold EP, Webster JR, Loose H, et al. Urodynamics of female incontinence factors influencing the results of surgery. Am J Obstet Gynecol 1973;117: 805–813.
21. Stanton SL, Cardozo LD. Results of the colposuspension operation for incontinence and prolapse. Br J Obstet Gynaecol 1979;86:693–697.
22. Cardozo LD, Stanton SL, Williams JE. Detrusor instability following surgery for genuine stress incontinence. Br J Urol 1979;51:204–207.
23. Steel SA, Cox C, Stanton SL. Long-term follow-up of detrusor instability following the colposuspension operation. Br J Urol 1985;58:138–142.
24. Khullar V, Salvatore S, Cardozo LD, Abbott D, Hill S, Kelleher CJ. Ambulatory urodynamics: a predictor of de-novo detrusor instability after colposuspension. Neurourol Urodyn 1994;13: 443–444.
25. Cardozo LD, Khullar V, Anders K, Hill S. Ambulatory urodynamics: a useful urogynaecological service? Presented at the Proceedings of 27th British Congress of Obstetrics and Gynaecology, Dublin, Ireland, 1995.

CHAPTER 15

Imaging Techniques for Evaluation of Bladder, Urethra, and Pelvic Floor

Stuart L. Stanton

Introduction

The variety and capability of imaging techniques have expanded enormously in the last 5 years. Radiology has diminished in importance for functional studies of the bladder, urethra, and pelvic floor to be superseded by ultrasound and magnetic resonance imaging (MRI). Computed tomography has more of a role in the investigation of anatomic abnormalities of the urogenital tract but not in the assessment of function. Part of the decline of radiology is radiation and cost. This chapter reviews the current role of imaging and its indications.

Intravenous Urogram

The intravenous urogram remains the primary investigative tool of the upper urinary tract for most urological patients, particularly those with hematuria, malignancy, calculi, or obstruction (1). Its importance to lower urinary tract disease is in the diagnosis of continuous incontinence and in the detection of ectopic ureter (Fig. 15.1), ureteric fistula, and tumor of the ureter or bladder. It has been used in combination with a flow rate measurement as an intravenous urodynamogram, but this combination now has relatively little application because no bladder pressures are recorded and although the technique enhances an intravenous urogram, it

does not replace cystometry as a basic urodynamic assessment.

Micturating Cystogram (MCG)

This is a dynamic method of radiological screening of bladder and urethra during bladder filling and voiding. No pressure recordings are taken and its main use is to demonstrate anatomic abnormalities, including vesicovaginal fistula, ureterocele, and diverticula.

Micturition cystography has been used to diagnose urethral diverticula. Bhatia et al. (2) showed that the diverticulum could be diagnosed by a biphasic urethral pressure profile, and this was confirmed by Summitt and Stovall (3), who used MCG, urethral pressure measurements, and cystoscopy to diagnose urethral diverticula. Urethral pressure profilometry confirmed the findings of cystoscopy and MCG and also diagnosed genuine stress incontinence, which was helpful in planning appropriate surgical treatment.

Lateral Bead Chain Urethrocystography

The position of the bladder neck is important in defining the cause of incontinence,

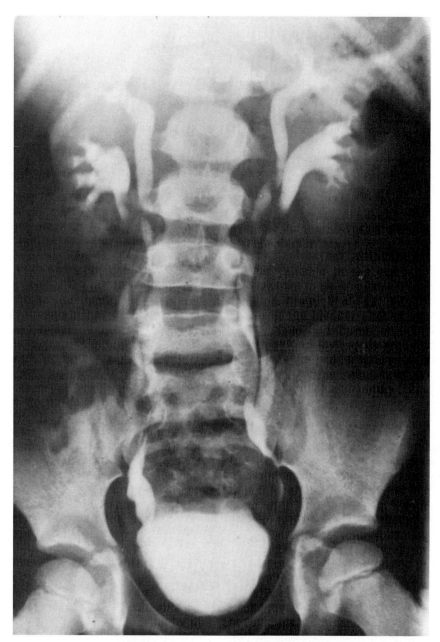

Figure. 15.1. Ectopic ureter. This intravenous urogram shows a duplex system on both sides. The ectopic ureter opens into the vagina, and the patient has had incontinence since birth.

in choosing the appropriate operation, and in determining the cause of failure. Lateral bead chain urethrocystography was first described by Hodgkinson (4), who imaged the bladder base, bladder neck, and proximal urethra using a flexible bead chain and lateral radiological screening. The imprecise nature, disadvantages of radiation, and the dependence on the department of radiology, however, led this procedure to be replaced by ultrasound using a Foley catheter to delineate the urethra and bladder neck. Gordon et al. (5) found this an accurate and practical alternative investigation. Grischke et al. (6) compared urethrocystometry, urethral pressure measurements, and uroflowmetry with lateral bead chain urethrocystography and found that although bead chain cystography had a high sensitivity (91%), it had a low specificity for stress incontinence. They concluded that ultrasound was preferable to radiology.

Colpocystodefecography

Because of the growing interest in prolapse and awareness of the increased importance of bowel symptoms, there is a challenge to assess simultaneously the function of the

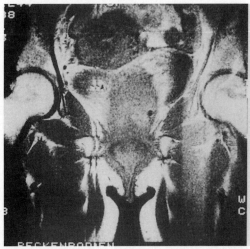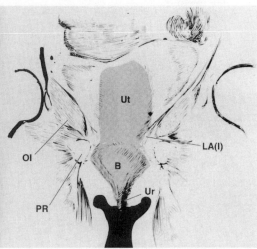

Figure. 15.2. Coronal MRI section of the female pelvis (Magnetom 1.0 T, TR 90 ms, TE 28 ms). *B*, bladder; *LA(I)*, levator ani muscle (iliococcygeus); *OI*, obturator internus muscle; *PR*, pubic rami; *Ur*, urethra; *Ut*, uterus. (From Diebus-Thiede G. Pelvic floor reeducation: principles and practice. London: Springer Verlag 1994.)

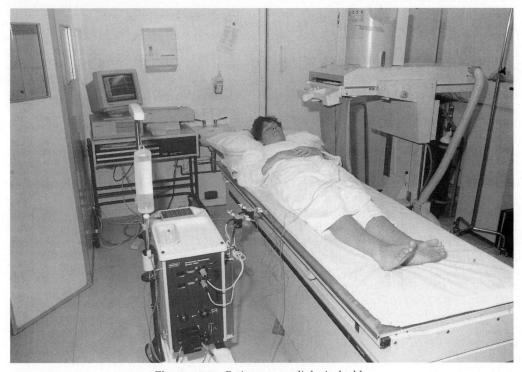

Figure. 15.3. Patient on a radiological table.

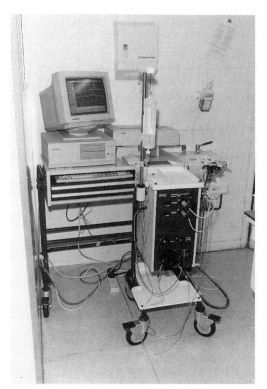

Figure. 15.4. ORMED twin-channel subtracted cystometric apparatus with color monitor, computer, and printer (Lectromed Limited, Garden City, Hertfordshire, U.K.).

pelvic floor and the organs it supports. Bethoux and Bory (7) introduced barium contrast into the bladder, vagina, and rectum and used a radiopaque marker in the uterus to enable them to x-ray the pelvis during maximum effort of contraction and then straining down. The technique has been modified by Hock et al. (8) and Altringer et al. (9) and now includes simultaneous fluoroscopy of small bowel, bladder, vagina, and rectum and screens the patient during defecation. Two hours before fluoroscopy, lower density barium sulfate suspension is ingested. At fluoroscopy, the bladder is catheterized and filled with 150–200 mL of water-soluble contrast. Thick barium paste is injected into the vagina and into the rectum. Two radiopaque markers are placed on the surface of the perineum so that the structures can be seen in relation to the perineal body. The patient then sits on an upright commode and views of the pelvis are then taken with the patient at rest, straining, and then squeezing the

sphincter muscles. The patient attempts to evacuate the contrast medium from bladder and rectum and rapid film sequences are taken at two frames per second. The examination takes up to 40 minutes. The clinicians claim that up to 75% of clinical diagnoses are changed after fluoroscopy. Altringer et al. (9) showed that where prolapse was diagnosed, between 25% and 36% of cystoceles, enteroceles, and rectoceles could not be visualized on defecography. However, where physical examination was negative, between 46% and 73% of patients were found to have cystoceles, enteroceles, and rectoceles. The disadvantages of this technique, namely its artificiality, exposure to irradiation, and ability to image prolapse, which may not be clinically relevant, have to be weighed against those situations where the prolapse has not been identified on clinical examination and needs to have treatment.

MRI

MRI is an accurate noninvasive, although expensive, method of imaging discrete structures. Devoid of ionizing radiation and more accurate than ultrasound, it is becoming an important investigation of the pelvic floor. However, it is expensive, and currently patients are imaged in the horizontal position. Also, those who are claustrophobic find passage through the machine quite difficult. Because of the magnetic field, it is difficult to use conventional systems for measuring intraabdominal and intravesical pressure changes. Klutke et al. (10) showed deficiencies in the muscle area around the urethra and descent of the bladder neck and were able to image the urethral submucosa. Kirschner-Hermanns et al. (11) and Diebus-Thiede (12) confirmed that degeneration of the levator ani could be seen in a number of women with genuine stress incontinence. Figure 15.2 shows a normal coronal section of the female pelvis.

Genital prolapse has been studied by Yang and colleagues (13, 14), who used fast imaging (eight shots in 12 seconds) under supine positions of relaxation, pelvic straining, and contraction. They were able to delineate si-

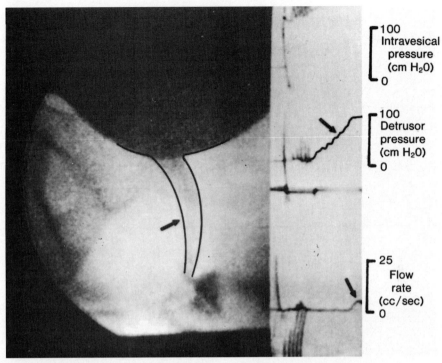

Figure. 15.5. Final video image showing normal micturition. The opaque medium opacifies the ure- thra (*arrow*). Notice the increased detrusor pressure and flow rate (*arrows*).

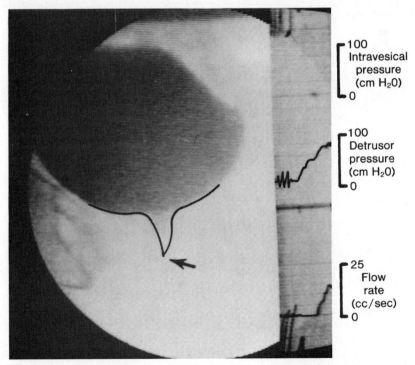

Figure. 15.6. Video image showing voluntary interruption of the micturition scheme at midurethra.

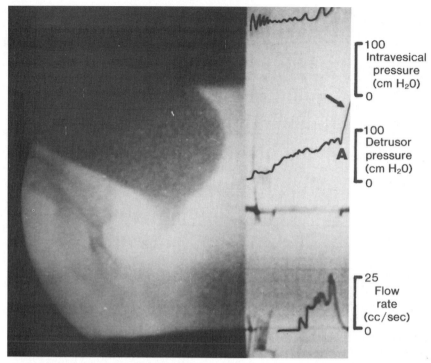

Figure. 15.7. Video image showing isometric detrusor contraction phase. At point A when the patient is asked to stop voiding, the extrinsic voluntary component of the sphincter mechanism contracts and closes the urethra before the detrusor begins to relax. This results in a marked increase in detrusor pressure (*arrow*) that gradually falls to the previoiding level once relaxation of the detrusor occurs. At the same time, the bladder neck gradually closes.

multaneously the anterior, middle, and posterior compartments but did not obtain good correlation with clinical findings and usually overdiagnosed prolapse. Monga et al. (15) used MRI to study pelvic floor function before and after sacrocolpopexy with specific reference to the effect of the operation on the anterior compartment and its role in the genesis of genuine stress incontinence. Although movement of both anterior and posterior portions of the middle compartment were noted, the prevalence of genuine stress incontinence was too small to allow any conclusions to be drawn about its cause.

Videocystourethrography

Videocystourethrography (VCU) combines all aspects of cystometry with fluoroscopy and simultaneous recordings of intravesical and intrarectal pressures and urine flow rates. It is regarded as the "gold standard" for assessment of bladder function and allows imaging of the upper urinary tract where reflux might occur and of the pelvic floor in relationship to the urethra and bladder.

The procedure is as follows. The patient is encouraged to attend with a full bladder and voids over a uroflowmeter in privacy to allow a free flow rate to be recorded. The urine volume is noted. The patient lies supine on a tilting radiological table. After measurement of the residual urine by sterile catheterization with a 12F Foley catheter (Fig. 15.3), the bladder is filled by gravity with 25% diodone at a rate of 100 mL/min. A weighing transducer measures the rate of filling. A 1-mm-diameter fluid-filled catheter is placed alongside the bladder filling catheter to measure the intravesical pressure. A 2-mm-diameter fluid-filled catheter protected by a finger cot is inserted a short distance into the rectum to measure the rectal (abdominal) pressure. Both are connected to pressure transducers. Electronic subtraction of the abdominal pressure from the intravesical pressure gives the detrusor pressure, which is an exact index of detrusor activity (Fig. 15.4). During bladder filling, the patient notes first sensation and then full bladder capacity. When the patient says that her bladder is full, the filling catheter is removed and the patient is stood upright and radiologically screened in the erect oblique position. She is asked to cough and leakage or bladder base descent is noted. The patient then voids, and when a satisfactory flow has been achieved, she is asked to interrupt her stream so that milkback can be observed. During this time, the maximum voiding pressure is being recorded. The patient resumes voiding until the bladder is empty and fluoroscopy reveals whether there is any residual urine. About 15% of women have difficulty voiding in the erect position, and the investigation may have to be conducted in the sitting position without fluoroscopy.

In the normal patient, as voiding begins, the pelvic floor relaxes, the urethral pressure falls, and the bladder neck opens, followed by a rise in detrusor pressure. This rise is usually below 70 cm of water, and peak flow rate should be in excess of 15 mL/s (Fig. 15.5). To determine whether the patient has voluntary control of micturition, she is asked to interrupt voiding, and this allows some evaluation to be made of the sphincter mechanism and the pelvic floor (Fig. 15.6). Milkback, which is the process by which the proximal urethra returns urine into the bladder, now occurs. The maximum voiding detrusor pressure may rise abruptly at this stage, which represents isometric contraction of the slow-acting detrusor in the presence of urethral closure (Fig. 15.7). This may or may not be related to the potential of the bladder to void under more difficult circumstances, such as after bladder neck surgery.

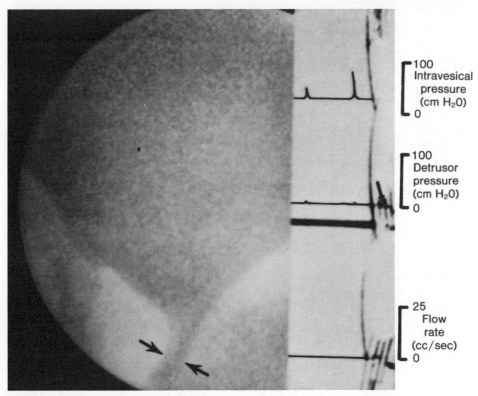

Figure. 15.8. Video image demonstrating incontinence due to urethral sphincter incompetence. The detrusor pressure is at zero, and after a cough, contrast media escapes via the bladder neck into the urethra (*arrow*).

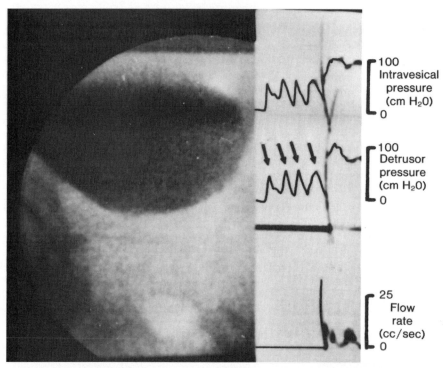

Figure. 15.9. Video image showing detrusor contraction on the detrusor pressure trace during bladder filling (*arrows*).

This examination confirms whether the patient leaks urine and under what circumstances leakage can occur. Any descent of the bladder neck and base may be noted. The technique exposes the patient to approximately 800 mrad, which is less than the exposure for an intravenous urogram.

In the patient with urethral sphincter incompetence (genuine stress incontinence) and without detrusor instability, the bladder fills normally without detrusor contractions and with a pressure rise of less than 15 cm H_2O. When the patient stands, the detrusor pressure rise remains less than 15 cm H_2O, and when she coughs, there is loss of contrast material through the urethra. The bladder neck often exhibits excess mobility and descent and when the patient is at rest may be open without a rise in detrusor pressure (Fig. 15.8). The patient may or may not be able to interrupt her urinary stream on command and subsequently voids to completion.

By contrast, in a patient with detrusor instability, there may be detrusor contractions or a steep detrusor pressure rise greater than 15 cm H_2O during filling and on standing (Fig. 15.9). Stress incontinence may occur on coughing and may trigger a detrusor contraction (Fig. 15.10). Often the contractions occur early during the filling phase before reaching full bladder capacity. Despite reports to the contrary, this author finds no relationship between the ability to voluntarily interrupt the urinary stream and the diagnosis of either urethral sphincter incompetence or detrusor instability (16).

Both Stanton et al. (17) and Benness et al. (18) reviewed the role of VCU in the assessment of lower urinary tract disorders. The former reviewed retrospectively 200 consecutive VCUs to discern whether the addition of radiology made any difference to management and found that radiology was diagnostic when a patient complained of postmicturition dribble or incontinence on standing. Two cases of urethral diverticulum were found, and in five cases screening during the erect position led to differentiation between sphincter incompetence and posture-induced detrusor instability. Benness et al. (18) carried out a prospective comparison with cystometry and found no significant difference in the diagnosis of genuine stress incontinence or detrusor instability, but when studies were negative, repeat investigation was recommended. Using a selective policy, they believed that just over half of the VCUs could have been avoided—an important cost and irradiation consideration.

Conclusion

For the spectrum of urogynecological disorders and, in particular, the variety of causes of incontinence, more and more reliance is being placed on several rather than one investigation. These must be dynamic rather than static. The investigator must be aware that bladder, pelvic floor, bowel, and relevant innervation may all need to be studied.

REFERENCES

1. Collie D, Paul A, Wild S. The diagnostic yield of intravenous urogram: a demographic study. Br J Urol 1994;73:603–606.
2. Bhatia N, McCarthy T, Ostergard D. Urethral pressure profiles of women with urethral diverticula. Obstet Gynecol 1981;58:375–378.
3. Summitt R, Stovall T. Urethral diverticula: evaluation by urethral pressure profilometry, cystourethroscopy and voiding cystourethrogram. Obstet Gynecol 1992;80:695–699.
4. Hodgkinson CP. Relationships of the female urethra and bladder in urinary stress continence. Am J Obstet Gynecol 1953;65:560–573.
5. Gordon D, Pearce J, Norton P, Stanton SL. Comparison of ultrasound and lateral chain urethrocystography in the determination of bladder neck descent. Am J Obstet Gynecol 1989;106:182–185.
6. Grischke E, Anton H, Stolz W, von Fournier D, Bastert G. Urodynamic assessment and lateral urethrocystography. Acta Obstet Gynaecol Scand 1991;70:225–228.
7. Bethoux A, Bory S. Les mécannismes statiques viscéraux pelviens chez la femme á la lumiére d'exploration fonctionelle du dispositif en position debout. Ann Chir 1962;16:887–916.

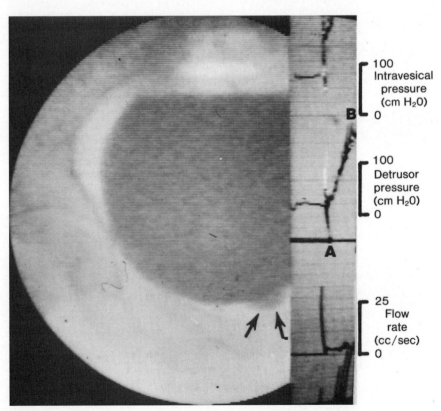

Figure. 15.10. Video image demonstrating rise in detrusor pressure on standing (*point A*). Coughing begins (*point B*) and the bladder neck partially opens (*arrow*).

8. Hock D, Lombard R, Jehaes C, et al. Colpocysto-defecography. Dis Colon Rectum 1993;36:1015–1021.

9. Altringer W, Saclardies T, Dominguez J, Brubaker L, Smith C. Four contrast defecography: pelvic "floor-oscopy." Dis Colon Rectum 1995;38:695–699.

10. Klutke C, Golomb J, Barbaric Z, Raz, S. Anatomy of stress incontinence: magnetic resonance imaging of the female bladder neck and urethra. J Urol 1990;143:563–566.

11. Kirschner-Hermanns R, Wein B, Neihans S, Schaefer W, Jakse G. Contribution of magnetic resonance imaging of the pelvic floor to the understanding of urinary incontinence. J Urol 1993;72:715–718.

12. Diebus-Thiede G. Magnetic resonance imaging of the pelvic floor. In: Schussler B, Laycock J, Norton P, Stanton SL, eds. Pelvic floor reeducation: principles and practice. London: Springer Verlag 1994:78–82.

13. Yang A, Mostin J, Rosenhein N, Zerhouni E. Pelvic floor descent in women: dynamic evaluation with fast magnetic resonance imaging and cinematic display. Radiology 1991;179:25–33.

14. Yang A, Mostwin J, Genadry R, Sanders R. Patterns of prolapse demonstrated with dynamic fast scan MRI: reassessment of conventional concepts of pelvic floor weaknesses. Neurourol Urodyn 1993;12:310–311.

15. Monga A, Heron C, Stanton SL. How does sacrocolpopexy affect bladder function and pelvic floor anatomy—a combined urodynamic and magnetic resonance imaging approach. Neurourol Urodyn 1994;13:378–380.

16. Cardozo L, Stanton SL. Genuine stress incontinence and detrusor instability. A review of 200 patients. Br J Obstet Gynaecol 1980;87:184–190.

17. Stanton SL, Krieger M, Ziv E. Videocysto-urethrography: its role in assessment of incontinence in the female. Neurourol Urodyn 1988;7:712–713.

18. Benness C, Barnick C, Cardozo L. Is there place for routine videocystourethrography in the assessment of lower urinary tract dysfunction? Neurourol Urodyn 1989;18:299–300.

CHAPTER 16

Ultrasound in Urogynecology

Heinz Koelbl

Introduction

Major improvements and technological advances in ultrasonic instrumentation have facilitated the establishment of ultrasound as a diagnostic tool in the management of female patients with upper and lower urinary tract disorders. Application of ultrasound in urogynecology is increasing, following the technical progress and development of sector scanning techniques and real-time ultrasonography.

Ultrasonic evaluation of the pelvis was originally described by Donald et al. in 1958 (1). Previously, assessment of the urinary bladder itself was limited primarily to determine gross changes, such as estimation of urine volume and the state of the bladder to other pelvic structures (2, 3).

Meanwhile, ultrasonographic evaluation of the upper urinary tract belongs to routine assessment in the pre- and posttherapeutic concept of urogynecology (4). Measurement of the kidneys and the calices complement detection of hydronephrosis, hydroureters, and parenchymal cysts of the kidneys in the diagnosis of upper urinary tract alterations. Ultrasound has also been suggested as an alternative source for imaging the urethrovesical anatomy (5). Although the clinical significance of various radiological parameters in patients with pelvic floor relaxation, especially associated with genuine stress incontinence (GSI), is controversial (6, 7), basic evaluation of its use was sufficient to justify introduction of sonography as an alternative to commonly used radiological procedures. Ultrasound has been used to detect anatomic alterations associated with GSI, to select the appropriate type of surgery, and to assess surgical results and postoperative complications. Moreover, ultrasound imaging is regarded as a conclusive investigation for the evaluation of pelvic floor muscle function (8). Movement of intrapelvic structures (e.g., urethrovesical junction [UVJ], bladder base) can be evaluated as a consequence of pelvic floor muscle contraction (Fig. 16.1).

Instrumentation

Ultrasound refers to sound energy with a frequency above 20,000 Hz. The sound waves are produced and received by piezoelectric crystals. The sound beam itself is propagated as a longitudinal wave through human soft tissue at a speed of 1.54 km/s. Penetration of tissue depends on the frequency of the sound waves. The higher the frequency, the shorter the wavelength and deeper the tissue penetration. Because frequency selection involves a compromise between better image resolution (high frequency) and deeper tissue penetration (low frequency), the decision must be based on the position of the organs to be examined.

There are various types of ultrasound transducers currently being used, each with an advantage in certain applications. The advantage of sector scanners include easy handling of the transducer head and a very small contact site. Linear-array scanners offer the improved handling of sector scanners without the limitations of narrow proximal field widths encountered with vaginal or rectal endoprobes.

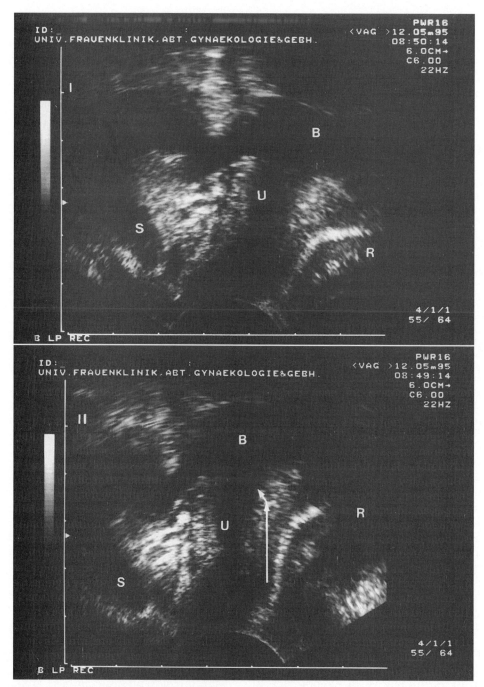

Figure 16.1. Demonstration of the bladder (*B*), the urethra (*U*), and the rectum with introital sonography (**I**). The bladder and the rectum (*R*) are lifted upward (*large arrow*) and forward (*small arrow*) behind the pubic symphysis during a voluntary and regular pelvic floor muscle contraction (**II**).

Real-time imaging is particularly suitable for examination of the bladder and the urethra. In these areas, it provides a mode of dynamic echography in which two-dimensional images are continuously updated. It allows the sonographer to scan the bladder and the urethra with speed and precision. Among the various real-time scanners available, the linear array and sector scanners have been recommended for patients with stress incontinence.

Vaginal and transrectal probes and sector scanners have overcome some of the difficulties associated with conventional linear array machines; they provide a sharper better-focused picture with good resolution. The endoprobe may be straight or flexible; however, it is commonly angulated up to 45° to facilitate visualization of the pelvic organs. This angulation also allows for less external movement of the probe and better patient comfort. A permanent record of the scan can be obtained by attaching a camera to the cathode ray tube. A videotape recorder is also useful for obtaining records for teaching of the patient and for future comparisons of results after treatment. Advanced technology of urodynamic instruments today allows direct sonographic and tonometric registration on single or double screens with a high reproducibility. Most of them are on-line with computers provided with improved software and picture-archiving systems. Thus, data storage of both tonometric and sonographic results essential for patient care and follow-up, scientific work, and for forensic reasons can be easily obtained.

With advanced technology, scanner size has become smaller and fulfills most of the needs for an acceptable investigation with high resolution. The ongoing development of microprobes will increase the knowledge about the physiology and pathophysiology of the relevant morphology. Small endoprobes have been used for demonstration of the sphincteric function of the urethra and intravesical ultrasound. Three-dimensional ultrasound has already become part of research in urogynecology.

For urogynecological investigation, commonly used frequencies for the transducers range from 2.4 to 5 MHz for transabdominal ultrasound; 5–7.0 MHz for endosonography, introital, and perineal techniques; and 20 MHZ for three-dimensional ultrasound.

ABDOMINAL ULTRASOUND

The use of ultrasound for the evaluation of the upper urinary tract has evolved from merely using the bladder as a transparent window to scan pelvic structures. As opposed to conventional radiological techniques, ultrasound is noninvasive, does not require contrast material, and does not expose the patient to ionizing radiation.

Ultrasound is used to evaluate the upper urinary tract, particularly for the detection of hydronephrosis and renal stones, and to assess renal parenchyma. In addition to measurement of the kidneys and the renal pelvis with its calices and detection of hydroureters, ultrasound is the relevant diagnostic modality in the detection of upper urinary tract lesions (9). It is quick and easy to perform and thus useful not only in the pre- and posttherapeutic assessment but also for the staging of gynecological malignancies (e.g., hydroureter in cervical cancer means Federation International de Gynecologie et Obstetrique stage IIIB). Difficulties exist in the differentiation between obstructive and nonobstructive patterns of hydroureters. Doppler ultrasound studies are capable of differentiating between these two entities. As yet, ultrasound study may detect hydronephrosis that is suggestive of ureteral damage, but it will not detect a ureter that has been injured and is leaking into the peritoneal cavity or one that is obstructed but has not yet produced calyceal dilatation. In addition, problems still occur in the complete visualization of the ureters due to its retroperitoneal course and to superimposed bowel contents. In the detection of genitourinary anomalies, like aplasia, hypoplasia, and horseshoe kidney, ultrasound diagnosis must be confirmed by radiological procedures.

Transabdominal ultrasound assessment primarily focuses on adynamic features such as residual urine, distortion of the bladder by pelvic pathology, and detection of bladder tumors (1). Bladder and postvoid residual volumes can be determined with transabdominal scanning, although accuracy is not reliable for volumes less than 50 mL. However, the unreliability at small bladder volumes is not much of a drawback because small residual urine volumes are generally not clinically significant. The bladder is scanned in two perpendicular planes (transverse and sagittal), and three diameters (height, width, and depth) are measured. Height corresponds to the greatest anteroposterior measurement. Both are obtained in sagittal plane scan. The simplest formula used to estimate volume is bladder volume (mL) = (H × W × D) × (0.7). The correction factor 0.7 is needed because the shape of the bladder is not circular until it is almost completely full. The same formula can be used for premicturition and postmicturition volume assessments. The error rate of this formula is approximately 21%. Recently, small portable ultrasound units have been developed. These portable units are easy to use and serve solely for the measurement of residual urine volumes, including special software to calculate bladder volume automatically. Meanwhile, a variety of successive models is available. Accuracy of these instruments has been found to be as good as catheter estimations of actual residual volume. The increasing availability of such units will make measurement of residual urine by ultrasound a routine procedure for inpatients and outpatients.

Numerous studies have demonstrated real-time ultrasonography to be useful to evaluate the anatomic relationship of the bladder, the UVJ, and the proximal urethra (4–6, 10). With careful observation, the changes in the shape and position of the vesical neck and the proximal urethra can be determined while the patient is performing a Valsalva maneuver or coughing. However, although the bladder neck can be seen on transabdominal ultrasound, it is occasionally hidden behind the symphysis pubis. The bladder neck is especially difficult to locate in obese patients and in women with severe genitourinary prolapse (11). This is the result of significant intervening tissue affecting sound wave penetration (attenuation) and acoustic shading from the symphysis. A urethral catheter may be needed to demonstrate the urethral axis. As a consequence, transabdominal ultrasound can be used to determine the extent of mobility of the bladder and urethra and to detect detrusor instability in some patients. However, the pitfalls of this technique to evaluate the urethrovesical anatomy should be considered.

Transabdominal ultrasound has also proven valuable in the evaluation of the urinary tract in neuromuscular bladder dysfunction. Brandt et al. (12) found that ultrasound of the bladder yielded significantly more diagnostic information than radiography in 27% of their study group. They also demonstrated bladder trabeculation and dilated ureters in neuromuscular dysfunction using abdominal sonography (12).

ENDOSONOGRAPHY

Vaginal or rectal ultrasound techniques involve probes of higher frequencies than transabdominal linear array scanners and, therefore, afford sharper better focused pictures with high resolution. The endosonographic probes avoid interference from the symphysis pubis and subcutaneous fat. Transrectal sonography produces a good view of the bladder, urethra, and the bladder neck, although the rectal probe can occasionally alter the alignment of the bladder neck movement during Valsalva maneuvers or coughing. They cannot be used in patients with significant pelvic relaxation.

VAGINAL ULTRASOUND

Vaginal ultrasound has been proposed as a suitable alternative to conventional radiological urethrocystography (13). This method is attractive because it is simple to perform, the equipment required is found in many gynecological units, and the risks of irradiation to patient and operator are removed (Fig. 16.2). Some concern exists that use of a transvaginal probe that lies in direct contact with the bladder neck may alter lower urinary tract anatomy and give erroneous results. Quinn et al. (13) described vaginal sonography in a series of 100 women with a range of urinary symptoms. The inferior border of the pubic symphysis was used as a "key landmark." A level mounted on the endoprobe ensured the maintenance of a horizontal position during scanning, thus avoiding any distortion of urethrovesical anatomy caused by the probe. In 19 of 23 patients with GSI, the UVJ was inferior to the level of the midsymphysis at rest, and in 18

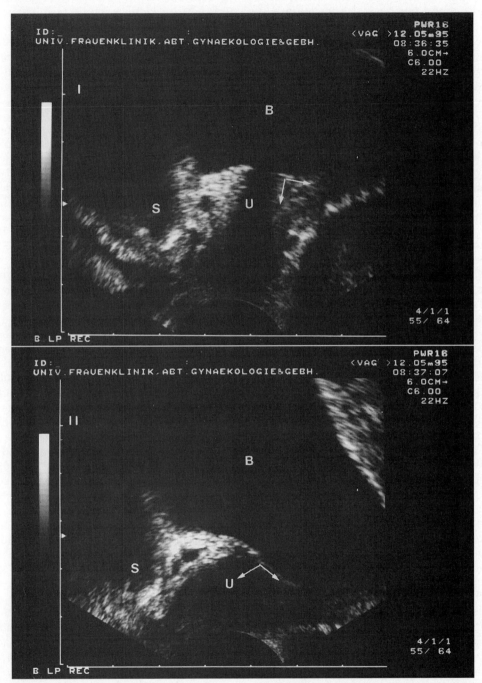

Figure 16.2. Sonographic urethrocystography with vaginal ultrasound in a patient with genuine stress incontinence showing the bladder (*B*), the urethra (*U*), and the pubic symphysis (*S*) at rest (**I**) and during stress (**II**) showing an increase of the retrovesical angle (*small arrows*), dislocation of the urethral axis, and displacement of the bladder base in a downward and posterior direction.

there was opening and descent of the bladder neck during coughing. Meanwhile, most studies report that vaginal ultrasound is an accurate method to record anatomic changes, especially the mobility of the bladder neck. In addition to its easy feasibility and reproducibility, Bergman and coworkers (6) reported that descent of the UVJ of more than 1 cm on straining correlated with the entity of stress urinary incontinence. On the other hand, a considerable overlap in the position of the bladder neck at rest and during straining and sneezing was observed by Carey and Dwyer (14). Hol and coworkers (15) used a Foley catheter and introduced it into the bladder with the balloon half-filled with soapy water. Thus, a recognizable fluid level, which is parallel to the horizontal axis of the patient, is produced and serves as a reference to assess mobility of the bladder neck during a standardized Valsalva force. Compared with a healthy control group, patients with GSI revealed a significantly lower and more posterior position of the bladder at rest and during straining and squeezing. However, there was a considerable interindividual overlap between the two groups for all parameters.

Alterations due to pelvic floor muscle contraction and straining can be evaluated by "still" pictures comparing the situation at rest with the extent of displacement at maximal effort. However, rapid movement of the urethrovesical unit (e.g., during coughing) can be measured only when a video recorder is attached to the ultrasound machine. Vaginal ultrasonography has been proposed as a suitable alternative to videocystourethrography. However, in a study of 44 women with urinary incontinence, Wise and coworkers (16) found an increase of the maximum urethral pressure and the functional urethral length and an improvement of the pressure transmission caused by the endoprobe inserted 2 cm into the vagina. The authors concluded that the use of a vaginal probe resulted in compression of the urethra and therefore reduced the likelihood of detecting incontinence of women with GSI or the severity of GSI diagnosed.

In addition to visualization of the bladder and urethra, vaginal scanning is also valuable in the assessment of urethral diverticula.

However, the diagnosis of this entity should be confirmed by cystoscopy and radiological procedures. Until recently, residual urines have been measured by transabdominal ultrasound only. However, it can be difficult to visualize low bladder volumes from the abdominal wall because of distortion and diffraction of the long ultrasonic beam. Haylen et al. (17) used a transvaginal linear-array ultrasound scanner to measure bladder volumes from 2 to 300 mL. The method is simple, atraumatic, and acceptable to patients, and a clear picture of the bladder is obtained (in the sagittal plane) even at low bladder volumes. From the maximum dimensions of the bladder in this plane (horizontal = H, vertical depth = D), an unknown bladder volume can be calculated from the formula bladder volume (mL) $- 5.9 \times H \times D - 14.6$.

Determination of bladder wall displacement and/or infiltration caused by cervical cancer is an essential part of the staging procedure. In a comparative study of computed tomography (CT), cystoscopic examinations, and magnetic resonance imaging (MRI), 21 women with stage Ib–IIIb cervical cancer were evaluated with vaginal ultrasound to diagnose invasion of the bladder wall. Moveability of the bladder wall against the vaginal ultrasound probe in the region of the anterior vaginal fornix was considered to exclude infiltration. This test showed an accuracy of 95%, whereas it was 76%, 86%, and 80% for CT, cystoscopy, and MRI, respectively (18). From these data, it appears that transvaginal ultrasonographic examination is a useful adjunct in detecting invasion of the bladder wall in patients with advanced cervical cancer.

RECTAL ULTRASOUND

Placing a linear-array transducer within the rectum to improve imaging of the bladder base and neck was described by Nishizawa and coworkers (19). The authors described how the technique may be used to replace X-ray cystography during urodynamic imaging. Shapeero et al. (20) used the same technique to visualize the bladder base and proximal urethra in the male suspected of having neuromuscular dysfunction of the bladder.

They performed sonographic and radiological voiding cystourethrography on all patients and concluded that the sonographic examination is as good, and occasionally better, than the radiographic method. The technique of using a transrectal probe for the investigation of women with urinary incontinence was introduced by Brown and coworkers (21). However, questions arose regarding endoprobe movement during straining maneuvers, thereby creating artifacts, attendant discomfort, and possible inhibition of bladder neck movement. Bergman and colleagues (10) established that insertion of the rectal probe did not alter urethral junction mobility as evaluated by the Q-tip angle change. Using the UVJ drop as a comparative parameter, they reported a sensitivity of 86% and specificity of 92% in the evaluation of women with GSI. However, the potential problems of endoprobe movement during straining were also noted by these authors.

CYSTOSONOGRAPHY

Similar to vaginal ultrasound, cystosonography is a helpful diagnostic intravesical procedure to scan the bladder wall, its wall displacement, and/or invasion from gynecological malignancies (22). This endosonographic method is performed with a rotation scanner with a range of 360° and a frequency of 6 MHZ. The scanner is introduced via a 24-Charrière resectoscope shaft. Cystosonography should be preceded by cystoscopy to avoid inadvertent bleeding (urethral strictures, bladder tumors). This type of endosonography is able to detect edema and/or tumor invasion of the bladder mucosa. Whereas cystoscopy is capable of demonstrating superficial changes of the bladder mucosa, cystosonography permits visualization of deeper layers of the bladder wall. Moreover, it is possible to obtain biopsy specimens under direct ultrasound control that cannot be detected by cystoscopy alone. Compared with transcutaneous sonography, the endosonographic evaluation of tumor spread is more precise, because of the short distance to the transducer head and the higher frequencies being applied (Fig. 16.3).

INTRAURETHRAL ULTRASOUND

Intraurethral ultrasound (IUUS) is a new endosonographic technique providing high resolution imaging (20 MHZ) of the urethra and the surrounding tissues. This technique is recommended for the diagnosis of diverticula and urinary incontinence, because other imaging methods provide little information on the sphincter itself. In a pilot study, Kirschner-Hermanns et al. (23) investigated the sphincteric region in women with IUUS. Examination of 44 stress-incontinent and healthy women revealed a negative correlation between the external urethral sphincter (area and circumference) and the grade of stress incontinence. In no patient with normal urinary continence was the sphincter reduced in size (23). The meaning of these findings in relation to urethral pressure measurements merits further evaluation because it could be helpful in the choice of treatment. Endoluminal ultrasound has also been applied during surgical treatment of urethral diverticula (24). Intraoperatively, the diverticula were well visualized by endoluminal ultrasound, which demonstrated improved identification of the size and orientation of urethral diverticula, sludge within the diverticula, the extent of periurethral inflammation, diverticular wall thickness, and the distance between the diverticular wall and urethral lumen compared with traditional imaging techniques.

PERINEAL AND INTROITAL SONOGRAPHY

Newer applications of sonography place the transducer on the perineum or just between the labia minora (introital sonography). These scanning techniques do not alter anatomic relationships, are not affected by patient straining, and can be used in patients even with severe genitourinary prolapse.

Ultrasound urethrocystography by perineal scanning for evaluation of female stress urinary incontinence was suggested by Kohorn and others (25). The procedure is carried out with the patient in a supine position with legs slightly abducted to allow access of the transducer to the perineum. A linear-array or curved-array transducer scanner is positioned in a sagittal orientation to visual-

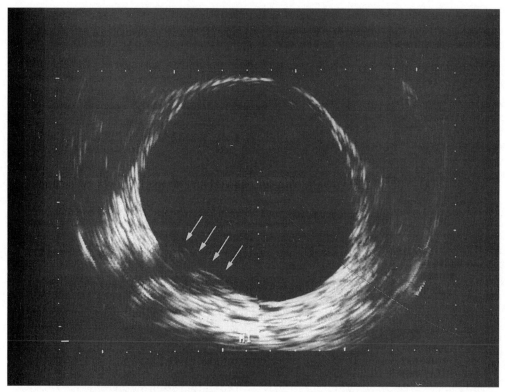

Figure 16.3. Cystosonography of a patient with stage IV cervical cancer showing bladder wall infiltration (*small arrows*).

ize the bladder, bladder base, UVJ, and the pubic symphysis (Fig. 16.4). Comparative results between radiological and perineal sonographic urethrocystography have been reported (26, 27). Perineal three-dimensional ultrasound scanning of the urethra, urethral sphincter, and bladder neck has been reported by Khullar and coworkers (28) describing a significantly smaller "rhabdosphincter" in women with urethral sphincter incompetence.

Regional distortion using vaginal or rectal endosonography, even with small endoprobes, was the reason for development of introital sonography (29). The technique involves placing a vaginal sector scanner to the vulva just underneath the external urethral orifice and visualizing the bladder, UVJ, urethra, and symphysis (Fig. 16.5). Modern vaginal probes are thin and give good visualization of the lower urinary tract when placed only a short distance into the vagina. Thus, this technique is devoid of any potential morphological artifact as a result of urethral or bladder neck distortion. Using introital

sonography, Hanzal et al. (30) prospectively determined the influence of transurethral catheters used for cystometry on bladder neck anatomy. This study revealed similar results for the assessment of bladder neck location and the posterior urethrovesical angle at rest and during straining, with and without a catheter in place. Urethral width was significantly greater with a catheter in situ. From these data, it appears that catheters used for urodynamic assessment increase urethral width but do not affect bladder neck location and urethral mobility. The exact location of microtip pressure transducers can easily be determined while visualizing the bladder neck and the urethra during filling (31). The voiding phase can also be evaluated even without the use of catheters. Micturition, and the patient's ability to stop voiding, which demonstrates the voluntary musculature and the urethral "milk-back" mechanism, can be visualized and evaluated. Wavelike detrusor contractions accompanied by bladder neck opening may be seen in patients with an unstable bladder. Inadequate emptying associated with urethral obstruction may be seen in patients after an overzealous urethropexy. Uncoordinated emptying may be seen in patients with detrusor-sphincter dyssynergia and can be verified by simultaneous EMG study. The location of the UVJ can be readily determined. Successful colposuspension is found to be associated with a urethrovesical location that is more anterior, although not necessarily more elevated (Fig. 16.5).

Discussion

Ultrasound has become an essential procedure in modern urogynecology to assess upper urinary tract lesions, morphological changes associated with female urinary incontinence, and pelvic floor relaxation. Its simplicity, cost effectiveness, and availability in gynecology endeavor its use as a basic urogynecological screening procedure, especially before and after conservative or surgical treatment. Meanwhile, ultrasound has become a potential alternative to conventional radiological procedures, and improve-

ments continue. As a consequence, a diagnostic regimen for the sequential use of ultrasound in urogynecology can be recommended as the result of scientific work (Table 16.1).

Exclusion of upper urinary tract lesions is carried out with the use of ultrasound, especially in patients undergoing gynecological surgery. However, there are difficulties in the recognition of congenital anomalies, and therefore radiology still has its place for selected indications. Surgical complications causing upper urinary tract lesions should be screened by ultrasound and completed by radiological procedures when indicated.

Many radiographic studies have been published in the evaluation of the mobility of the bladder base, the UVJ, urethra, and support of the surrounding soft tissues in women thought to have an anatomic defect as the basis for stress urinary incontinence. Presently, cinefluoroscopy is still in routine use, although urinary incontinence can be visualized only insufficiently by means of static methods such as the lateral urethrocystogram. Therefore, ultrasound is particularly suitable for dynamic examination of

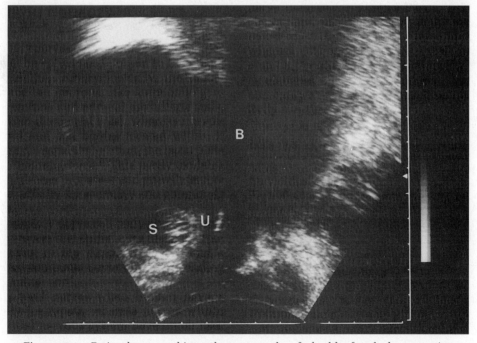

Figure 16.4.   Perineal sonographic urethrocystography of a healthy female demonstrating the bladder (*B*), the urethra (*U*), and the pubic symphysis (*S*).

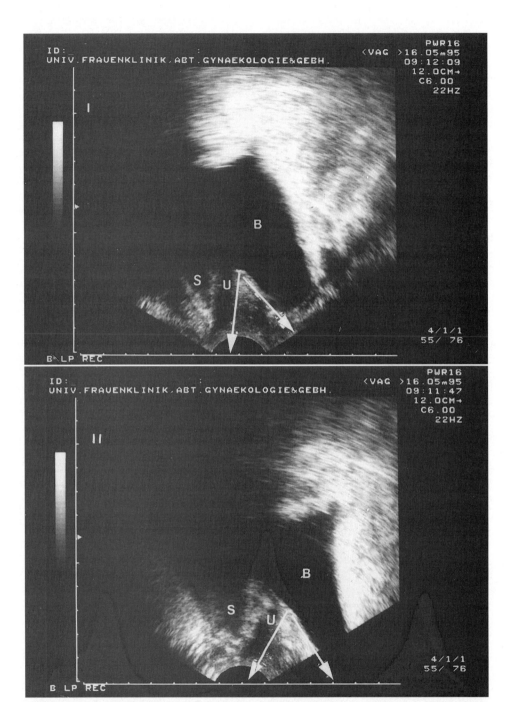

Figure 16.5. Urethrocystography with introital sonography demonstrating the bladder (*B*), the urethra (*U*), and the pubic symphysis (*S*) of a continent patient after colposuspension at rest (**I**) and during stress (**II**). There is minimal movement of the urethrovesical junction during stress in a downward and posterior direction. The retrovesical angle (*arrows*) remains unchanged.

Table 16.1. Sonographic Assessment in Urogynecology

Sonography of the upper urinary tract
  Kidney size
  Renal pelvis
  Ureters
Sonography after spontaneous micturition to assess
  The emptied bladder
  Residual volume
  Neighboring areas (uterus, adnexal region, pubic symphysis)
Sonography during filling cystometry to assess
  The filling bladder
  Bladder neck (opening, funneling, mobility)
  Urethra (mobility, axis, angles)

the bladder and the urethra without time limit, especially because of the lack of side effects. Compared with transvaginal and transrectal endosonographic methods, perineal scanning and introital sonography are less invasive. Moreover, demonstration of the urethra does not necessarily require catheterization.

Ultrasound evaluation of the bladder neck and urethra provides a wide range of information for the urogynecologist. Moreover, neighboring structures can be visualized at the same time, giving more complex information. The position of the bladder neck in the relaxed state and the degree of displacement with reference to the symphysis pubis can be measured. This information can be helpful in determining the type of surgical procedure. Surgical correction of the anatomic defect can be assessed. Application of visualization techniques to demonstrate the urethrovesical anatomy in patients with GSI relates to one of the aims of antiincontinence bladder surgery: to elevate the bladder neck to a position within the abdominal cavity. Conversely, failure of adequate bladder neck elevation is a factor leading to recurrent GSI after surgery. Thus, the ability to measure objectively the descent of the bladder neck pre- and postoperatively is important. Although intraoperative use of ultrasound to assess these changes has challenged some urogynecologists, its definite clinical value and feasibility during antiincontinence surgery has not yet been proven. Detrusor contractions with concomitant funneling of the bladder neck are occa-

sionally detected during scanning. Finally, postoperative voiding difficulties can be evaluated sonographically to determine the location of obstruction and the volume of residual volume.

Rapid development, especially the application of higher frequencies with small transducers, and the availability of ultrasound instruments in gynecology, the cost-effectiveness, and the lack of radiation without the necessity of lead shielding meet the aims of urogynecologists as a favorable diagnostic procedure. Moreover, there is no limit of investigation time and no contrast media reaction that favor its clinical application. Compared with radiology, the increasing number of comparable results and the technical developments of smaller endoprobes and three-dimensional scanners will increase the diagnostic field in urogynecology, resulting in a better understanding of the relevant functions and dysfunctions due to the responsible structures.

Ultrasound in urogynecology is on its way to replacing conventional radiological procedures. However, until now and similar to conventional radiology, it does not yet appear to provide conclusive and discriminatory diagnostic information but supplies complementary data to be used in conjunction with other diagnostic tools (32).

REFERENCES

1. Donald I, MacVican J, Brown T. Examination of abdominal masses by pulsed ultrasound. Lancet 1958;1:1188–1191.
2. Orgaz RE, Gomez AZ, Ramirez CT. Application of bladder ultrasonography I. Bladder content and residue. J Urol 1981;125:174–176.
3. Henriksson L, Marsal K. Bedside ultrasound diagnosis of residual urine volume. Arch Gynecol Obstet 1982;231:129–133.
4. Benson JT, Sumners JE. Ultrasound evaluation of female urinary incontinence. Int Urogynecol J 1990;1:7–11.
5. White RD, McQuown D, McCarthy TA, Ostergard DR. Real time ultrasonography in evaluation of urinary stress incontinence. Am J Obstet Gynecol 1980;138:235–237.
6. Bergman A, Koonings P, Ballard CA. Ultrasonic prediction of stress urinary incontinence development in surgery for pelvic floor relaxation. Gynecol Obstet Invest 1988;26:66–72.
7. Drutz HP, Shapiro BJ, Mandel F. Do static cysturethrograms have a role in the investigation of female incontinence? Am J Obstet Gynecol 1978;130:516–520.

8. Schüssler B, Norton P, Laycock B, Stanton S, eds. Ultrasound. In: Pelvic floor reeducation. Berlin: Springer-Verlag, 1994:64–74.

9. Ellenbogen PH, Scheible FW, Talner LB. Sensitivity of gray scale ultrasound in detecting upper urinary tract obstruction. Am J Roentgenol 1978; 130:731–736.

10. Bergman A, Vermesh M, Ballard AC, Platt LD. Role of ultrasound in urinary incontinence. Urology 1989;33:443–444.

11. Bernascheck G, Spernol R, Wolf G. A comparative study of ultrasound and urethrocystography. Geburtshilfe Frauenheilkd 1981;41:339–342.

12. Brandt TD, Harrey N, Calenoff L, Greenberg M, Kaplan P, Nanninga J. Ultrasound evaluation of the urinary system in spinal chord injury patients. Radiology 1981;141:473–478.

13. Quinn MJ, Beynon J, McMortensen NUJ, Smith PJB. Transvaginal endosonography: a new method to study the anatomy of the lower urinary tract in urinary stress incontinence. Br J Urol 1988;62:414–417.

14. Carey M, Dwyer PL. Position and mobility of the urethrovesical junction in continent and stress incontinent women before and after successful surgery. Aust NZ J Obstet Gynaecol 1991;31:279–284.

15. Hol M, VanBolhuis C, Vierhout ME. Vaginal ultrasound studies of bladder neck mobility. Br J Obstet Gynaecol 1994;74:47–53.

16. Wise BG, Burton G, Cutner A, Cardozo L. Effect of vaginal ultrasound probe on lower urinary tract function. Br J Urol 1992;70:12–16.

17. Haylen BT, Frazer MI, Sutherst JR, West CR. Transvaginal ultrasound in the measurement of bladder volumes in women: preliminary report. Br J Urol 1989;63:152–154.

18. Iwamoto K, Kigawa J, Minagawa Y, Miura H, Terakawa N. Transvaginal ultrasonographic diagnosis of bladder wall invasion in patients with cervical cancer. Obstet Gynecol 1994;83:217–219.

19. Nishizawa O, Takada H, Sakamoto F. Combined urodynamic and ultrasonic techniques: a new diagnostic method for the lower urinary tract. Tohoku J Exp Med 1982;136:231–232.

20. Shapeero LG, Friedland GW, Perkash I. Transrectal sonographic voiding cystourethrography: studies in neuromuscular bladder dysfunction. Am J Radiol 1983;141:83–90.

21. Brown MC, Sutherst J, Murray A. Potential use of ultrasound in place of X-ray fluoroscopy in urodynamics. Br J Urol 1985;57:88–90.

22. Koelbl H, Bernaschek G. Cystosonography: a diagnostic adjunct for the staging of advanced gynecologic malignancies. Obstet Gynecol 1988;72:951–954.

23. Kirschner-Hermanns R, Klein HM, Muller U, Schaefer W, Jakse G. Intra-urethral ultrasound in women with stress incontinence. Br J Urol 1994;74:315–318.

24. Chancellor MB, Liu JB, Rivas DA, Karasick S, Bagley DH, Goldberg BB. Intraoperative endoluminal ultrasound evaluation of urethral diverticula. J Urol 1995;153:72–75.

25. Kohorn EI, Scioscia AL, Jeanty P. Ultrasound cystourethrography by perineal scanning for the assessment of female stress urinary incontinence. Obstet Gynecol 1986;68:269–272.

26. Koelbl H, Bernaschek G, Wolf G. A comparative study of perineal ultrasound scanning and urethrocystography in patients with genuine stress incontinence. Arch Obstet Gynecol 1988;244:39–45.

27. Gordon D, Pearce M, Norton P, Stanton S. Comparison of ultrasound and lateral chain urethrocystography in the determination of bladder neck descent. Am J Obstet Gynecol 1989;160:182–185.

28. Khullar V, Salvatore S, Cardozo LD, Hill S, Kelleher CJ. Three dimensional ultrasound of the urethra and urethral sphincter—a new diagnostic technique. Neurourol Urodyn 1994;13:352–354.

29. Koelbl H, Bernaschek G. A new method for sonographic urethrocystography and simultaneous pressure-flow measurements. Obstet Gynecol 1989;74:417–422.

30. Hanzal E, Joura EM, Häusler G, Koelbl H. Influence of catheterization on the results of sonographic urethrocystography in patients with genuine stress incontinence. Arch Gynecol Obstet 1994;255:189–193.

31. Koelbl H, Bernaschek G, Deutinger J. Assessment of female urinary incontinence by introital sonography. J Clin Ultrasound 1990;18:370–374.

32. Koelbl H. Ultraschalldiagnostik. In: Fischer W, Koelbl H, eds. Urogynäkologie in Praxis und Klinik. DeGruyter: Berlin, 1955:65–76.

CHAPTER 17

Clinical Neurophysiological Techniques in Urinary and Fecal Incontinence

J. Thomas Benson

Urinary and fecal storage and elimination processes are complex and involve the entire nervous system. Reflex interactions occur at local and spinal levels for "quasi-automatic" activity, and supraspinal levels of activity add the dimension of conscious control.

The basic unit of the nervous system is the nerve cell. The nerve cell is intended to last the lifetime of the organism in contrast to other cells such as the red blood cell, which lasts only for months. The nerve cell is dynamic, constantly reorganizing, restructuring, and regrowing to retain function. It is composed of a nerve cell body and a process (axon) that may be 5000 times as long as the nerve cell body. The chief function of the nerve cell is to transmit "signals" referred to as action potentials to an effector (e.g., muscle) or to another neuronal structure. The transmission within the nerve cell process is ionic (electrical), using protein "channels" in the axon membrane that allow passage of sodium, potassium, and chloride ions. This process is "all or none," whereas at the neuroeffector site or synapse, the transmission is chemical and graded, depending on neurotransmitters acting on receptors. The chemical agents acting as neurotransmitters and microtubules and neurofilaments used for axonal restructuring are synthesized in the nerve cell body, which is a very highly differentiated secretory cell with prominent nucleolus and rough endoplasmic reticulum (Nissl's). The axon lacks ribosomes and en-

doplasmic reticulum and cannot synthesize essential constituents. Therefore, a process of axonal transport from nerve cell body throughout the axon, acting both anterograde and retrograde, is vital for the nerve cell's function and survival. Any process that interferes with axonal transport will stop the axons ability to transmit action potentials.

The axon is surrounded by endoneurium (Fig. 17.1), which is largely composed of myelin, secreted by Schwann's cells in peripheral nerves and by oligodendrocytes within the spinal cord and brain. Evolutionary development has led to myelin sheaths around nerves with periodic interruptions of the myelin at nodes of Ranvier, where sodium channels are numerous. This allows increased rates of conduction without requiring massive size of nerves—so-called "saltatory conduction." Nerve sizes are dependent, then, on the degree of myelination and are functionally related to size, with action potential transmission faster in larger size nerves (Table 17.1). A collection of various sized axons surrounded by perineurium, a firm protective structure composed of alternating layers of epithelial cells and basement membranes, constitutes a nerve fascicle. Blood vessels supplying the axons traverse the perineurium at angles, subject to obstruction with nerve stretching. Groups of fascicles are surrounded by loose connective tissue, the epineurium, and constitute the nerve proper.

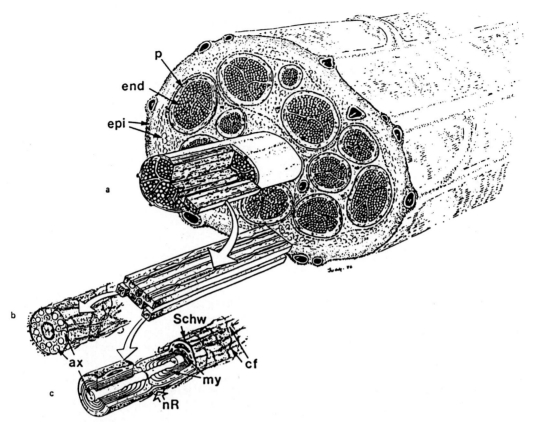

Figure 17.1. Microanatomy of a peripheral nerve trunk and its components. (**a**) Fascicles surrounded by a multilaminated perineurium (*p*) are embedded in a loose connective tissue, the epineurium (*epi*). The outer layers of the epineurium are condensed into a sheath (**b** and **c**) and illustrate the appearance of unmyelinated and myelinated fibers, respectively. *Sch,* Schwann cell; *my,* myelin sheath; *ax,* axon; *nR,* node of Ranvier. (From Lundburg G. Nerve injury and repair. New York: Churchill Livingstone, 1988.)

The nervous system is divided into the central nervous system, composed of spinal cord and brain, and the peripheral nervous system, composed of cranial and spinal nerves connecting the central system to the periphery. Peripheral nerves are formed by dorsal (sensory) and ventral (motor) nerve roots joining together near their exiting site of the vertebral column (Fig. 17.2).

The sacral peripheral nerves supplying the pelvis have features that are clinically significant, making them particularly vulnerable: the cauda equina, the pelvic plexus, and the pudendal nerves. The cauda equina is formed by descent of lumbosacral nerve roots from their origin in the spinal cord to their respective vertebral column exits. Such descent is caused by the spinal cord growing disproportionately to the vertebral column so that in the adult, the cord ends at about the first lumbar vertebra (Fig. 17.3). The roots of the cauda equina do not have the firm protection of the perineurium and are subject to traumatic disease. After the roots meet at the sacral exit foramina, they split into posterior rami, innervating episacral cartilaginous and ligamentous structures, and anterior rami. The anterior rami course around and through overlying muscle, forming the lowermost components of the lumbosacral plexus. Branches of the lumbosacral plexus meet with small visceral nerves and form the pelvic plexus. The pelvic plexus overlies and invests in the pelvic muscular floor, thus supplying pelvic floor muscles from a "superior" aspect, and surrounds and supplies the pelvic viscera. The pelvic plexus is subject to trauma from obstetric delivery or pelvic surgery.

The pudendal nerve is formed in the lower

division of the lumbosacral plexus. It leaves the pelvis through the greater sciatic foramen, wraps around the ischial spine, and is firmly invested in obturator fascia (Alcock's canal). It then courses back into the pelvis through the lesser sciatic foramen to provide muscular innervation to the pelvic floor from an "inferior" aspect. The area of fascial investment of the nerve locks it in place, subjecting it to stretch injury when the pelvic floor descends.

Therapies of neuronal dysfunctions are developing rapidly as knowledge of protein channels, neurotransmitters, and receptors increases. With increased availability of therapeutic intervention, diagnosis and localization of pathophysiological processes is assuming greater importance. The pathological entities interfering with pelvic neuronal processes are voluminous. To achieve diagnosis and localization of abnormality, a systemic approach may be used consisting of evaluating for somatic motor (efferent), somatic sensory (afferent), visceral motor, and visceral sensory activity with full real-

ization that most situations clinically are admixtures. Much of the information necessary for diagnosis may be obtained by careful history and physical examination. When necessary, this information may be supplemented by other measurements of somatic or visceral efferent or afferent activity including urodynamics, dynamic cystoproctography, anal manometry, and electrodiagnostic techniques, which are explained in this chapter.

Somatic Motor

Somatic motor nerves supply skeletal muscle, have their nerve cell body in the anterior gray matter of the spinal cord, and a single axon from each cell goes to the effector organ (muscle). Most skeletal muscles are supplied by a large motor axon from an alpha motor neuron cell that goes to extrafascial muscle fibers and a smaller axon from a "gamma" motor neuron cell that goes to intrafascial muscle fibers (spindles)

Table 17.1. Classification of Nerve Fibers

Sensory and Motor Fibers	Sensory Fibers	Largest Fiber Diameter	Fastest Conduction Velocity (m/s)	General Comments
A-α	Ia	22	120	Motor: The large alpha motoneurons of lamina IX, innervating extrafusal muscle fibers Sensory: The primary afferents of muscle spindles
A-α	Ib	22	120	Sensory: Golgi tendon organs, touch and pressure receptors
A-β	II	13	70	Motor: The motoneurons innervating both extrafusal and intrafusal (muscle spindle) muscle fibers Sensory: The secondary afferents of muscle spindles, touch and pressure receptors, and pacinian corpuscles (vibratory sensors)
A-γ		8	40	Motor: The small gamma motoneurons of lamina IX, innervating intrafusal fibers (muscle spindles)
A-δ	III	5	15	Sensory: Small, lightly myelinated fibers; touch, pressure, pain, and temperature
B		3	14	Motor: Small, lightly myelinated preganglionic autonomic fibers
C	IV	1	2	Motor: All postganglionic autonomic fibers (all are unmyelinated) Sensory: Unmyelinated pain and temperature fibers

THE PERIPHERAL NERVOUS SYSTEM

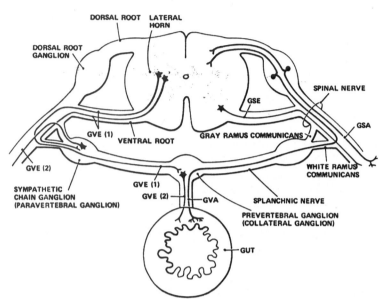

Figure 17.2. Functional components of a spinal nerve. General somatic afferent (GSA), general visceral afferent (GVA), and general somatic efferent (GSE) fibers and their origin are illustrated on the right and are arbitrarily separated, for clarity, from the general visceral efferent fibers and cells (GVE) (1) and (GVE) (2) on the left. The autonomic (GVE) structures diagrammed here belong to the sympathetic division. (From Gilman S, Gilman SW, eds. Manter and Gatz's essentials of clinical neuroanatomy and neurophysiology. Philadelphia: FA Davis, 1992.)

(Fig. 17.4). Using sensory axons, the spindles act in a "somatic muscle reflex" to control the muscle activity and "balance" antagonistic muscle action. The somatic motor supply to the urethral and anal sphincter skeletal muscle, however, is different. There are no spindles in the urethral sphincter and relatively few in the anal sphincter, so the segmental skeletal reflex system is supplemented by other reflex activities. The sphincters, unlike muscles with abundant spindles, have no antagonist muscle to limit "stretch." They have profuse connective tissue, and length-tension curves are steeper (i.e., the muscle is "stiffer"), perhaps because of the lack of antagonist.

The group of cell bodies in the spinal cord that give rise to the motor axons supplying the sphincters are collectively called "Onuf's nucleus." They are somewhat smaller than alpha anterior horn cells. Unlike other motoneurons, these sacral motoneurons have reciprocal inhibitory interactions with sacral parasympathetic neurons and receive input not only from somatic upper motor neuron pathways but also from the hypothalamus and other autonomic regions. They are also frequently less involved in disease processes affecting other anterior horn cells (e.g., amyotrophic lateral sclerosis or polio).

The sacral somatic motor activity of the pudendal nerve and somatic nerves through the pelvic plexus use acetylcholine as the chief neurotransmitter, acting via nicotinic receptors as do most of the body's skeletal muscles. However, there is increasing evidence of striated sphincter muscle having neuromuscular transmission by chemical processes usually seen only with smooth muscle. Hence, the sacral motoneurons have distinct properties, unlike other somatic motoneurons.

SOMATIC MOTOR NERVE PATHOLOGY

Nerve damage may occur at any point from the anterior horn cell to the root (radiculopathy), plexus (plexopathy), peripheral nerve (neuropathy), neuromuscular junction, or muscle fibers.

Anterior horn cell diseases typically do not involve Onuf's nucleus, reflecting the unique properties of these neurons.

Lumbosacral radiculopathies commonly involve bladder and bowel dysfunction. In fact, bladder and bowel involvement is a clinical marker to separate radiculopathy from anterior horn cell disease. The S2–4 nerve roots going to the pelvis originate in the small terminal portion of the spinal cord (conus medullaris) and constitute the central portion of the cauda equina. Conus medullaris lesions may be produced by ankylosing spondylitis, ependymomas, lipomas, dermoid cysts, transverse myelitis, arteriovenous malformations, and congenital meningomyelocele with cord tethering. It is a fairly common complication of abdominal aortic aneurysm surgery secondary to prolonged aortic clamping.

Cauda equina lesions are very common. Central disc protrusion can affect the bladder and bowel nerve roots, and many clinicians consider bladder and bowel involvement to be a chief indication for surgical treatment of disc protrusion. Cauda equina lesions are seen with congenital caudal aplasia (from diabetic mothers) and congenital and acquired spinal stenosis (pseudoclaudication syndrome). Ankylosing spondylitis, schwannomas, primary and metastatic malignancies, lymphomas, meningiomas, neurofibromas, chordomas, AIDS, and cytomegalovirus infection are other causes of cauda equina disease. Damage may also occur with distal aortic occlusive disease. Cauda equina lesions secondary to arachnoiditis are seen in episodic fashion, suggesting contamination of epidural agents. Arachnoiditis is also seen with injections of alcohol, phenol, or with very high dosages of intrathecal penicillin therapy. Diabetic lumbosacral radiculopathies most commonly involve the L3–4 roots and are bilateral in half of all cases. These may occur without evidence of diabetic peripheral neuropathy. Radiculopathy should

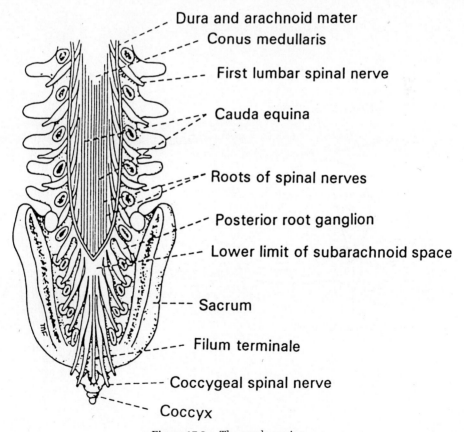

Dura and arachnoid mater
Conus medullaris
First lumbar spinal nerve
Cauda equina
Roots of spinal nerves
Posterior root ganglion
Lower limit of subarachnoid space
Sacrum
Filum terminale
Coccygeal spinal nerve
Coccyx

Figure 17.3. The cauda equina.

be considered before investigating visceral pathology in diabetics with chronic truncal pain. Patients with hereditary motor sensory neuropathies (type I) have increased vulnerability of the cauda equina.

Lumbosacral plexus lesions are most commonly associated with malignancies (cervical, rectal, lymphoma), radiation damage, or hematomas. EMG is useful in distinguishing plexopathy due to radiation from plexopathy due to recurrence of malignancy, as myokymia (see section on Needle EMG) may be seen with radiation damage.

Mononeuropathies occur frequently in pelvic nerves secondary to injury that may be mechanical, thermal, electrical, radiation, vascular, granulomatous, or from primary or metastatic neoplastic lesions. The leading cause of pelvic mononeuropathy is the mechanical effect (compression and stretching) of labor and delivery. Mechanical compressive nerve damage of permanent nature has been shown to occur with 80 mm Hg

pressure for 8 hours. Because second stage of labor forces normally reach maximums of 240 mm Hg pressure (1), it is not surprising to see nerve lesions. Stretch has been shown to cause nerve demyelination if the nerve is stretched 15% of its length (2). The pudendal nerve is stretched 15% with only 1.35 cm descent of pelvic floor during labor. Thus, pudendal stretch injury is also not surprising.

Pelvic nerve damage that is diffuse and bilaterally symmetric suggests polyneuropathy. Diabetes and alcoholism are likely the leading causes, but polyneuropathies may result from toxicity, metabolic deficiency, immune disorders, or hereditary diseases (Table 17.2). Generally, motor, sensory, and autonomic functions all are affected to some degree. Neuromuscular junction disorders (e.g., myasthenia gravis or myasthenic syndrome) typically have minor effects on sphincters.

Upper motor neuron lesions may have a

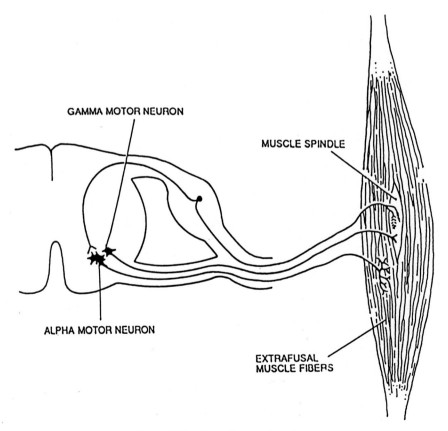

Figure 17.4. Somatic muscle reflex.

Table 17.2.   Motor > Sensory Polyneuropathy

Acromegaly
Acute inflammatory polyradiculoneuropathy
   (Guillain-Barré syndrome)
AIDS
Angiofollicular lymph node hyperplasia
Arsenic polyneuropathy
Carcinoma
Chronic inflammatory polyradicuoneuropathy
Cryoglobulinemia
Diphtheria
Glue sniffer's neuropathy
Hereditary neuropathy
Hypothyroidism
Leprosy
Lyme disease
Lymphoma
Monoclonal gammopathy
Motor neuron disease
Multiple demyelinating neuropathy with
   consistent conduction block
Osteosclerotic myeloma
Pharmaceuticals
   Amiodarone
   Perhexiline
   Suramin
   Lead
   Dapsone
   Didanosine
   Taxol
   Vincristine
Porphyria
Spinal muscular atrophy
Systemic lupus erythematosus
Ulcerative colitis
Waldenstrom's macroglobulinemia

profound effect on motor nerves to sphincters as well as on motor neurons to the bladder and bowel. Upper motor neuron control of lower motor neuron skeletal muscle activity is both stimulatory and inhibitory with the latter predominating. With loss of upper motor neuron control, there is exaggeration of skeletal muscle activity, reflected in increased reflexes. Urodynamically, increased skeletal activity with loss of coordination with visceral activity is typically seen with lesions below the integration center in the pons and is typified by contractions occurring in the sphincter skeletal muscles simultaneous with involuntary vesical contraction (detrusor sphincter dyssynergia). Cerebral lesions lead to loss of voluntary relaxation of sphincter skeletal activity; hence, a common symptom is hesitancy.

DIAGNOSIS OF SOMATIC MOTOR DYSFUNCTION

Somatic motor nerve loss as it reflects bladder or bowel function is related to skeletal muscle activity at the urethra or the anal canal. Rectal examination reveals a loss of "squeeze," but resting tone may be relatively normal because it is constituted chiefly (80%) by smooth muscle. Augmenting the physical examination is anal manometry, which can quantitate the squeeze pressure, and dynamic cystoproctography, which can demonstrate loss of puborectalis contraction effect on the anorectal angle. The typical history with pure somatic motor loss is inability to squeeze to prevent passage of flatus or liquid bowel content and an inability to squeeze to relocate solid content back into the rectal reservoir.

As for the bladder, loss of somatic motor activity in the urethra leads to symptoms of stress incontinence, and on urodynamics, typical diagnostic features of genuine stress urinary incontinence (vesical pressure exceeding urethral pressure during increased abdominal pressure in the absence of a detrusor contraction) may be seen. On physical examination, pelvic floor muscular weakness may be evident. Reflexes are helpful clinically for localization of lesions. Conus medullaris lesions have more symmetric bilateral loss of clitoral–anal reflex with S2–4 dermatomal sensory changes. Cauda equina lesions may demonstrate varying symmetry in sensory dermatome testing and clitoral–anal reflex and may have absent knee (L3–4) reflexes and hyperactive Achilles (S1) reflexes with higher lesions or loss of Achilles reflex with lower lesions.

Electrodiagnostic Features of S2–4 Somatic Motor Loss

The surface EMG (see section on EMG) reflects total muscle fiber activity, and as such gives information of total functioning mass when carefully standardized (Fig. 17.5).

Pudendal and perineal compound muscle action potentials (see section on Pudendal Nerve Motor Conduction) have reduced amplitude and prolonged distal latencies, reflecting the degree of axonal loss and demyelination, respectively. The changes are

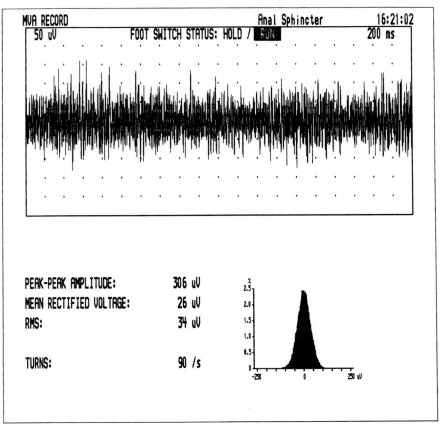

Figure 17.5. Maximum voluntary activity (MVA) with amplitude histogram of anal sphincter with squeeze. Peak-peak amplitude: amplitude from highest to lowest displayed point on trace. Mean rectified voltage: mean amplitude of rectified waveform. RMS: root mean square value of recorded trace. Turns: calculated number of peaks exceeding 100 μV normalized to equivalent time base of 1 second. Machine parameters: 200-ms time base, 50-μV gain, 10-kHz and 20-Hz high and low cut filters, respectively.

bilaterally symmetric with conus lesions, have variable bilaterality with cauda equina lesions, and are unilateral with peripheral mononeuropathies. Sensory conduction studies are normal with radiculopathies, even with clinical sensory loss, because the disease process is proximal to the dorsal root ganglion; hence, the distal axon (one being tested) is not affected (see Diagnosis of Somatic Sensory Dysfunction). In plexus or peripheral neuropathy, sensory studies are abnormal. Sphincter needle examination (see Needle EMG) acutely (0–7 days) shows reduced recruitment; at 7–15 days, insertional activity will increase and fibrillation begins to appear. After months, motor unit potential morphology reflects reinnervation by developing increased phases, duration, and amplitude. Those changes are related to the severity and the duration of the neuropathic process and hence are helpful adjuncts to determine prognosis.

Sacral Reflex Studies

Both clitoral–anal and urethral–anal reflex studies are abnormal with conus, cauda equina, or peripheral motor lesions, the abnormality being limited to the affected sides in unilateral radicular or peripheral nerve lesions. Pelvic plexus lesions may be suggested by abnormal urethral–anal reflex with normal clitoral–anal reflex.

Supportive evidence for somatic motor involvement with lumbosacral radiculopathy, plexopathy, or peripheral neuropathy is gained by performing lower extremity conduction studies (e.g., peroneal and tibial motor nerve conduction studies and sacral and peroneal sensory nerve conduction studies) and needle examination of lower extremity and lumbosacral paraspinal muscles. In fact, such studies are necessary to allow correct interpretation of the pelvic nerve studies.

Diagnosis of upper motor neuron lesions can be assisted electrodiagnostically by studying recruitment with needle EMG. Another important sign of upper motor neuron disorder is sacral reflex studies demonstrating loss of volitional abolition of the clitoral–anal and urethral–anal reflex during voiding.

Somatic Sensory

Sensory nerves have their nerve cell bodies outside the spinal cord proper, in the dorsal root ganglion. Embryologically, the dorsal root ganglion neurons, like autonomic ganglion neurons and adrenal medullaris cells, arise from the neural crest, whereas the spinal cord and cell bodies located within it arise from a separate location, the basal plate of the "neural groove." This partly explains certain disease processes and growth factors with an affinity for secretory and autonomic nerves.

The sensory nerve cell body gives rise to a single process that splits into a distal component going to the peripheral nerve and a proximal component entering and ascending in the spinal cord.

Peripheral nerves when injured have a capacity for repair, whereas nerves within the central nervous system have much less. Hence, the distal process of a sensory nerve may regenerate after injury, but if the proximal branch of the secretory nerve is damaged, it is capable of regeneration up to its junction with the central nervous system only.

SOMATIC SENSORY NERVE PATHOLOGY

Sensory effects are possible with involvement of the central nervous system conducting the impulses to the cerebral cortex, involvement of proximal axon of the sensory ganglion, such as with radiculopathy, involvement of the nerve cell (neuronopathy), or involvement of the distal axon by plexopathy or neuropathy. Hence, all of the condi-

tions affecting somatic motor axons beyond the central nervous system may also affect somatic sensory. Certain processes, however, have predilection for predominantly sensory neuronal and axonal involvement (Table 17.3). Of particular gynecological interest is paraneoplastic sensory involvement associated with ovarian cancer. If sensory nerve and cerebellar disease are present in patients demonstrating anti-Purkinje cell antibodies, 80% have ovarian cancer (3).

The type of sensory involvement relates to the nerve fibers affected. By physical size principles alone, larger fibers are more affected than smaller with focal peripheral nerve damage. Friedrich's ataxia, B_{12} deficiency, and occasionally subacute sensory neuropathies tend to produce large fiber loss, whereas predominantly small fiber loss is seen in hereditary sensory neuropathy (type I), diabetes, leprosy, amyloidosis, Tangier's and Fabry's disease, and congenital insensitivity to pain.

Table 17.3. Sensory Neuronopathy or Neuropathy

AIDS
Amyloidosis
B_{12} deficiency
Biliary cirrhosis
Crohn's disease
Drugs
    Cis platinum
    Vincristine
    Aromatic hydrocarbons
    Isoniazid
    Hydralazine
    Nitrofurantoin
    Metronidazole
    Misonidazole
    Pyridoxine toxicity
    Thalidomide toxicity
    Taxol
    Didanosine
    Zalcitibine
Fabry's
Friedreich's ataxia
Hereditary sensory neuropathy
Leprosy
Paraneoplastic
Porphyria
Reef fish poisoning
Spinocerebellar degeneration
Tangier's
Vasculitic neuropathy
Vitamin E deficiency

DIAGNOSIS OF SOMATIC SENSORY DYSFUNCTION

Somatic sensory loss to the urethra or anal canal results in the patient not recognizing passage of urine through the urethra or passage of material through the anal canal. The many physiological reflexes dependent on such somatic sensation are abnormal. The resulting clinical incontinence is difficult to treat, and surgery has disappointing results.

Physical examination may show sensory deficits in S2, S3 and S4 dermatome testing; such loss is not seen with pelvic plexus sensory neuropathy.

Adjuncts to diagnosis include anal manometry wherein the patient does not perceive filling of the anal canal balloon. Normally, rectal distention leads to internal anal sphincter relaxation by an intrinsic gut reflex, the rectal anal inhibitory reflex. This reflex is an intrinsic enteric reflex and tends to be preserved with most sensory neuropathies and lost principally with myenteric plexus loss as in Hirschsprung's disease. However, when somatic sensation is lost, there is a failure of the external anal sphincter to contract to replace content to the rectum for storage, and incontinence occurs without sensation. This can be demonstrated on anal manometry with concomitant surface and sphincter EMG. Likewise, when urine passes into the urethra (without attempt to void), reflex periurethral skeletal muscle activity occurs unless blocked centrally (as during urination). This reflex may be lost with somatic sensory loss.

Electrodiagnostic Adjuncts to Diagnosis for Somatic Sensory Loss

Clitoral–anal reflex testing includes determining the level of sensory perception of pudendal afferents para clitorally (see Clitoral–Anal Reflex). With complete sensory loss, the reflex is absent. Current perception threshold for different sensory nerve fiber types may also be performed.

If small fiber sensory afferents are affected, urethral–anal reflex may have elevated sensory threshold (see Urethral–Anal Reflex). If the visceral sensory pathway is still intact, the reflex will not be absent. With pure sensory loss, sphincter motor activity is preserved, and with surface or needle sphincter EMG, conscious regulation (e.g., suppressing activity by trying to void) remains intact without evidence of denervation, but reflex activity depending on the somatic sensory loop is absent. In conditions with clinical sensory loss, abnormalities of sensory nerve action potentials would be present if the process is at the dorsal root ganglion or distal. In radiculopathy, the sensory nerve function distal to the dorsal root ganglion cell body is preserved. Sacral reflexes may be completely normal in patients with complete loss of sensation if the lesion is above the conus medullaris. A generalized process will be suggested by abnormalities in other sensory studies (e.g., sural and superficial peroneal) or upper extremity nerve conduction studies.

Somatosensory evoked potentials (see Cortical Evoked Potentials) are useful in demonstrating and localizing disease process. If pelvic reflexes and the peripheral component of pudendal or posterior tibial evoked potential studies are normal with loss or delay in cervical or cerebral potentials, the disease process may be localized to the spinal cord or supraspinal areas.

Visceral Motor

The visceral motor or autonomic nervous system controls bladder and anorectal smooth-muscle activity. It exerts influences that are more continuous and generalized than the somatic system. The continuous "tonic" activity of visceral motor efferents is due to spontaneous discharge of reticular "pacemaker" neurons in the brainstem. The visceral motor system, unlike the somatic, is a two-neuron pathway with at least one synapse in the autonomic ganglia. It is separated morphologically and functionally into sympathetic and parasympathetic divisions. The preganglionic autonomic neurons occupy the visceral motor column of the cord (intermediolateral cell column), with sympathetic ones from T1 to L3 segments of the spinal cord and pelvic parasympathetic neurons from S2 to S4 segments. These neurons originate from the basal plate of the neural groove and use acetylcholine as principle neurotransmitters. They also synthesize nitric oxide and some release enkephalin or neurotensin. Their axons leave the cord as small myelinated fibers and synapse with autonomic ganglion neurons.

The autonomic ganglion neurons affect transmission of preganglionic inputs into postganglionic neurons and use acetylcholine with fast excitation (nicotinic receptors), slower excitation (muscarinic receptors), and late slow response mediated by neuropeptides (e.g., substance P). The postganglionic axons are unmyelinated and release acetylcholine (parasympathetic) or norepinephrine (sympathetic) and neuropeptides and ATP (purine) cotransmitters. Sympathetic postganglionic receptors are alpha and beta adrenergic. Postganglionic parasympathetic receptors are chiefly muscarinic.

Unlike skeletal muscle, smooth muscle cells have properties of automatism, adaptation, and intramural conduction. Automatism is the ability to sustain rhythmic contractions in the absence of innervation, adaptation is the ability to modify rhythmicity and contractility in response to mechanical factors (e.g., distention), and intramural conduction is the ability to transmit electrical inputs between syncytial fibers, usually by gap junctions. Whereas the main consequence of denervation in skeletal muscle is paralysis and atrophy, the main consequence of autonomic denervation is denervation supersensitivity, involving upregulation of postjunctional receptors. An excellent example of this is detrusor instability occurring as a consequence of postganglionic parasympathetic denervation.

There are basic functional differences in sympathetic and parasympathetic activity. The sympathetic responds to stress, is more diffuse, and effects have longer duration. The parasympathetic locally controls organs, and its effects are of shorter duration. Most organs have dual sympathetic and parasympathetic control, but the latter predominates in the lower urinary and gastrointestinal tracts.

Pelvic preganglionic sympathetic axons from L1 to L3 exit via ventral roots and pass by white rami communicants (white because they are myelinated) of the corresponding spinal nerve to reach the paravertebral chain. At this level, some run rostrally and caudally. Other synapse and postganglionic axons return to peripheral nerves via gray (unmyeli-nated) rami communicants and travel with the nerves, such as the pudendal and pelvic somatic nerves. Some pass through the paravertebral chain without synapsing to follow vessels (lumbar splanchnic nerves) to synapse on inferior mesenteric (presacral) ganglia that provide postganglionic input to hypogastric and pelvic plexuses to innervate pelvic and perineal organs and glands.

Preganglionic parasympathetic fibers arise from S2 to S4 spinal cord segments, exit via ventral roots, and join the pelvic plexus by direct branches (nervi erigentes) to synapse at the ganglia. The ganglia are located within the visceral walls, so postganglionic fibers are very short.

COLORECTAL EFFECTS

The smooth muscle of the gut has intrinsic (myogenic) and neuronal control. The intrinsic gut myogenic activity is coordinated with excitatory and inhibitory motoneurons for peristalsis control and with secretomotoneurons for gastrointestinal exocrine secretion. Generally, sympathetic activity, centered chiefly at the L3 and L4 cord levels, acts to reduce gut mechanosensitivity, except at the internal anal sphincter, where noradrenergic activity increases contractility.

The parasympathetic axons act throughout the gut to increase contractility (doing so through the vagus nerve for most of the gastrointestinal tract with S2–4 parasympathetic supply going to the descending colon and rectum). At the internal anal sphincter, however, parasympathetic activity promotes relaxation. Under sacral parasympathetic influence, colon compliance is promoted similarly to the parasympathetic effect on bladder compliance.

BLADDER EFFECTS

Sympathetic outflow to the bladder acts on alpha receptors to contract the outlet (especially in males, presumably to protect against retrograde ejaculation) and relax the detrusor, acting on beta receptors. Parasympathetic effects act to contract the detrusor. Sympathetic loss may lead to decreased proximal urethral smooth muscle "tone" and speculatively may have some association with loss of detrusor "relaxation." Parasympathetic effects are much more pronounced, leading frequently to loss of effective coordinated detrusor contraction (areflexia); hence, cystometric studies are of value. Coordination of bladder visceral efferent and somatic activity is chiefly a function occurring in the pons. Central nervous system lesions above the pons, then, are characterized by "coordinated" loss of control (uninhibited detrusor contractions), whereas those below the pons have detrusor sphincter dyssynergia.

VISCERAL MOTOR NERVE PATHOLOGY

There are generalized autonomic syndromes also involving bladder and bowel dysfunction. The most common neurological cause of detrusor areflexia is diabetes. Syndromes of "pure cholinergic dysfunction" exist characterized by bladder atony, Adies' pupil, alacrima, constipation, dry mouth, hyperpyrexia, cardiovagal failure, and impotency. Etiologies include Lambert-Eaton (myasthenia syndrome, frequently associated with malignancies) and neuromuscular junction toxicity from organic phosphates in insecticides or botulinus toxin in improperly canned food. In acute inflammatory demyelinating polyradiculoneuropathy (Guillain-Barré syndrome), urinary retention early in the course of the disease is an early predictor of severity as over 80% will require ventilatory assistance later (4). Acute intermittent porphyria is an autosomal dominant disease that generally presents in the third or fourth decade with premenstrual abdominal pain, constipation, voiding dysfunction, quadriparesis, and bathing trunk dysthesia. Generalized sympathetic disorders tend to be length dependent and are characterized by postural hypotension and overactivity early with cold sweaty feet and loss of activity later with red, swollen, anhidrotic distal extremities. Disease processes primarily affecting autonomic nerves are listed in Table 17.4.

DIAGNOSIS OF VISCERAL MOTOR DYSFUNCTION

Most nerve conduction and EMG studies evaluate large nerve fiber activity and hence may not be sensitive to small fiber autonomic dysfunction. When the autonomic process is generalized, quantitative testing is available.

Table 17.4. Predominantly Autonomic

Acute inflammatory demyelinating poly-
  radiculoneuropathy
Amyloid
Diabetes
Pandysautonomia
Paraneloplastin
Perhexiline
Porphyria
Riley-Day syndrome
Shy-Drager syndrome
Thallium
Vincristine

Distal small fiber neuropathy is frequently not associated with electrodiagnostic abnormalities but is associated with distal sudomotor abnormalities of either quantitative sudomotor axon reflex (QSART) (see Autonomic Tests) or the thermoregulatory sweat test in over 80% of cases (5).

Various tests of systemic vasoconstrictor (sympathetic) and cardiovagal (parasympathetic) function are available and helpful in generalized autonomic dysfunction.

The best available test of sacral parasympathetic function remains the cystometric study, and ambulatory cystometrics will improve the poor sensitivity of this test.

Visceral Sensory

Volume and tension receptors distributed throughout the bladder muscle wall are carried chiefly by the pelvic nerve to the sacral cord; bladder base pain receptors are in the submucosa and are carried by hypogastric nerve pathways to the L1–3 portion of the cord. Proximal urethral sensations are carried by both visceral afferent pathways, and sphincter muscle proprioception is also carried by pudendal pathways.

Enteric afferents are in submucosal plexus and mesenteric plexus. Splanchnic nerves carry enteric afferent input to the prevertebral ganglia that act to integrate local reflexes with the organs. The chief afferent neurotransmitters are vasointestinal polypeptide and acetylcholine with neurotensin (facilitating) and enkephalin (inhibiting) cotransmitters. The afferents course through the dorsal roots, directly through the sacral pelvic splanchnics or indirectly via white rami communicants to lumbar levels, to the nerve cell body. The nerve cell body, just as for somatic afferents, is located in the dorsal root ganglion.

The pelvic visceral afferents are A-delta and C fibers. Sensation of filling, fullness, desire to micturate, urgency, and pain can be elicited at different degrees of bladder filling. Anorectally, the ability to distinguish gas, liquid, and solid exists in addition. Most painful sensations are carried in the pelvic and not the hypogastric nerve, and frequency and urgency can be relieved by selective neurectomy of S3 (6). The sensation that micturition is imminent arises from the bladder neck. Sensory endings are often perivascular. Parasympathetic efferents can excite bladder afferent receptors similar to the way somatic gamma efferents excite muscle spindle afferents. Spinal transmissions of pelvic organ sensation is found in dorsal columns (1° afferents, touch, pressure), lateral columns (temperature, fullness, desire to micturate, sexual sensations), and ventral columns (pain, touch).

VISCERAL SENSORY PATHOLOGY

All neuropathic processes involving small sensory and autonomic nerves may lead to visceral afferent dysfunction. The most commonly involved process is diabetes.

DIAGNOSIS OF VISCERAL SENSORY DYSFUNCTION

History of Loss of Sensation with Anorectal or Urinary Tract Filling or Passage

Cystometric testing of the urinary tract may reveal delay of first sensation of filling or of maximum capacity. This is frequently associated with overflow incontinence. On anal manometry, loss of sensation with rectal balloon filling is noted until exaggerated levels may be seen. Mega colon or bladder may be seen on visual studies.

Electrodiagnostic Testing

Sacral reflexes and delay of sensation (increased threshold) with electrical stimuli may be seen when the proximal urethra is stimulated in the urethral–anal reflex test.

Clitoral–anal reflex is also tested to assist with cauda equina localization. If the reflex is present with normal latency, the sensory loss is assumed to be suprasacral. Evoked potentials from the proximal urethra can trace the sensory afferent pathway completely to the cortex.

Visceral afferent dysfunction may be part of a generalized picture of autonomic or peripheral neuropathy, and ancillary testing of the peripheral nerves and autonomic nerves may be helpful.

The Tests

EMG

EMG is the recording of electrical potentials generated by the depolarization of muscle fibers. In most skeletal muscles of the body, the muscle can be voluntarily relaxed to the point of absent electrical activity, but the sphincters are only electrically quiet during voiding.

Surface electrodes are of great value in pelvic function studies, recording skeletal muscle activity over a relatively large area. They are used to monitor voluntary muscle contraction during kinesiological studies such as with urodynamics or anal manometry. Surface electrodes are generally square or round metal plates made of platinum or silver and come in different sizes, most commonly 1 × 1 cm. Reduction of resistance between skin and electrode generally requires cleansing with alcohol and scraping the surface corneum and using electrode conductive cream. Surface electrodes are also used to record evoked compound nerve or muscle action potentials or to stimulate peripheral nerves. They are also used as reference or ground electrodes.

Surface electrodes may be applied to a Foley catheter to record or stimulate from the bladder base or proximal urethra. Various types of surface electrodes on anal plugs or vaginal "sponges" exist. Reproducibility and standardization requires use of specific types of electrodes, and electrode type and size is important to be included when establishing laboratory values. Quantification of surface EMG activity in the proximal urethra and anal canal in normal subjects is given in Table

17.5. This has been helpful in diagnosing patients with intrinsic sphincter deficiency (those patients who respond poorly to standard urethropexy therapy and may require sling or other management) as they typically have loss of urethral skeletal muscle activity. Quantification is more exact, however, if needle electrodes are used.

NEEDLE EMG

Placing a needle in a muscle has certain advantages over surface EMG recording. The source of the electrical activity is more certain and more sensitive testing is possible. Needle EMG can give information concerning denervation, reinnervation, upper and lower motor neuron function, and activity and time course of neurological disease. There are various types of needles, for example, monopolar, concentric, bipolar, macro, and single fiber, which vary in recording surface, pickup areas, and expense. Most studies today are done with concentric needles because data obtained tends to be more reliable with the fixed electrode, and newer disposable needles are arguably as comfortable and inexpensive as monopolar needles. Features studied with needle EMG include insertional activity, spontaneous activity, recruitment, and motor unit potential characteristics.

Insertional activity is the electrical activity created by movement of the needle through muscle fibers. Normally, this activity lasts less than 500 ms. This activity is increased in early denervation states and decreased in conditions of muscle degeneration and replacement with fatty or collagenous tissue.

Spontaneous activity occurs involuntarily. In most skeletal muscles at rest, there is absence of electrical activity except for "spontaneous" activity. Sphincter needle EMG studies are preceded by local applica-

tion (for 20 minutes) of lidocaine 2.5% and prilocaine 2.5% cream. The constant firing of activity in the sphincter makes spontaneous activity assessment more difficult but still possible with experience. Spontaneous activity can be normal or abnormal. Normal spontaneous activity is activity at the end plate of the muscle (area of nerve innervation) and is due to muscle fibers firing because the nerve terminal to that fiber is irritated. Abnormal spontaneous activity is composed of fibrillations, fasciculations, myotonia, myokymia, neuromyotonia, and complex repetitive discharges. There are distinctive patterns for each and fairly distinct associations of pathophysiological states with each. An example is a form of complex repetitive discharge (pseudomyotonia) seen in the urethral skeletal muscle in many cases of urinary retention.

The motor unit action potentials observed with activation of the muscle follow sequential patterns of increasing the rate of firing and acquiring additional motor units when the force of contraction is increased. The type of "recruitment" can be measured with needle EMG and follow generally distinctive patterns in normal, neurogenic, or myogenic disease states.

The motor unit action potentials reflect the electrophysiological "view" of the motor unit, which is defined as anterior horn cell, its axon, and all the muscle fibers innervated by that given axon. In disease states characterized by denervation, active "reinnervation" occurs, if possible, by adjacent axons sending spouts to reinnervate the denervated muscle fibers. This leads to different morphology of the existing motor unit that is reflected in the motor unit action potential viewed by the exploring needle. Quantifiable features of the motor unit action potential includes rise time (time for potential to go from extreme location positive or negative to the opposite, indicates proximity of the

Table 17.5. Sphincter Maximum Voluntary Activity in 12 Subjects Aged 35–65

	Peak-Peak (µV)	Mean Rectified Voltage	Root Mean Squared
EAS rest	96 ± 47 (41–191)	5 ± 4 (1–11)	8 ± 4 (3–17)
EAS squeeze	341 ± 165 (125–620)	25 ± 13 (9–40)	35 ± 17 (12–64)
Urethra rest	26 ± 10 (15–50)	2 ± 1 (1–3)	2 ± 1 (1–4)
Urethra squeeze	70 ± 40 (25–166)	6 ± 3 (1–13)	8 ± 5 (2–18)
Urethra rest (needle EMG)		9 ± 3 (6–4)	14 ± 4 (10–22)

Values are means ± SD with ranges in parentheses.

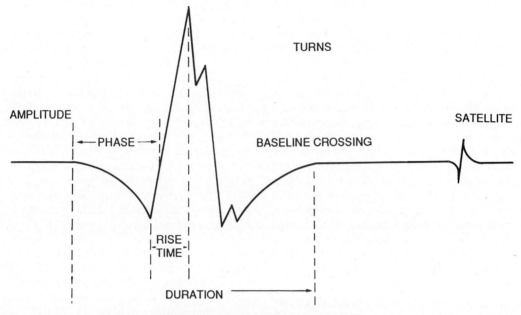

Figure 17.6. Motor unit action potential.

Table 17.6. **Automatic Decomposition Electromyelography of Sphincter Muscles in Asymptomatic Female Subjects Aged 33–45 (n = 10)**

	Urethral			Anal		
	Rest	Squeeze	Cough	Rest	Squeeze	Cough
Duration (ms)	5.6 ± 3.1	6.7 ± 3.9	4.8 ± 1.3	4.0 ± 1.7	4.7 ± 1.0	4.6 ± 1.5
Amplitude (ms)	58 ± 24	55 ± 16	54 ± 15	39 ± 19	49 ± 7	58 ± 16
Firing rate (Hz)	12.7 ± 10.5	11.1 ± 3.9	14.8 ± 7.5	27.1 ± 12.1	28.9 ± 12.1	19.2 ± 13.8

needle to the source of the electrical activity), amplitude, duration, and number of phases (Fig. 17.6).

The conversion of analog to digital needle examination data and the availability of low-cost fast microcomputers are leading to the development of automated techniques of evaluating motor unit action potentials. These techniques have the possible benefits of examining later acquired potentials (those present with increased muscle force); reducing examiner bias; and improving accuracy, reliability, and result comparisons. Automatic decomposition electromyography is one such method developed by Dorfman et al. (7). Using this methodology, we found the data on sphincter studies in volunteer subjects as presented in Table 17.6. These techniques are as yet problematic, but the potential for development of objective testing with much more uniform application is great.

Needle EMG shows some abnormality virtually anytime there is an organic component of neuromuscular disorder that is significant enough to be symptomatic. Besides urethral and anal sphincters, other pelvic floor muscles (e.g., puborectalis and pubococcygeus) may be examined. Because nerve supply to the puborectalis and external anal sphincter varies, we found it clinically helpful to select the "healthiest" portion of the anal sphincter closure mechanism to use in sphincter repair. Previously performed needle EMG "mapping" of the external anal sphincter has now been replaced by anal ultrasound.

NERVE CONDUCTION STUDIES

Nerve conduction studies can test the integrity of a nerve, the integrity of the muscle supplied by the nerve, and the integrity of the neuromuscular junction. Neuropathies may be categorized as focal or diffuse, root, plexus, nerve, branch, or neuromuscular junction. Time course (e.g., acute, subacute, or chronic) can be depicted and fiber type involvement (e.g., sensory, motor, or autonomic) can be suggested. Lower extremity nerve conduction studies are performed in conjunction with pelvic floor studies because status of the cauda equina, lumbosacral plexus, and generalized neuropathy (which is typically length dependent) are all in part measurable with such studies. Furthermore, interpretation of the pelvic nerve studies must be in the context of the given patient's general neuronal status. Hence, peroneal motor and sensory studies, tibial motor studies, and sural sensory studies are useful as screens when evaluating pelvic neuronal status with pudendal studies.

PUDENDAL NERVE MOTOR CONDUCTION

The pudendal nerve can be stimulated at the level of the ischial spine. Such stimulation may be performed with probes or with electrodes attached to the examiners finger tip. The latter is preferred because the ischial spine may be located more comfortably and reliably if the examiner has the feedback from the finger. The St. Mark's disposable electrode (Fig. 17.7) provides an excellent vehicle for fingertip stimulation of the pudendal nerve. The response to the pudendal nerve stimulation is recorded by 9-mm silver chloride electrodes placed 1 cm lateral (G1) and 1 cm posterior (G2) to anal opening when testing the inferior hemorrhoidal branch of the pudendal nerve or by electrodes on the Foley catheter when recording the perineal (urethral) branch of the pudendal nerve. The resulting waveform obtained is a compound muscle action potential (CMAP) and measurable quantities include latency, amplitude area, and wave form (Fig. 17.8). The latency reflects the time involved for nerve conduction from the ischial spine to the muscle, the transmission across the neuromuscular junction, and the resulting muscle fiber contractions, summating to form the CMAP. The latency is somewhat prolonged with loss of large fast conducting axons but even more influenced by processes of demyelination. The latency itself correlates little with strength and hence with clinical muscle

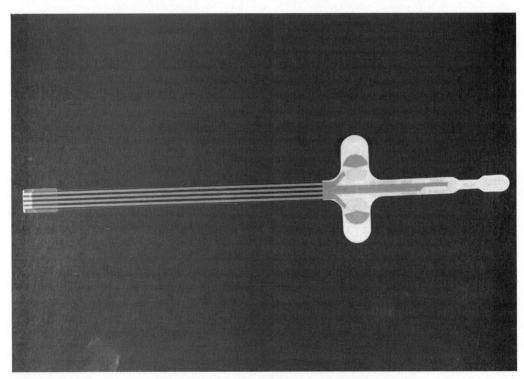

Figure 17.7. St. Mark's pudendal electrode.

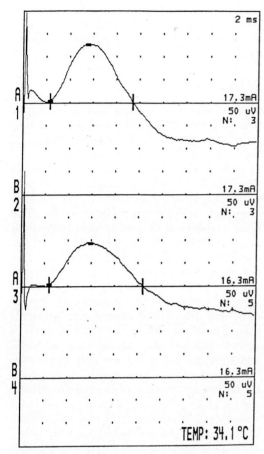

Figure 17.8. Compound muscle action potentials with pudendal nerve stimulation (pudendal nerve terminal motor latency study). **A1,** Right pudendal stimulation and right anal recording; **A3,** left pudendal stimulation and left anal recording. Machine parameters: 2-ms time base, 50-µV gain, 0.05-ms pulse duration, 1-Hz repetition rate, 10-kHz and 10-Hz high and low cut filters, respectively.

Table 17.7. Comparison of Pudendal Motor Nerve Conduction Methodologies in 12 Female Subjects Aged 34–46

	Standard - St. Mark's[a]	Modified Methodology[b]
Latency (ms)		
Mean ± SD	2.1 ± 0.3	2.2 ± 0.4
Range	1.5–2.7	1.6–2.9
Interrater variability (%)	4	1
Amplitude (µV)		
Mean ± SD	432 ± 160	99 ± 44
Range	190–760	34–182
Interrater variability (%)	34	1

[a]Stimulation site, ischial spine via rectal approach. Recording, electrodes at base of examiner's finger.
[b]Stimulation site, ischial spine via vaginal approach. Recording, paraanal surface electrodes.

force. The amplitude reflects maximal stimulation, wherein the amount of stimulation of the nerve is increased to the level where no further increases in amplitudes of the CMAP is obtainable. The amplitude is related to the total axonal content of the nerve and hence has more relationship clinically with resulting muscle strength. Most processes involving nerve damage have both demyelination and axonal loss so latency and amplitude have considerable but not invariable direct relationship.

Most pudendal nerve conduction studies in the literature have used latency as the principal determinant, whereas amplitude is

more meaningful. The problem has been one of reproducibility. The standard St. Mark's pudendal technique involves stimulating the nerve at the ischial spine intrarectally, and the pickup electrodes at the base of the examiner's finger records the activity of the external anal sphincter (EAS). Interobserver latency determinations have been consistent, but amplitude observations have been variable (Table 17.7). This is apparently due to variations in location of the recording electrode relative to the EAS, depending on the examiners finger size. With standard positioning of the recording electrodes on paraanal skin, much more consistency in amplitude has been gained, allowing this valuable parameter to be useful clinically.

Another great advantage of this technique modification is that the nerve can now be stimulated vaginally instead of rectally, a comfortable alternative for most women. The pudendal conduction study has other limitations. Conduction blocks cannot be determined because of the inability to stimulate the nerve above and below a possible lesion. Sacral root stimulation can be accomplished, but it is difficult to know in any given patient that total pudendal root supply has been adequately stimulated. Obtaining proximal motor nerve values by F waves (recording "rebound" motor axon potentials occurring by impulse traveling to the anterior horn cell and returning to the muscle being recorded) is difficult technically because the short section of nerve under study prevents recording of the rebound event.

Another limitation of pudendal nerve studies is failure, in many studies, to use age-matched control values. Pudendal motor terminal latencies have age-related normal values, apart from the effects of parity (Table 17.8).

Despite these limitations, pudendal nerve conduction studies provide an important and helpful determinant that when used in conjunction with other parameters can be very helpful in increasing understanding of pelvic neuropathy.

Obtaining sensory nerve conduction studies on the pudendal nerve has been technically very difficult.

Current perception threshold studies represent another modality of sensory testing. This test is performed by applying surface electrodes and delivering stimuli at 2 KHz, 250 Hz, and 5 Hz. The relative amount of constant current allowing perception of the stimuli is determined. Normal data have been collected for stimulation of the pelvic floor (Table 17.9).

SACRAL REFLEXES

Sacral reflexes are reflex contractions of striated muscle structures of the pelvic floor, occurring in response to stimulation of the perineum or other pelvic visceral sites. The two used most commonly in our laboratory are the clitoral–anal and urethral–anal reflexes.

Clitoral–Anal Reflex

This reflex may be obtained clinically by touching the clitoral region with a cotton swab and observing contraction in the external anal sphincter. Approximately 10% of neurologically normal females do not have the reflex clinically, although it is present with electrodiagnostic testing, a method first suggested by Rushworth in 1967 (8). The reflex tests the afferent and efferent pudendal nerve pathways and hence the roots of the cauda equina and the conus medullaris. The reflex has two components, the first occurring at a 30- to 50-ms latency and the second at 60–70 ms. Hence, the response is polysynaptic with the second component representing suprasacral reflexes. In some normals, a paired stimulus may be required, with the test stimulus applied 5 ms after the conditioning stimulus. The response is recorded by the anal electrodes as described for pudendal nerve terminal motor latency study (see section on this technique) and may selectively be recorded on the left and right sides. Stimulation likewise may be done on either the left or right side of the clitoris. Single

Table 17.8. Normative Data for Pudendal Motor Nerve Conduction Studies

	Pudendal Motor Terminal Latency (ms)	Perineal Motor Terminal Latency (ms)
Subjects (*n* = 20) nulliparous, ages 16–30 (mean 23)	2.0 ± 0.3 (1.4–2.4)	2.3 ± 0.3 (1.7–2.9)
Subjects (*n* = 13) nulliparous, ages 35–65 (mean 46)	2.3 ± 0.4 (1.5–3.5)	2.4 ± 0.4 (1.7–3.8)
Amplitude (µV)	92 ± 51 (34–182)	155 ± 127 (21–466)
Subjects (*n* = 28), parous, ages 35–66 (mean 43)	2.3 ± 0.4 (1.8–3.3)	2.6 ± 0.4 (2.0–3.1)
Amplitude (µV)		52 ± 27 (26–99)

Table 17.9. Perineal Current Perception Thresholds in 15 Subjects Aged 23–57

Sensory Nerve Fiber Type	Stimulus Frequency	Right Paraclitoral[a]	Left Paraclitoral[a]	Right Paraanal[a]	Left Paraanal[a]
Aβ	2kHz	1.62 ± 0.38 (1.08–2.33)	1.75 ± 0.34 (1.13–2.23)	1.42 ± 0.44 (0.53–2.08)	1.13 ± 0.36 (0.58–1.88)
Aδ	250Hz	0.34 ± 0.19 (0.08–0.63)	0.41 ± 0.23 (0.13–0.98)	0.40 ± 0.18 (0.08–0.58)	0.40 ± 0.20 (0.03–0.78)
C	5Hz	0.19 ± 0.15 (0.03–0.58)	0.20 ± 0.13 (0.05–0.48)	0.25 ± 0.17 (0.07–0.58)	0.29 ± 0.28 (0.03–0.93)

[a]Values are means ± SD with ranges in parentheses.

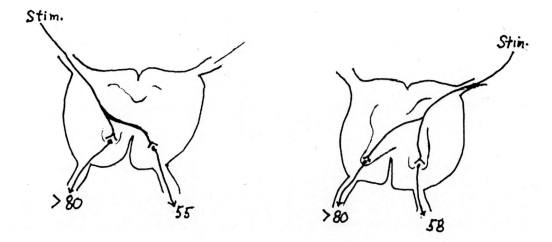

Lateralization Study of Clitoral Anal Reflex

Herniated disc L4-L5 compressing right motor (anterior) roots.

Stimulate at sides of clitoris.

Response with concentric needle at 3 o'clock (left) and 9 o'clock (right) anal sphincter.

Figure 17.9. Surface electrodes (instead of concentric needle).

responses are recorded and compared because averaging works poorly due to slight variability in response latency. Localized lesions may be indicated as being either afferent or efferent and right or left (Fig. 17.9). This reflex is suppressed during voiding. Failure of such suppression has been found to be highly sensitive in detecting spinal cord lesions above the sacral level (9).

The intensity of stimulation used for the response is three to four times the intensity at perception threshold, which is generally less than 9 mA of constant current stimulation.

Urethral–Anal Reflex

Using a catheter mounted ring electrode for stimulation, a reflex response may be obtained at the right and left external anal sphincter with repeated single epochs of stimulation as with the clitoral–anal reflex response. This technique is termed "urethral electromyelography" by Bradley (10). This reflex has a long latency of 60–90 ms because the very proximal urethral response is carried by small myelinated or unmyelinated pelvic and hypogastric nerves and the path-

way is multisynaptic. The sensory threshold for this reflex is generally less than 13 mA, and the reflex usually requires a stimulus intensity three times the sensory threshold. The reflex is suppressed during voiding, and this is useful as a test of upper motor neuron function. Disease processes involving the proximal urethral afferent nerves or the pelvic plexus may have abnormal urethral–anal reflex activity, and this test has been found to be a sensitive electrodiagnostic test for patients with voiding dysfunction after radical pelvic surgery (see Table 17.10).

CORTICAL EVOKED POTENTIALS

Any type of synchronizable stimulus reaching the cortex can be studied electrophysiologically. With electrodes at the scalp or over the spinal columns, potentials representing the algebraic summation of electrical activity that is "time-locked" to a select stimulus delivered via a predetermined sensory pathway are recorded. The evoked potentials are very small and can only be separated from random electrical "noise" in the body by the computer process of "averaging."

Table 17.10. Electrodiagnostic Test Results in Patients With Voiding Dysfunction After Radical Hysterectomy

	Age (y)	PNTML (ms)		PeNTML (ms)		Urethral Anal Reflex (ms)		Urethral Sensory Threshold (ms)	Clitoral Anal Reflex (ms)		Lt Clitoral Anal Reflex		Rt Clitoral Anal Reflex		Clitoral Sensory Threshold		Needle EMG Anal Sphincter	Needle EMG Urethra
		Rt	Lt	Rt	Lt	Rt	Lt		Rt	Lt	Rt	Lt	Rt	Lt	Rt	Lt		
Pt 1	39	2.1	2.4	NR*	NR*	NR*	NR*	>100mA*	40	40	40	40	50	60	6.3	6.3	Normal	CRD*
Pt 2	50	2.2	NR*	NR*	NR*	226*	NR*	>100mA*	93	NR*	93	NR*	56	NR*	11.8*	11.8*	L. Abn*	CRD*
Pt 3	52	2.3	2.6	3.6*	3.6*	63	78	9.4	55	72	55	72	48	69	5.5	6.3	Normal	Reinnervation*
Pt 4	32	3.0*	3.3*	2.8	3.4*	NR*	NR*	>100mA*	81*	66*	81*	66*				7.1	Normal	Reduced insertional*
Pt 5	40	3.1*	2.7	2.7	NR*	NR*	NR*	8.6	61*	67*	61*	67*				5.5		CRD*

PNTML, pudendal nerve terminal motor latency; PeNTML, perineal nerve terminal motor latency; NR, no response; CRD, complex repetitive discharge; *, abnormal.

Hundreds or even thousands of stimuli must be averaged for the specific time-locked response to be recorded. The evoked potentials have early cortical peaks (40 ms or less) produced from large diameter afferent sensory impulses traveling rostrally through ipsilateral spinal dorsal columns, synapsing at cervicomedullary and ventroposterolateral thalamic nuclei, and activating contralateral primary somatosensory cortex organized in accordance with the classical homunculus. Later responses (over 70 ms) embody smaller diameter nerve fibers ascending via anterolateral columns. The lower extremity and the pudendal and bladder afferents activate medial regions of the contralateral hemisphere; hence, recording electrodes are best placed in the midline with an electrode at the nasion (Fz site) and one just posterior to the scalp vertex (Cz1). The ground may be placed over the chin or elsewhere between stimulus and response. Recording is done over the spinal column with one electrode over L1 vertebra and the second over the iliac crest or alternatively over L5 vertebra. This arrangement produces a response at the area where the impulses reach the spinal cord and represents the "peripheral" component of the evoked potential test. The "central" component, then, is represented in the impulse transmission from the cord to the cortex.

PUDENDAL NERVE SOMATOSENSORY EVOKED POTENTIAL

The stimulus may be applied to right or left clitoral region with the anode lateral and cathode adjacent to the clitoris. Three times the sensory threshold current is applied and must be at a comfortable level. The patient must be totally relaxed with eyes closed. Resistance at recording electrodes must be below 3 kΩ; hence, very careful skin preparation is necessary. The pudendal nerve afferents at this region are cutaneous sensory only, and achieving reproducible responses over the spinal cord is not usually possible in women, but cortical responses are reliably obtainable. If the pudendal nerve is stimulated at the ischial spine, where muscle afferents are also present, more reproducible spinal column potentials are recordable. The latency to the cortex generally occurs with the first positive peak deflection be-

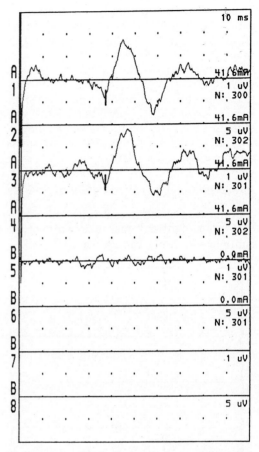

Figure 17.10. **A1,** Cortical evoked potential from left pudendal (clitoral branch) stimulation with marker at 37 ms. **A3,** Response replicated. **B5,** Control series without stimulation. Machine parameters: 10-ms time base, 1-μV gain, 0.1-ms pulse duration, 2.5-Hz repetition rate, 1.5-kHz and 3-Hz high and low cut filters, respectively.

tween 35 and 43 ms, a value very similar to the somatosensory evoked potential when stimulating the posterior tibial nerve at the ankle (Fig. 17.10). In view of the much longer distance traveled by impulses with ankle stimulation, the similar cortical latencies are theorized to represent somewhat slower cord conduction of pudendal afferents relative to tibial nerve afferents.

PROXIMAL URETHRAL EVOKED POTENTIALS

Stimulating via a ring electrode on a Foley catheter (see Pudendal Nerve Motor Conduction) can produce recordable potentials over the scalp, using the same electrode placement as with pudendal somatosensory evoked potentials. The latency is longer (around 50 ms to the first positive peak), suggesting that only visceral afferents are stimulated by this method. The responses are very small (Fig. 17.11), and absence may be of uncertain clinical significance because such absence may well be technical. However, obtaining a response with normal latency is very valuable in excluding a subpontine neurogenic bladder disorder (11).

Interpretation of Evoked Potential Studies

Comparing absolute and interpeak latencies to standardized data or to uninvolved contralateral study can be used to localize

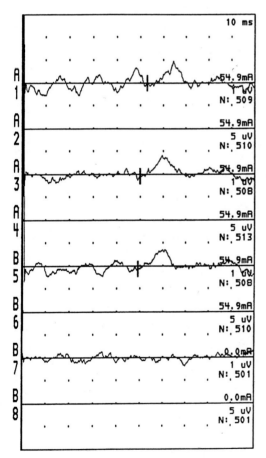

Figure 17.11. A1, Cortical evoked potential from bladder base stimulation with marker at 53 ms. **A3,** Response replicated with marker at 50 ms. **B5,** Response replicated with marker at 49 ms. **B7,** Control series without stimulation. Machine parameters: 10-ms time base, 1-μV gain, 0.1-ms pulse duration, 2.5-Hz repetition rate, 1.5-kHz and 3-Hz high and low cut filters, respectively.

problems causing conduction delay, whereas amplitude variations can reflect loss of axonal content. Careful analysis is required, and a study should never be considered abnormal without knowing the state of the peripheral nervous system. Hence, evoked potential studies may suggest peripheral neuropathy, demyelinating disease, radiculopathies, cortical disorders, or other myelopathies (cord disorders) presenting with visceral or sphincter dysfunction.

AUTONOMIC TESTS

Most electrophysiological testing evaluates larger fiber nerve activity. Tests selective for the small myelinated or unmyelinated autonomic nerves include QSART, sympathetic skin response, orthostatic blood pressure (BP) and heart rate (HR) responses to tilt, HR response to deep breathing and beat to beat BP responses to Valsalva maneuver, tilt, and deep breathing.

QSART

Acetylcholine is iontophoresed into skin, and the impulse travels antidromically to a branch point and then orthodromically to release acetylcholine from the nerve terminal. At the terminal, neuroglandular transmission and binding to muscarinic receptor on eccrine sweat glands evokes a sweat response that ceases secondary to acetylcholinesterase activity in subcutaneous tissue. The recordable response has latency of 1–2 minutes, returning to baseline in 5 minutes, and sites are standardized (foot, proximal and distal leg, and forearm). Excessive or persistent responses is often seen in painful neuropathies and florid reflex sympathetic dystrophy (12). Absent response indicates failure of postganglionic sympathetic sudomotor axon and is length dependent so that distal anhidrosis is commonly seen in peripheral neuropathies. A present reflex with anhidrosis present with core temperature rise suggests preganglionic lesions occurring anywhere along the sympathetic efferent neuraxis.

Sympathetic Skin Response

A suprabulbar somatosympathetic reflex may be recorded in response to stimuli (e.g.,

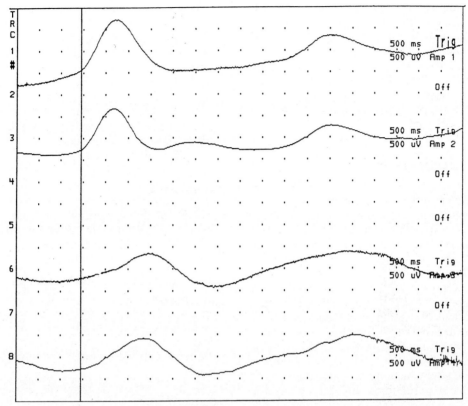

Figure 17.12. Sympathetic skin responses (SSR) at 1440 ms after single stimulation to right hand at 23 mA. *Trace 1,* SSR from right perineum. *Trace 2,* SSR from left perineum. *Trace 6,* SSR from right foot. *Trace 8,* SSR from left foot. Machine parameters: 500 ms, 500 μV, 0.1-ms pulse duration, 100-Hz and 0.2-Hz high and low cut filters, respectively.

electrical), a loud noise, or skin stroking. The source of the response is electrical activity in sweat glands. Typically recorded over palms or soles, it can also be recorded over the perineum (Fig. 17.12). The test correlates with QSART, although it is not as sensitive. The variability of the test precludes its general use clinically.

Systemic Vasoconstrictor Function

During upright tilt, normal individuals undergo transient reduction in BP, recovering within 1 minute. Patients with adrenergic failure have more reduction and less recovery.

HR Response to Deep Breathing. Afferent and efferent pathways are vagal. A Valsalva ratio, the maximal HR divided by the minimal HR response within 30 seconds of the peak HR, may be obtained while the patient is undergoing controlled Valsalva expiration. The ratio primarily reflects cardiovagal function but is also dependent on cardiac sympathetic function.

Response to Standing. Upon standing, resultant tachycardia occurs that is maximal at the 15th heart beat after standing and relative bradycardia around the 30th beat. The RR interval at beat 30 divided by the RR interval at beat 15 can be used as an index of cardiovagal function.

Autonomic testing is indicated when distal small fiber neuropathy is suspected or when generalized autonomic disorders including postural hypotension, sympathetically maintained pain, or bladder and bowel dysfunction is present.

BETHANECHOL TEST FOR VESICAL DENERVATION

A cystometrogram (CMG) (gas filling acceptable) is recorded as a baseline control, recording pressure, and volume at 100 mL. Bethanechol chloride 0.03 mg/kg is injected subcutaneously and postinjection CMGs are collected at 10, 20, and 30 minutes, performed in the same manner as the control CMG. A positive test is an intravesical pressure increase of > 15 cm H_2O over the control CMG at 100-mL bladder volume.

Conclusions

Bladder and bowel dysfunction can accompany neuromuscular disease, metabolic problems, and orthopedic difficulties. With increasing willingness to discuss and seek help for such problems, associated with a vast improvement in therapeutic choices, there is more need for thorough evaluation. Information derived from clinical neurophysiological testing is unique in that it relates to function. It therefore acts complementary to imaging studies so that clinical decisions regarding treatment of anatomic disorders may be more properly made.

Patients particularly helped by electrophysiological testing include those being evaluated for anal sphincter repair, those with voiding disorders, detrusor sphincter dyssynergia, overflow incontinence, stress incontinence (especially where intrinsic sphincter deficiency is suspected), spinal myelopathies, peripheral or autonomic neuropathies, diabetics with bladder or bowel symptoms, pelvic floor trauma from childbirth or other, sacral injuries, and patients with unexplained perineal numbness or pain or with failure of diagnosis on standard evaluations for bladder or rectal dysfunction.

Algorithm for Pelvic Neurology Study

BASELINE

Lower Extremity Motor

Peroneal nerve: response at extensor digitorum brevis (EDB) or tibialis anterior if EDB

is absent. Stimulate ankle, knee, and F waves.

Tibial nerve: response at abductor halluces brevis with stimulation at ankle, knee, and F waves.

Lower Extremity Sensory

Sural nerve sensory action potential: superficial peroneal sensory or other sensory nerves if sural absent.

Needle EMG

Pelvic girdle, paraspinal, and extremity muscles if indicated by physical findings and/or nerve conduction studies.

SOMATIC MOTOR ABNORMALITIES

Anal–Rectal

Manometry with rectal–anal inhibitory reflex.

Balloon expulsion test for constipation disorders.

Imaging

Ultrasound for sphincteroplasty.

Dynamic cystoproctography for pubococcygeus function.

External anal sphincter surface EMG—resting and maximum voluntary activity.

Pudendal (inferior hemorrhoidal) motor conduction study—latency, amplitude.

Clitoral–anal reflex: latency, suppressibility, threshold.

Needle EMG anal sphincter, puborectalis, and pubococcygeus if clinically indicated.

Urethral

Manometry: cystometrics with urethral lead for pressure and surface EMG.

Urethral pressure profile and/or leak point pressures.

Urethral surface EMG—resting and maximum voluntary activity.

Perineal motor conduction study—latency, amplitude.

Sacral reflexes

Urethral–anal: threshold, latency, suppressibility.

Clitoral–anal: threshold, latency, suppressibility.

Needle EMG: periurethral skeletal muscle.

SOMATIC SENSORY ABNORMALITIES

Anal–Rectal

Rectal and anal canal balloon distention test.

Manometry with rectal–anal inhibitory reflex testing.

If mixed nerve (motor and sensory) abnormality suspected, repeat motor algorithm for motor.

Clitoral–anal reflex: threshold, latency, suppressibility.

Current perception threshold: paraanal.

Pudendal and/or posterior tibial somatosensory evoked potentials.

Urethral

Cystometrics: includes urethral pressure profile and surface EMG.

If mixed nerve (motor and sensory) abnormality is suspected, repeat motor algorithm for motor sacral reflexes.

Clitoral–anal: threshold, latency, suppressibility.

Urethral–anal: threshold, latency, suppressibility.

Current perception threshold: paraclitoral.

Proximal urethral evoked potentials: if abnormal or if unobtainable, pudendal somatosensory evoked potentials.

VISCERAL MOTOR

Anal–Rectal

If clinical indications are present:
  Balloon expulsion test.
  Dynamic proctography.
  Anal manometry with rectal-anal inhibitory reflex.
  Colon transit studies.
Sacral reflexes
Urethral–anal: threshold, latency, suppressibility.
Clitoral–anal: threshold, latency, suppressibility.
Autonomic studies added adjunctively if clinically indicated.

Lower Urinary Tract

Cystometry study, voiding study.

Bethanechol stimulation test if no detrusor contraction on urodynamics.

Sacral reflex

Urethral–anal: threshold, latency, suppressibility.

Clitoral–anal: threshold, latency, suppressibility.

Autonomic tests added adjunctively if clinically indicated.

VISCERAL SENSORY

Anal–Rectal

Visceral motor studies plus balloon distention studies.

Evoked potential studies.

Pudendal and/or posterior tibial.

Paraanal current perception threshold studies plus urethral evoked potentials.

Sacral reflexes.

Lower Urinary Tract

Visceral motor studies plus urethral evoked potentials.

Paraclitoral current perception threshold.

Sacral reflexes.

REFERENCES

1. Rempen A, Kraus M. Measurement of head compression during labor. J Perinatal Med 1991;19: 115–120.
2. Lundberg G. Nerve injury and repair. New York: Churchill Livingstone, 1988:54.
3. Hetzel DJ, Stanhope CR, O'Neill BP, Lennon VA. Gynecologic cancer in patients with subacute cerebellar degeneration predicated by antipurkinje cell antibodies. Mayo Clinic Proc 1990; 65:1558–1563.
4. Ropper AH, Wijdicks EFM, Truaz BT. Guillain-Barré syndrome. Contemporary Neurology Sciences. Philadelphia: FA Davis, 1991.
5. Stewart JD, Low PA, Fealey RD. Distal small fiber peripheral neuropathy: results of tests of sweating and autonomic cardiovascular reflexes. Muscle Nerve 1992;15:661–665.
6. Torens MJ, Hald T. Bladder denervation procedure. Urol Clin North Am 1979;6:283–284.
7. Dorfman LJ, Howard JE, McGill KC. Influence of ADEMG analysis. J Neurol Sci 1988;86:125–136.
8. Rushworth G. Diagnostic value of the electromyographic study of reflex activity in man. Electro-

encephalogr Clin Neurophysiol 1967;25(suppl): 65–73.

9. Dyro FM, Yalla SV. Refractoriness of urethral striated sphincter during voiding: studies with afferent pudendal reflex arc stimulation. J Urol 1986;135:732–736.

10. Bradley WE. Urethral electromyelography. J Urol 1972;108:563–564.

11. Fowler CJ. Methods in clinical neurophysiology. Denmark: Dantec Elektronik, 1991:1–17.

12. Low PA. Autonomic nervous system function. J Clin Neurophysiol 1993;10:14–27.

CHAPTER 18

Pad Testing, Nursing Interventions, and Urine Loss Appliances

Charon A. Pierson

Introduction

Noninvasive tests for urinary incontinence can provide valuable evidence for the clinician, either as an adjunct to extensive urodynamic testing or as a preliminary assessment tool to determine whether a problem of incontinence truly exists. Such tests serve three purposes: to assess the quantity of urine loss, to assess the impact of incontinence on daily activities, and to determine the frequency of episodes of incontinence.

These tests do not diagnose the cause of incontinence; however, certain patterns from the results of these tests may suggest a direction for further testing. Included in the category of noninvasive tests are the voiding diary (frequency and volume charts), the 1-hour office pad test, the 12-hour home pad test, the use of dyes to color the urine, and the electronic recording nappies. These noninvasive interventions are a useful adjunct to medical and surgical interventions. They can also be used as the principle management plan for selected cases of incontinence or for patients who are not suitable candidates for more invasive treatments. The goals of such interventions are to educate patients about normal bladder function, to assist patients in dealing with incontinence on a daily basis, to prevent worsening of the problem, and to prevent development of complications from incontinence.

In some cases, these interventions are suf-ficient to manage the problem adequately; in other cases, they are only a part of the total management plan. These interventions include the use of various environmental aids, pads, or pants; Kegel exercises; vaginal cones; regular toileting schedules; dietary counseling; catheters; obstructing devices; and collecting devices.

Noninvasive Tests

VOIDING DIARY

A voiding diary is a useful tool in the assessment of incontinence and may even have therapeutic value in outpatient populations. The voiding diary (Fig. 18.1, *A* and *B*) is a record of the frequency and volume of intake and output during a 24-hour period, along with a record of the frequency and estimated volume of incontinence. The use of a 1-week diary has been shown to be a reliable method for assessing diurnal and nocturnal micturition frequency and the number of incontinent episodes (1). Other notations such as urge to urinate and patient activities may prove useful in differentiating stress from urge incontinence. Anecdotal evidence suggests that some patients will modify their behavior after becoming aware of activities and behaviors that seem to be associated with their incontinence. Patients' sleeping hours should also be noted to differentiate noctur-

This chart is a record of your voiding (urinating) and leakage (incontinence) of urine for a one-week period. Please complete this according to the following instructions prior to your visit to our office. Choose a time period to keep this record when you can conveniently measure every voiding and begin your record with the first voiding upon arising as in the sample below.

EXAMPLE

PATIENT VOIDING DIARY

(1) Time	(2) Amount Voided	(3) Amount Intake	(4) Type of Intake	(5) Leakage 1 = Damp 2 = Wet 3 = Soaked	(6) Activity at Time of Leakage

(1) Record time of all voidings, leakage, and intake of liquids.
(2) Measure all intake and output in ml or oz (1 oz = 30 ml).
(3) Record the amount of all liquid intake in either ml or oz (1 cup = 8 oz = 240 ml).
(4) Record the type of intake (OJ, coffee, H_2O, beer, etc).
(5) Estimate the amount of leakage according to the following scale:
    1 = damp, few drops
    2 = wet underwear or pad
    3 = soaked or emptied bladder
(6) Describe the activity you were performing at the time of leakage. If you were not actively doing anything, record whether you were sitting, standing, or lying down.

Figure 18.1. A. Patient instructions for the voiding diary.

PATIENT VOIDING DIARY

Time	Amount Voided	Amount Intake	Type of Intake	Leakage 1 = Damp 2 = Wet 3 = Soaked	Activity at Time of Leakage

Figure 18.1—*continued* **B.** Patient recording sheet for the voiding diary.

nal frequency and incontinence. The voiding diary also provides concrete evidence to the clinician of the impact of incontinence on the patient's life.

The chart also allows the clinician to total the intake and output to rule out excessive intake as a factor in the incontinence. Output greatly in excess of intake suggests further investigation for diabetes insipidus. Finally, the type of intake, such as caffeine or alcohol, might be noted to coincide with incontinence episodes.

ONE-HOUR OFFICE PAD TEST

A method of quantifying urine loss was reported by Sutherst et al. (2) in a study of 100 incontinent women and 50 continent controls. Each subject wore a series of six preweighed sanitary pads for 1 hour (10 minutes per pad). The pads were weighed again after use, with the pad weight increase assumed to be urine loss. Mean pad weight increase for the continent controls was 0.26 g (range, 0–2.1 g), which was assumed to be discharge or perspiration. Mean pad weight

increase for the incontinent group was 12.2 g (range, 0–252.4 g). The authors concluded that a pad weight increase of >1 g/h is abnormal and requires further investigation. The reproducibility and the reliability of this test have been demonstrated by other investigators (3–5), and the test procedure has been standardized by the International Continence Society (ICS) for research purposes (6). The ICS recommends the use of nonparametric statistics for the analysis of pad test results.

A diagrammatic representation of the test schedule and interpretation as developed by the ICS is presented in Figure 18.2, *A* and *B*. The activity schedule may be modified according to the patient's abilities; however, variations should be noted. If the pad becomes completely saturated before the hour is over, it is removed and replaced with a clean one, and the total weight of the two pads is used to determine the total amount of urine lost. Pads are worn inside waterproof pants or have a waterproof backing. The test is terminated by a measured voiding and should be considered invalid if it is termi-

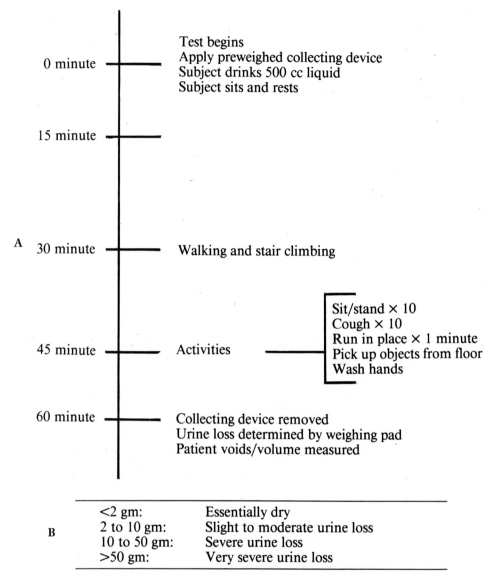

A.

0 minute — Test begins
Apply preweighed collecting device
Subject drinks 500 cc liquid
Subject sits and rests

15 minute —

30 minute — Walking and stair climbing

45 minute — Activities — Sit/stand × 10
Cough × 10
Run in place × 1 minute
Pick up objects from floor
Wash hands

60 minute — Collecting device removed
Urine loss determined by weighing pad
Patient voids/volume measured

B.

<2 gm:	Essentially dry
2 to 10 gm:	Slight to moderate urine loss
10 to 50 gm:	Severe urine loss
>50 gm:	Very severe urine loss

Figure 18.2. **A.** Diagrammatic representation of the complete schedule for a 1-hour pad test. **B.** Interpretation of findings for the 1-hour pad test.

nated prematurely without any demonstrated urine loss. No observations about the triggering events for urine loss can be made with this version of the test, but a rough grading of the severity of incontinence can be made.

TWELVE-HOUR HOME PAD TEST

A study reported by Ali et al. (7) compared the 1-hour office pad test with a 12-hour home pad test and showed nearly 100%

correlation between the two. The principle of the longer test is the same as that of the 1-hour test, except that the patient is sent home with the 12 preweighed pads individually sealed inside clearly marked and numbered plastic bags. The patient performs the test at home, using one pad per hour, and seals the used pads back in the individual bags. In this study, evaporation loss was tested and found to be minimal: 0.2 g after 24 hours and up to 0.8 g after 6 days. Instructions for the test and a data recording sheet are shown in

Figure 18.3, *A* and *B*. When the patient returns the 12 pads to the office, they are weighed individually, and the difference in dry and wet weights is computed.

The advantages of the longer 12-hour home pad test include the following: (*a*) the patient is in familiar surroundings and may react more normally than in an office testing situation, (*b*) the results give some idea of the impact of incontinence on the life of the patient, (*c*) patterns of incontinence may be observed by correlating the activities with the quantities of urine loss, (*d*) the results may provide opportunities for teaching the patient about caffeine-triggered incontinence, and (*e*) the results may provide the clinician with clues to suggest other appropriate interventions. The major disadvantage is the lack of control for an investigator, so the 1-hour office test might be more suitable for research purposes.

COLORING OF URINE WITH DYE

Perhaps the simplest test to differentiate urine loss from excessive vaginal discharge is to color the urine with a harmless dye and watch the pad or panties for the colored stain. Phenazopyridine is given orally and colors the urine orange. The stain, if it gets onto underclothes, is permanent, so a pad should be worn. The bladder should be full, and the patient is encouraged to perform any activities that normally cause her to lose urine. The major disadvantage to this test is that no quantification of urine loss is possible.

This test is designed to measure the amount of urine leakage (incontinence) that you experience during a 12 hour period at home, during your normal routine of daytime activities. Do not try to do this on the same day as the Time and Amount Chart—choose a separate day for each test. Try to do this test the day prior to your visit to this office.

Your kit contains 12 preweighed, numbered sanitary pads in individual Zip-loc bags. The important points to remember are:

1. Use the pads in order as they are numbered (from 1 to 12).
2. Wear each pad for 1 hour only.
3. Record the time the pad was in place (see example below).
4. After removing each pad, store it in its original bag and seal the Zip-loc carefully.
5. Store the used pads in a cool dry place after they have been sealed.
6. Return all bags and pads to this office the next day.
7. Record any unusual activities in the last column, or summarize your routine activities.
8. Remember to begin the test early since it lasts for 12 hours. If you begin at noon you will not finish until midnight!

EXAMPLE

Pad	Time	Dry Wt. (gm)	Wet Wt. (gm)	Diff. (gm)	Activity
1	8–9 A.M.				A.M. exercise—aerobics
2	9–10:05 A.M.				Light housework

Figure 18.3.   **A.** Patient instructions for the home pad test.

Pad	Time	Dry Wt. (gm)	Wet Wt. (gm)	Diff. (gm)	Activity
1					
2					
3					
4					
5					
6					
7					
8					
9					
10					
11					
12					

Figure 18.3—*continued*   **B.** Patient recording sheet for the voiding diary.

ELECTRONIC RECORDING NAPPIES

This electronic recording device was developed in Great Britain for the purpose of recording the frequency and quantity of incontinence episodes in a controlled environment (8). The equipment consists of disposable absorbent pads (nappies) impregnated with dry electrolyte. Strips of aluminum electrodes are placed on each pad, and the nappie is connected to a recording monitor by a 2-meter-long cable. Contact with urine changes the electrical capacitance in the electrodes, and this is recorded automatically on the monitor. The patient performs various activities that trigger incontinence, and notation is made by an observer of the activity each time leakage is recorded. The frequency of leakage is fairly reproducible; however, Eadie et al. (9), Rowan et al. (10), and Stanton (11) found problems with reproducibility of volume measurement up to 35%.

PSYCHOSOCIAL EVALUATION

Researchers who work with incontinent individuals are struck by the variety of coping responses to the social implications of urine loss on the part of the patients (12).

Some are devastated by one incontinence episode and rush to the nearest medical center demanding surgery, whereas others are only mildly inconvenienced by nearly continuous dribbling of urine for many years. Wyman et al. (13) demonstrated a small but significant correlation between a psychosocial impact score and the number of incontinence episodes and amount of urine lost as measured by a pad test. It seems that a complex relationship exists between the severity of incontinence and the psychosocial parameters that can be measured. At the very least, the conscientious clinician will ask a few direct questions of the incontinent patient and/or her caregivers about how they are coping with the problem of incontinence.

In the elderly, incontinence is often the cause of social isolation and admission to nursing homes. Sometimes the decaying mental status of the patient is a contributing factor in the development of the problem, and a mini-mental status examination is indicated for anyone who appears to be cognitively impaired. Early interventions, such as teaching the caregivers principles of timed voidings in the home situation, may help families cope with the incontinence and prevent unnecessary admissions to nursing homes.

Increased life stress as measured by the Holmes and Rahe scale was found to correlate with detrusor instability in one study (14). In this same study, self-reported depression did not correlate with either stress or urge incontinence. In place of written tests for stress and depression, the clinician may include several questions during the interview to determine the presence of unusual life stress, anxiety, and depression. If detected, appropriate intervention should be instituted.

Two national resources for consumers are Help for Incontinent People (HIP) and the Simon Foundation. Both organizations offer newsletters and other publications to guide the consumer in locating services for the incontinent person. They can be contacted at the following locations: HIP, P.O. Box 544, Union, SC 29739; and The Simon Foundation, Box 815, Wilmette, IL 60091.

Nursing Interventions

ENVIRONMENTAL CONSIDERATIONS

Arranging the environment, especially for the elderly and disabled, to allow easy access to toilets can prevent some problems with incontinence. Toilets should be clearly marked with unambiguous signs in public places so that the individual does not spend time searching for bathroom facilities. Field (15) reported that, on the average, the elderly ambulatory patient can walk 15 meters to a toilet after the urge to void has been noted. Toilets must also be of the proper height, with hand grips to facilitate rapid and comfortable seating. Wall railings, walking aids, foot coverings that provide traction on floors, and adequate lighting make the trip to the toilet a safe one for the elderly or disabled. Institutions that care for the elderly or disabled should be designed with this in mind. Easy-to-remove clothing for these patients also saves time once the toilet is reached.

Conventional toilets may be as low as 36 cm from the floor, and the elderly person with arthritic hips and knees or the person transferring from a wheelchair is more comfortable with a seat 42–46 cm high. Seat raisers

are available to convert a low toilet, but they must be evaluated for sturdiness and comfort. A combination commode with a variable seat height is available. This can be used at the bedside at night and can be used as a seat raiser during the day by removing the collecting pan and placing it directly over the toilet seat.

Bedside commodes for nighttime voiding can reduce the incidence of incontinence and the occurrence of serious falls on the way to a distant toilet. Milne et al. (16), in a study of the elderly in a community in Edinburgh, found that 55% rose up at least once during the night to urinate and 25% rose two or more times. Brink and Wells (17) reported that as many as 30% of falls in the elderly occur in toilet areas and 43% are associated with activities surrounding bathroom use. Commodes can reduce time and distance to toilets, thus decreasing risk of falls. Commodes come in a variety of styles and sizes, and many of them are disguised to look like normal household furniture when not in use. Reimbursement from Medicare and from other types of insurance plans varies, but frequently some payment is made when the appliance is prescribed. National health services of many European countries provide these articles to the patients.

Ideally, assessment is made of the patient's environment by a trained nurse, and recommendations are made to make the facilities in the home as safe and convenient as possible. The patient and the family also benefit from the nurse's teaching and support. Incontinence is frequently a hidden problem, with the patient and the family too ashamed or embarrassed to admit the distress it often causes.

REGULAR TOILETING

Regular toileting schedules for bedridden or mentally confused patients depend on the behavior of the caregivers rather than on the behavior of the patient. Continence necessitates an awareness of the passage of time, knowledge of the appropriate location to void, and the ability to reach that location in a timely manner. Bedridden or confused patients may lack any or all of these. The establishment of a functional toileting schedule requires an observation period of 1–2 weeks. During this period, the patient must be checked hourly for incontinence and offered the bedpan or commode at least every 2 hours. All intake and output are measured and recorded, as is an estimate of the volume of leakage. Careful study of the chart after this assessment period reveals voiding patterns, and a schedule can be made to accommodate this natural pattern. Also, fluid intake frequently needs to be controlled, especially in the confused patient.

DIETARY COUNSELING

Some patients consume an excessive amount of fluids in the belief that this keeps the kidney "flushed out." Frequently, these are the patients who have a long history of recurrent urinary tract infections. They have been cautioned in the past to drink "a lot of liquids" and have carried that practice to excess, sometimes consuming 3–4 liters of fluid per day. An adequate fluid intake for a normal adult is 1.5–2.0 liters per day, and only during an acute infection is it necessary to increase that to 2.5–3.0 liters. Restricting fluids after the dinner hour can prevent problems with nocturia and enuresis; however, when taken to excess, fluid restriction can lead to dehydration in elderly or infirm patients.

Anecdotal evidence suggests that weight loss reduces incontinence in some women. This has not been adequately investigated to date.

Caffeine is a regular part of the diet of most people throughout the world. Because its use is so pervasive, a concerted effort must be made if caffeine is to be eliminated from the diet. Caffeine acts as a diuretic and may overload the bladder with urine, thus triggering incontinence. It also has a direct stimulatory effect on the bladder itself, causing bladder contraction. Elimination of caffeine from the diet should be a first step in any management plan for the incontinent patient. A list of the caffeine content of beverages, foods, and drugs can be found in Tables 18.1–18.3.

An average cup of brewed American-style coffee contains 100 mg of caffeine and an average cup of tea contains 70 mg. Recently, gourmet coffees and varieties of brewing techniques have made calculation of caffeine content somewhat confusing. In general, the more expensive arabica blends and darker roasts (gourmet coffees) have less caffeine than the less expensive and lighter roasts. It is possible to brew gourmet coffees with as little as 50 mg of caffeine per cup, and of course, decaffeinated coffees, with as little as 2–5 mg per cup, are more widely available. A demitasse cup of coffee can contain as much as double the amount of caffeine, depending on the blend of coffee used.

KEGEL EXERCISES

Kegel exercises were developed by Dr. Arnold Kegel to restore function to perineal musculature after vaginal delivery (18). He found that restoration of tone and function to lax or atrophied perineal muscles required 20–40 hours of dedicated exercise over a period of 20–60 days. Directions for performing the exercise are found in Figure 18.4. Kegel found that the best results were obtained when patients were followed weekly and checked for progress with a perineom-

Table 18.1. Caffeine Content of Selected Foods

Item	Caffeine (mg)	
	Average	Range
Coffee (5 oz)		
Brewed, drip method	115	60–180
Brewed, percolator	80	40–170
Instant	65	30–120
Powdered, flavored	51	25–73
Decaffeinated, brewed	3	2–5
Decaffeinated, instant	2	1–5
Tea (5 oz)		
Brewed, major U.S. brands	40	20–90
Brewed, imported brands	60	25–110
Instant	30	25–50
Iced (12 oz)	70	67–76
Cocoa beverage (5 oz)	4	2–20
Chocolate milk beverage (8 oz)	5	2–7
Milk chocolate (1 oz)	6	1–15
Dark chocolate, semisweet (1 oz)	20	5–35
Baker's chocolate (1 oz)	26	26
Chocolate-flavored syrup (1 oz)	4	4

Source: Food and Drug Administration (FDA), Food Additive Chemistry Evaluation Branch. Data are based on evaluations from existing literature on caffeine levels.

Table 18.2.   Caffeine Content of Selected Beverages

Item	Caffeine (mg per 12 oz)
Sugar-Free Mr. PIBB	58.8
Mountain Dew	54.0
Mello Yellow	52.8
TAB	46.8
Coca-Cola	45.6
Diet Coke	45.6
Shasta Cola	44.4
Shasta Cherry Cola	44.4
Shasta Diet Cola	44.4
Mr. PIBB	40.8
Dr. Pepper	39.6
Sugar-Free Dr. Pepper	39.6
Big Red	38.4
Sugar-Free Big Red	38.4
Pepsi-Cola	38.4
Aspen	36.0
Diet Pepsi	36.0
Pepsi Light	36.0
RC Cola	36.0
Diet Rite	36.0
Kick	31.2
Canada Dry Jamaica Cola	30.0
Canada Dry Diet Cola	1.2

Source: Institute of Food Technologists (IFT), April 1983. Data are based on information from the National Soft Drink Association, Washington, D.C. IFT also reports that there are at least 68 flavors and varieties of soft drinks produced by 12 leading bottlers that have no caffeine.

Table 18.3.   Caffeine Content of Selected Prescription and Nonprescription Drugs

	Caffeine (mg)
Prescription drugs	
Cafergot (for migraine headache)	100
Fiorinal (for tension headache)	40
Soma Compound (pain relief, muscle relaxant)	32
Darvon Compound (pain relief)	32.4
Nonprescription drugs	
Weight control aids	
Codexin	
Dex-A-Diet II	200
Dexatrim, Dexatrim Extra Strength	200
Dietac capsules	200
Maximum Strength Appedrine	100
Prolamine	140
Alertness tablets	
No Doz	100
Vivarin	200
Analgesic/pain relief	
Anacin, Maximum Strength Anacin	32
Excedrin	65
Midol	32.4
Vanquish	33
Diuretics	
Aqua-Ban	100
Maximum Strength Aqua-Ban Plus	200
Permathene H2 Off	200
Cold/allergy remedies	
Coryban-D capsules	30
Triaminicin tablets	30
Dristan Decongestant tablets and Dristan-AF Decongestant tablets	16.2
Duradyne-Forte	30

Source: FDA, National Center for Drugs and Biologics.

eter (a pneumatic apparatus inserted into the vagina and attached to a manometer by a rubber tube). Significant clinical results were seen when the perineometer readings exceeded 60 mm Hg. The ability to achieve that level varied with diligence of practice and with age, with younger patients generally achieving the best results. It is essential to teach women how to perform pelvic muscle exercises and reinforce the instructions at each visit (19). Many women will report that they have been doing the exercise for years with no improvement. It is essential to go over the technique in a systematic manner during the pelvic examination and provide feedback to the patient because many women have never learned the proper technique and may, in fact, Valsalva instead of contract the pelvic muscles. There is evidence in the literature that a sustained contraction of 10 seconds, followed by a rest period of equal length, should form the basic exercise program. Some clinicians also advocate per-

forming several sets of fast, short, maximal strength contractions, which mimic the power contractions needed in cases of extreme exertion (20). Henderson (21) showed that women who were taught Kegel exercises in prenatal classes achieved significantly higher readings on the perineometer by the first postpartum visit than did a control group of women who had no structured instruction. Kegel exercises should be taught to all female patients, especially in the prenatal and postpartum periods, to help prevent the development of incontinence. The exercises alone may not cure major problems of incontinence

KEGEL EXERCISES

What are Kegel exercises?

These exercises were originally developed by Dr. Arnold Kegel to help women with problems controlling urination. They are designed to strengthen and give you voluntary control of a muscle called the pubococcygeus (or P.C. for short). The P.C. muscle is part of a sling of muscle stretching from your pubic bone in front to your coccyx, or tailbone, in back. The muscle encircles not only the urethra (urinary opening) but also the vaginal opening and the rectum.

Why do Kegel exercises?

1. To help control loss of urine brought on by such things as laughing, coughing, or sneezing.
2. To improve muscle tone in the vaginal area, especially before and after childbirth.

How do you identify the P.C. muscle?

Sit on the toilet. Spread your legs apart. See if you can stop and start the flow of urine without moving your legs. If you can stop and start the stream, you are using the P.C. muscle. If you don't succeed the first time, keep trying until you have identified the muscle.

How do you do Kegel exercises?

Tighten the P.C. muscle as you did to stop your urine. Hold it for a slow count of ten. Relax it for a slow count of ten. Do your exercises three times a day, gradually working up to 50 to 75 contractions three times a day. If you lose count, do your exercises for 15 to 20 minutes each time, which should give you enough time to achieve the same results. You may not notice any improvement until you have been exercising regularly for three to six months.

Several times a day you should practice short, powerful contractions to prepare yourself for those times when you exert maximum stress to lift, cough, or sneeze. Do not hold these contractions for more than a second or two. A good time to practice these power "flicks" is when you feel a sensation of fullness in your bladder. This will most closely mimic the kind of situations where you need this extra strength in real life.

When can you do Kegel exercises?

You can do these exercises any time during the day; however, unless you establish regular practice times, you are likely to forget to do them. Therefore, it is helpful to have specific times during the day that you set aside for exercising. The exercises can be done lying, sitting, or standing, but it is helpful to do them in the standing position at least once a day. Most likely, you experience the greatest urine loss in the standing position, and doing the exercises in the standing position may be more realistic to you. If you do not see improvement after several months of exercise, consult your clinician for further evaluation.

Figure 18.4. Patient instructions for Kegel exercises.

and genital relaxation, but they can be a valuable adjunct to therapy in most cases.

VAGINAL CONES

A simple biofeedback device called the vaginal cone can be used to train women to contract the pelvic floor more effectively. Plevnik (22) designed a set of cone-shaped weights of equal shape and volume that gradually increase in weight (Fig. 18.5). When a cone of appropriate weight is placed in the vagina, it tends to slip out unless the pelvic floor contracts in an effort to retain the cone. The feeling of losing the cone is the stimulus that causes the patient to contract her pelvic floor muscles. Additionally, any increase in abdominal pressure will tend to force the cone out of the vagina, thus increasing the biofeedback effect. This sensory feedback ensures reliable contraction and thus adequate exercise of the pelvic floor for a prescribed period of time each day.

In contrast, some perineometers are unable to differentiate between increased pubococcygeous strength and increased intraabdominal pressure, because both cause an elevation in readings. This may actually make the problem worse by training the woman to Valsalva at the time when she most needs to contract the pelvic floor. Other biofeedback devices are only suitable for office treatment and require urethral and vaginal or anal probes to feedback data to the patient.

In a study of 30 women with urodynamically proven stress incontinence, Peattie et al. (23) found a 70% cure or improvement after 1 month of vaginal cone therapy. Because of the encouraging response, 63% opted to delay surgery and continue therapy with the cones, whereas 37% elected to undergo incontinence surgery. In a comparison of cone therapy versus physiotherapy (i.e., Kegel exercises), the same authors (24) found 100% compliance in the cones group and 67% in the physiotherapy group. Although the numbers of patients in the study were too small to show any significant difference between the two groups, both groups improved satisfactorily. Ten of 15 in the cones group and 5 of 9 in the physiotherapy group no longer required bladder suspension surgery. Cone therapy at this point appears to be a useful alternative to surgery; however, long-term studies are still needed to document lasting effectiveness.

The protocol (23) for use of the vaginal cones is as follows:

1. At the first office/clinic visit, the patient inserts the lightest cone into her vagina and walks for 1 minute. Repeat this exercise with increasingly heavier cones until the patient finds that she must consciously contract her pelvic floor muscles to retain the cone. The heaviest weight retained without voluntary holding is called the *passive weight* and represents resting pelvic floor tone.
2. The patient is then prescribed a set of cones and is instructed to begin her therapeutic regimen with the passive weight cone. The daily regimen requires the patient to walk for 15 minutes twice a day while retaining the cone in the vagina.
3. The patient is instructed to increase to the next heaviest weight after she is successful in retaining the cone during two consecutive training periods. NOTE: If the pelvic floor tone is so poor that even the lightest cone will not remain in the vagina, pelvic floor stimulation can be used at first

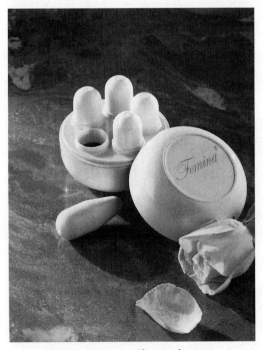

Figure 18.5. Set of vaginal cones.

to increase strength and allow the therapy to begin.

This new form of treatment for incontinence appears promising; however, more studies need to be done on long-term effectiveness. The cones are available without prescription from Dacomed Corporation (1701 East 79th Street, Minneapolis, MN 55425, telephone 800-328-1103). Insurance reimbursement for the cones is variable, and the clinician usually must provide additional justification and product literature to the insurance carrier. Patient instructions and a training video are also available from the company.

VAGINAL FISTULA CUP

A vaginal fistula cup is a temporary solution to the problem of urinary incontinence caused by a vesicovaginal fistula. It is a soft-rubber cup-shaped apparatus that fits into the vagina, with the rubber tubing connected to a leg bag (Fig. 18.6). The best results with this device are obtained when the fistula is located high in the vaginal vault and when the vault has at least some tone to help hold the device in place. The patient can be taught to manage this device fairly easily, as insertion is similar to placing a diaphragm. The tubing can be cut to the proper length to fit comfortably into the top of a leg bag.

If the fistula is lower in the vault, for example, at the bladder neck, the fistula cup may prevent leakage when it is used in conjunction with an indwelling catheter. The catheter must be seated firmly at the urethrovesical junction and attached to a leg bag on the opposite leg.

This device has also been used successfully to deal with leakage from a rectovaginal fistula in women who have had pelvic irradiation. The caliber of the tubing is large enough to allow passage of semiliquid stool (Stowe B, personal communication, 1984).

URETHRAL OBSTRUCTING DEVICES

Urethral obstructing devices are usually best suited to short-term problems, for example, the woman who has adequate control under normal circumstances but who requires extra help for her 1-hour exercise class or for a tennis match. The principle is to introduce something into the vagina that is large enough to exert pressure on the midurethra to augment normal control. A super tampon (or two) is sometimes enough to do this. A large diaphragm is often helpful for the woman who has a concomitant genital prolapse. It must be fitted very snugly behind the pubic bone and should not be left in place for extended periods, because it may inhibit voiding or cause irritation of the anterior vaginal wall. An inflatable pessary (Fig. 18.7) is also used the same way, and patients, when properly instructed, can manage these quite well. The advantage to this type of pessary is the ease of removal for cleaning, thus eliminating the possible odor or infection that can accompany the use of a pessary. This pessary

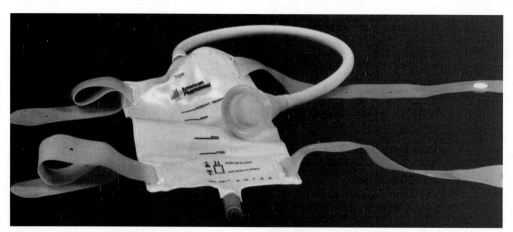

Figure 18.6. Kay's vaginal fistula cup connected to a leg bag. (Reproduced courtesy of Shield Health Care Centers, Inc., 4085 Tweedy Blvd., South Gate, CA 90280.)

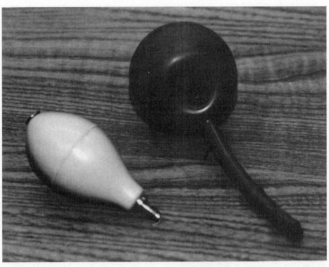

Figure 18.7. Inflatable pessary.

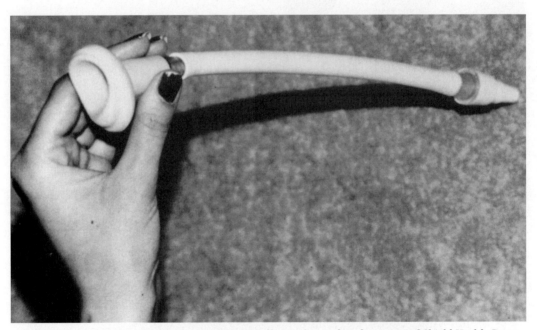

Figure 18.8. Misstique Female External Urine Collector. (Reproduced courtesy of Shield Health Care Centers, Inc., 4085 Tweedy Blvd., South Gate, CA 90280.)

can be inflated to a size that comfortably fits any vagina and can be adjusted at any time by the patient.

EXTERNAL COLLECTING DEVICES

A suitable collecting device for the female requires a good seal around the urethral meatus; to date, this has been a problem. Re-search has continued, however, and two new products are available. The first, called Misstique, uses stoma adhesives to achieve a suitable seal around the meatus, along with a special valve to prevent backflow of urine (Fig. 18.8). Application of the Misstique collector requires a reasonable amount of dexterity, but it has been successful in some women (Stowe B, personal communication, 1984).

The newest product (Female Urinary Incontinence System, Hollister, Inc.) is made of soft silicone and is designed to encompass the urethral meatus with a form-fitting pericup (Fig. 18.9). This design funnels urine away from the meatus, even if the meatus is located in the vaginal introitus. The device provides a secure fit without the need for adhesive products. It comes in two sizes, along with a fitting device, tubing, support pants, and collecting bag. Initial studies by the manufacturer found the product acceptable, easy to use, and comfortable (Hollister, Inc., technical literature, 1988) in selected ambulatory patients.

Certainly no external collector is suitable for all patients, and selection criteria must be developed, based on clinical trials, for each device. The prospect of external collecting devices is appealing in our current medical reimbursement system in the United States, because durable medical equipment is a reimbursable expense, whereas disposable products such as pads are often not.

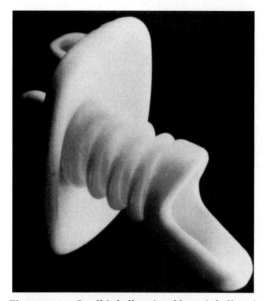

Figure 18.9. Small (2 bellows) and large (4 bellows) Female Urinary Device. (Reproduced courtesy of Hollister Incorporated, 2000 Hollister Drive, Libertyville, IL 60048.)

PADS, PANTS, AND PROTECTIVE SHEETS

Of the many styles and sizes of pads and pants available today, there are five basic types of pants: (*a*) completely rubberized pants to be worn over regular pants or cloth diaper, (*b*) a close fitting or elastic brief to be worn with a specially designed waterproof pad (Fig. 18.10), (*c*) a marsupial pants that has a plastic backed pouch in the front to hold

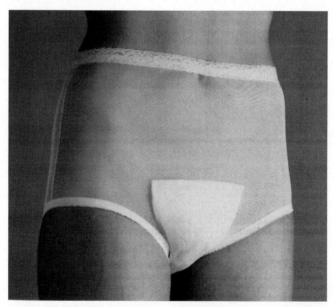

Figure 18.10. DEPEND Shield: absorbent, adhesive-backed pad to insert into ordinary underwear. (Reprinted courtesy of Kimberly-Clark Corporation, Retail Sales, Neenah, WI and Institutional Sales, Roswell, GA. All rights to copyright in photographs owned by Kimberly-Clark Corporation.)

a specially designed pad (Fig. 18.11), (*d*) an absorbent undergarment worn in place of pants (Fig. 18.12), and (*e*) disposable diapers, which look very much like disposable baby diapers (Fig. 18.13).

Available pads and protective sheets are of three basic types: (*a*) those made of washable reusable materials such as cotton, (*b*) those made of synthetic disposable materials with

a waterproof backing, and (*c*) those made with a central core of a gelling material that expands as it absorbs urine (Fig. 18.14).

In the United States, most women seen in an outpatient setting seem to prefer sanitary pads for mild incontinence, perhaps because they are accustomed to using them during menstruation. In general, these pads are rarely adequate for containing leakage but are

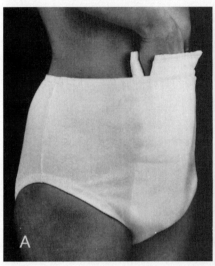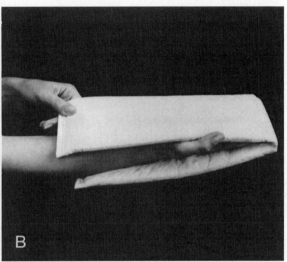

Figure 18.11. **A.** Dignity incontinence pants with extra absorbent pads inserted into vinyl-lined pocket. **B.** Extra absorbent pads to be used with Dignity incontinence pants. (Courtesy of ConvaTec—a Squibb Company.)

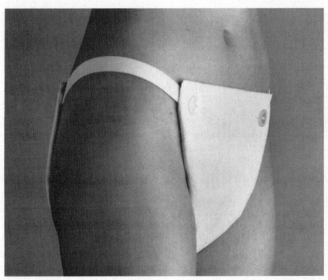

Figure 18.12. DEPEND undergarment: absorbent undergarment worn like underwear and held in place with button-on elastic straps. (Reprinted courtesy of Kimberly-Clark Corporation, Retail Sales, Neenah, WI, and Institutional Sales, Roswell, GA. All rights to copyright in photographs owned by Kimberly-Clark Corporation.)

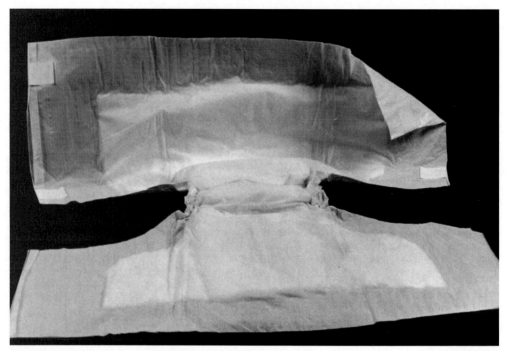

Figure 18.13. Adult-sized disposable diapers.

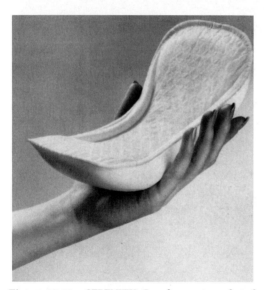

Figure 18.14. SERENITY Guards: contoured pad made of a superabsorbent powder, which turns into gel on contact with urine. (Courtesy of Johnson & Johnson Personal Products Division.)

probably more acceptable to some women than specially designed incontinence clothing. Facial and toilet tissues are another frequently used protective measure, although they are usually quite inadequate.

Recently, specially designed incontinence products have been marketed on television and in the print media in the United States, which has created tremendous growth in the industry. In 1972, the sale of disposable pads and diapers was a $99 million market; in 1987 that market has increased to $496 million (19).

In counseling a patient on the use of special incontinence pads or pants, it is very helpful to have the results of a 12-hour home pad test as an indicator of the degree of absorbency required for adequate protection and the pattern of urine loss. Several pads are available in regular and super absorbency. Many pads and pants available are not adequate to absorb large amounts of urine lost suddenly, as occurs in the patient with detrusor instability, for example. Clinicians should become familiar with the products available locally and should suggest several options to each patient on a trial basis. In some cases, private insurance will provide incontinence supplies to patients with a written prescription or a letter justifying the need. It is very helpful to cultivate a good rapport with personnel in a local home-care supply store who have current knowledge of the products available and of insurance reimbursement.

It is very important to consider the psychological implications of incontinence when counseling incontinent women on the availability of incontinence products. Incontinence implies loss of control, and a return to wearing protection much like a baby diaper can be psychologically devastating. Appearance of the pads and pants, as well as comfort and absorbency, must be considered. In some patients, complete protection from visible leakage may be sacrificed for the sake of appearance and comfort. An assessment must be made on an individual basis, taking into account the above factors and the patient's lifestyle, mobility, manual dexterity, and coexisting problems such as skin sensitivity or fecal incontinence.

CATHETERIZATION

Urethral catheters have been available for 5000 years, with the earliest record of their use depicted in Egyptian hieroglyphics. In the 1930s, Foley developed the latex balloon catheter, which was the first significant design improvement over those early Egyptian catheters made of reeds, bronze, and tin. Today, catheters are of two different types based on use: the long-term indwelling catheter is used for intractable urinary incontinence and the intermittent self-inserted catheter is used for urinary retention and for some neurogenic-type bladder dysfunctions.

The use of an indwelling catheter for any extended period of time generally produces problems such as pain and spasm from mucosal irritation, leakage around the catheter, blockage from urinary sediment and debris, and inevitable infection. Kennedy (25) found that most problems with spasm and leakage around the catheter were related to the large diameter catheters, and Mandelstam (26) suggested that the most suitable size for indwelling catheters is 16–18 French with no more than 5–10 mL in the balloon.

The ambulatory patient requires a closed drainage system that is portable and concealable for daytime use and a nighttime system that will hold large amounts of urine. For daytime use, the small leg bag (Fig. 18.6) that straps to the thigh can be concealed easily under skirts or pants. The outlet valve pic-

tured here is the "push-pull" type, which is very easy to operate and adequately prevents leakage. The older variety with "pull off" covers over the outlet valve always results in urine spillage. The rubber straps that hold the bag in place are adjustable; however, they are frequently uncomfortable. A stretch brief with a pocket to hold the bag on the front of the thigh is available in Great Britain and is reported to be quite comfortable (26). Leg straps made of other types of materials, such as fabric-backed foam rubber, are also available.

The small capacity of the leg bag is not sufficient for nighttime volumes, so this system must be changed to a large capacity bag or bottle for sleep. The daily opening of the closed drainage systems leaves the patient more vulnerable to infection. This has led many to favor the technique of intermittent catheterization.

Indwelling catheters should not be used as a convenience for caregivers. Suitable candidates are those who are terminally ill and in pain when moved about for changing or toileting. An indwelling catheter may also be a short-term solution in patients with decubiti that will not heal.

CLEAN INTERMITTENT CATHETERIZATION

Clean intermittent catheterization has been shown to be a safe and effective treatment (27) for select voiding dysfunctions. Candidates for this procedure should have adequate manual dexterity to handle the catheter safely, adequate mental capacity to perform the procedure as directed, a bladder capacity of 100 mL or more, and an intact urethra, without strictures.

The most important principle in this technique is the frequency of catheterization. Patients are taught to catheterize themselves frequently enough so that the volume of urine in the bladder is never greater than 300 mL. This prevents overdistention of the bladder, which decreases the blood supply to the tissues, thus rendering them more susceptible to infection. The cleanliness of the technique is secondary, and patients must be cautioned never to delay catheterization for lack of a clean environment or equipment. A small caliber catheter, 8–14F size, and

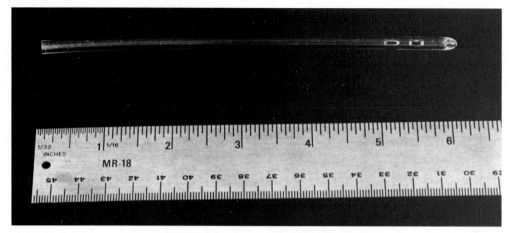

Figure 18.15. Female disposable catheter, size 14F.

adequate lubrication make the procedure more comfortable and reduce trauma to the urethra.

It is sometimes recommended that patients are given antibacterial medication for the first 2–3 weeks while they adjust to the procedure. They do not require continuous suppression to maintain sterile urine. If frequent infections become a problem, the most likely cause is overdistention of the bladder or incomplete emptying (27).

The equipment to perform clean intermittent catheterization includes a supply of clear plastic female catheters, which are about 7 inches long (Fig. 18.15), and lubricant. These can be carried in a plastic bag, a cosmetic case, or anything similar. No sterilization is necessary. The patient is instructed to wash her hands and the catheter with ordinary hand soap and to rinse with water; however, she should never omit the procedure for lack of soap and water. During the learning process, the patient will need a mirror to locate the urethra; in time, however, she will be able to do this by touch.

The patient is instructed to catheterize every 3 hours during the day and once or twice during the night for the first 2 weeks. During this time, a careful record is maintained of all volumes and times. With use of this record as the database, a schedule is established to keep the volume of urine below 300 mL at all times. This may entail controlling intake in some individuals. Antibiotics are given for 2–3 weeks, and some patients also require an-

ticholinergic medications to control bladder spasms.

If the patient is unable to perform the procedure herself, a family member or the principle caregiver can be instructed to do it for her. Young children can be taught the procedure when they are old enough to tell time and have the motor skills necessary to handle the catheter safely.

Conclusions

One of the first steps in the assessment of the incontinent patient should be a voiding diary, followed by a pad test to determine whether a significant problem with incontinence really exists. Caffeine or alcohol intake should be investigated. Kegel exercises should be taught on the initial examination and should be reinforced on each visit thereafter. For the elderly or disabled patient, a home visit should be made by a nurse to evaluate the living environment and facilitate easy access to the toilet. Other aids such as vaginal cones, collecting devices, pads, pants, catheterization, and obstructing devices should be prescribed after medical and nursing assessments have been completed.

REFERENCES

1. Wyman J, Choi S, Hawkins, S, Wilson M, Fantl AJ. The urinary diary in evaluation of incontinent women: a test-retest analysis. Obstet Gynecol 1988;71:812–817.

2. Sutherst J, Brown M, Shaner M. Assessing the severity of urinary incontinence in women by weighing perineal pads. Lancet 1981;23:1128–1131.
3. Klarskov P, Hald T. Reproducibility and reliability of urinary incontinence assessment with a 60 min test. In: Proceedings of the 2nd joint meeting of the ICS/UDS. Aachen, West Germany: International Continence Society and Urodynamic Society, 1983;II:512–514.
4. Murray A, Price R, Sutherst J, Brown M. Measurement of the quantity of urine loss in women by weighing perineal pads. In: Proceedings of the 12th meeting of the ICS. Leiden, The Netherlands: International Continence Society, 1982:243–244.
5. Wood P, Murray A, Brown M, Sutherst J. Reproducibility of a one hour urine loss test (pad test). In: Proceedings of the 2nd joint meeting of the ICS/UDS. Aachen, West Germany: International Continence Society and Urodynamic Society 1983;II:515–517.
6. International Continence Society. Quantification of urine loss. In: Fifth report on the standardization of terminology. Aachen, West Germany: International Continence Society, 1983.
7. Ali K, Murray A, Sutherst J, Brown M. Perineal pad weighing test: comparison of one hour ward pad test with twelve hour home pad test. In: Proceedings of the 2nd joint meeting of the ICS/UDS. Aachen, West Germany: International Continence Society and Urodynamic Society, 1983;I:380–382.
8. James E, Flack F, Caldwell K, Martin M. Continuous measurement of urine loss and frequency in incontinent patients. Br J Urol 1971;43:233–237.
9. Eadie A, Glen E, Rowan D. The Urilos recording nappy system. Br J Urol 1983;55:301–303.
10. Rowan D, Doohan D, Glen E. Detection of urine loss using the exeter recording nappy and other similar devices. Urol Int 1976;31:70–77.
11. Stanton S. Urilos: the practical detection of urine loss. Am J Obstet Gynecol 1977;128:461–463.
12. Norton C. The effects of urinary incontinence in women. Int Rehabil Med 1982;4:9–14.
13. Wyman J, Hawkins S, Choi S, Taylor J, Fantl JA. Psychosocial impact of urinary incontinence in women. Obstet Gynecol 1987;70:378–381.
14. Pierson C, Meyer CB, Ostergard DR. Vesical instability: a stress related entity. In: Proceedings of the International Continence Society. London: International Continence Society, 1985.
15. Field M. Urinary incontinence in the elderly: an overview. J Gerontol Nurs 1979;5:12–19.
16. Milne J, Williamson J, Maule M, Wallace E. Urinary symptoms in older people. Mod Geriatr 1972;2:198–212.
17. Brink C, Wells T. Environmental support for geriatric incontinence. Clin Geriatr Med 1986;2:829–840.
18. Kegel A. Progressive resistance exercise in the functional restoration of the perineal muscles. Am J Obstet Gynecol 1948;56:238–248.
19. Agency for Health Care Policy and Research, Public Health Service. Urinary incontinence panel: urinary incontinence in adults: clinical practice guidelines. AHCPR Publication no. 92–0038. Rockville, MD: U.S. Government Printing Office, 1992.
20. Wyman J. Level 3: comprehensive assessment and management of urinary incontinence by continence nurse specialists. Nurse Pract For 1994;5:177–185.
21. Henderson J. Effects of a prenatal teaching program on postpartum regeneration of the pubococcygeal muscle. J Obstet Gynecol Neonat Nurs 1983;12:403–408.
22. Plevnik S. New method for testing and strengthening of pelvic floor muscles. In: Proceedings of the International Continence Society. London: International Continence Society, 1985.
23. Peattie A, Plevnik S, Stanton S. Vaginal cones: a conservative method of treating genuine stress incontinence. Br J Obstet Gynaecol 1988;95:1049–1053.
24. Peattie A, Plevnik S. Cones versus physiotherapy as conservative management of genuine stress incontinence [abstract]. Neurourol Urodyn 1988;7:265–266.
25. Kennedy A. Incontinence advice. I. Long-term catheterization. Nurs Times 1983;27:91–92.
26. Mandelstam D. Disability and incontinence. Int Rehabil Med 1982;4:3–7.
27. Horsley J, Crane J, Reynolds M. Clean intermittent catheterization. New York: Grune and Stratton, 1982.

SUGGESTED READINGS

Jester K, Faller N, Norton C. Nursing for continence. Philadelphia: WB Saunders, 1990.
Morishita L (ed). A systematic approach to promoting urinary continence. Nurse Pract For 1994;5:121–195.

CHAPTER 19

Effect of Drugs on the Lower Urinary Tract

Joseph M. Montella and Cindy J. Wordell

To fully appreciate the effects of drugs on the lower urinary tract, one must have a basic knowledge of the neurophysiology of this area. Although this was covered in depth in Chapter 4, a brief review is essential to understanding both the therapeutic effects of medication used to control stress and urge incontinence and the potential effects of other medications commonly used by patients with urinary incontinence. This chapter reviews the mechanism of drug action on the lower urinary tract, the medications most commonly used to treat symptoms and their potential drug interactions, and the side effects on the continence control mechanism of some commonly prescribed medications.

The lower urinary tract is innervated by both the somatic and autonomic nervous systems, the latter composed of the sympathetic and parasympathetic divisions. The somatic nervous system is chiefly responsible for the innervation of the levator ani and the striated external urethral sphincter and is involved in the volitional control of urination.

The sympathetic and parasympathetic divisions are chiefly responsible for the storage and emptying functions of the bladder, respectively. Both divisions are composed of preganglionic and postganglionic fibers. The preganglionic fibers of the sympathetic system that innervate the bladder arise primarily from nerve roots T11 through L2 and terminate in the sympathetic ganglia located adjacent to the spinal cord. The postganglionic fibers then travel through the hypogastric nerve plexus to terminate at the detrusor

muscle, bladder neck, and the smooth muscle of the urethra. The preganglionics of the parasympathetic system arise from nerve roots S2 through S4 and travel in the pelvic splanchnic nerves. They then join with the sympathetic postganglionic fibers to form the hypogastric plexus of Frankenhauser and terminate in the parasympathetic ganglia located within the bladder itself. The postganglionic fibers, which are extremely short, terminate in the detrusor muscle (1).

The neurotransmitter acetylcholine is present in the preganglionic fibers of both systems; the postganglionics of the parasympathetic system also use acetylcholine as its neurotransmitter. Cholinergic receptors found in the lower urinary tract are predominantly muscarinic receptors that can be blocked by atropine; nicotinic receptors do not appear to found in appreciable amounts. The location of these cholinergic muscarinic receptors is predominantly in the detrusor muscle in the body of the bladder, the trigone, and the bladder neck.

Postganglionic fibers of the sympathetic system use the neurotransmitter norepinephrine, which affects adrenergic receptors. These are further divided into alpha-adrenergic receptors and beta-adrenergic receptors. Alpha receptors regulate smooth muscle contraction and vasoconstriction, whereas beta receptors control smooth muscle relaxation. These receptors are also located in different concentrations in different areas of the bladder; detrusor muscle predominantly has beta receptors with few alpha receptors, whereas the bladder neck

Table 19.1. General Action of Drugs

Drugs acting on the bladder
  Parasympathetic agents
    Cholinergic (parasympathomimetic)
      agents
    Anticholinergic (parasympatholytic)
      agents
  Musculotropic relaxants
  Tricyclic antidepressants
  Calcium-channel blockers
  Beta-adrenergic agonists
Drugs acting on the urethra
  Alpha-adrenergic agonists
  Alpha-adrenergic blockers
  Beta-adrenergic blockers
  Estrogen

and urethra have alpha receptors with few beta receptors. Stimulation of alpha receptors therefore would cause urethral and bladder neck contraction, and stimulation of beta receptors would cause detrusor muscle relaxation, leading to continence or urinary retention. Conversely, alpha-receptor blockade would produce relaxation of the urethral and bladder neck and beta-receptor blockade would cause detrusor muscle contraction, leading to incontinence (2).

Because the bladder is composed of smooth muscle, medication designed to prevent contraction of the muscle by either direct relaxant activity or via blocking of calcium-mediated contractions can be used to treat forms of detrusor instability.

The effects of drugs on the lower urinary tract can be divided into those that act primarily on the bladder and those that act on the urethra. Table 19.1 lists the general classes of medication and their sites of action.

Drugs Acting on the Bladder

PARASYMPATHETIC DRUGS

Cholinergic (Parasympathomimetic) Agents

Parasympathomimetic drugs are of three types, each exerting its influence by an alteration of the action of the naturally occurring neurotransmitter, acetylcholine. The first type exerts its effect through a direct stimulation of the end organ by actual substitution for the naturally occurring neurotransmitter. These drugs are chemically similar to acetylcholine. The second type prevents the destruction of acetylcholine by inactivating its degrading enzyme, acetylcholinesterase. These drugs are anticholinesterases. The third group directly stimulates the acetylcholine receptor sites to produce their parasympathomimetic effects; however, they are not chemically related to acetylcholine. These drugs have as their primary effect on the lower urinary tract a stimulation of detrusor contractility while causing increased urethral resistance (3). Table 19.2 lists those drugs that have therapeutic importance in urogynecology. These drugs stimulate vesical contraction in patients with urinary retention secondary to vesical hypotonia, but their effects are limited to acute cases and the results of using these medications are controversial (4).

Anticholinergic (Parasympatholytic) Drugs

Anticholinergic (parasympatholytic) drugs directly antagonize the effect of acetylcholine at the end organ providing a competitive blockade of muscarinic receptors at postganglionic parasympathetic receptor sites (3). Atropine is the classical prototype in this group, and its primary effect on the lower urinary tract is to relax the detrusor muscle but has little effect on the urethra. It can also be useful as an antidote for acetylcholinomimetics and anticholinesterases secondary to its competitive blockade. Table 19.3 lists the anticholinergic medications that are therapeutically useful for urge incontinence and detrusor instability (5–15). Propantheline is recommended as the agent of choice in this class of medication secondary to evidence of its usefulness in controlled trials and in uncontrolled case series (16, 17).

Although hyoscyamine and other oral anticholinergics are known to be clinically useful for the treatment of detrusor instability, there are no studies that adequately compare the effects of this medication to placebo.

Musculotropic Relaxants (Antispasmodics)

These agents exert a direct depressant effect on smooth muscle at a site that is metabolically distal to the cholinergic receptor mechanism (18). They have a papavarine-like relaxant activity in addition to variable antimuscarinic and local anesthetic actions (19). The most effective medication in this group is oxybutynin, because randomized controlled studies of its use demonstrated its superiority to placebo in treatment of urge incontinence (20–24). Although flavoxate is widely used, four randomized controlled studies have not demonstrated its superiority to placebo in treatment of urge incontinence (22, 25–27). Table 19.4 lists commonly used agents of this class.

Dicyclomine hydrochloride also has anti-cholinergic and smooth muscle relaxant properties. Studies are limited as to its effectiveness, and no studies exist comparing this with other anticholinergics.

Tricyclic Antidepressants

These agents exert complex pharmacological actions that include anticholinergic effects, direct smooth muscle relaxation, antihistamine, and local anesthetic effects on the detrusor muscle (19, 28). In addition, they can increase alpha-receptor stimulation by blocking norepinephrine reuptake at the adrenergic nerve terminal, thereby increasing urethral closure pressure. These drugs can be effective in reducing bladder contractility and may be used for combined cases of urge and stress incontinence; however, limited research on the use of tricyclic antidepressants is available. Table 19.5 lists medications of this type.

Calcium Channel Blockers

These agents stop the influx of extracellular calcium required for the contractile process of the detrusor and also prevent the mobilization from intracellular calcium stores with resultant inhibition of excitation contraction coupling (29). They are mainly used in the treatment of angina because of their ability to prevent intracellular movement of calcium through the slow channel in a membrane; however, investigators have used these drugs in the treatment of detrusor instability because uninhibited bladder contractions have been shown to be dependent on calcium influx. No controlled studies for nifedipine, diltiazem, or verapamil have been performed, and their use for urge incontinence is not recommended at this time. Terodiline, an agent that possesses both calcium channel blocking and anticholinergic properties, has shown in vivo activity in

Table 19.2. Cholinergic (Parasympathomimetic) Agents

Drug Name	Dosage Forms	Dosage (tid to qid)
Bethanechol (Urecholine®)	Tabs 5, 10, 25, 50 mg	10–50 mg
Neostigmine (Prostigmin®)	Injectable 0.5 mg/mL	0.5–1.0 mg IM or SQ

Table 19.3. Anticholinergic Agents

Drug Name	Dosage Forms	Dosage[a]
Hyoscyamine (Levsin®)	Tabs 0.125 mg	0.125–0.25 mg
	Timecaps 0.375 mg	One bid
Methantheline (Banthine®)	Tabs 50 mg	50–100 mg
Propantheline (Probanthine®)	Tabs 7.5, 15 mg	7.5–15 mg + 30 mg qhs

[a]Dosages are tid to qid unless otherwise noted.

Table 19.4. Combined Anticholinergic Agents and Musculotropic Relaxants

Drug Name	Dosage Forms	Dosage (tid to qid)
Dicyclomine (Bentyl®)	Tabs 10, 20 mg	20 mg
	Syrup 10 mg/5 mL	
Flavoxate (Urispas®)	Tabs 100 mg	100–200 mg
Oxybutynin (Ditropan®)	Tabs 5 mg	5–10 mg
	Syrup 5 mg/5 mL	

Table 19.5. Tricyclic Antidepressants

Drug Name	Dosage Forms	Dosage (tid to qid)
Doxepin (Sinequan®)	Caps 10, 25, 50, 75 mg	10–25 mg
Imipramine (Tofranil®)	Tabs 10, 25, 50 mg	25–50 mg
Nortriptyline (Pamelor®)	Tabs 10, 25, 50 mg	25 mg

Table 19.6. Alpha Adrenergic Stimulators

Drug Name	Dosage Forms	Dosage
Phenylephrine/antihistamine (Comhist LA®)	Caps	One capsule bid
Phenylpropanolamine/antihistamine (Entex LA®, Ornade®)	Tabs	One tab bid
Phenylpropanolamine/phenylephrine/antihistamine (Entex®)	Caps	One capsule qid
Pseudoephedrine/antihistamine (Entex PSE®, Deconamine SR®)	Tabs	One tab bid

controlling detrusor contractions, but patients had polymorphic ventricular tachycardia (torsades de pointes) when used in high doses. A randomized double-blind trial of terodiline using 25 mg twice a day showed a 70% reduction in incontinence over placebo, with no cardiovascular side effects (30). Further investigation of other calcium channel blockers with fewer cardiovascular side effects continues.

Beta-Adrenergic Agents

Because the bladder wall also has beta-adrenergic receptors (which control smooth muscle relaxation), beta-agonist therapy should theoretically be therapeutically useful for urge incontinence and detrusor instability. The role of these agents and the sympathetic nervous system in general in controlling micturition is unclear, and therefore these agents are not clinically useful in controlling the aforementioned disorders.

Drugs Acting on the Urethra

ALPHA-ADRENERGIC AGONISTS

These agents have been shown to be the most clinically useful in their actions on the urethra to increase urethral sphincteric tone and reduce stress incontinence by increasing outlet resistance (3). Table 19.6 lists clinically useful medications, the alpha-agonist component combined with an antihistamine in all commercially available preparations to be safely used for urinary incontinence.

Three prospective randomized controlled studies of middle-aged normotensive women with stress incontinence using phenylpropanolamine revealed a 9–14% cure and a 19–60% decrease in incontinence over placebo (31–33). In addition, imipramine can be clinically useful for stress incontinence through its action on alpha receptors.

ALPHA-ADRENERGIC BLOCKING AGENTS

These agents block the alpha-adrenergic receptors, relaxing the urethral sphincter and causing symptoms of stress incontinence (3). These agents have therapeutic usefulness in the patient who has spasm of the urethral sphincteric mechanism, the relief of which will diminish symptoms of urgency, frequency, and especially urinary retention. Two drugs, prazosin and phenoxybenzamine, have been demonstrated to decrease the contractility of the smooth muscle component of the urethral sphincter and relax the surrounding vascular bed (34–36). Because alpha-adrenergic blockade leaves beta receptors unopposed, thereby producing hypotension and tachycardia, caution must be exercised when using these drugs. In patients with marked cerebral or coronary atherosclerosis or with renal insufficiency secondary to reduced perfusion, their use is not recommended (15).

BETA-ADRENERGIC BLOCKING AGENTS

Because beta-adrenergic stimulation causes relaxation of the urethral sphincter, beta-blocking agents theoretically could be useful in patients with mild degrees of stress incontinence. Blockade of the beta-adrenergic neurons allows the alpha-adrenergic neurons to function more efficiently in the maintenance of continence. Beta blockers are not used to treat stress incontinence at this time.

ESTROGEN

Because the vagina and urethra are of similar embryologic origin, the effects of estrogen on the vaginal mucosa can be extrapolated to the urethra. It is postulated that estrogen supplementation in postmenopausal women may improve urethral mucosal coaptation and increase vascularity, tone, and the responsiveness to alpha-adrenergic stimulation. Two studies using estriol show a maximum of 14% dryness and 29% improvement over controls in treating incontinence (32, 37). A metaanalysis from six randomized controlled trials and 17 uncontrolled clinical series revealed a favorable effect of estrogen on incontinence in postmenopausal women (38). The recommended dose is conjugated estrogen orally (0.3–1.25 mg daily) or vaginally (1–2 g daily).

Side Effects of Commonly Used Medications

The preceding discussion focused on drugs used to treat urinary incontinence, but there are numerous medications that act on the lower urinary tract to produce the symptoms of frequency, urinary retention, and urinary incontinence. Table 19.7 lists commonly used medications that may produce these symptoms. The clinician who treats patients with these complaints must do a full medication history to determine whether the complaints correlate with their usage of these medications. Before adjusting them, however, discussion with the clinician who prescribed them is germane.

Drug Interactions

Caution must be exercised in the pharmacological manipulation of the lower urinary

Table 19.7.   Side Effects of Commonly Used Medications

Generic Name	Brand Name
Drugs causing urinary frequency	
Calcitonin	Calcimar, Miacalcin, Cibacalcin
Carteolol	Cartrol
Cisapride	Propulsid
Cyclizine	Marezine
Cyproheptadine	Periactin
Dantrolene	Dantrium
Doxorubicin	Adriamycin
Edrophonium	Tensilon, Enlon
Fluoxetine	Prozac
Gabapentin	Neurontin
Leuprolide	Lupron, Lupron Depot
Ofloxacin	Floxin
Omeprazole	Prilosec
Paroxetine	Paxil
Phendimetrazine	Adphen
Phenmetrazine	Preludin
Phensuximide	Milontin Kapseals
Prazosin	Minipress
Procarbazine	Matulane
Protriptyline	Vivactil
Selegiline	Eldepryl
Trimeprazine	Temaril
Drugs causing urinary retention	
Dicyclomine	Bentyl
Disopyramide	Norpace
Hyoscyamine	Levsin
Isoproterenol	Isuprel
Methantheline	Banthine
Methscopolamine	Pamine
Mexiletine	Mexitil
Orphenadrine	Norflex
Oxybutynin	Ditropan
Paroxetine	Paxil
Selegiline	Eldepryl
Trazodone	Desyrel
Tridihexethyl chloride	Pathilon
Drugs causing urinary incontinence	
Baclofen	Lioresal
Bromocriptine	Parlodel
Cisapride	Propulsid
Demecarium	Humorsol
Echothiophate	Phospholine Iodide
Felbamate	Felbatol
Fluoxetine	Prozac
Gabapentin	Neurontin
Guanfacine	Tenex
Leuprolide	Lupron, Lupron Depot
Sertraline	Zoloft

tract because potentially dangerous drug interactions may occur with medications that the patient is currently taking for other conditions. The following discussion serves to alert the clinicians to some of the more common interactions that may be found in the urogynecological population.

PARASYMPATHOMIMETIC DRUGS

Bethanechol is the primary parasympathomimetic agent used in the neuropharmacological management of the lower urinary tract, especially in cases of acute urinary retention. Although few drug interactions have been reported with bethanechol, quinidine and procainamide, both class IA antiarrhythmics, have been reported to potentially antagonize the cholinergic effects. However, this has not been well documented (39).

Tacrine (Cognex®, Parke-Davis), used in the treatment of Alzheimer's disease, is a cholinesterase inhibitor. Concomitant use with bethanechol can result in additive or synergistic cholinergic activity resulting in adverse effects such as vomiting or diarrhea. The onset of this effect is rapid, although the clinical severity of this interaction is minor (40).

PARASYMPATHOLYTIC DRUGS

In contrast to cholinergic agents, drugs with anticholinergic properties have been reported to have many more drug interactions. All drugs with clinically important anticholinergic activity decrease gastrointestinal motility, resulting in delayed absorption, increased time to peak serum concentration, or increased area under the serum-concentration time curve of concurrently administered drugs. This can be attributed to a prolonged absorption phase (41–43). This interaction may be significant when a drug with a narrow therapeutic serum concentration range, such as digoxin, is used.

Antacids have been reported to interfere with the absorption of dicyclomine and hyoscyamine, making it important to avoid concurrent administration of an antacid with one of these products (44, 45).

Many commonly used therapeutic agents, including antihistamines, phenothiazines,

tricyclic antidepressants, amantadine, type IA antiarrhythmics, and butyrophenones, have anticholinergic activity that may increase the therapeutic activity or adverse events when used in combination with one of the drugs listed in Tables 19.3 and 19.4. The tricyclic antidepressants, imipramine and nortriptyline, when used in combination with an anticholinergic agent may cause urinary retention, adynamic ileus or clinical manifestation of chronic glaucoma (46).

Cholinergic drugs, such as pilocarpine ocular system (Ocusert®), pilocarpine drops (Pilocar® and Isopto Carpine®), and carbachol drops (Isopto Carbachol®), are used to control intraocular pressure in the management of glaucoma. Systemic administration of anticholinergic agents may antagonize the effect of these cholinergic drugs (44).

TRICYCLIC ANTIDEPRESSANTS

Oral anticoagulants, in particular, dicumarol and bishydroxycoumarin, have been reported to interact with nortriptyline. This interaction probably results from decreased metabolism of the anticoagulant, causing a prolonged half-life. Although this interaction is not reported to occur with warfarin, close monitoring of the prothrombin time is warranted when a tricyclic antidepressant is added to warfarin therapy (47, 48).

The antihypertensive effect of the centrally acting agents guanethidine, clonidine, and guanfacine have been reported to decrease when therapy is initiated with a tricyclic antidepressant, such as nortriptyline or imipramine. Concomitant administration of clonidine with a tricyclic antidepressant resulted in dangerous elevations in blood pressure and hypertensive crisis (49). A loss of blood pressure control was reported during concurrent administration of guanfacine (Tenex®) and a tricyclic antidepressant (50). Guanethidine requires uptake into the adrenergic neuron to exert its antihypertensive effect. Tricyclic antidepressants block this uptake, decreasing the antihypertensive effect of guanethidine (51, 52).

The tricyclic antidepressants have also been reported to interact with the anticonvulsants carbamazepine and phenytoin. Concurrent administration of carbamazepine, with either nortriptyline or imipramine, has resulted in a significant decrease in the serum level of the tricyclic compound (53, 54). Clinically, this interaction may result in a loss of the tricyclic effectiveness. In contrast to concurrent administration with carbamazepine, administration of imipramine with phenytoin resulted in decreased phenytoin metabolism and increased phenytoin serum levels (55). When imipramine is added to a regimen that includes phenytoin, the phenytoin serum concentration should be monitored to ensure that phenytoin toxicity does not develop.

Tricyclic antidepressant metabolism is inhibited by concurrent administration of the histamine-2 receptor antagonist cimetidine. This has resulted in prolonged half-life and elevated tricyclic serum concentrations. Clinically, this may be evident as heightened anticholinergic effects, including urinary retention, blurred vision, and dry mouth (56). Ranitidine has less effect on the metabolism of the tricyclic compounds, offering a potentially safer alternative (57).

Some of the selective serotonin reuptake inhibitors have been documented to have an interaction with tricyclic antidepressants, including imipramine and nortriptyline. Addition of fluvoxamine or fluoxetine to a regimen that includes imipramine results in a significant increase in imipramine serum levels, primarily through deceased metabolism (58–60). The effect of fluvoxamine on imipramine metabolism may also be bidirectional, with fluvoxamine increasing imipramine serum concentration and imipramine increasing fluvoxamine serum levels (61). Fluoxetine has also been reported to increase nortriptyline serum levels (60, 62). Clinically, this may be evident as heightened anticholinergic effects, including urinary retention, blurred vision, and dry mouth.

Administration of a monoamine oxidase inhibitor with a tricyclic antidepressant prompted reports of serious drug interactions, including excitation, hyperpyrexia, convulsions, and potentially death. This interaction has been attributed to altered catecholamine uptake and metabolism (63, 64). Several alternative agents with anticholinergic effects are available for management of urological disorders (Tables 19.3 and 19.4), making it possible to avoid this interaction. Monoamine oxidase inhibitors include tranylcypromine, phenelzine, isocarboxazid, and selegeline (Eldepryl®). The antibiotic furazolidone also has been reported to have MAO inhibitor (MAOI) properties (3).

Amphetamines and methylphenidate both exert their therapeutic effects by releasing biogenic amines from storage at the nerve terminals (3). Because the tricyclic antidepressants act by blocking reuptake at the nerve terminal, concurrent administration may result in increased blood pressure (65).

Concurrent administration of norepinephrine, particularly by the intravenous route, with a tricyclic antidepressant has resulted in a significant increase in the occurrence of arrhythmias and tachycardia. This interaction has also been reported when phenylephrine or pseudoephedrine are administered concurrently with a tricyclic antidepressant (66, 67).

Several drugs have been noted to decrease the clearance of imipramine, resulting in increased serum levels and an increased potential for anticholinergic adverse effects. Drugs that have been reported to do this include diltiazem, labetalol, propranolol, quinidine, and verapamil (68–71).

ALPHA-ADRENERGIC ANTAGONISTS

Clinically, these drugs are known to cause tachycardia, which is largely mediated through beta-adrenergic stimulation. When a beta blocker is administered concurrently, this compensatory increase in heart rate is suppressed, resulting in an exaggerated postural hypotensive response to the first dose (72).

Administration of an alpha-beta agonist, such as epinephrine, has been noted to enhance the beta-mediated tachycardia and peripheral vasodilation due to unopposed beta stimulation during treatment with phenoxybenzamine (73). In a case report, concurrent administration of methyldopa for treatment of hypertension, with phenoxybenzamine for Raynaud's disease, resulted in total urinary incontinence. The drug interaction recurred on rechallenge (74).

When the calcium channel blocker verapamil was added to a regimen containing the alpha blockers terazosin or prazosin, a substantial increase in the area under the serum concentration time curve of the alpha blocker was noted along with a significant decrease in blood pressure (75–77).

ALPHA-ADRENERGIC AGONISTS

Phenylpropanolamine stimulates both alpha and beta receptors. Phenylephrine is a very potent alpha-receptor stimulator with less effect on the beta receptors in the heart (3). Concurrent use of a beta-adrenergic agonist, such as albuterol, is not recommended because of the potential for additive adrenergic stimulation (78). Concurrent administration of a beta-adrenergic antagonist, such as propranolol, has different effects for the alpha-adrenergic agonists. Concurrent administration with phenylephrine has been shown to enhance the pressor response to phenylephrine, probably due to unopposed alpha-adrenergic stimulation (79). In contrast, concurrent administration of propranolol with phenylpropanolamine has been reported to decrease the blood pressure response to phenylpropanolamine (80).

Guanethidine has been reported to interact with systemically administered sympathomimetic amines, such as phenylephrine (81, 82). A severe hypertensive reaction has been reported to occur when phenylpropanolamine is administered with methyldopa, although the patient was also receiving a beta blocker (83).

Concomitant use of phenylephrine or phenylpropanolamine with an monoamine oxidase inhibitor has resulted in hypertensive severe reactions. Headache, vomiting, elevated blood pressure, and palpitations have all been reported from concurrent administration (84). The clinician must remember that drugs with MAOI activity include selegeline (Eldepryl®), which is used in the treatment of Parkinson's disease. There has been a report of enhanced pressor response to tyramine in a patient taking selegeline, making a reaction with other sympathomimetic amines theoretically possible (85).

Administration of a tricyclic antidepressant with alpha-adrenergic agonists was discussed previously.

Conclusions

Drugs can affect the lower urinary tract both positively and negatively. Parasym-

patholytics and tricyclic antidepressants can be used alone or in combination with behavioral therapy to treat micturition disorders such as detrusor instability. Alpha-agonists and estrogen can be used in combination to improve stress continence. Commonly used medications can cause the symptoms of urgency, retention, and incontinence, and by altering these medications, the clinician may be able to treat patients with these problems. Finally, the clinician must be aware of potential drug interactions, especially among elderly patients who may be using a variety of medications. By understanding the usefulness and the side effects of drugs, the clinician can control the life-altering problem of incontinence.

REFERENCES

1. Fletcher TF, Bradley WE. Neuroanatomy of the bladder and urethra. J Urol 1978;119:153–160.
2. Kluck P. The autonomic innervation of the human urinary bladder, bladder neck and urethra: a histochemical study. Anat Rec 1980;198:439–447.
3. Gilman AG, Rall TW, Nies AS, Taylor P, eds. Goodman and Gilman's the pharmacological basis of therapeutics. 8th ed. New York: Pergamon Press, 1990.
4. Sourander LB. Treatment of urinary incontinence: the place of drugs. Gerontology 1990;36:19–26.
5. Awad SA, Bryniak S, Downie JW, Bruce AW. The treatment of the uninhibited bladder with dicyclomine. J Urol 1977;117:161–163.
6. Benson GS, Sarshik SA, Raezer DM, Wein AJ. Bladder muscle contractility: comparative effects and mechanisms of action of atropine, propantheline, flavoxate, and imipramine. Urology 1977;9:31–35.
7. Diokno AC, Hyndman CW, Hardy DA, Lapides J. Comparison of action of imipramine (Tofranil) and propantheline (Probanthine) on detrusor contraction. J Urol 1972;107:42–43.
8. Diokno AC, Lapides J. Oxybutynin: a new drug with analgesic and anticholinergic properties. J Urol 1972;108:307–309.
9. Draper JW, Zorgniotti AW. The effect of banthine and similar agents on the urinary tract. NY State J Med 1954;54:77–83.
10. Gregory JG, Wein AJ, Schoenberg HW. A comparison of the action of Trofanil and Pro-Banthine on the urinary bladder. Invest Urol 1974;12:233–235.
11. Kohler FP, Morales PA. Cystometric evaluation of flavoxate hydrochloride in normal and neurogenic bladders. J Urol 1968;100:729–730.
12. McGrath WR, Lewis RE, Kuhn WL. The dual mode of the antispasmodic effect of dicyclomine hydrochloride. J Pharmacol Exp Ther 1964;146:354–358.

13. Stewart BH, Banowsky LHW, Montague DK. Stress incontinence: conservative therapy with sympathomimetic drugs. J Urol 1976;115:558–559.

14. Thompson IM, Lauvetz R. Oxybutynin in bladder spasm, neurogenic bladder, and eneuresis. Urology 1976;8:452–454.

15. Whitfield HN, Doyle PT, Mayo ME, Poopalasingham N. The effect of adrenergic blocking drugs on outflow resistance. Br J Urol 1976;47:823–827.

16. Dequeker J. Drug treatment of urinary incontinence in the elderly. Controlled trial with vasopressin and propantheline bromide. Gerontol Clin 1965;7:311–317.

17. Zorzitto ML, Jewett MAS, Fernie GR, Holliday PJ, Bartlett S. Effectiveness of propantheline bromide in the treatment of geriatric patients with detrusor instability. Neurourol Urodyn 1986;5:133–140.

18. Finkbeiner AE, Welch LT, Bissada NK. Uropharmacology: direct acting smooth muscle stimulators and depressants. Urology 1978;12:231–235.

19. Appelbaum SM. Pharmacologic agents in micturitional disorders. Urology 1980;16:555–568.

20. Tapp AJ, Cardozo LD, Versi E, Cooper D. The treatment of detrusor instability in postmenopausal women with oxybutynin chloride: a double-blind placebo controlled study. Br J Obstet Gynaecol 1990;97:521–526.

21. Holmes DM, Montz FJ, Stanton SL. Oxybutynin versus propantheline in the management of detrusor instability: a patient-regulated variable dose trial. Br J Obstet Gynaecol 1989;96:607–610.

22. Zeegers AGM, Kiesswetter H, Kramer AEJL, Jonas U. Conservative therapy of frequency, urgency and urge incontinence: a double-blind clinical trial of flavoxate hydrochloride, oxybutynin chloride, emepronium bromide and placebo. World J Urol 1989;5:57–61.

23. Riva D, Casolati E. Oxybutynin chloride in the treatment of female idiopathic bladder instability. Clin Exp Obstet Gynecol 1984;11:37–42.

24. Moore KH, Hay DM, Imrie AE, Watson A, Goldstein M. Oxybutynin hydrochloride (3 mg) in the treatment of women with idiopathic detrusor instability. Br J Urol 1990;66:479–485.

25. Meyhoff HH, Gerstenberg TC, Nordling J. Placebo—the drug of choice in female motor urge incontinence? Br J Urol 1983;55:34–37.

26. Robinson JM, Brocklehurst JC. Emepronium bromide and flavoxate hydrochloride in the treatment of urinary incontinence associated with detrusor instability in elderly women. Br J Urol 1983;55:371–376.

27. Chapple CR, Parkhouse H, Gardener C, Millroy EJ. Double-blind, placebo controlled, crossover study of flavoxate in the treatment of idiopathic detrusor instability. Br J Urol 1990;66:491–494.

28. Wein AJ. Receptor function and drug action in the lower urinary tract. Semin Urol 1988;8:121–130.

29. Andersson KE, Sjogren C. Aspects on the physiology and pharmacology of the bladder and urethra. Prog Neurobiol 1982;19:71–89.

30. Norton P, Karram M, Wall LL, Rosenzweig B, Benson JT, Fantl JA. Randomized double-blind trial of terodiline in the treatment of urge incontinence in women. Obstet Gynecol 1994;84:386–391.

31. Hilton P, Tweddell AL, Mayne C. Oral and intravaginal estrogens alone and in combination with alpha-adrenergic stimulation in genuine stress incontinence. Int Urogynecol J 1990;1:80–86.

32. Walter S, Kjaergaard B, Lose G, et al. Stress urinary incontinence in postmenopausal women treated with oral estrogen (estriol) and an alpha-adrenoceptor-stimulationg agent (phenylpropanolamine): a randomized double-blind placebo-controlled study. Int Urogynecol J 1990;1:74–79.

33. Ek A, Andersson KE, Gullberg B. Ulmsten U. The effects of long-term treatment with norephedrine on stress incontinence and urethral closure pressure profile. Scand J Urol Nephrol 1978;12:105–110.

34. Khanna OP, Gonick P. Effects of phenoxybenzamine hydrochloride on canine lower urinary tract: clinical implications. Urology 1975;6:323–330.

35. Krane RJ, Olsson CA. Phenoxybenzamine in neurogenic bladder dysfunction. II. Clinical considerations. J Urol 1973;710:653–656.

36. Mobley DF. Phenoxybenzamine in the management of neurogenic vesical dysfunction. J Urol 1976;116:737–738.

37. Samsioe G, Jansson I, Mellstrom D, Svanborg A. Occurrence, nature and treatment of urinary incontinence in a 70-year-old female population. Maturitas 1985;7:335–342.

38. Fantl JA, Cardozo L, McClish DK, et al. Estrogen therapy in the management of urinary incontinenc in postmenopausal women: a meta-analysis. First report of the hormones and urogenital therapy committee. Obstet Gynecol 1994;83:12–18.

39. Hansten PD, Horn JR. Drug interactions and updates. Vancouver, WA: Applied Therapeutics, Inc., 1993.

40. Product Information. Cognex(R), tacrine. Morris Plains: Parke-Davis, 1993.

41. Brown DD, Schmid J, Long RA, et al. A steady-state evaluation of the effects of propantheline bromide and cholestyramine on the bioavailability of digoxin when administered as tablets or capsules. J Clin Pharmacol 1985;25:360–364.

42. Regardh CG, Lundborg P, Persson BA. The effect of antacid, metoclopramide and propantheline on the bioavailability of metoprolol and atenolol. Biopharm Drug Dispos 1981;2:79–87.

43. Kanto J, Allonen H, Jalonen H, et al. The effect of metoclopramide and propantheline on the gastrointestinal absorption of cimetidine. Br J Clin Pharmacol 1981;11:629–631.

44. Product Information. Bentyl®, dicyclomine. Cincinnati: Lakeside Pharmaceuticals, 1995.

45. Product Information. Levsin®, hyoscyamine sulfate. Milwaukee: Schwarz Pharma, 1991.

46. Hansten PD, Horn JR. Drug interactions. Philadelphia: Lea and Febiger, 1992.

47. Pond SM, Graham GG, Birkett DJ, et al. Effects of tricyclic antidepressants on drug metabolism. Clin Pharmacol Ther 1975;18:191–199.

48. Vesell ES, Passananti GT, Greene FE. Impairment of drug metabolism in man by allopurinol and nortriptyline. N Engl J Med 1970;283:1484–1488.

49. Hui KK. Hypertensive crisis induced by interaction of clonidine with imipramine. J Am Geriatr Soc 1983;31:164.

50. Buckley M, Feely J. Antagonism of antihypertensive effect of guanfacine by tricyclic antidepressants [letter]. Lancet 1991;337:1173–1174.

51. Meyer JF, McAllister CK, Goldberg LI, et al. Insidious and prolonged antagonism of guanethidine by amitriptyline. JAMA 1970;31:1487–1488.

52. Mitchell JR, Arias L, Oates JA. Antagonism of the antihypertensive action of guanethidine sulfate by desipramine hydrochloride. JAMA 1967;202:973–976.

53. Brosen K, Kragh-Sorensen P. Concomitant intake of nortriptyline and carbamazepine. Ther Drug Monit 1993;15:258–260.

54. Brown CS, Wells BG, Cold JA, et al. Possible influence of carbamazepine on plasma imipramine concentrations in children with attention deficit hyperactivity disorder. J Clin Psychopharmacol 1990;10:359–362.

55. Perucca E, Richens A. Interaction between phenytoin and imipramine. Br J Clin Pharmacol 1977;4:485–486.

56. Miller DD, Macklin M. Cimetidine-imipramine interaction: a case report. Am J Psychiatry 1983;140:351–352.

57. Wells BG, Pieper JA, Self TH, et al. The effect of ranitidine and cimetidine on imipramine disposition. Eur J Clin Pharmacol 1986;31:285–290.

58. Aranow RB, Hudson JI, Pope HG Jr, et al. Elevated antidepressant plasma levels after addition of fluoxetine. Am J Psychiatry 1989;146:911–913.

59. Goodnick PJ. Influence of fluoxetine on plasma levels of desipramine [letter]. Am J Psychiatry 1989;146:552.

60. Spina E, Pollicino AM, Avenoso A, et al. Effect of fluvoxamine on the pharmacokinetics of imipramine and desipramine in healthy subjects. Ther Drug Monit 1993;15:243–246.

61. Hartter S, Wetzel H, Hammes E, et al. Inhibition of antidepressant demethylation and hydroxylation and fluvoxamine in depressed patients. Psychopharmacology 1993;110:302–308.

62. Von Ammon Cavanaugh S. Drug-drug interactions of fluoxetine with tricyclics. Psychosomatics 1990;31:273–276.

63. Lockett MF, Milner G. Combining the antidepressant drugs [letter]. Br Med J 1965;1:921.

64. Schuckit M, Robins E, Feighner JP. Tricyclic antidepressants and monoamine oxidase inhibitors. Combination therapy in the treatment of depression. Arch Gen Psychiatry 1971;24:509–514.

65. Flemenbaum A. Hypertensive episodes after adding methylphenidate (Ritalin®) to tricyclic antidepressants. Psychosomatics 1972;13:265–268.

66. Boakes AJ, Laurence DR, Teoh PC, et al. Interactions between sympathomimetic amines and antidepressant agents in man. Br Med J 1973;1:311–315.

67. Ghose K. Assessment of peripheral adrenergic activity and its interaction with drugs in man. Eur J Clin Pharmacol 1980;17:233–238.

68. Hermann DJ, Krol TF, Dukes GE, et al. Comparison of verapamil, diltiazem, and labetalol on the bioavailability and metabolism of imipramine. J Clin Pharmacol 1992;32:176–183.

69. Gillette DW, Tannery LP. Beta blocker inhibits tricyclic metabolism. J Am Acad Child Adolesc Psychiatry 1994;33:223–224.

70. Brosen K, Gram LF. Quinidine inhibits the 2-hydroxylation of imipramine and desipramine but not the demethylation of imipramine. Eur J Clin Pharmacol 1989;37:155–160.

71. Steiner E, Dumont E, Spina E, et al. Inhibition of desipramine 2-hydroxylation by quinidine and quinine. Clin Pharmacol Ther 1988;43:577–581.

72. Elliott HL, McLean K, Sumner DJ, et al. Immediate cardiovascular responses to oral prazosin—effects of concurrent beta-blockers. Clin Pharmacol Ther 1981;29:303–309.

73. Product Information. Dibenzyline®, phenoxybenzamine. Philadelphia: Smith Kline and French Laboratories, 1990.

74. Fernandez PG, Sahni S, Galway BA, et al. Urinary incontinence due to interaction of phenoxybenzamine and a methyldopa. Can Med Assoc J 1981;124:174–175.

75. Varghese A, Lenz M, Locke C, et al. Combined terazosin and verapamil therapy in essential hypertension: hemodynamic interactions [abstract]. Clin Pharmacol Ther 1991;49:146.

76. Lenz ML, Varghese A, Pool JL, et al. Combined terazosin and verapamil therapy in essential hypertension: hemodynamic interactions [abstract]. Clin Pharmacol Ther 1991;49:146.

77. Elliott HL, Meredith PA, Campbell L, et al. The combination of prazosin and verapamil in the treatment of essential hypertension. Clin Pharmacol Ther 1988;43:554–560.

78. Product Information. Ventolin®, albuterol. Glaxo, Inc., Research Triangle Park, 1989.

79. Adler AG, McElwain GE, Merli GJ, et al. Systemic effects of eye drops. Arch Intern Med 1982;142:2293–2294.

80. Pentel PR, Asinger RW, Benowitz NL. Propranolol antagonism of phenylpropanolamine-induced hypertension. Clin Pharmacol Ther 1985;37:488–494.

81. Gulati OD, Dave BT, Gokhale SD, et al. Antagonism of adrenergic neuron blockade in hypertensive subjects. Clin Pharmacol Ther 1966;7:510–514.

82. Ober KF, Wang RIH. Drug interactions with guanethidine. Clin Pharmacol Ther 1973;14:190–195.

83. McLaren EH. Severe hypertension produced by interaction of phenylpropanolamine with methyldopa and oxprenolol. Br Med J 1976;2:283–284.

84. Harrison WM, McGrath PJ, Stewart JW, et al. MAOIs and hypertensive crisis: the role of OTC drugs. J Clin Psychiatry 1989;50:64–65.

85. Schulz R, Antonin KH, Hoffman E, et al. Tyramine kinetics and pressor sensitivity during monoamine oxidase inhibition by selegiline. Clin Pharmacol Ther 1989;46:528–536.

SECTION IV

Pathology and Treatment of Lower Urinary Tract Abnormalities

CHAPTER 20

Pathogenesis of Stress Urinary Incontinence: The Role of Connective Tissue

Peggy A. Norton

Introduction

Stress urinary incontinence (SUI) and pelvic organ prolapse often coexist and share many risk factors: childbirth, aging, hormonal status, and chronic increased intraabdominal pressure. The etiology of SUI and pelvic organ prolapse is likely to be multifactorial but certainly includes abnormalities in the muscular components of the pelvic floor, the innervation of pelvic floor, and the connective tissue of this region. This chapter discusses what is known about the function and anatomy of pelvic connective tissue and its role in the pathogenesis of SUI and pelvic organ prolapse.

Connective Tissue and the Pelvic Floor

In the pelvis, three types of connective tissue structures are important: suspensory ligaments, tendinous insertions of the muscular components into the pelvic sidewall and other pelvic structures, and fibrous sheets in the anterior and posterior vaginal walls. The cardinal and uterosacral ligaments are suspensory structures because they originate from the lateral sacrum and greater sciatic foramen cephalad to their insertion into the uterus, cervix, and up-per vagina. The cardinal and uterosacral structures are not ligaments in the classic sense. They consist of an irregular mesh-like arrangement of collagen and elastin fibrils, with interspersing smooth muscle fibers. Additionally, the fibrous attachments of the upper vagina to the pelvic sidewall should be viewed as suspensory. Some of the strength of these structures may arise in the perivascular connective tissue of these structures. The fibrous connective tissue often seen ventral to the bladder neck in the space of Retzius is well developed in many women and has been termed the pubourethral ligaments by some authors. DeLancey (1) termed this connective tissue the paravaginal fascial attachments, whose role is probably stabilization rather than suspension.

Muscle fibers act by shortening their length but require a connection to a fixed source (often bone) to exert force. This connection is usually in the form of tendon, a confluence of the fascial sheath into dense regular connective tissue. This connective tissue consists mostly of collagen fibers in dense regular configurations, that is, the fibers are lined up along the major direction of strain. In the pelvis, this type of connective tissue is seen in the arcus tendineus fasciae pelvis and arcus tendineus levator ani. The attachments of the upper vagina to the lateral pelvis may be classified in this manner, although these attachments have some features of the suspensory ligaments described above. If this connective tissue attachment is attenuated or broken, muscle contraction has no function in the pelvis. Lateral wall or paravaginal defects are good examples of tendinous connections that have been disrupted (2).

Surgeons are familiar with a fibrous sheet of fascia in the anterior vaginal wall that is used in the repair of cystocele. A similar tissue is recognized as the female equivalent of Denonvilliers fascia in the posterior wall and is termed rectovaginal fascia (3). Anteriorly, the pubocervical fascia attaches the middle third of the vagina to the pelvic sidewall and creates a "plate" on which the bladder rests. Posteriorly, the rectovaginal fascia also attaches the vagina to the pelvic sidewall and prevents the rectum from prolapsing forward. These fibrous sheets have been described as fascia, although this is actually the vaginal wall and its lateral connective tissue attachments to the pelvic sidewall. Histologically, they consist of some smooth muscle fibers with a preponderance of collagen fibers in a loose irregular configuration which is well suited to support a structure against forces with multiple direction vectors. Some investigators have suggested that this tissue should be described as the "muscular layer" of the vagina, but this is as imprecise as the term "fascia." The finding of smooth muscle in varying degrees along with collagen, elastin, and vascular elements makes this a fibromuscular layer, whose role is largely supportive.

Connective Tissue Components

Some important characteristics of connective tissue structure and biology must be identified. Three fibrous proteins make up the macrostructure of connective tissue: collagen, elastin, and reticulin. These proteins are produced by fibroblasts and smooth muscle cells and may be expressed in unique combinations to suit the mechanical needs of the tissue. For example, structures such as skin need to be able to stretch and are composed of elements in a criss-cross orientation, whereas strength structures such as tendon are oriented longitudinally.

Collagen is responsible for much of the mechanical strength in tissues. In some forms, collagen has a tensile strength similar to that of fine steel wire, with the tenacity of glue and the toughness of leather. Although there are up to 20 collagen types described, two types are important in the pelvic floor. Type I collagen aligns in large fibers, is composed of two $alpha_1(I)$ chains and one $alpha_2(I)$ chain, and is the form of collagen found in mature tissues. Type III collagen is formed from three $alpha_1(III)$ chains and is found in various combinations with type I collagen. Type III collagen is found in tissues requiring more flexibility than strength, such as uterine wall, vascular walls, and skin. It should be regarded as a collagen with less mechanical strength than the ubiquitous type I. In some fibers, combinations of collagen types may be seen. The existence of so many collagen types attests to the concept that by varying the ratios of collagen types, cells can control the parameters of fiber formation such as length, diameter, and orientation (4).

Elastin is the matrix component that allows a structure to stretch to a limited degree and then return to its original shape. Elastin fibers orient along the direction of a stretch and then allow restoration along the original orientation with release. If stretched beyond its limits, elastin will break and not return the structure to its original contour. Reticulin is a background matrix that coexists with ground substance, the "filler" protein between larger fibrous proteins. The microfibrillar system is a related protein that appears to connect the matrix to the basement membrane structures, imparting strength and mechanical stability to these structures. The abnormality in the matrix responsible for Marfan's syndrome appears to be in the fibrillin gene on chromosome 15. Fibronectin and laminin are additional components that seem to be important in the formation and stabilization of collagen fibrils.

Pregnancy is a state of pronounced changes in collagen biochemistry. The amount of collagen in the uterus increases eightfold during gestation (6), and cervical "ripening" is actually the action of collagenase to break down cervical collagens in hours to days (7). The suspensory cardinal and uterosacral ligaments insert into the cervix, and the effect of collagenase on these nearby structures during cervical ripening is unknown. Abnormalities in the amount of collagen relative to muscle can dramatically alter the mechanical strength of such tissue; cervical incompetence has been related to decreased amounts of collagen, whereas protracted labor and inadequate cervical dilation may be due to insufficient remodeling of uterine and cervical tissue during pregnancy and parturition (8).

Collagen seems to be constantly remodeled in response to tissue needs. Collagen synthesis in one part of the body can be suppressed in favor of wound healing in another part of the body, especially in the acute phase response. Ihlberg and associates (9) created small skin wounds before laparotomy; although wound healing was initiated in the experimental incisions, the process was interrupted in favor of healing of the larger abdominal wound, and no further maturation of the experimental scars occurred. During normal wound healing, type III is the initial type of collagen produced, oriented in a haphazard fashion. Tensile strength develops over weeks to months with the replacement of type III collagen with the stronger type I collagen.

A good example of collagen remodeling is scurvy. This vitamin C deficiency led to bruising, gum bleeding, impaired wound healing, and disruption of old scars in British sailors on long voyages. The Scottish surgeon James Lind corrected the deficiency with citrus fruit, which resulted in British sailors being nicknamed "limeys." Ascorbic acid is essential for collagen synthesis, and the disruption of previously healed wounds in scurvy demonstrates the fact that collagen is constantly undergoing remodeling in the body. Total collagen content from skin biopsies has been shown to decrease 40% in the first few years after menopause and is fully reversible with hormone replacement therapy (10). In particular, type III collagen content in skin is significantly increased after subcutaneous estradiol treatment (11). In a study of the estrogen receptors of the pelvic floor, receptors were detected in the nuclei of connective tissue cells and striated muscle cells, suggesting that the action of estrogen is through these target tissues (12). Therefore, collagen may be amenable to pharmacological, hormonal, or even dietary manipulation.

Connective Tissue and Stress Incontinence

What is known about the role of connective tissue in the pathogenesis of stress incontinence? The major risk factors in stress incontinence each have an association with connective tissue as discussed above: pregnancy, aging, and hormonal status. Ulmsten and coworkers (13) found that women with SUI had 40% less total collagen in the round ligament and incisional skin compared with continent women. They proposed that decreased collagen led to a weakness in the urogenital suspensory apparatus and increased bladder neck hypermobility. These workers also pointed out the prevalence of abdominal hernias, lower leg varices, and uterine prolapse in women with SUI and suggested that connective tissue analyses might identify women at risk for developing prolapse or incontinence. Rechsberger and colleagues (14) found a similar reduction in total collagen, along with increased estrogen receptor concentration in these tissues. In a separate study, fibroblast cultures established from women with SUI accumulated 30% less collagen than cultures from continent women.

Kondo and colleagues (16) examined the biophysical properties of fascia by measuring the shear strength (amount of force required to penetrate the tissue with a standardized Stamey needle). Women with stress incontinence had lower shear strength in both rectus fascia and anterior vaginal wall than controls, irrespective of age. They concluded that some women suffering from SUI may have a hereditary disorder involving the biophysical properties of tissues. Versi and colleagues (17) measured the total collagen from skin biopsies and found that higher collagen content was associated with higher resting and dynamic urethral pressures. However, these studies were performed when definitions of incontinence did not distinguish between hypermobile and intrinsic sphincter deficient types of stress incontinence. These researchers suggested that the increase in skin collagen seen with hormone replacement therapy may have implications for the role of estrogen in the treatment of SUI.

Connective Tissue and Pelvic Organ Prolapse

Even less is known about the relationship between connective tissue and a condition closely related to SUI: pelvic organ prolapse. Norton and coworkers (18) reported that clinically significant stages of genital prolapse were associated with joint hypermobility in women and concluded that a generalized "stretchiness" of connective tissue may be etiological.

Conclusions

What are the implications for clinical practice and future research? It is still unknown whether the connective tissue abnormalities are intrinsic or induced, stretches or breaks, systemic or isolated. Likewise, the interaction between neuromuscular damage and connective tissue damage is unclear: a defect in one system may produce abnormalities in the related system. Prevention and treatment of stress incontinence will require research that considers these interactions between connective tissue abnormalities and neuromuscular injury.

REFERENCES

1. DeLancey, JO. The pubovesical ligament, a separate structure from the urethral supports. Neurourol Urodyn 1989;8:53.
2. Richardson AC, Edmonds PV, Williams NL. Treatment of stress urinary incontinence due to a paravaginal fascial defect. Obstet Gynecol 1981; 57:357.
3. Richardson AC. The rectovaginal septum revisited: its relationship to rectocele and its importance in rectocele repair. Clin Obstet Gynecol 1993;36:976–983.
4. Burgeson R. New collagens, new concepts. Annu Rev Cell Biol 1987;4:551–577.
5. Lee B, Godfrey M, Vitale E, et al. Linkage of Marfan syndrome and a phenotypically related disorder to two different fibrillin genes. Nature 1991;352:330–334.
6. Woessner J, Brewer T. Formation and breakdown of collagen and elastin in the human uterus during pregnancy and postpartum involution. Biochem J 1963;89:75–82.
7. Rechsberger T, Uldbjerg N, Oxlund H. Connective tissue changes in the cervix during normal pregnancy and pregnancy complicated by cervical incompetence. Obstet Gynecol 1988;7:563–567.
8. Granstrom L, Ehrman G, Ulmsten U, et al. Changes in the connective tissue of corpus and cervix uteri during ripening and labor in term pregnancy. Br J Obstet Gynaecol 1989;96:1198–1202.
9. Ihlberg L, Haukipuro K, Risteli L, Oikarinen A, Kairaluoma M, Risteli J. Collagen synthesis in intact skin is suppressed during wound healing. Ann Surg 1993;217:397–403.
10. Brincat M, Moniz C, Studd J, et al. The long-term effects of the menopause of administration of sex hormones on skin collagen and skin thickness. Br J Obstet Gynaecol 1985;92:256–259.
11. Savvas M, Bishop J, Laurent G, Watson N, Studd J. Type III collagen content in the skin of postmenopausal women receiving estradiol and testosterone implants. Br J Obstet Gynaecol 1993; 100:154–156.
12. Smith P, Heimer G, Norgren A, Ulmsten U. Localization of steroid hormone receptors in the pelvic muscles. Eur J Obstet Gynecol Reprod Biol 1993; 50:83–85.
13. Ulstem U, Ekman G, Giettz G, Malmstrom A. Different biochemical composition of connective tissue in continent and stress incontinent women. Acta Obstet Gynecol Scand 1987;66: 455–457.
14. Rechsberger T, Donica H, Baranowski W, Jakowicki J. Eur J Obstet Gynecol Reprod Biol 1993; 49;187–191.
15. Falconer C, Ekman G, Malmstrom A, Ulmsten U. Decreased collagen synthesis in stress incontinent women. Obstet Gynecol 1994;84;583–586.
16. Kondo A, Narushima M, Yoshikawa Y, Hayashi H. Pelvic fascia strength in women with stress urinary incontinence in comparison with those who are continent. Neurourol Urodyn 1994;13: 507–513.
17. Versi E, Cardozo L, Brincat M, Cooper D, Montgomery J, Studd J. Correlation of urethral physiology and skin collagen in postmenopausal women. Br J Obstet Gynaecol 1988;95: 147–152.
18. Norton P, Baker J, Sharp H, Warenski J. Genitourinary prolapse and joint hypermobility in women. Obstet Gynecol 1995;85:225–229.

CHAPTER 21

Diagnosis and Management of Congenital Urological Abnormalities of Importance to the Gynecologist

David E. Hald, Sherrie A. Hald, and Allan M. Shanberg

Introduction

Congenital anomalies of the genitourinary system represent an intellectually challenging clinical entity. The embryogenesis of the urinary and genital systems are closely associated. Subsequently, a congenital anomaly in one system is often associated with a congenital anomaly in the other. The presenting signs and symptoms of these anomalies can range from the most subtle to the obvious. Because of their varied anatomy and functional complexity, congenital anomalies of the genitourinary system do not lend themselves to simple management algorithms. The clinician confronted with these abnormalities must be familiar with a multiplicity of clinical presentations, radiological appearances, and management options available in each case. Therefore, the management of these patients includes combined medical and surgical approaches.

Embryologically and anatomically, the genital and urinary systems are intimately intertwined; however, functionally they can be divided to facilitate our understanding of these complex organ systems. A genuine understanding of medical embryology greatly facilitates recognition of the significance and rationale for managing many of these anomalies. Such familiarity is not of esoteric interest because congenital anomalies involving the genitourinary system occur in 10% of live births (1).

Although the content of this textbook is primarily dedicated toward lower urinary tract dysfunction, the expanding role of the gynecologist in the primary care setting, the frequency with which congenital upper tract disorders occur, and their significance to all pelvic surgeons necessitates inclusion of these conditions within this chapter. A comprehensive and sensitive approach in managing patients with these congenital anomalies results in improved functional outcome and can help to minimize the emotional crisis for the patient and involved family members.

Embryology of the Upper Urinary Tract

The upper urinary tract consists of the kidneys and ureters. The kidneys develop as three successive renal systems. The original system, termed the pronephros, forms in the cervical region and is nonfunctional. The mesonephros forms in the thoracic and lumbar regions and is characterized by simple excretory units that drain into their own collecting system, the mesonephric or Wolf-fian duct. The mesonephric ducts persist in males and serve as the genital ducts. In females, the mesonephric ducts regress and form vestigial remnants, whereas the para-mesonephric or Mullerian ducts persist.

The metanephros represents the perma-nent kidney and begins to form in the 5-week embryo. This functional unit actually forms from two distinct sources: the ureteric bud and the metanephric blastema. The ureteric bud originates as a diverticulum on the ter-minal mesonephric duct and gives rise to the entire collecting system. Proper connection to the excretory portion, derived from the metanephric blastema, is essential or renal agenesis or congenital cystic renal disease can occur. Furthermore, early division of the ureteric bud or an abnormal location on the mesonephric duct can lead to a duplicated collecting system, an ectopic ureter, or vesi-coureteral reflux.

RENAL AGENESIS

Fortunately, bilateral renal agenesis that is incompatible with postnatal life is a rare phenomena. However, the unilateral absence of a kidney is not infrequent, occurring once in every 1200 births (2). This anomaly is believed to arise when the ureteric bud fails to develop or does not reach the metanephric tissue, resulting in failure in the proliferation of the excretory tubules and the absence of a kidney. This entity is usually discovered incidentally during radiological evaluation because the functioning contralateral kidney is able to perform the necessary excretory role.

Associated urinary tract anomalies in-clude the complete absence of the ipsilateral ureter in most cases or presence of an atretic or maldeveloped ureter in the remaining cases. On cystoscopic examination, a hemi-trigone is usually visualized when the ureter is completely absent. Because of a separate embryological origin from the metanephros, ipsilateral adrenal agenesis is rarely encoun-tered.

Associated internal genital anomalies are observed in over 50% of females with renal agenesis. These include unicornuate uterus with absence of the ipsilateral horn and fallopian tube, bicornuate uterus with primi-tive development of the horn on the affected side, and didelphic uterus with a single or duplicated cervix. Also, reported in the pres-ence of renal agenesis is the absence or duplication of the vagina (3). The close asso-ciation of these internal genital anomalies with renal agenesis mandates a thorough urological survey in this patient population.

Clinically, the absence of one renal unit mandates protection of the remaining kid-ney. Subsequently, patients with an identi-fied solitary kidney are advised to avoid contact sports. The problem with the solitary kidney occurs when the functioning renal unit becomes diseased. In these patients, acute renal insufficiency can be observed with any renal insult; therefore, the primary care physician must follow these patients closely to prevent or minimize nephron loss from urological or medical renal disease. Obstetric care in a patient with a solitary kidney requires special attention, especially to prevent nephrolithiasis and avoid urinary tract obstruction. Nonetheless, the overall prognosis for these patients is excellent.

RENAL ECTOPIA AND HORSESHOE KIDNEY

The estimated incidence of renal ectopia is 1 in 1300 patients and may occur bilaterally in 10% of cases (4). Ectopic kidneys may be found in various locations, but of importance to the gynecologist are those ectopic kidneys found in the pelvic and iliac positions. These ectopic kidneys may be of varying sizes and shapes and are frequently associated with malrotation. Their blood supply is highly variable, and an ectopic kidney may be mis-taken for a mass during pelvic operations.

Initially, the kidneys lie in the pelvis, but with differential caudal growth and rotation they come to lie in their characteristic ana-tomic position within the retroperitoneum. During ascension, the kidney must traverse the umbilical arterial web and the blood supply of the kidney continually changes. When a kidney fails to bypass these vessels, it remains in a caudal or ectopic position.

The pelvic kidney is the most common ectopic location and usually is present below the bifurcation of the abdominal aorta and adjacent to the sacrum. A lumbar kidney is situated in the iliac fossa anterior to the iliac vessels. The ureter of an ectopic kidney usually enters the bladder in a normal location. However, the renal pelvis is often anteriorly displaced because of malrotation, and this may predispose the ectopic kidney to ureteropelvic junction obstruction, urinary tract infection, and stone formation.

Clinically, the ectopic kidney is usually asymptomatic and therefore requires no special intervention. However, it is at an increased risk for traumatic injury because of its low-lying position and lack of protection from the rib cage. Urinary tract obstruction and infection should be treated in an appropriate manner when observed in these kidneys.

A striking feature of renal ectopia is the frequent association with genital anomalies. The incidence ranges from 45 to 70% in female patients. The most common abnormalities described are bicornuate or unicornuate uterus, rudimentary or absent uterus, absence of the proximal or distal vagina, and vaginal duplication (5).

To our knowledge, no deaths have been attributed to the presence of an ectopic kidney. However, case reports describing the mistaken removal of a solitary ectopic kidney, thought to represent a pelvic malignancy, have been noted with disastrous results (6). This should not occur today with the widespread availability of imaging techniques to accurately diagnose this entity. If any intraoperative concern arises, then ultrasonography or a high-dose (2 mL/kg up to 150 mL maximum) intravenous infusion pyelogram can be performed rapidly in the operating room to confirm the presence or absence of a functioning ectopic kidney. Often, oblique films are useful in distinguishing a renal mass from the underlying bony pelvis.

Renal fusion anomalies are not infrequent, and horseshoe kidney is the most common entity, with a reported incidence of approximately 1 in every 400 live births (7). The etiology is believed to be the fusion of the lower poles of the two metanephros before rotation and ascension. This results in the presence of an isthmus, usually with its own blood supply, connecting the two renal units. The inferior mesenteric artery serves as a stopping point for ascension of this linked renal unit and thus accounts for a horseshoe kidney's usual position being at the third or fourth lumbar vertebral level.

The most commonly encountered clinical problems associated with a horseshoe kidney include ureteropelvic junction obstruction, vesicoureteral reflux, nephrolithiasis, and urinary tract infection. As with renal ectopia, management of urological disease in the horseshoe kidney is administered as indicated. Pregnancy is not typically affected by the presence of a horseshoe kidney because it is superior to the pelvic inlet. Overall, the long-term prognosis for patients with a horseshoe kidney is excellent.

CONGENITAL CYSTIC KIDNEY DISEASE

Renal cysts are present in a wide array of renal diseases that the obstetrician-gynecologist may encounter. Simple renal cysts are quite common in the adult population and usually are of no significance. A cystic kidney is a kidney with three or more cysts. Renal cystic disease is a heterogeneous group of disorders, and by convention the term polycystic kidney disease refers to two inheritable conditions: autosomal recessive polycystic kidney disease and autosomal dominant polycystic kidney disease. A third cystic kidney disease increasingly encountered by the obstetrician because of widespread use of antenatal ultrasonography is unilateral multicystic dysplastic kidney disease. This is a noninheritable form of cystic disease.

Unilateral multicystic dysplastic kidney disease is one of the most frequent forms of cystic disease seen in childhood. In contrast to the dilation of normal renal elements as is seen in both the genetic forms of polycystic kidney disease, the multicystic kidney is entirely dysplastic and composed of immature stroma. The multicystic kidney is usually a unilateral lesion in which the entire kidney is replaced with cysts of varying size (Fig. 21.1). These kidneys rarely have functional parenchyma, and the ipsilateral ureter is usually atretic at the ureteropelvic junction. Sonographically, the multicystic kidney can be difficult to distinguish from massive hydronephrosis. A renal scan demonstrating absence of renal function is the confirmatory test in the diagnosis of multicystic dysplastic kidney disease.

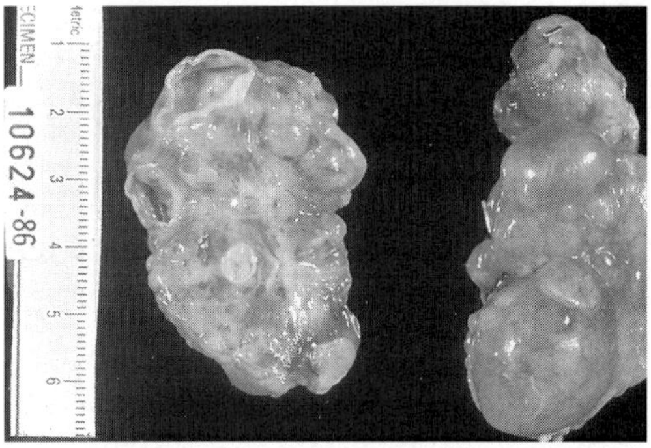

Figure 21.1. Gross specimen of unilateral multicystic dysplastic kidney.

When not identified antenatally, these kidneys classically present as an abdominal or flank mass. Commonly associated with the multicystic kidney is the presence of vesicoureteral reflux and ureteropelvic junction obstruction in the contralateral kidney. Treatment options for these kidneys include laparoscopic and open nephrectomy or observation with serial imaging. In fact, serial ultrasonography has revealed that the natural history of multicystic kidney disease is generally one of spontaneous involution. However, there have been associated case reports of hypertension, Wilms' tumor, and renal cell carcinoma occurring within or due to unilateral multicystic kidney disease (8, 9).

Congenital polycystic kidney disease encompasses two distinct clinical entities. They differ in their mode of inheritance and their pathological characteristics. Common to both, however, is the presence of bilateral renal cysts and a lack of renal dysplasia. Both forms may occur in children, but the recessive form is much more prevalent in a pediatric population and has therefore been commonly called infantile polycystic kidney disease. For simplicity, and to promote a more precise terminology, these two forms are now classified as autosomal recessive polycystic kidney disease and autosomal dominant polycystic kidney disease.

Autosomal recessive polycystic kidney disease is a rare disorder occurring in 1 of every 10,000–40,000 births (10). These kidneys contain multiple bilateral small cysts that histologically represent renal collecting duct dilation. Associated hepatic involvement is always present, and this disease usually presents at birth with large palpable bilateral flank masses. The earlier the age of onset, the worse the prognosis. Previously, this entity had a dismal prognosis with most subjects dying in the neonatal period. However, with improved neonatal intensive care, the survival rate for those presenting in the neonatal period is nearly 50% at 15 years of age (11). The ultimate long-term prognosis depends on the level of renal function, because the liver manifestations can usually be managed successfully. Unfortunately, almost all of these patients will develop end-stage renal disease by adulthood. Adult polycystic kidney disease is also a hereditary disorder but with an autosomal dominant transmission. The penetrance is nearly 100%, and the gene responsible for its transmission has been localized to the short arm of chromosome 16. The incidence is approximately 1 in every 1000–2500 live births, and patients with polycystic disease account for 5–10% of the current population with end-stage renal disease (12). This entity represents a systemic disease because these patients have cystic lesions within the pancreas, liver, and spleen and a high incidence of cerebral berry aneurysms and mitral valve prolapse. Like the recessive form of polycystic kidney disease, the earlier the age of onset, the worse the prognosis.

Classically, autosomal dominant polycystic kidney disease presents during the fourth or fifth decade. The presenting signs and symptoms for polycystic kidney disease include hypertension, flank pain, symptomatic urinary tract infection, nephrolithiasis, gross hematuria, and palpable masses. Hypertension is a common finding in this patient population and should be aggressively treated to minimize end-organ damage. Of importance to the urogynecologist is recognition of the increased risk for iatrogenic urinary tract infection and subsequent sepsis in this patient population. These patients all require appropriate antibiotic prophylaxis before instrumentation of the urinary tract.

For the clinician managing patients with autosomal dominant polycystic kidney disease, it is often difficult to distinguish pyelonephritis from an infected cyst. Failure to respond to lipid-soluble antibiotics remains the best clinical indicator of cyst infection. In the past, cyst aspiration was used to treat these infected cysts. However, this is not currently advised, given the great number of cysts and the potential to infect adjacent uninfected cysts. In cases of intractable cyst infection, a simple nephrectomy may be required with an extraperitoneal approach preferred to avoid intraperitoneal contamination. Finally, pregnancy is not contraindicated in this patient population as long as renal function is normal.

Ureteral Abnormalities

ECTOPIC URETER

An increasing number of urological abnormalities, including ectopic ureters, are being diagnosed by prenatal ultrasonography. The appearance of these conditions is one of hydronephrosis. The benefit of antenatal recognition has been a reduced incidence of urosepsis because these neonates are placed immediately on prophylactic antibiotics. Also, earlier diagnostic imaging and the institution of appropriate medical and surgical management has led to improved functional outcome.

The normal anatomic location of the ureteral orifice is on the interureteric ridge of the bladder trigone. An ectopic ureter is simply one that inserts elsewhere. This clinical condition is more frequently found in females, and although it can occur in a single renal system, it is usually associated with a duplicated renal system in female cases. In the female patient, the ectopic ureter commonly inserts into a more caudal position on the bladder trigone, bladder neck, or the female urethra.

Embryologically, the ectopic ureter is the result of an abnormally located ureteral bud on the terminal mesonephric duct. At 4 weeks of gestation, the ureteral bud develops from the terminal mesonephric duct, and this is the location of the future ureteral orifice. That portion of the duct distal to the ureteral bud will become the trigone of the bladder. If the ureteral bud arises too distally on the mesonephric duct, the ureteral orifice with longitudinal rotation will end up in a more cranial and lateral position in the bladder wall. These orifices are prone to reflux because they have less of a submucosal tunnel

within the bladder wall, and this is discussed later in this chapter.

On the other side, if the ureteral bud arises in a more proximal position on the mesonephric duct, then with rotation it will ultimately end up with an ectopic orifice more caudal to the bladder trigone. These ureters can insert into the vestigial remnants of the mesonephric duct, including the epoophoron, oophoron, and Gartner's duct. It is theorized that these ectopic ureters subsequently rupture into the adjacent female structures and therefore drain into the fallopian tubes, uterus, upper vagina, and vestibule.

An important anatomic relationship exists between the two orifices of a duplicated renal system. In a duplicated renal system, the ureter draining the upper pole system will invariably insert in a caudal and medial position relative to the insertion of the ipsilateral lower pole ureter that is more cranial and lateral. This constant anatomic relationship is the so-called Weigart-Meyer rule (13).

The classic presentation of total urinary incontinence in females with an ectopic ureter is explained by the embryology discussed earlier. The ectopic location of the ureteral orifice is commonly distal or outside the realm of the female urinary sphincter and patients therefore leak (Fig. 21.2). This also explains why some patients present with vaginal discharge. If the ureter terminates in the urethra, it can be mistakenly diagnosed as a urethral diverticulum. Finally, many patients still present with urinary tract infections that prompt a radiographic workup.

The diagnostic workup for an ectopic ureter involves several radiographic studies, including renal and bladder ultrasonography, intravenous pyelography, voiding cystourethrography, and nuclear renal scans as indicated. In addition, vaginoscopy and cystourethroscopy are sometimes helpful in locating the ectopic ureteral orifice. However, the diagnosis of an ectopic ureteral insertion site can be difficult because the orifice is often difficult to distinguish in the normal folds of the vaginal mucosa or uterus. In addition, an upper pole duplication may not visualize well because of obstruction with subsequent poor renal function and can be difficult to read on an ultrasound. In the event of suspicion of this type of duplication, we have found magnetic resonance imaging to be quite helpful (Fig. 21.3). If the upper pole can be seen on an ultrasound or intrave-nous pyelogram yet the ectopic ureteral orifice location cannot be determined, then the upper pole segment can be percutaneously accessed with antegrade injection of contrast dye to delineate the insertion site of the ectopic ureter (Fig. 21.4).

Bilateral single-system ectopic ureters are a rare entity that most commonly occur in females. However, this has profound consequences as both ectopic ureters usually drain into the female urethra. This inhibits the proper development of the bladder trigone and bladder neck. These patients present with incontinence and have an open bladder neck with poor tone. The lack of resistance at the bladder outlet leads to formation of only a rudimentary bladder as illustrated in Figures 21.5 and 21.6. These children require urinary diversion at birth with cutaneous ureterostomies to preserve renal function. Generally, when these children are preschool age, they can be reconstructed with simultaneous bladder augmentation with intestine and bilateral ureteral reimplantation.

Surgical correction of ectopic ureters can

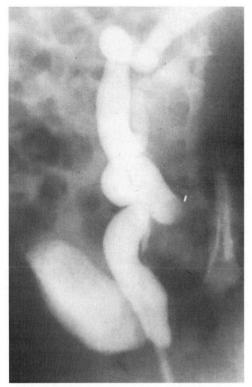

Figure 21.2. Ectopic ureter from upper pole duplicated system entering into the vagina.

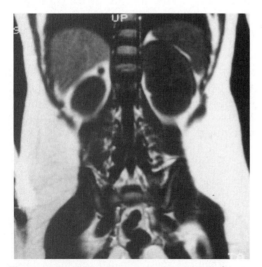

Figure 21.3. Magnetic resonance imaging demonstrating a small atrophic duplicated right upper pole segment from an ectopic ureter inserting into the upper vagina.

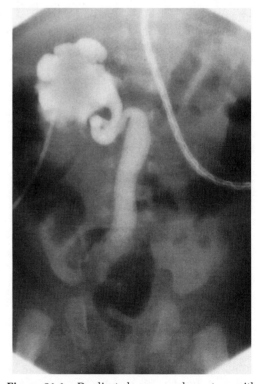

Figure 21.4. Duplicated upper pole system with antegrade injection of contrast dye to demonstrate the insertion site of the dilated ectopic ureter.

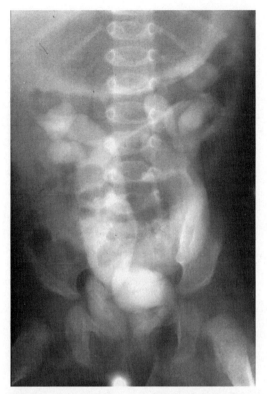

Figure 21.5. Intravenous pyelogram demonstrating bilateral ectopic ureters inserting into the urethra.

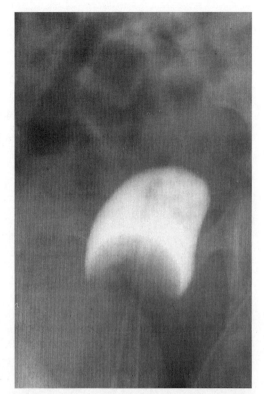

Figure 21.6. Cystogram in the same child demonstrating a rudimentary bladder with a 3.0-mL Foley catheter balloon occupying one half of the bladder.

involve anything from partial upper pole heminephrectomy of a nonfunctioning upper pole segment to ureteroureterostomy for a functioning upper pole segment to salvage additional renal function. Simultaneous removal or ligation of the remaining ureteral segment is performed depending on the presence or absence of vesicoureteral reflux. Occasionally, the ectopic ureter can simply be reimplanted into the bladder to salvage a functioning renal segment.

Sometimes after partial nephrectomy, the distal ureter cannot be safely removed for fear of jeopardizing the blood supply to the normal ipsilateral ureter. In addition, if the ectopic ureter passes through the urethral sphincter area, removal can be precluded by fear of damaging the urinary sphincter mechanism. In these situations, we found it helpful to gently fulgurate the ureteral mucosa using a Bugbee electrode. This allows the ectopic ureter to fibrose and become atretic, without damaging the sphincter mechanism (14).

URETEROCELE

A ureterocele is a cystic dilation of the terminal end of the ureter upon its insertion either into the bladder or ectopically into the urethra. Ureteroceles have a predilection for female gender with an observed ratio of occurrence of 4:1 female to male. In addition, most of ureteroceles arise from a duplicated renal system. There has been a great deal of controversy with respect to their nomenclature and their embryological development. Therefore, The American Academy of Pediatrics, Section on Urology, proposed a standardized simplified terminology for ectopic ureters and ureteroceles. In this system, a ureterocele is either intravesical if it is entirely located within the bladder or ectopic if a portion is located at the bladder neck or urethra.

Today, many ureteroceles are diagnosed through postnatal workup for fetal hydronephrosis identified by the obstetrician on prenatal ultrasonography. Despite early detec-

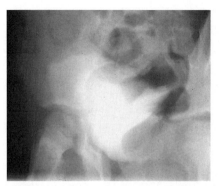

Figure 21.7. Ureterocele filling defect in the bladder on a cystogram.

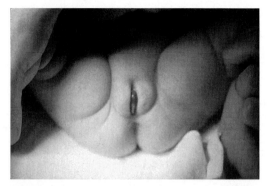

Figure 21.9. Ureterocele prolapsing through the bladder neck and urethra in a female child.

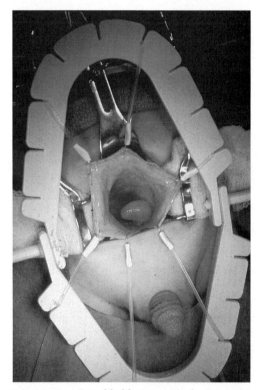

Figure 21.8. Open bladder view of a large ureterocele in a male child.

tion, postnatal diagnosis of ureteroceles still occurs with the most common presentations being urinary tract infection or urosepsis in an infant or child. Asymptomatic ureteroceles can be discovered incidentally as a filling defect within the bladder on an intravenous pyelogram and must be distinguished from bladder neoplasia (Fig. 21.7).

As demonstrated in Figure 21.8, at open surgery of a ureterocele in a male child, these

cystic dilations can achieve a very large size and are capable of obstructing the bladder neck opening, resulting in urinary retention. They also can cause obstruction of the normal contralateral ureteral orifice or the associated ipsilateral duplicated ureter. Ectopic ureteroceles in female patients can present with total incontinence if the orifice lies distal to the sphincteric mechanism or the large size of the cystic dilation inhibits proper closure of the bladder neck.

Occasionally, ureteroceles in female children can prolapse through the urethra and present as a mass protruding through the introitus (Fig. 21.9). This lesion must be differentiated from other known causes of interlabial masses, including congenital paraurethral cyst, urethral prolapse, imperforate hymen, or a solid dermoid midline tumor in the female child. Ultrasonography is extremely helpful in differentiating these lesions, and the ureterocele can usually be identified by its typical round smooth-walled appearance and characteristic cystic presence within the bladder. In cases of ureterocele prolapse, a critically septic infant can be managed by a simple transverse incision of the ureterocele at the level of the vaginal introitus. Rapid decompression allows for recovery of the septic patient, and a subsequent thorough diagnostic workup can then be performed to ensure proper management.

Management of ureteroceles varies from simple observation in the asymptomatic adult or child without upper tract obstruction to the simple endoscopic incision of the ureterocele, as described by Tank (15). If endoscopic incision should fail or if there is a massive prolapsing ureterocele or massive vesicoureteral reflux, then open surgical reconstruction of the ureterocele and reimplantation of the ureters becomes necessary. If the ureterocele should be associated with a dysplastic or nonfunctional upper pole renal system, then partial upper pole nephrectomy is performed with ligation or excision of the remaining ureter depending on the presence or absence of vesicoureteral reflux (16).

An unfortunate side effect of reconstructive surgery for ureteroceles repaired in infancy is urinary incontinence, which is seen as the patient becomes older. In the female patient, this usually results from damage to the sphincteric mechanism during the reconstructive surgery of the bladder neck and proximal urethra. A contributing factor to the incontinence seen with bilateral high-grade obstructing systems is a lack of concentrating ability in the renal tubules and subsequent polyuria.

VESICOURETERAL REFLUX

Vesicoureteral reflux, which is the reversal of urine flow up the ureters, is a very common problem in pediatric urology, with a female predilection. The etiology of congenital or primary reflux is due to the lateral and cranial displacement of the ureteral orifice in the bladder, a consequence of the ureteral bud arising too distal on the mesonephric duct. This results in a shortened submucosal bladder tunnel and predisposes the renal system to the backup of urine.

Reflux is graded from grade 1 (minor ureteral only) to grade 5 (severe intrarenal with distention of the collecting system and loss of the papillary impression on the calyces) (Fig. 21.10). Both host and pathogen factors play a key role in the ultimate outcome of patients with vesicoureteral reflux. Reflux can be transient when associated with severe cystitis or can be congenital. The latter is of importance to the gynecologist and is frequently associated in the adult female with recurrent urinary tract infection, pyelonephritis, reflux nephropathy, and hypertension.

Congenital reflux has been more highly associated with renal scarring and damage and, interestingly enough, is identified in about one third of siblings screened for reflux (17). Vesicoureteral reflux has also been associated with dysfunctional voiding patterns, distal obstruction, detrusor sphincter dysynergia, or detrusor hyperreflexia. In these cases, treatment should be directed toward the etiology of the disease process and not toward the ureterovesical junction, unless the underlying etiology has been previously corrected. The diagnosis of reflux is straightforward with the voiding cystourethrogram used for the initial grading of the reflux and follow-up may be performed with nuclear renal scans to limit the radiation exposure. Cystoscopically, the refluxing ureteral orifice is usually enlarged and laterally displaced.

In neonates and children with low and intermediate grades of reflux, medical management by antibiotic prophylaxis is the treatment of choice. With growth, the bladder wall and the submucosal tunnel may thicken and lengthen, respectively, thereby explaining the resolution seen in patients managed with chemoprophylaxis alone. In fact, mild to moderate grades of reflux spontaneously resolve in 50–80% of cases (18). However, high-grade reflux is unlikely to resolve with medical management and long-term surveillance of all reflux patients, but even those cured are essential.

In the adult or child that has failed conservative management, the treatment of choice is surgical reimplantation of the ureter with creation of an antireflux valve mechanism. Surgical procedures used today are extremely successful, with approximately 98–99% success rates, low perioperative morbidity, and a very low incidence of postoperative obstruction at the implantation site (19). The endoscopic subtrigonal injection

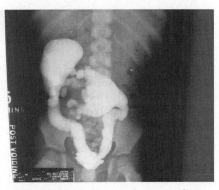

Figure 21.10. Voiding cystourethrogram demonstrating high-grade reflux in a female child with an associated horseshoe kidney.

"STING" of Teflon or collagen has been used with moderate success. However, the superior success rates of open surgery and the risk of Teflon migration have precluded its use in the United States. Long-term results with collagen injections are currently being investigated, and this may prove to be a reasonable treatment alternative.

Finally, there is little evidence at present that the presence of reflux alters the course of a pregnancy or the outcome of the fetus, although there is a chance for proteinuria and hypertension if reflux nephropathy is present with pregnancy.

URETEROPELVIC JUNCTION OBSTRUCTION

Ureteropelvic junction obstruction is the blockage of the ureter at the renal pelvis-proximal ureteral junction. This congenital obstruction is a condition that is frequently found during antenatal ultrasonography. In fact, it is the most common cause of antenatal hydronephrosis.

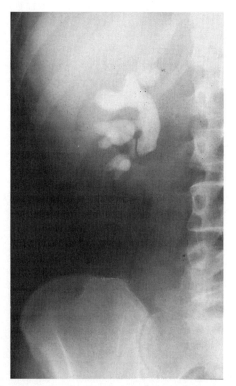

Figure 21.11. Intravenous pyelogram demonstrating ureteropelvic junction obstruction.

In adults, this is a frequently misdiagnosed entity. Adults often present with vague gastrointestinal complaints, flank pain with diuretic consumption, or recurrent urinary tract infection. This congenital anomaly is thought to arise as a consequence of disorganization in the in utero canalization of the renal pelvis and proximal ureter. This disorganization of smooth muscle leads to poor ureteral peristalsis with deposition of collagen and subsequent narrowing at this site.

The workup of a patient suspected of having a ureteropelvic junction obstruction usually includes an intravenous pyelogram with delayed films to ascertain the level of the obstruction (Fig. 21.11). Retrograde ureteropyelography is performed when the intravenous pyelogram is inconclusive. The success of open surgical repair and percutaneous endoscopic management are both quite high in adults, and therefore patients are given a choice in management. In children, an open dismembered pyeloplasty is the technique most often used. This technique is chosen because of the better long-term success noted compared with endoscopic correction in the pediatric patient population.

Embryology of the Lower Urinary Tract

During the fourth to seventh weeks of development, the cloaca is divided by the urorectal septum into the anorectal canal and the urogenital sinus. The primitive urogenital sinus can be divided into three components: a vesical, upper, and larger component that becomes the urinary bladder; the middle or pelvic portion; and a caudal phallic portion. Initially, the bladder is continuous with the allantois, and in normal development this lumen is obliterated and becomes the cord-like urachus. The adult derivative of the urachus is the median umbilical ligament. Persistence of all or a portion of the allantois leads to the urachal anomalies seen in adults, including urachal fistula, urachal sinus, urachal diverticulum, and urachal cyst.

The entire female urethra is derived from the vesical portion of the primitive urogenital sinus. The associated connective tissue and smooth muscle are derived from the adjacent splanchnic mesenchyme. Although rare, congenital anomalies of the female urethra occur, including female hypospadias and congenital urethral diverticulum. Abnormalities in the development of the lower abdominal wall give rise to the various exstrophy anomalies, including classic bladder extrophy, cloacal exstrophy, and female epispadias.

URACHAL MALFORMATIONS

The urachus lies in the retropubic space and is located anatomically between the peritoneum and the transversalis fascia. It extends from the apex of the bladder to the umbilicus and is termed the median umbilical ligament in adults. Although disorders of the urachus are rare, serious complications of urachal abnormalities have been reported. These include a high incidence of infection in urachal cyst and sinus anomalies, peritonitis by rupture of an infected cyst, and neoplasia. Thus, when an accurate diagnosis has been established, removal of the urachal remnant is advised.

Abnormalities of the normal disintegration of the urachus include a patent urachus or urachal fistula that typically presents after birth with the drainage of urine from the umbilicus. Diagnosis can be confirmed with a fistulogram documenting continuous flow into the bladder. Patent urachus may be associated with bladder outlet obstruction in neonates and adults, and therefore an intravenous pyelogram and voiding cystourethrogram are performed to rule out these conditions. Early treatment of a patent urachus is advised to prevent the development of urinary tract infection and sepsis. The treatment of choice is the extraperitoneal removal of the urachus within its umbilicovesical fascia with excision of a bladder cuff to prevent the subsequent development of adenocarcinoma in the vesical portion of urachal remnant.

A urachal sinus is a blind ending opening at the umbilicus or bladder that may drain mucus intermittently. It arises when the umbilical or vesical portion of the urachus fails to involute. The diagnosis of urachal sinus can be made with a sinogram, demonstrating incomplete communication of contrast for the length of the urachus. Again, treatment is

total excision of the urachal remnant with a cuff of normal bladder.

Urachal diverticulum may predispose a patient to recurrent urinary tract infections and is often associated with bladder outlet obstruction. This congenital abnormality is occasionally noted incidentally during cystoscopy and may be associated with the formation of a stone within the diverticulum. Located at the apex of the bladder, urachal diverticulum should be removed if symptomatic. Asymptomatic diverticula do not require intervention.

Urachal cysts are encountered when a segment of the urachus fails to obliterate. These cysts frequently become infected and should be considered in the differential diagnosis of midline abdominal or pelvic pain. Computed tomography scan is the diagnostic study of choice. Empiric antibiotic therapy is indicated because cases of perforation into the peritoneum have been reported with subsequent systemic sepsis. Treatment options include incision and drainage, percutaneous drainage with antibiotics, and extraperitoneal excision with a cuff of bladder. The latter is preferred because of the high incidence of recurrent infection if the urachal remnant is not completely excised.

Urachal tumors are an uncommon entity but can be identified during routine cystoscopic examination of the bladder by the gynecologist. Generally, symptoms associated with these tumors include gross hematuria, dysuria, and the presence of an abdominal or pelvic mass. Histologically, they usually represent poorly differentiated adenocarcinomas and are sometimes associated with mucous secretion. They should be considered in all cases of bloody umbilical drainage and can be diagnosed with cystoscopy and transurethral biopsy of the lesion at the apex of the bladder. The entire urachal lumen is at risk for the development of adenocarcinoma; however, most urachal tumors arise in the bladder. Supravesical tumors may attain considerable size before they give rise to symptoms.

The primary treatment of urachal carcinoma has been wide surgical excision of the urachus within its umbilicovesical fascia and a partial cystectomy. For supravesical cases, it may be necessary to remove the umbilicus and a portion of the posterior abdominal wall if the lesion is locally extensive. In general, the prognosis for urachal adenocarcinoma is grave, and no study has demonstrated a clear survival advantage with more aggressive surgical therapy such as anterior pelvic exenteration (20).

CONGENITAL BLADDER ANOMALIES

Congenital anomalies of the bladder are exceedingly rare and include diverticula and duplication anomalies. Because most diverticula are actually acquired, their presence mandates evaluation for possible bladder outlet obstruction. The exception is the congenital periureteral diverticula of Hutch associated with vesicoureteral reflux. These diverticula are a consequence of weakening of the hiatus near the ureteral orifice and therefore are located cystoscopically near the ureteral orifice. Most Hutch diverticula are small and occur equally in both sexes. The diagnosis is established with a voiding cystourethrogram, and treatment is offered if symptoms associated with infection or stones develop. Repair is based on the treatment of the reflux.

The complete duplication of the bladder has been reported and is more common in males. With bladder duplication, there is an increased association with duplication of the external genitalia and the gastrointestinal tract. These rare cases typically present with two bladder halves, each with an associated ureter and urethra. Spinal duplication and fistulas between the rectum, vagina, and urethra are other commonly associated findings in these rare cases (22). In addition, complete bivalving of the bladder is seen in female children with cloacal extrophy (Fig. 21.12).

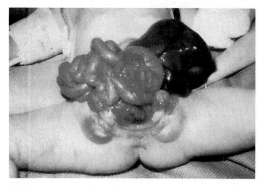

Figure 21.12. Cloacal exstrophy in a female child.

URETHRAL ABNORMALITIES

Disorders of the female urethra are quite rare, and their clinical presentation is usually due to stress or total incontinence. These disorders include congenital urethral diverticulum, female hypospadias, and subsymphyseal epispadias. In general, these diagnoses come to the attention of the clinician who carries out a careful urogenital history and thorough physical examination.

Of these disorders, congenital urethral diverticulum is the most common entity. This condition may present as postvoid dribbling in the female patient with associated infection, dyspareunia, or an anterior vaginal wall mass. Voiding cystourethrography in a standing position is a useful diagnostic test. When this does not identify a suspected diverticulum, then endovaginal ultrasonography or retrograde pressure urethrography with double occlusion balloon technique may be helpful. Surgical management options for this disorder include endoscopic techniques, marsupialization of the diverticulum, or open diverticulectomy.

A rare disorder of the female urethra is hypospadias. A patient with this disorder may be completely asymptomatic or present with incontinence. A careful physical examination of the urethra can usually aid in the diagnosis. The ventral urethra is shortened, and the urethra may be difficult to catheterize. Surgical elongation of the urethra can often cure the incontinence if present. This congenital condition is believed to result from a poorly developed urogenital sinus.

Subsymphyseal epispadias is also a rare condition encountered in older female children presenting with incontinence. This entity represents a variant of the extrophy-epispadias complex and is associated with a patulous poorly developed dorsal urethra. There is also a defect in the pubic hair at the midline. Surgical reconstruction of the urethra is mandatory to treat this form of congenital incontinence.

EXSTROPHY COMPLEX AND VARIANTS

Exstrophy of the bladder represents a spectrum of abnormalities in which there may be defects in the abdominal wall, umbilicus, pubis, bladder, external genitalia, and intes-

tines. Common to all the exstrophic abnormalities is the increased incidence in the
male population. However, recognition of
these entities in the female population is
important to the urogynecologist and the
obstetrician.

Exstrophy is probably caused by a failure
of the cloacal membrane to retract. The cloacal membrane covers the midlower abdomen
in the first weeks of gestation. In the fourth
week of gestation, the membrane retracts
caudally, allowing the medial migration of
mesoderm on the lateral borders of the membrane to produce the abdominal wall and roll
the bladder into a spherical structure. If the
membrane persists inappropriately, then this
portion of the abdominal wall fails to develop, and when the cloacal membrane ruptures, the bladder is left exposed and everted
(Fig. 21.13).

Associated anomalies include vesicoureteral reflux in almost all patients, inguinal
hernias, and epispadias with a widely separated pubis always being present. Classic
bladder exstrophy is the most commonly
seen condition in this complex, whereas
cloacal exstrophy represents the most serious
form of this entity. Cloacal exstrophy results
from premature rupture of the cloacal membrane before separation. This results in two
halves of an extrophied bladder separated by
an exstrophied ileocecal segment of bowel.

The initial management of the exstrophied
bladder should be to protect the mucosa of
the bladder from injury by simply covering
this with plastic wrap. Care should be taken
by the pediatrician and obstetrician to protect the bladder mucosa from diaper irritation and the umbilical cord clamp. Primary
bladder closure is usually performed in the
first few days of life when the pelvic ring is
more flexible, presumably from the presence
of maternal relaxin. After the bladder is
closed, no initial attempt is made to tighten
the bladder neck. Bilateral iliac osteotomies
are often performed to bring the pubic rami to
the midline, anterior to the bladder, allowing
for a more secure bladder closure.

Epispadias repair and female genitoplasty
are then performed at 6–18 months of age
before the sexual identity stage of psychosocial development. This is followed by a separate bladder neck reconstructive procedure
for developing continence with simulta-

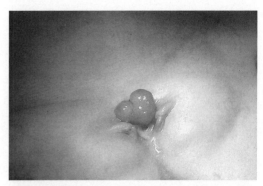

Figure 21.13. Subsymphyseal epispadias in a female newborn with exstrophy.

neous bilateral ureteral reimplantation to
prevent vesicoureteral reflux. The most common reason for failure of a bladder neck
constructive procedure is the presence of a
small-capacity noncompliant bladder. This
can be corrected with an augmentation cystoplasty. If persistent leakage occurs because
of low outflow resistance, then collagen injection or placement of an artificial urinary
sphincter may be undertaken. An alternative
solution is the performance of a continent
cutaneous urinary diversion.

The significance of the exstrophic conditions for the obstetrician are the high incidence of cervical and uterine prolapse after
pregnancy in this patient population. Cesarean section is often recommended in continent patients to avoid damage to the previously reconstructed bladder neck. In addition, these patients have a very high incidence of fetal malpresentation.

The least severe form of this complex is isolated female epispadias. These patients have
a characteristic clinical examination with depressed mons, bifid clitoris, ill-developed
labia minora, patulous urethra, and an un-
formed bladder neck (Fig. 21.14). Pubic dia-
stasis is also present and can aid in the diagnosis in the less severe forms of female
epispadias. In addition to genitoplasty, these
patients usually require bladder neck reconstruction for treatment of incontinence and
bilateral ureteral reimplantation for correction of vesicoureteral reflux. Recognition of
this entity is important to the urogynecologist because a bladder neck suspension will
fail as the treatment of incontinence if this is
the only surgical therapy used.

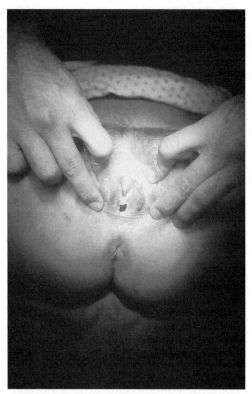

Figure 21.14. Subsymphyseal epispadias in an adult female without extrophy demonstrating depressed mons, bifid clitoris, and a patulous urethra.

Embryology of the External Genitalia

The female external genitalia arise from the genital tubercle, genital swellings, and the urogenital folds. Although indifferent at 6–7 weeks, the external genitalia in the absence of androgen stimulation and the presence of maternal estrogens, produced by the placenta and the mother, develop into the female structures seen in adult life. The genital tubercle becomes the clitoris and the urogenital folds become the labia minora. The genital swellings enlarge and become two folds of skin termed the labia majora.

CLITORAL ANOMALIES

Congenital clitoral anomalies include bifid clitoris and clitoral hypertrophy. A bifid clitoris is seen in association with the exstrophy-epispadias complex and is associated with total urinary incontinence. The most common cause of an enlarged clitoris in the newborn is prematurity. With differential growth, this will resolve without intervention. In a term infant, the presence of clitoral enlargement should suggest the possibility of an intersex abnormality. Although there are many intersex disorders, congenital adrenal hyperplasia is most commonly encountered clinically.

CONGENITAL ADRENAL HYPERPLASIA (FEMALE PSEUDOHERMAPHRODITISM)

This is a disorder of glucocorticoid synthesis in the adrenal gland secondary to a hereditary defect in the enzymes necessary for glucocorticoid production. Defects in 21-hydroxylase, 11-hydroxylase, and, rarely, 3β-dehydrogenase are the most common enzyme abnormalities found in these chromosomally normal females that may have completely virilized external genitalia.

Secondary to this block in the production of hydrocortisone, corticotropin production increases. This increases androgen production, which then virilizes the external genitalia of these otherwise normal female patients (Fig. 21.15). The tragedy of this syndrome is that if unrecognized, these children may either die from adrenal insufficiency or, because of the development of female secondary sex characteristics at puberty, may be diagnosed as female after having been reared as males (22). Therefore, in the neonatal period, any child with ambiguous genitalia and bilateral nonpalpable testes should be suspected of having an intersex abnormality until proven otherwise.

Female pseudohermaphroditism can also occur secondary to maternal ingestion of progestational agents in the first trimester of pregnancy or in infants born to mothers with virilizing tumors during pregnancy.

Satisfactory genital reconstruction can occur in the neonatal period and is encouraged during this time period to prevent the psychological trauma to the parents that can result from sending the female child home with a fully developed phallus (Fig. 21.16).

LABIAL ANOMALIES

The most frequently seen congenital labial anomalies are labial ectopia and fusion. The ectopic labia are rare entities but have been associated with renal agenesis. Labial fusion anomalies are more frequently seen and may be asymptomatic or present with recurrent urinary tract infections or postvoid dribbling. The congenital fusion of the labia represents union of the urogenital folds, and this anomaly is best repaired with surgical separation (Fig. 21.17). The presence of chronic inflammation can lead to labial adhesions that can mimic this congenital anomaly. These acquired adhesions can be treated with topical estrogen cream. If unsuccessful, then surgical separation of the labia is indicated for labial adhesions as well.

Embryology of the Internal Genitalia

The vagina forms after the solid tip of the paramesonephric ducts, termed the mullerian tubercle, has joined with the urogenital sinus. Two solid outpouchings named the sinovaginal bulbs grow cranially from the sinus, whereas the mullerian tubercle grows caudally. Eventually after proliferation is completed, canalization produces the vagina. In this manner, the upper one third of the vagina is paramesonephric in origin, whereas the lower two thirds originate from the urogenital sinus. The hymen represents the point of origin of the sinovaginal bulbs from the urogenital sinus.

UTERINE ANOMALIES

Development of the uterus depends on normal fusion of the paired paramesonephric ducts, with subsequent resorption of the medial portions. Failure of lateral fusion or of recanalization results in uterine malformation. Uterine malformations occur with an incidence of approximately 1 per 600 women. They range from minor fusion and recanalization defects, such as arcuate uterus

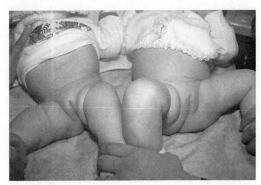

Figure 21.16. Twin female children with adrenogenital syndrome 1 year after genital reconstruction.

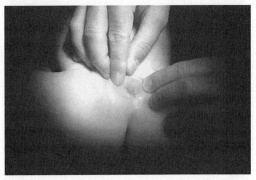

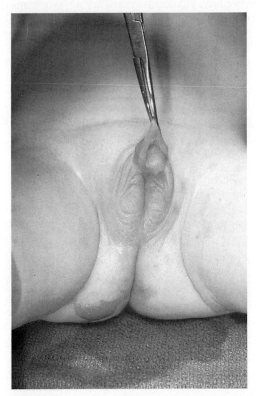

Figure 21.15. Female child with congenital adrenal hyperplasia with masculinized external genitalia.

Figure 21.17. Congenital fusion abnormality of the labia.

and uterine septum, to major malformations, including unicornuate uterus and uterine duplication with or without communication.

The developing mullerian and mesonephric systems are intimately associated. Proper development of one system is interdependent on the other; therefore, arrested or aberrant development in one system adversely affects the other. Approximately 30% of these patients with a major uterine malformation will have an associated urinary tract anomaly (23). In general, most symmetric communicating uteri are associated with a normal urinary system. However, virtually all cases of communicating uteri with an obstructive hemivagina have an associated renal anomaly, primarily ipsilateral renal agenesis. Unicornuate uterus is virtually always associated with ipsilateral renal agenesis (24, 25). Consequently, women with these major anomalies should be evaluated radiographically for concomitant urological anomalies.

HYDROMETROCOLPOS

Patients with hydrometrocolpos or hydrocolpos usually present in infancy with a large abdominal mass, which is fluid distention of the vagina (colpo) and uterus (metro). The mass can displace the intestines upward and can cause significant hydronephrosis from obstruction of the ureters (Fig. 21.18). The cause is usually imperforate hymen, transverse vaginal septum, or vaginal atresia.

A variant of hydrometrocolpos may frequently be seen in female children with an imperforate anus or other cloacal-type abnormalities. In these children with cloacal abnormalities, the external genitalia may be confused with an intersex abnormality, as demonstrated in Figure 21.19, which shows a female child with a single perineal orifice (cloaca) and hypertrophy of the clitoral folds. The obstruction to both the urethra and the vagina can result in massive dilation of the vagina as it fills with urine from the bladder. This has frequently been termed a urine-storing vagina (Fig. 21.20).

The treatment of hydrometrocolpos in the neonatal period should be urgent and aggressive because of the risk of neonatal sepsis. In cases of vaginal atresia or a single perineal orifice from an imperforate anus or cloacal anomaly, the surgical treatment is complicated. If possible, ideal treatment consists of a perineal pull-through procedure separating the urethra and the vagina. Unfortunately, this is not technically feasible in some small neonates. In such cases, consideration is given to temporarily diverting the urinary tract and the vagina. This can be accomplished by diverting both the bladder and vagina to the skin temporarily at the same time as the colostomy is performed. A simple alternative we have found useful is to place the child on clean intermittent catheterization through the cloaca. This may be contin-

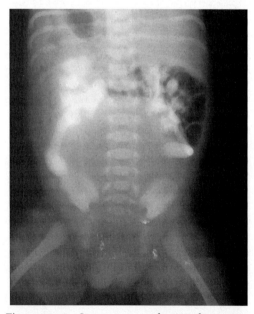

Figure 21.18. Intravenous pyelogram demonstrating upward displacement of intestinal gas pattern by a large pelvic mass in a newborn with hydrometrocolpos.

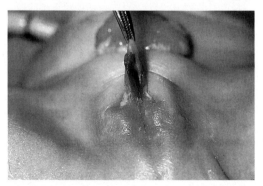

Figure 21.19. Female child with a single perineal orifice secondary to cloacal abnormality.

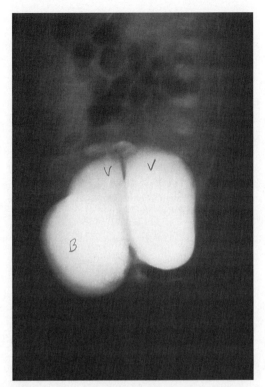

Figure 21.20. Urine-storing duplicated vagina in a female child with a cloacal abnormality.

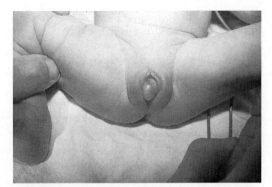

Figure 21.21. Imperforate hymen with bulging hydrometrocolpos in a newborn.

ued until the child is large enough to perform a definitive pull-through procedure.

IMPERFORATE HYMEN

When vaginal canalization terminates before the origin of the sinovaginal bulbs, imperforate hymen develops. This condition most often presents at the onset of puberty with cyclic abdominal pain and amenorrhea. Occasionally, imperforate hymen presents in infancy or childhood with an abdominal mass secondary to hydro-or mucocolpos. Examination reveals a bulging membrane at the introitus that is often bluish or purple in color (Fig. 21.21). When identified, treatment should never be undertaken by simple needle aspiration. Expedient drainage with a cruciate incision is the preferred intervention. Imperforate hymen is not associated with urological anomalies.

TRANSVERSE VAGINAL SEPTUM

Failure of complete canalization of the vagina results in a transverse vaginal septum.

This occurs in approximately 1 of 75,000 female births (26). Although this also presents with primary amenorrhea and hematometrocolpos, unlike imperforate hymen, this is associated with an increase in urinary tract anomalies. Most frequently reported is unilateral renal agenesis.

VAGINAL AGENESIS

Agenesis of the vagina (atresia) is primarily associated with the Mayer-Rokitansky-Kuster-Hauser syndrome. Although primarily a chance occurrence, an autosomal recessive form has been described by McKusick and associates (27). This condition consists of congenital absence or malformation of the vagina, cervix, and uterus. Usually, the ovaries and fallopian tubes are present and normal. Presentation is one of primary amenorrhea and possibly an abdominal mass. This maldevelopment of the paramesonephric system is associated with a 25–50% incidence of renal anomalies, most commonly renal agenesis and pelvic kidney (28, 29). Although ovarian function can usually be documented, it is worthwhile to obtain karyotyping because of the phenotypic similarity to the androgen insensitivity syndrome in which urinary anomalies are rare, but the gonads (testes) are abnormal and should be removed after puberty due to the risk of gonadoblastoma.

TURNER SYNDROME

This syndrome, also known as gonadal dysgenesis, is the most common cause of primary amenorrhea seen by the gynecologist. These patients also have associated short stature, webbed neck, multiple congenital anomalies, underdeveloped external genitalia, and bilateral streak gonads with a genotype missing a portion or all of the X chromosome. Between 33 and 60% of all patients with Turner syndrome have either structural or positional abnormalities of the kidneys (30). The most common abnormalities described are horseshoe kidney, double collecting systems, absence of a kidney, malrotation, and adult onset silent hydronephrosis.

Conclusions

Congenital anomalies of the genitourinary system are frequently encountered in clinical practice. Many clues to these diagnosis are subtle; however, the close association of the genital and urinary systems mandates a thorough evaluation of each system in these patients. Because of the diversity of clinical presentations and embryological possibilities, the management of these congenital anomalies requires individualized care after extensive radiological and endoscopic evaluation. Although many of these conditions are rare isolated events, recognition of these conditions can facilitate proper patient referral and minimize morbidity. With this in mind and meticulous operative technique, the functional outcome in patients with these complex problems can be optimized.

REFERENCES

1. Vaughn ED Jr, Middleton GW. Pertinent genitourinary embryology. Review for the practicing urologist. Urology 1975;6:139–149.
2. Shieh CP, Hung CS, Wei CF, Lin CY. Cystic dilatations within the pelvis in patients with ipsilateral renal agenesis or dysplasia. J Urol 1990;144:324–327.
3. D'Alberton A, Reschini E, Ferrari N, Candiani P. Prevalence of urinary tract abnormalities in a large series of patients with uterovaginal atresia. J Urol 1981;126:623–624.
4. Thompson GJ, Pace JM. Ectopic kidney: a review of 97 cases. Surg Gynecol Obstet 1937;64:935–943.
5. Wiersma AF, Peterson LF, Justema EJ. Uterine anomalies associated with unilateral renal agenesis. Obstet Gynecol 1976;47:654–657.
6. Downs RA, Lane JW, Burns E. Solitary pelvic kidney: its clinical implications. Urology 1973;1:51–56.
7. Glenn JF. Analysis of 51 patients with horseshoe kidney. N Engl J Med 1959;261:684.
8. Susskind MR, Kim KS, King LR. Hypertension and multicystic kidney. Urology 1989;34:362–366.
9. Birken G, King D, Vare D, Lloyd T. Renal cell carcinoma arising in a multicystic dysplastic kidney. J Pediatr Surg 1985;20:619–621.
10. Zerres K, Volpel MC, Weiss H. Cystic kidneys: genetics, pathologic anatomy, clinical picture and prenatal diagnosis. Hum Genet 1984;68:104–135.
11. Gagnadoux M, Habid R, Levy M, Brunelle F, Broyer M. Cystic renal diseases in children. Adv Nephrol 1989;18:33–57.
12. Glassberg KI, Stephans FD, Lebowitz RL, et al. Renal dysgenesis and cystic disease of the kidney: a report of the committee on terminology, nomenclature and classification, Section on Urology, American Academy of Pediatrics. J Urol 1987;138:1085–1092.
13. Meyer R. Development of the ureter in the human embryo: a mechanistic consideration. Anat Rec 1946;96:355–371.
14. Ehrlich RM, Shanberg AM, Koyle MA. A technique for ureteral stump ablation. J Urol 1988;140:1240–1241.
15. Tank ES. Experience with endoscopic incision and open unroofing of ureteroceles. J Urol 1986;136:241–242.
16. Decter RM, Roth DR, Gonzales ET. Individualized treatment of ureteroceles. J Urol 1989;142:535–537.
17. Noe HN. The long-term results of prospective sibling reflux screening. J Urol 1992;148:1739–1742.
18. Arant BS. Medical management of mild and moderate vesicoureteral reflux: follow-up studies of infants and young children. A preliminary report of the southwest pediatric nephrology study group. J Urol 1992;148:1683–1687.
19. Duckett JW, Walker RD, Weiss R. Surgical results: international reflux study in children—United States branch. J Urol 1992;148:1674–1675.
20. Pode D, Fair WR. Urachal tumors. AUA Update Series 1991;10:34–39.
21. Kossow JH, Morales PA. Duplication of bladder and urethra and associated anomalies. Urology 1973;1:71–73.
22. New IN, Dupont B, Grumbach K, Levine LS. Congenital adrenal hyperplasia and related conditions. In: Stanbury JB, Wyngaarden JB, Frederickson DS, Goldstein JL, Brown MS, eds. Metabolic basis of inherited disease. 5th ed. New York: McGraw-Hill, 1983:973–1000.
23. Semmens J. Congenital anomalies of female genital tract: functional classification based on review of 56 personal cases and 500 reported cases. Obstet Gynecol 1962;19:328.
24. Toaff ME, Lev-Toaff AS, Toaff R. Communicating uteri: review and classification with introduction of two previously unreported types. Fertil Steril 1984;41:661–679.

25. Wiersma AF, Peterson LF, Justema EJ. Uterine anomalies associated with unilateral renal agenesis. Obstet Gynecol 1976;47:654–657.
26. Stenchever MA. Congenital abnormalities. In: Herbst AL, Mishell DR, Stenchever MA, Droegemueller W, eds. Comprehensive gynecology. 2nd ed. St. Louis: Mosby, 1992:255–270.
27. McKusick VA, Bauer RL, Koop CE, Scott RB. Hydrometrocolpos as a simple inherited malformation. JAMA 1964;1989:813–816.
28. Tarry WF, Duckett JW, Stephens FD. The Mayer-Rokitansky syndrome: pathology, classification and management. J Urol 1986;136:648–652.
29. Fore SR, Hammond CB, Parker RT, Anderson EE. Urologic and genital anomalies in patients with congenital absence of the vagina. Obstet Gynecol 1975;46:410–416.
30. Hall JC, Gilchrist DM. Turner syndrome and its variants. Pediatr Clin North Am 1990;37:1421–1435.

CHAPTER 22

Urinary Tract Dysfunction in Adolescents and Young Women

Robert W. Lobel and Peter K. Sand

Female adolescents are affected by both the residual urogenital disorders of childhood and those inherent to the young sexually active woman. Even if present since early childhood, many disease states first reach the attention of a physician during adolescence. This is especially true of the abnormal voiding states that are found in this age group. Many of these voiding disorders are the same as those found in the adult; however, their etiology, evaluation, and treatment are often quite different. Neat compartmentalization of these disorders is difficult. For example, lower urinary tract infections (UTIs) can cause voiding dysfunction and vesicoureteral reflux, and vice versa. Because of the proximity of the lower urinary tract to the vulva, vagina, rectum, and anus, any inflammatory or irritative process, infectious or not, in one of these organs can produce urinary tract symptoms and dysfunctional voiding.

Urogenital Tract Infections

Urogenital tract infections are probably the most common etiology underlying urogynecological complaints in the adolescent or young woman. Clinicians treating any aspect of urogynecological disorders should have a heightened awareness and suspicion for these infections. Trichomonal, monilial, herpetic, and gonococcal infections of the lower genital tract may often directly involve the urethra, causing symptoms of dysuria, urgency, frequency, or retention. Even if the urethra is not directly involved, these lower urinary tract symptoms may be noted secondary to the generalized afferent sensation from the pudendal nerve, which innervates both the vulva and urethra.

LOWER UTI

Lower UTI is covered in detail in Chapter 28. However, there are several issues that are unique to this disease in children and adolescents. Pyelonephritis, renal scarring, hypertension, and end-stage renal failure are clearly linked to UTIs acquired early in life. These sequelae underlie the value of early accurate diagnosis, treatment, and prevention of recurrence or relapse. Because of their shorter urethra with lower urethral pressure, girls are more susceptible to UTI than boys, with enteric bacterial ascent from the rectum and perineum being the main portal of entry. Multiple studies have documented that, on routine screening, significant bacteriuria in clean voided specimens ($>10^5$ colonies/mL) has been found in up to 3% of schoolgirls. Viral UTI is less common, but acute hemorrhagic cystitis may sometimes be secondary to type 11 and, less commonly, type 21 adenovirus. Viral UTI is manifest by sudden pain and hematuria that lasts 2 to 7 days. Papovavirus has also been implicated as a cause of this syndrome.

Symptoms of lower UTI (dysuria, fre-

Table 22.1. Risk Factors for Urinary Tract Infection in Adolescents and Young Women

Vesicoureteral reflux
Younger age
Poor toileting habits
Voiding dysfunction
Sexual activity
Limited immune status

quency, urgency, suprapubic pain, incontinence) are the same in the adolescent as in the adult but may be absent in up to one third of all initial infections in young adolescents. The symptoms of urgency and frequency may also be absent in some recurrent infections, which makes diagnosis difficult. The absence of symptoms in some of these recurrent cases does not make these infections any less destructive.

Risk factors for the development of UTI are listed in Table 22.1. Vesicoureteral reflux has been consistently found in about 40% of girls with more than one infection. In one study, more than one third of voiding cystourethrograms demonstrated reflux in girls with only one episode of infection. Radiologic evaluation (primarily with ultrasound) is generally recommended for girls with UTI who are under the age of 5, who have pyelonephritis, or who have a recurrent UTI.

In the presence of a normal radiographic evaluation of the urinary tract, other factors must be considered. Infants have heavy periurethral colonization of *Escherichia coli* and other enterobacteriaceae as well as enterococci (1). The etiology is unknown, but colony counts usually decrease significantly after the first year of life. Poor toileting habits (e.g., infrequent micturition, constipation, and the use of avoidance maneuvers) are present in 90% of children with UTI who have normal imaging studies (2). Similarly, any voiding disorders that cause urinary retention (e.g., detrusor-sphincter dyssynergia) can result in UTI. Detrusor instability in young women without incontinence may also increase the risk of recurrent UTI from backwash of urethral bacteria into the bladder with activation of the guarding reflex (levator ani contraction) to prevent leakage. The risk of UTI rises with the onset of sexual intercourse, presumably by the entry of periurethral bacteria into the bladder at the time

of coitus. Finally, girls with recurrent UTI have lower levels of urinary IgA. This may impair their host response to infection.

Diagnosis of UTI in children and adolescents is established by a urine culture that grows greater than 10^5 colonies on a voided specimen or 10^2 colonies on a catheterized specimen. Most patients can obtain a clean catch specimen reliably, but sometimes catheterization or suprapubic aspiration may be necessary to rule out contamination. Antibiotic therapy should be individualized. In most patients with a normal urinary tract, a 3-day course of antibiotics is as effective as a longer course and has the advantage of causing fewer side effects, less bacterial resistance, and better patient compliance.

Because of the risk of silent upper UTI and renal scarring, patients should be screened for asymptomatic bacteriuria after active infections have been cleared. If persistent bacteriuria is found, consideration should then be given to evaluation of the upper tract for urolithiasis, malformation, and scarring. Routine cystoscopy and intravenous pyelography in girls with uncomplicated UTIs have a very low diagnostic yield and are to be discouraged.

RECURRENT UTI

Recurrent infections (at least two in a 6-month period) should be treated with appropriate antibiotics until culture confirms cure. A course of low-dose antibiotic prophylaxis usually prevents subsequent recurrent infections. This type of treatment is not curative, however, and most patients return to their baseline state of increased susceptibility when the prophylaxis ends. A different approach to recurrent infections involves having the patient screen her own urine for bacteriuria on a weekly basis. The most popular rapid screen, the Greiss nitrite reagent (a combination of sulfanilic acid and alpha-naphthalene), is available in several commercially available test kits. Given enough contact time (4 hours), most urinary tract bacteria convert normal urine nitrate to nitrite. The reagent undergoes diazotization with nitrites to form a red azo dye, effecting a color change on the dipstick. Because of this time requirement, the first morning voided specimen is most suitable. Specificity is excellent (92–100%), but the sensitivity of this test is poor (3).

Three decades ago, urethral dilatation, urethrotomy, and Y-V urethroplasty were commonly performed on those rare patients with normal urinary tracts who did not respond to antibiotics. Although it has been demonstrated that the urethral caliber of girls with recurrent cystitis is not reduced and that their urethras may even be larger than those of controls, a few authors demonstrated remarkable cure rates of up to 90% with dilatation (4). Although the external urethral sphincter is not a physical obstruction in most of these girls, it may act as a functional obstruction in the presence of detrusor-sphincter dyssynergia or pseudodyssnergic syndromes. Increased sensory afferent activity from an inflamed urethra may lead to discoordination between the detrusor and the external sphincter in some girls with symptomatic infections. This dyssynergic voiding pattern may persist long after the infection is cured and lead to distal urethrovesical reflux (backwash) and further infection. Dilatation may act to eliminate the afferent stimulation by treating the underlying inflammatory process. In one prospective trial, 78% of patients treated by urethrotomy plus antibiotics compared with only 29% of girls treated with antibiotics alone was shown to be free of infection 2 years later (5). In addition, reflux was resolved in 50% of the patients treated by urethrotomy. However, convincing prospective trials have shown no superiority of dilatation or urethrotomy over antibiotics alone (6). This lack of superior efficacy, as well as the complications of bleeding, vesicovaginal fistula, decreased urethral closure pressure (7), and subsequent incontinence, has caused these procedures to fall into disfavor by many.

COITUS-RELATED UTIs

The onset of sexual activity will presage coitus-related urinary symptoms in many adolescents and young women. "Honeymoon cystitis" is well known to gynecologists as a syndrome that now often precedes the honeymoon in young women. This is a condition where first coitus, coitus with a new partner, or coitus in a new position results in the symptoms of UTI. These irritative symptoms may be secondary to UTI or urethritis as discussed below. The entry of periurethral bacteria at the time of intercourse may be affected by anatomic changes of the introitus, and nulliparas are at increased risk compared with multiparas. Bacteriuria may be found in up to 30% of women normally after intercourse (8). One study found that recent vaginal intercourse was the most significant risk factor for developing infection of the lower urinary tract (9). Diaphragm use also contributed significantly to these young women's chances of developing UTI. Oral contraceptive use, tampon use, and the direction of wiping after a bowel movement were not found to be significant risk factors on multivariate analysis. Postcoital voiding was found to be protective against developing symptomatic infection. A more recent investigation found that a single act of vaginal intercourse increased the risk of UTI by 90% (10). Vaginal intercourse using a condom increased the risk of UTI by an additional 43%. Sexually transmitted diseases, as discussed below, can also cause urinary tract symptomatology.

URETHRITIS

When investigation of lower urinary tract symptoms reveals no obvious pathology, urethritis should be considered, particularly in young women and adolescents who are sexually active. Most investigators believe that infection is the major cause of urethritis. However, bacterial cultures are usually negative. Although *Chlamydia, Mycoplasma,* and *Ureaplasma* have garnered much attention for their possible roles in urethritis, we and others (11) have found little evidence of these organisms, even with special cultures and the newer polymerase chain reaction tests. Other pathogens, such as *Candida, Trichomonas,* and human papilloma virus, can also cause urethritis. The urethral syndrome is discussed in detail in Chapter 24.

VULVOVAGINITIS

Patients with severe vulvovaginitis of any etiology can present with dysuria, frequency, urgency, and incontinence, as well as the more common vaginal complaints of discharge, odor, and itching. The most common infectious causes are bacterial vaginosis, *Candida,* and *Trichomonas.*

Nonspecific vulvovaginitis is the most common type of genital inflammation in prepubertal girls. The vulva and vagina are erythematous, but discharge is rare. Wet mount and cultures fail to identify pathogens. Treatment consists of meticulous perineal care (e.g., sitz bathes, otherwise only plain water contact with perineum, no wiping but patting the perineum dry with cotton rolls, protective layer of zinc oxide) and the removal of potential vulvar allergens or irritants.

Herpes simplex and herpes zoster virus infections, when they affect the vulva and perineum, can cause detrusor-sphincter dyssynergia and urinary retention. It is unclear whether this is secondary to acute pain and involuntary guarding, to inflammation of the sacral nerve roots, or both. The patient should be treated symptomatically and may require catheterization.

ACQUIRED IMMUNODEFICIENCY SYNDROME

The incidence of human immunodeficiency virus (HIV) and acquired immunodeficiency syndrome (AIDS) in adolescents and young women is increasing more rapidly than in men. In 1994, 58,448 women aged 13 years or older were reported to be infected with HIV; 14,081 of these had AIDS. This represents 18% of all AIDS patients reported in that year. Women aged 15–44 years account for 84% of these cases. Most of these women are black or Hispanic (77%) and live in the northeast and south (80%). Transmission to the female primarily occurs from sexual contact with an infected male or from intravenous drug abuse (12). The genitourinary tract is frequently involved in AIDS, and the urogynecologist can expect to treat more cases of AIDS-related urinary tract dysfunction in the future. HIV-associated nephropathy, in the form of proteinuria and rapidly progressive irreversible renal failure, has been found in up to 35% of patients and is more common in blacks and intravenous drug abusers (13). The most common microscopic finding is focal segmental glomerulosclerosis. Computed tomography reveals diffusely enlarged kidneys without scarring or hydronephrosis. Up to 68% of AIDS patients demonstrate azotemia, hematuria, proteinuria, or pyuria at some point of their illness.

There is an increased incidence of not only common but also unusual and polymicrobial UTIs in AIDS patients. Dysuria, frequency, urgency, and hematuria with negative routine cultures in the HIV-infected woman may be secondary to acid-fast bacilli, cytomegalovirus, or herpes. Chancroid, syphilis, chlamydia, and herpes simplex virus 2 are found to be associated with HIV transmission more commonly than gonorrhea and trichomonas. Genitourinary malignancies often diagnosed include Kaposi's sarcoma, non-Hodgkin's lymphoma, and cervical dysplasia or carcinoma.

Thirty-nine percent of AIDS patients have neurologic complications, centrally, peripherally, or both (14). In a study evaluating AIDS patients with bladder dysfunction, urinary retention was the presenting symptom in 55% (15). Urodynamic evaluation revealed an acontractile detrusor in 36%, detrusor hyperreflexia in 27%, and an underactive detrusor in 18% of these patients. Toxoplasmosis was present in 4 of 11 patients.

Noninfectious Inflammatory Conditions

Vulvodynia is less of a diagnosis than a symptom that describes chronic vulvar pain and burning with no discernible abnormalities. Possible etiologies are listed in Table 22.2. Lower urinary tract symptoms may arise from the increased sensory afferent activity from the site of inflammation, which in turn may lead to discoordination between the detrusor and the external urethral sphincter in some girls with vulvar or vaginal pain.

Table 22.2. Etiology of Vulvodynia

Vulvar vestibulitis
Causalgia
Postherpetic neuralgia
Subclinical human papilloma virus infection
Chronic candidiasis
Sjögren disease

Vulvar vestibulitis is characterized by entry dyspareunia, vestibular erythema, point-tenderness to cotton-swab pressure within the vestibule, and no other discernible etiology. Treatment can be difficult. Sitz baths, topical or injectable steroids, analgesics, interferon injections, and tricyclic antidepressants have all been used with varying degrees of success. Laser ablation or vestibulectomy may be effective in patients refractory to medical management (16).

Trauma to the lower urogenital tract (most commonly motor vehicle accidents, straddle injuries, and vigorous intercourse) may cause abrasions, lacerations, or hematoma formation with the subsequent development of pain and hematuria.

Anatomic Disorders

VESICOURETERAL REFLUX

Vesicoureteral reflux is typically a problem that presents in early childhood (the peak incidence is at ages 3–5 years), but it can be responsible for significant morbidity in the adolescent female. The patient with vesicoureteral reflux may present with recurrent UTIs, pyelonephritis, or radiating flank pain during micturition. Reflux, usually in association with a UTI, may result in irreversible kidney damage. Reflux nephropathy (kidney damage secondary to reflux) is a long-term risk factor for hypertension and end-stage renal disease (17, 18).

Reflux occurs because of anatomic abnormalities of the ureterovesical junction. Primary reflux is congenital and occurs when the intramural ureteral length is relatively too short. Secondary reflux is associated either with anomalies such as a duplex collecting system or, more commonly, functional disorders producing high bladder pressures such as detrusor instability (without leakage or with high outlet resistance), detrusor sphincter dyssynergia, and nonneurogenic neurogenic bladder (Hinman syndrome). By itself, a high voiding pressure will not cause reflux if the ureterovesical junction is normal. However, the chronic urinary tract obstruction resulting from these disorders will cause bladder hypertrophy, bladder diverticula and saccules, and alterations of the

ureterovesical junction (19). These anatomic changes, in turn, can lead to incompetence of laterally placed ureteral orifices, which are susceptible because of their short intramural ureters. Once the ureterovesical "valve" has been damaged, even low bladder pressures can force urine across it. Nearly 75% of patients with reflux in one study were found to have one of these high-pressure disorders. The International Reflux Study in Children tried to exclude patients with voiding dysfunction so that it could study pure reflux, but 18% of these patients were found to have some type of voiding dysfunction (20).

The prevalence of reflux is unknown but has been estimated to be as high as 1%. One third of the siblings of these patients has reflux. Parent-to-child inheritance may be even higher, with up to 66% of children of affected mothers having reflux (17). Seventy-five percent of these siblings and children whose reflux are detected by family screening is asymptomatic. There are also racial differences in the prevalence of reflux, with only one tenth as many blacks affected as whites (21). These patterns suggest a genetic predisposition that is probably related to the length of the intramural ureter. This length is indirectly proportional to the evolution of ureterovesical incompetence and reflux.

Diagnosis is usually based on voiding cystourethrography, which determines the grade of disease and, hence, the chance of spontaneous resolution (Table 22.3). Isotope cystograms, having the advantage of less radiation exposure, may be used in follow-up studies and in screening for familial reflux. Ultrasound may be used in young children as a screen for reflux. If the upper urinary tract is not dilated, cystourethrography is unnecessary. Ultrasound is also valuable in fetal evaluation, where hydronephrosis may be caused by reflux in 10% of cases (22). Eighty percent of infants with reflux diagnosed antenatally are male.

The age of the patient at onset and initial grade of disease are inversely proportional to the rate of spontaneous remission. Because of this, medical management is typically the first treatment option. Medical management centers around prevention of UTIs. Sterile reflux generally will not cause significant kidney damage except in association with high-pressure voiding states. Patients with

Table 22.3. Grade (International System) and Prevalence of Vesicoureteral Reflux (VUR) (From the International Reflux Study in Children)

Grade	Voiding Cystourethrography Findings	All Cases of VUR (%)	Spontaneous Resolution (%)
I	Enters ureter (not renal pelvis)	5–8	90
II	Enters renal pelvis (no distension)	35	75
III	Fills collecting system (no distortion)	25–35	50
IV	Blunting of calyces, tortuous ureter	15–25	40
V	Huge dilation of collecting system, no visible papillary impression, very tortuous ureter	5	5

reflux not on prophylactic antibiotics have progressively worse renal scarring than those on long-term prophylaxis (17). Isotope cystogram, serum creatinine, urinalysis, and urine culture should be performed on a routine basis to monitor the reflux. Patients should be evaluated for dysfunctional voiding states (detrusor instability, detrusor-sphincter dyssynergia), which, if present, should be treated appropriately.

Reflux is unlikely to resolve spontaneously beyond the age of 11, although some children with grade I or II reflux have had resolution as late as age 14 or 15. Endoscopic treatment, consisting of subureteral injection of artificial collagen, dextranomer, or autologous fat, has been reported to cure reflux (up to grade IV) in over 70% of cases (23, 24). Surgical repair (ureteroneocystotomy) is reserved for patients who have grade V reflux or have failed medical or endoscopic management (i.e., breakthrough UTIs, worsening of reflux, or renal disease). In these refractory cases, most investigators believe that surgery is essential to prevent continuing renal cortical damage. However, new renal scarring develops in approximately 20–25% of patients with high-grade reflux, whether treated surgically or medically (25). Initial reports from the International Reflux Study in Children show that ureteroneocystotomy eradicates reflux in over 97% of cases. Ureteral obstruction, the main postoperative complication, occurs in 2–4% of patients (26, 27).

UROLITHIASIS

The incidence of urinary tract stones in children is between 1 in 1000 and 1 in 7600 (28). Predisposing factors for urolithiasis (e.g., genitourinary anomalies, metabolic abnormalities) are found in 75% of these patients, underscoring the need for thorough evaluation and testing for these factors (29). Although calcium stones are the main source of calculus disease in the adult, struvite stones account for up to 72% of cases in children (30). These stones are often asymptomatic until they break loose from the renal papilla and pass into the ureter, causing hematuria and pain.

Struvite Calculi

Struvite calculi or "infection stones" are composed of magnesium ammonium phosphate. This triple salt precipitates to form a crystal lattice that often fills the renal pelvis, forming a staghorn calculus. Formation of these stones in girls usually follows infection with urea-splitting organisms such as Proteus. The bacteria act as a nidus and stimulate local struvite supersaturation, with formation of the stone around the bacteria. This allows for continued bacterial seeding of the urine and makes eradication of infection without removal or passage of the calculus nearly impossible. In symptomatic patients, treatment now usually consists of lithotripsy or ureteroscopic removal of the stones. Open surgical excision of the stones is necessary in only 2–4% of patients (31). Antibiotic suppression is also indicated to limit the growth of these stones.

Cystine Calculi

Cystinuria is an autosomal recessive disorder of intestinal and renal transport of cystine, lysine, ornithine, and arginine. The onset of this disease is in childhood, and recurrences are frequent. Staghorn calculi are common. Treatment consists of reducing the cystine concentration by hydration and by prevention of an acidic urine pH (which would favor crystallization) with oral alkali. For those patients in whom this treatment is unsuccessful, D-penicillamine or alpha-mercaptopropionylglycine may be used, but these agents are associated with a significant number of toxic side effects.

Uric Acid Calculi

Urate stones are radiolucent and tend to form staghorns. Normally, uric acid is a sodium salt. With dehydration, acidification of the urine (pH < 5.5), or hyperuricosuria, the urate is freed, which leads to crystallization due to the lower solubility of the free urate. Treatment consists of hydration and alkalinization with oral citrate to raise the urine pH to 6.0. Allopurinol may be used when conservative therapy is unsuccessful.

Calcium Calculi

Calcium stones affect 0.5% of adults but are rare in adolescents. Recurrence is as high as 50% within 5 years. The most common cause is idiopathic hypercalciuria, which is found in 5% of the population. It has been proposed that this hypercalciuria is secondary to either increased intestinal absorption or decreased renal tubular reabsorption. Other causes of calcium stones are primary hyperparathyroidism, hyperuricemia, renal tubular acidosis, and hyperoxaluria.

Therapy for idiopathic hypercalciuria is administration of thiazide diuretics, which cause a more than 10-fold reduction in subsequent disease. Cellulose phosphate, which chelates intestinal calcium, has been successful in reducing the incidence of recurrent disease. A single parathyroid adenoma is the cause of hypercalciuria in 85% of those patients with primary hyperparathyroidism. Hyperplasia is the cause in the other 15%. Primary treatment of these patients is lithotripsy when possible and extirpative surgery to treat the parathyroid adenoma or hyperplasia.

URETHRAL ABNORMALITIES

Urethral disorders causing lower tract dysfunction in adolescents and young women are rare but include urethral prolapse, para-urethral cysts, urethral diverticula, ectopic ureterocele, trauma, and urethral strictures (32). Patients with urethral prolapse may present with hematuria, vaginal spotting, dysuria, and a mass. Physical examination reveals a circumferential congested mass protruding from the urethral meatus, reflecting eversion of the urethral mucosa. It is rarely found in estrogen-producing women. Treatment consists of vaginal estrogen cream. Paraurethral cysts are similarly rare but can result in discomfort and abscess formation. Excision is rarely required with urethral prolapse and paraurethral cysts. In contrast, symptomatic urethral diverticula require surgery and are fully discussed in Chapter 25. Ectopic ureterocele refers to a cystic dilatation of the distal ureter extending beyond the urethrovesical junction. Most girls with a ureterocele have a duplex collecting system, and 10% present with prolapse from the urethra. Urethral trauma most commonly occurs in conjunction with straddle injuries to the perineum from falls.

Urethral strictures presenting in adolescence are usually iatrogenic in nature, following endoscopy, traumatic catheterization, dilation, or surgery (33). Difficulty voiding, retention, dribbling, and incontinence are common complaints. The incidence of inflammatory strictures secondary to urethritis increases with the onset of sexual activity and related diseases. In the female, urethral dilation may be appropriate initial treatment because most of the strictures are short. Fifty percent of patients respond to a single dilation. Formal repair should be considered when dilation is unsuccessful.

Voiding and Storage Abnormalities

Initially, infants void reflexively after small increases in bladder pressure from distension with urine, which stimulate reflex detrusor contractions with reciprocal urethral relaxation. Micturition occurs frequently during the first year of life, approximately 20 times a day (34). Although reflex voiding continues for about 2 years, it becomes less frequent because of increasing bladder capacity. After the initiation of toilet training, an intermediate stage is reached during which the child is able to prevent urine loss by voluntarily contracting the external urethral sphincter (usually by age 3). Eventually, the child learns to suppress the spontaneous detrusor contractions voluntarily after the maturation of numerous neurological pathways that modulate inhibition of the detrusor. Thus, the child attains an adult voiding pattern, with voluntary initiation and inhibition of detrusor contractions in coordination with reciprocal urethral relaxation by the age of 4 years. This pattern may be disrupted by physical or emotional disorders. When the process is disrupted or delayed, numerous voiding abnormalities may result. Most of these are functional disorders, but some are anatomic.

ANATOMIC DISORDERS

Spinal dysraphism (Table 22.4) is the most common primary cause of neurogenic bladder dysfunction in children, with a prevalence of 0.1% (35). Most of these disorders are manifest at birth and require immediate neurosurgical intervention. Because of advanced medical care, many of these patients now reach adolescence and adulthood. Also, occult spinal dysraphism may present later in life with new onset of urinary tract symptoms (incontinence, infection, or changes in voiding patterns) and is associated with a cutaneous marker in 75% of patients (36). Some girls will lose continence after spinal or pelvic trauma or surgery. Secondary tethered cord most frequently occurs from postsurgical scarring. The bladder dysfunction in patients with anatomic disorders may be secondary to central disease and present with detrusor sphincter dyssynergia and uninhibited involuntary detrusor contrac-

Table 22.4. Types of Spinal Dysraphism

Cystic or Open Defects	Noncystic or Closed Defects
Meningocele	Intradural lipoma
Myelomeningocele	Diastematomyelia
Lipomeningocele	Dermoid cyst or sinus
Myeloschisis	Cauda equina tumor
Rachischisis	Anterior sacral meningocele
	Tethered cord
	Syringomyelia

tions or may be due to peripheral lesions and may be associated with a large flaccid bladder, urinary retention, and overflow incontinence.

Relative urethral hypospadias is associated with frequency, nocturia, dyspareunia, and UTI. A recent study found this anomaly in 39.7% of young women attending a family planning clinic (37).

Müllerian fusion anomalies have associated urinary tract abnormalities in approximately 40% of cases. Many of these conditions do not present until adolescence or pregnancy. The most recognized of these is the didelphic uterus with unilateral renal agenesis. In a recent study, two adolescents presenting with acute urinary retention were found to have uterine didelphys, unilateral hematocolpos, and ipsilateral renal agenesis (38). Difficult micturition, frequency, UTI, and stress incontinence have also been reported in up to 10% of patients with this triad of findings.

As with spinal dysraphism, advancements in medical care have resulted in greater longevity for patients with cerebral palsy. Younger patients often present with urinary incontinence, frequency, and urgency, usually secondary to detrusor hyperreflexia (39). When voiding difficulty is present, it is usually due to hypertonicity of the pelvic floor, probably related to the pyramidal or spastic type of cerebral palsy. Older patients more often present with urinary hesitancy, stranguria, and retention (40).

MEDICAL DISORDERS

Diabetes mellitus and diabetes insipidus are well-known causes for excessive thirst, polydipsia, and polyuria. Adolescents and young women may present with urinary urgency and frequency but rarely have autonomic neuropathy. Thus, voiding and storage dysfunctions are rarely manifested in these adolescent patients. When these symptoms are present, however, detrusor hyperreflexia is actually a more common etiology than the classic diabetic bladder (decreased bladder sensation, detrusor areflexia, and overflow incontinence) (41). A small study of asymptomatic diabetic adolescents found an increase in both the time to first sensation and maximum capacity but no voiding abnormalities or retention (42).

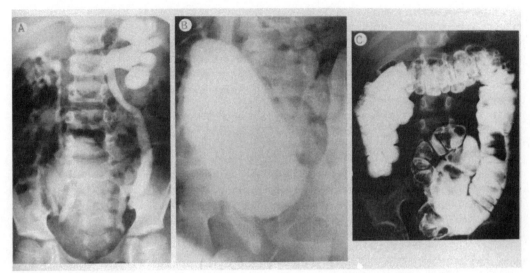

Figure 22.1. Classic radiologic findings in patients with the nonneurogenic neurogenic bladder. **A.** Intravenous pyelogram with dilated upper urinary tracts. **B.** Cystogram with "Christmas tree" bladder. **C.** Barium enema with dilated colon and feces. (Reprinted from Hinman F, Baumann FW. Vesical and ureteral damage from voiding dysfunction in boys without neurologic or obstructive disease. J Urol 1973;109:727–732, with permission.)

Patients with hyperthyroidism may present with urgency, frequency, incontinence, and/or retention in up to 7% of cases (43). Nocturnal enuresis has been noted as well in women with hyperthyroidism. Urinary tract dysfunction resolves with successful treatment of the thyroid.

Idiopathic hypercalciuria, well known for causing urolithiasis, more frequently causes incontinence, present in a quarter of all patients with this metabolic disorder (44). Hematuria, frequency, and urgency are other common complaints, presumably secondary to bladder irritation from calcium crystals.

Sickle cell disease is accompanied by nocturnal enuresis in about a third of cases. The reason for this relationship is unknown but speculated to be secondary to diabetes insipidus caused by renal medullary damage from the sickling episodes. Many of these patients do not view the incontinence as a problem and decline treatment (45).

FUNCTIONAL DISORDERS

Nonneurogenic Neurogenic Bladder (Hinman Syndrome)

The nonneurogenic neurogenic bladder, originally described by Beer in 1915 (46), has only become appreciated in the past 25 years as a common and serious voiding disorder that, if not corrected, can lead to renal failure (47). Hinman and Baumann (48) originally described 14 neurologically intact boys presenting with nocturnal and diurnal enuresis, encopresis, UTI, upper tract dilatation (Fig. 22.1), and "failure personalities." Subsequently, Allen (49) reported similar findings in a predominantly female population. The key steps leading to disease are failure to inhibit the detrusor reflex and overcompensation by the external sphincter. The patient, having ignored the warnings of impending detrusor contraction, must respond with a strong urethral contraction to avoid incontinence. Momentary embarrassment with incontinence is avoided at the expense of the upper urinary tract. Uroflowmetry will reveal an intermittent and interrupted flow. Voiding pressure studies combined with periurethral electromyography reveal the pattern of detrusor-sphincter dyssynergia in these neurologically normal girls indistinguishable from that found in patients with spinal cord trauma (50).

In almost all cases, the Hinman syndrome is preceded by a dysfunctional family unit or disruption of the patient's emotional or social equilibrium. In response to these stresses, patients with this disorder use the external urethral sphincter to delay or interrupt normal micturition (51). However, in some cases, a painful stimulus (e.g., urethritis or UTI) and residual dysuria can cause the patient to guard against bladder contractions with sphincter contraction and, in time, elicit the syndrome. Early stages of the disease may present only with complaints of incomplete voiding, retention, recurrent UTI, or chronic pelvic pain. During voiding pressure studies, these latter patients are also found to have a failure of complete urethral relaxation that mimics detrusor-sphincter dyssynergia (Fig. 22.2). The overwhelming functional obstruction that evolves with prolonged disease may lead to bladder trabeculation and vesicoureteral reflux as well as urethrovesical backwash with eventual detrusor decompensation. The vesicoureteral reflux, el-

evated residual urine, and urethrovesical backwash lead to recurrent infection, which further inflames the distal urethra. The inflamed urethra may be a source of increased afferent pudendal stimulation, which causes further external sphincter spasm. Treatment of concurrent urethritis with antibiotics, urethral suppositories, or dilation is sometimes helpful.

The nonneurogenic neurogenic bladder is best treated by bladder education and retraining, supplemented by relaxation techniques, intermittent catheterization, biofeedback, short-term pharmacological treatment of both detrusor instability and detrusor-sphincter dyssynergia, and, rarely, psychological or psychiatric referral (52–54). Concurrent treatment for constipation and encopresis is often necessary.

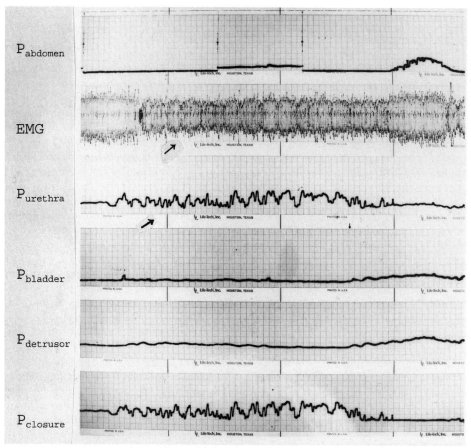

Figure 22.2. Voiding pressure-flow study of a 23-year-old woman presenting with urinary frequency, urgency, and retention. Failure of urethral relaxation (*large arrow*) and increased EMG activity (*small arrow*) are noted.

Detrusor-Sphincter Dyssynergia

True detrusor-sphincter dyssynergia is a neurological disorder involving the loss of reciprocal coordination between the detrusor and the external urethral sphincter. The clinical picture in the adolescent is identical to the transitional phase found in the infant being toilet trained. Patients commonly present with retention, difficulty emptying, recurrent UTIs, and incontinence.

In contrast to the Hinman syndrome, in which neurological disease is absent, the dyssynergic voiding pattern of true detrusor-sphincter dyssynergia represents a neurological disorder and is involuntary. Treatment in the adolescent is similar to that in the adult. Intermittent self-catheterization helps prevent infection and deterioration of the upper urinary tract. Diazepam and baclofen may be used in some to aid in the relaxation of the external urethral sphincter. Some patients may benefit from decreasing involuntary urethral resistance with alpha-adrenergic blockers (e.g., prazosin or terazosin) or the smooth muscle relaxant phenoxybenzamine.

Sexual Abuse

In a school-based sample, 13% of 8- and 10-grade girls reported forced sexual intercourse (55). In a telephone survey of 958 girls aged 10–16, 15% reported a history of sexual abuse (56). The incidence of sexual abuse is relatively consistent among income groups. Sexually abused children and adolescents have an increased frequency of anxiety, depressive, and aggressive disorders as well as problems with sex roles and sexual functioning (57). Recently, Ellsworth et al. (58) noted an association between sexual abuse and voiding dysfunction. They focused on 18 of approximately 300 patients with voiding dysfunction. This subset (6%) encompassed those reporting a history of sexual abuse. Enuresis (89%), history of UTIs (44%), and constipation (67%) were common complaints. This supports prior work finding an increase in voiding symptoms, enuresis, and encopresis in children evaluated for sexual abuse (59). In our own practice, we have also anecdotally noted a relationship between painful bladder symptoms and a history of

Table 22.5.   Causes of Urinary Urgency and Frequency in Young Patients

Infectious	Medical
Urinary tract	Diabetes
infection	Hypocalciuria
Urethritis	Hypothyroidism
Vulvovaginitis	Dysfunctional voiding
AIDS	Hinman syndrome
Pain syndromes	Detrusor-sphincter
Vulvodynia	dyssynergia
Interstitial cystitis	Detrusor instability
Urethral syndrome	Sensory urgency
Reflex sympathetic	Other
dystrophy	Medications
	Sexual abuse

sexual abuse in young women, but this association has not been explored scientifically for causality versus the coincidental concurrence of two prevalent conditions in these patients.

In any case, it seems possible that sexual abuse may produce lower urinary tract symptomatology. The clinician evaluating such symptoms should be alert to other evidence of sexual abuse that may arise in the history and physical examination. Discrete referral to a specialist in sexual abuse (usually either a pediatrician or pediatric gynecologist) should be considered if the index of suspicion is high, because reporting of abuse is mandatory in most states. Ancillary testing and treatment of specific disease states should follow usual decision-making pathways, but the patient's heightened wariness of further manipulation of her urogenital tract should be sensitively considered and may require alternative strategies for evaluating her symptoms. Supplementing standard treatment with psychological or psychiatric counseling may prove to be invaluable.

Urgency/Frequency Syndrome

Helping the young patient who presents with urinary urgency, frequency, and suprapubic pain often requires considerable diagnostic and treatment skills (Table 22.5). Painful bladder conditions such as interstitial cystitis and urethral syndrome are discussed elsewhere in the text. The presence of nocturia can be easily elicited during the patient history and may direct further inquiry. Patients with interstitial cystitis commonly have marked nocturia, whereas those with urethral syndrome do not. Reflex sympathetic dystrophy is a poorly understood chronic pain syndrome usually characterized by severe burning pain in an extremity after injury to the extremity. The pain is constant and exacerbated by emotional stress and may continue well after the initial insult has resolved. Excess sympathetic activity acting on damaged nerves is the likely etiology. Applying this concept to bladder symptoms is logical in situations where nerve damage can be confirmed and may even be a factor after chronic inflammation of perivascular sympathetic afferents from infectious and inflammatory insult to the lower urinary tract. Treatment consists of sympathetic blockade and physiotherapy.

Sensory urgency from supratentorial habituation to frequent voiding may also cause this syndrome in young women. The frequent voiding pattern creates a vicious cycle with the adolescent gradually decreasing her functional bladder capacity. This may be effectively treated with bladder drill and pelvic floor stimulation. Isolated urinary frequency has been reported as a side effect of terfenadine, a nonsedating antihistamine commonly prescribed for allergic rhinitis (60).

Urinary Retention

Urinary retention in the adolescent most often occurs acutely after a strong emotional or physical trauma. Drugs (e.g., alpha-adrenergics, anticholinergics, and central nervous system stimulants), anesthesia, and childbirth, especially in association with any previously existing detrusor sphincter dyssynergia or urethral inflammation, may also cause acute retention. Establishing bladder drainage with an indwelling catheter or intermittent catheterization and "tincture of time" is usually the only treatment needed for acute conditions. Detrusor-sphincter dyssynergia should be treated according to its etiology. Retention may also result from physical obstruction, as with traumatic bladder rupture, significant hematuria, or a large neoplasm.

Occasionally, acute retention becomes a chronic condition, which in this age group is most often associated with a very large capac-

ity bladder and underactive detrusor, euphemistically known as a "lazy bladder" (61). This condition is similar to the bladder dysfunction associated with a peripheral lesion and is found predominantly in girls under 6 years of age but may continue into adolescence. The underlying pathological process is habitual neglect of voiding. This neglect, if not initially triggered by an acute cause of retention, is frequently associated with a fear of voiding in school bathrooms or with the desire to imitate maternal patterns. Recurrent UTIs and incontinence (overflow) are common complaints.

Cystometry reveals a large-capacity high-compliance bladder. An underactive detrusor and Valsalva effort are usually seen on voiding pressure studies. The voiding cystourethrogram reveals a large smooth-walled bladder, with reflux occurring in more than 75% of these patients. Treatment consists of long-term antibiotic prophylaxis and clean intermittent self-catheterization. Pharmacological intervention is rarely effective.

INCONTINENCE

Nocturnal Enuresis

Although there is no formal consensus on the definition of nocturnal enuresis, it may be defined as the involuntary leakage of urine at least two nights per month, beyond the age at which bladder control is normally obtained (4–6 years of age) in the absence of congenital or acquired defects of the urinary tract (62, 63). It is the most common functional urinary tract disorder in children, affecting up to 20% of 5 year olds. The prevalence falls to 1–2% in 15 year olds, with a 3:2 male predominance. More than 80% of enuretics wet only at night, and most of these patients have no obvious pathology (62). The etiology of nocturnal enuresis is unknown but likely involves neural detrusor immaturity, nocturnal vasopressin insufficiency, and immature nocturnal arousal (64).

Initial evaluation consists of a thorough history, physical examination, voiding diary, uroflowmetry, urinalysis, and urine culture. The history should concentrate on other urinary tract symptoms and psychosocial factors such as the parents' attitudes. The abdomen, urogenital tract, and lower back should be examined, and the lumbosacral nerve roots should be screened. Positive findings in any of the above areas should warrant further investigation.

On the other hand, if the evaluation finds an anatomically intact child with exclusively nocturnal enuresis, treatment can be initiated without further testing. The cornerstone of therapy must be education and reassurance for the patient and parents alike. Some will elect to not treat the enuresis, being comfortable to wait for spontaneous remission. For girls under age 7, this is a reasonable option, but older patients will likely desire treatment.

Behavior modification such as urinary alarms will be effective in up to 82% of girls and is usually the initial treatment (10). The typical system uses a signal alarm that when stimulated by moisture, awakens the patient at the beginning of micturition. Success is optimized with education, close follow-up, and the continuation of treatment until a 4-week dry period is attained. Alarms can be disruptive, especially when the patient shares a room with siblings. Motivational therapy, in the form of positive reinforcement and the cessation of punitive measures, may enhance behavior modification techniques but by itself is effective in only 25% of cases.

Beyond the age of 14, pharmacotherapy offers the best hope for treatment. Imipramine was first used to treat enuresis in 1960 (65) and is effective in up to 50% of patients. It may be added to behavior modification to aid in the maintenance of continence. Its mechanism of action for nocturnal enuresis is unclear, and patients may find the anticholinergic side effects intolerable. More recently, desmopressin acetate (DDAVP) has become the preferred pharmacological treatment of nocturnal enuresis. Available as a nasal spray, DDAVP has a half-life of 24 minutes to 4 hours (66). It has fewer side effects than imipramine but is far more expensive. Improvement is noted in up to 91% of cases, but only 25% of patients on DDAVP achieve complete dryness (67). With either agent, relapse is common when the drug is withdrawn. Monda and Husmann (68) prospectively compared observation, imipramine, DDAVP, and alarm systems in a recent study. One year after beginning the

study, 16% of patients in the observation arm were dry. Patients on imipramine or DDAVP were continent in 36% and 68% of cases, respectively, while on medication, but this fell to 16% and 10% when treatment was discontinued. Behavior modification with an enuresis alarm was curative in 56% of patients 6 months after treatment was discontinued.

Genuine Stress Incontinence

Stress incontinence is commonly thought to be rare in adolescents and young women; however, in one study, 52% of nulliparous college students reported at least occasional episodes of stress incontinence (69). In a questionnaire survey of all varsity athletes at a large university, 28% reported at least one episode of urinary incontinence while participating in their sport (70). Gymnastics and basketball elicited significantly more incontinence than volleyball, swimming, softball, and golf. Interestingly, 42% of the athletes reported at least one episode of incontinence during other daily activities. Bo et al. (71) recently tried to correlate the symptoms of stress incontinence in college physical education majors with urodynamic findings and the diagnosis of genuine stress incontinence. Although stress incontinence was reported by 38% of the students, pad testing was negative in four of seven symptomatic women. However, these four did demonstrate pressure equalization during the cough urethral closure pressure profile. Electromyography was normal in all subjects. Another study examined 29 young nulliparous women with transvaginal ultrasound and found that at a volume of at least 200 mL, the bladder neck was open in 21% of these women at rest (72). This suggests that the underlying anatomic defect associated with poor urethral pressure transmission and genuine stress incontinence may already be present in many women long before childbirth or before any symptoms appear.

When genuine stress incontinence is diagnosed in this age group, we strongly advocate nonoperative treatment for a number of reasons. Although operative intervention offers the highest initial success rate, there is scant data on the management of subsequent pregnancies and other stressful activities in young women after surgery for incontinence. In addition, although successful retropubic urethropexies may be found to be still functional at 2 and 5 years, we again have little data regarding success in these women 20 and 30 years later. When operative treatments are used, the patient must be given thorough counseling.

More importantly, the highest success rates of nonsurgical therapy are in young women with intact pelvic floors. Pelvic floor exercises with or without biofeedback, pelvic floor stimulation, and weighted vaginal cones are good first choices in these young women, offering cure or improvement in up to 76% of patients (73). We prefer to avoid the use of medications because of side effects and the need for continuous therapy.

Detrusor Instability

Detrusor overactivity has already been discussed in relationship to detrusor-sphincter dyssynergia, the nonneurogenic neurogenic bladder, and vesicoureteral reflux. When an adolescent presents with uncomplicated detrusor instability, appropriate intervention may prevent these sequelae. The condition often is discovered at the time of a urogenital tract infection. In patients under age 12, it may be secondary to delayed maturation of cortical inhibition. Encouragingly, treatment with anticholinergics, tricyclic antidepressants, and bladder drill are successful in more than 90% of patients. Surgical intervention with augmentation cystoplasty is rarely necessary in these girls.

Coitus-Related Incontinence

Incontinence during coitus may also be seen in this age group and may be the only urinary complaint in some young women. The timing of this incontinence may help direct further investigation and treatment. Urine leakage during orgasm is usually secondary to unsuppressed involuntary detrusor contractions at a moment of decreased cortical inhibition. However, leakage during intercourse before orgasm may be due to genuine stress incontinence secondary to straining and strenuous physical activity. This may also represent overactive detrusor function from transvaginal manipulation of

the bladder floor by the penis. Urodynamic studies with or without masturbation can be done to confirm the presumptive diagnosis, but these are often unable to duplicate the clinical setting and thus miss the underlying pathology.

REFERENCES

1. Dairiki-Shortliffe LM. The management of urinary tract infections in children without urinary tract abnormalities. Urol Clin North Am 1995;22: 67–73.
2. Wan J, Kaplinsky R, Greenfield S. Toilet habits of children evaluated for urinary tract infection. J Urol 1995;154:797–799.
3. Lowe FC, Brendler CB. Evaluation of the urologic patient. In: Walsh PC, Retik AB, Stamey TA, Vaughan ED Jr, eds. Campbell's urology, 6th ed. Philadelphia: WB Saunders 1992:319.
4. Hendry WF, Stanton SL, Williams DI. Recurrent urinary infections in girls: effects of urethral dilation. Br J Urol 1973;45:72–83.
5. Vermillion CD, Halverstadt DB, Leadbetter GW. Internal urethrotomy and recurrent urinary tract infection in female children. II. Long-term results in the management of infection. J Urol 1971;106: 154–157.
6. Kaplan GW, Sammons TA, King LR. A blind comparison of dilatation, urethrotomy, and medication alone in the treatment of urinary tract infection in girls. J Urol 1973;109:917–919.
7. Kessler R, Constantinou CE. Internal urethrotomy in girls and its impact on the urethral intrinsic and extrinsic continence mechanisms. J Urol 1986;136:1248–1253.
8. Buckley RM, McGuckin M, MacGregor RR. Urine bacterial counts after sexual intercourse. N Engl J Med 1978;298:312–324.
9. Strom BL, Collins M, West SL, Kreisberg J, Weller S. Sexual activity, contraceptive use, and other risk factors for symptomatic and asymptomatic bacteriuria: a case-control study. Ann Intern Med 1987;107:816–823.
10. Foxman B, Geiger AM, Palin K, Gillespie B, Ostergard JS. First-time urinary tract infection and sexual behavior. Epidemiology 1995;6: 162–168.
11. Bump RC, Copeland WE. Urethral isolation of the genital mycoplasmas and *Chlamydia trachomatis* in women with chronic urologic complaints. Am J Obstet Gynecol 1985;152:38–41.
12. Update: AIDS among women—United States, 1994. MMWR 1995;44:81–84.
13. Kwan DJ, Lowe FC. Genitourinary manifestations of the acquired immunodeficiency syndrome. Urology 1995;45:13–27.
14. Levy RM, Bredesen DE, Rosenblum ML. Neurological manifestations of acquired immunodeficiency syndrome (AIDS): experiences at UCSF and review of the literature. J Neurosurgery 1985; 62:475–495.

15. Khan Z, Singh VK, Yang WC. Neurogenic bladder in acquired immune deficiency syndrome (AIDS). Urology 1992;40:289–291.
16. Reid R, Omoto KH, Precop SL, et al. Flashlamp-excited dye laser therapy of idiopathic vulvodynia is safe and efficacious. Am J Obstet Gynecol 1995;172:1684–1701.
17. Belman AB. A perspective on vesicoureteral reflux. Urol Clin North Am 1995;22:139–150.
18. Chantler C, Carter JE, Bewick M, et al. 10 years' experience with regular haemodialysis and renal transplantation. Arch Dis Child 1980;55:435–445.
19. Koff SA. Relationship between dysfunctional voiding and reflux. J Urol 1992;148:1703–1705.
20. van Gool JD, Hjalmas K, Tamminen-Mobius T, Olbing H. Historical clues to the complex of dysfunctional voiding, urinary tract infection, and vesicoureteral reflux. J Urol 1992;148:1699–1702.
21. Askari A, Belman AB. Vesicoureteral reflux in black girls. J Urol 1982;127:747–748.
22. Elder JS. Commentary: importance of antenatal diagnosis of vesicoureteral reflux. J Urol 1992;148:1750–1754.
23. Frey P, Lutz N, Jenny P, Herzog B. Endoscopic subureteral collagen injection for the treatment of vesicoureteral reflux in infants and children. J Urol 1995;154:804–807.
24. Stenberg A, Lackgren G. A new bioimplant for the endoscopic treatment of vesicoureteral reflux: experimental and short-term clinical results. J Urol 1995;154:800–803.
25. Olbing H, Claesson I, Ebel K, et al. Renal scars and parenchymal thinning in children with vesicoureteral reflux: 5-year report of International Reflux Study in Children (European branch). J Urol 1992;148:1653–1656.
26. Hjalmas K, Lohr G, Tamminen-Mobius T, et al. Surgical results in the International Reflux Study in Children (Europe). J Urol 1992;148:1657–1661.
27. Duckett JW, Walker RD, Weiss R. Surgical results—International Reflux Study in Children: US branch. J Urol 1992;148:1674–1675.
28. Gearhart JP, Herzberg GZ, Jeffs RD. Childhood urolithiasis: experiences and advances. Pediatrics 1991;87:445–450.
29. Milliner DS, Murphy ME. Urolithiasis in pediatric patients. Mayo Clin Proc 1993;68:241–248.
30. Diamond DA, Rickwood AMK, Lee PH, Johnston JH. Infection stones in children: a twenty-seven-year review. Urology 1994;43:525–527.
31. Smith LH, Segura JW. Urolithiasis. In: Kelalis PP, King LR, Belman AB, eds. Clinical pediatric urology, 3rd ed. Philadelphia: WB Saunders, 1992:1327–1352.
32. Elder JS. Congenital anomalies of the genitalia. In: Walsh PC, Retik AB, Stamey TA, Vaughan ED Jr, eds. Campbell's urology, 6th ed. Philadelphia: WB Saunders, 1992:1920.
33. Scherz HC, Kaplan GW. Etiology, diagnosis, and management of urethral strictures in children. Urol Clin North Am 1990;17:389–394.
34. Goellner MH, Ziegler EE, Foman SJ. Urination during the first three years of life. Nephron 1981;28:174–178.
35. Sutherland RS, Mevorach RA, Baskin LS, Kogan BA. Spinal dysraphism in children: an overview and an approach to prevent complications. Urology 1995;46:294–304.
36. Bauer SB. Genitourinary problems in adolescence. J Reprod Med 1984;29:385–390.
37. Sand PK, Ostergard DR. Urethral-hymenal fusion: effects on urinary symptomatology. Int Urogynecol J 1994;5:370.
38. Broseta E, Boronat F, Ruiz JL, Alonso M, Osca JM, Jimenez-Cruz JF. Urological complications associated to uterus didelphys with unilateral hematocolpos. Eur Urol 1991;20:85–88.
39. Reid CJD. Lower urinary tract dysfunction in cerebral palsy. Arch Dis Child 1993;68:739–742.
40. Mayo ME. Lower urinary tract dysfunction in cerebral palsy. J Urol 1992;147:419–420.
41. Kaplan SA, Te AE, Blaivas JG. Urodynamic findings in patients with diabetic cystopathy. J Urol 1995;153:342–344.
42. Barkai L, Szabo L. Urinary bladder dysfunction in diabetic children with and without subclinical cardiovascular autonomic neuropathy. Eur J Pediatr 1993;152:190–192.
43. Goswami R, Taneja R, Shah P, Ammini AC, Wadhwa SN. Micturition disturbances in hyperthyroidism. Br J Urol 1995;75:678–679.
44. Vachvanichsanong P, Malagon M, Moore ES. Urinary incontinence due to idiopathic hypercalciuria in children. J Urol 1994;152:1226–1228.
45. Figueroa TE, Benaim E, Griggs ST, Hvizdala EV. Enuresis in sickle cell disease. J Urol 1995;153:1987–1989.
46. Beer E. Chronic retention of urine in children. JAMA 1915;65:1709–1712.
47. Phillips E, Uehling DT. Hinman syndrome: a vicious cycle. Urology 1993;42:317–320.
48. Hinman F, Baumann FW. Vesical and ureteral damage from voiding dysfunction in boys without neurologic or obstructive disease. J Urol 1973;109:727–732.
49. Allen TD. The non-neurogenic neurogenic bladder. J Urol 1977;117:232–238.
50. Allen TD, Bright TC. Urodynamic patterns in children with dysfunctional voiding problems. J Urol 1978;119:247–249.
51. Allen TD. Commentary: voiding dysfunction and reflux. J Urol 1992;148:1706–1707.
52. Hinman F. Nonneurogenic neurogenic bladder (the Hinman syndrome)—15 years later. J Urol 1986;136:769–777.
53. Wennergren H, Oberg B. Pelvic floor exercises for children: a method of treating dysfunctional voiding. Br J Urol 1995;76:9–15.
54. Kjolseth D, Knudsen LM, Madsen B, Norgaard JP, Djurhuus JC. Urodynamic biofeedback training for children with bladder-sphincter dyscoordination during voiding. Neurourol Urodyn 1995;12:211–221.
55. Nagy S, Adcock AG, Nagy MC. A comparison of risky health behaviors of sexually active, sexually abused, and abstaining adolescents. Pediatrics 1994;93:570–575.
56. Finkelhor D, Dziuba-Leatherman J. Children as victims of violence: a national survey. Pediatrics 1994;94:413–420.

57. Wissow LS. Child abuse and neglect. N Engl J Med 1995;332:1425–1431.

58. Ellsworth PI, Merguerian PA, Copening ME. Sexual abuse: another causative factor in dysfunctional voiding. J Urol 1995;153:773–776.

59. Bloom DA. Editorial: sexual abuse and voiding dysfunction. J Urol 1995;153:777.

60. Jonides L, Dumont A, Rudy C, Walsh S. Urinary frequency in an adolescent female. J Pediatr Health Care 1993;7:42–52.

61. Bauer SB, Retik AB, Colodny AH. The unstable bladder of childhood. Urol Clin North Am 1980; 7:321–336.

62. Mark SD, Frank JD. Nocturnal enuresis. Br J Urol 1995;75:427–434.

63. Butler RJ. Establishment of working definitions in nocturnal enuresis. Arch Dis Child 1991;66: 267–271.

64. Bloom DA, Faerber G, Bomalaski MD. Urinary incontinence in girls. Urol Clin North Am 1995; 22:521–538.

65. MacLean REG. Imipramine hydrochloride (Tofranil) and enuresis. Am J Psychiatry 1960;117:551.

66. Norgaard JP, Jonler M, Rittig S, Djurhuus JC. A pharmacodynamic study of desmopressin in patients with nocturnal enuresis. J Urol 1995;153: 1984–1986.

67. Moffatt ME, Harlos S, Kirshen AJ, Burd L. Desmopressin acetate and nocturnal enuresis: how much do we know? Pediatrics 1993;92:420–425.

68. Monda JM, Husmann DA. Primary nocturnal enuresis: a comparison among observation, imipramine, desmopressin acetate, and bed-wetting alarm systems. J Urol 1995;154:745–748.

69. Nemir A, Middleton RP. Stress incontinence in young nulliparous women. Am J Obstet Gynecol 1954;68:1166–1168.

70. Nygaard IE, Thompson FL, Svengalis SL, Albright JP. Urinary incontinence in elite nulliparous athletes. Obstet Gynecol 1994;84:183–187.

71. Bo K, Stein R, Kulseng-Hanssen S, Kristofferson M. Clinical and urodynamic assessment of nulliparous young women with and without stress incontinence symptoms: a case-control study. Obstet Gynecol 1994;84:1028–1032.

72. Chapple CR, Helm CW, Blease S, Milroy EJG, Rickards D, Osborne JL. Asymptomatic bladder neck incompetence in nulliparous females. Br J Urol 1989;64:357–359.

73. Bo K, Hagen RH, Kvarstein B, Jorgenson J, Larsen S. Pelvic floor muscle exercise for the treatment of female stress urinary incontinence. III. Effects of two different degrees of pelvic floor muscle exercises. Neurourol Urodyn 1990;9:489–502.

CHAPTER 23

The Urinary Tract in Pregnancy

Robert W. Lobel, Peter K. Sand, and Larry W. Bowen

During pregnancy, the urinary tract undergoes many morphological and physiological changes. These changes can cause many symptoms and pathological conditions that may affect the fetus and the mother. Some of these conditions may persist long after the pregnancy is over. In this chapter, we review these alterations and examine their pathophysiological consequences.

Morphological and Physiological Changes

URETHRA

The urethral mucosa appears hyperemic and congested as pregnancy progresses. The transitional epithelium becomes more squamous in character because of increased estrogen levels. The urethra passively lengthens as the bladder is drawn further cephalad and anterior by the enlarging uterus. Several investigators have documented an increase in the total urethral length of 4–7 mm and an average increase in functional length of 5 mm. Both total and functional length decrease slightly below the first trimester values after vaginal delivery but not after cesarean section. Iosif et al. (1) showed the urethral closure pressure to increase from 61 to 73 cm H_2O, a total of 12 cm H_2O, a change that promotes continence in pregnancy. However, to explain the wide prevalence of stress incontinence in pregnancy, some investigators have suggested that progestational effects in the urethra may inhibit estrogen-induced changes and in some way negatively influence the pressure transmission capacity of the urethra during increases in intraabdominal pressure. Pregnant rabbit bladder bases were recently shown to have decreased responsiveness to alpha agonists (2). The resulting relaxation of the urethrovesical junction may help to further explain the stress incontinence associated with pregnancy.

BLADDER

As noted above, the urinary bladder is displaced anteriorly and superiorly as pregnancy progresses, becoming more an abdominal organ than a pelvic organ by the third trimester. The base of the bladder enlarges, and the trigone appears convex rather than concave. The detrusor hypertrophies with the increased estrogen stimulation of pregnancy. Progesterone causes hypotonia of the detrusor, leading to an increased bladder capacity, over 1 L in some studies (3). With engagement of the fetal head, bladder capacity often decreases, only to rise again in the early postpartum period (4). In one postpartum study, 86% of the patients had reduced bladder sensation and tone associated with volumes greater than 865 mL (5). Despite the progesterone-induced hypotonia, bladder pressure increases from 9 cm H_2O in early pregnancy to 20 cm H_2O at term and then returns to normal levels postpartum (1).

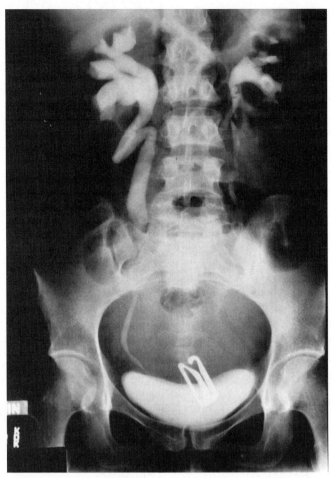

Figure 23.1. Hydroureter in the first trimester. Physiological dilation of the right ureter and renal pelvis above the pelvic brim at 12 weeks gestation before physical compression by the gravid uterus.

URETER

Hydroureter is the most dramatic anatomic response of the urinary tract to pregnancy. Dilatation usually has abrupt onset after 21 weeks gestation (6) but can be seen as early as the first trimester (Fig. 23.1). Physiological dilation is restricted to the renal pelvis and the upper two thirds of the ureters. The ureters are also displaced laterally and become more tortuous in appearance. Both hormonal and physical factors contribute to this dilation. Progesterone inhibits ureteral motility by its hypotonic effects on smooth muscle but mechanical compression by the enlarging uterus probably accounts for most of the dilation (7). Almost 90% of patients has some degree of ureteral dilation at term, with the right ureter affected more than the left in 86% of cases (6). This asymmetry is probably due to the cushioning effect of the sigmoid colon on the left, dextrorotation of the uterus, and the greater potential for obstruction of the right ureter by the right ovarian vein and iliac vessels.

Ureteral dilation is associated with a large increase in ureteral volume (50–200 mL). This reservoir effect, together with decreased ureteral motility, leads to nearly a fivefold delay in excretion from the right ureter. Ureteral changes resolve by 4 weeks postpartum in most patients (Fig. 23.2).

KIDNEY

Dilation of the renal pelvis, calyces, and parenchyma lengthen the kidney by 1.5 cm during pregnancy. Contributing factors include those outlined above for hydroureter as well as a 40–50% increase in the glomerular filtration rate (GFR) and 60–80% increase in the effective renal plasma flow (ERPF)(8).

The GFR increases steadily during pregnancy and normalizes in the puerperium (9). The ERPF increases to a greater degree and then falls abruptly in the last month of pregnancy. It may remain depressed for up to 6 months after delivery. Thus, the filtration fraction (GFR/ERPF) remains slightly elevated after the first trimester and the amount of solute filtered by the kidney increases dramatically while reabsorptive capacity remains constant. The net effect is an increased loss of many solutes. Both the blood urea nitrogen and serum creatinine fall 30% below their normal values. The mean serum urea nitrogen in the pregnant woman is 8.7 mg/dL and the mean plasma creatinine is 0.46 mg/dL (10). Increased excretion of glucose and amino acids can lead to physiological glycosuria and aminoaciduria. There is some resolution of these changes later in pregnancy (9). Significant proteinuria (≥300 mg/24 hours) is not seen in normal pregnancy.

Despite the increase in GFR, tubular reabsorption of salt and water increase, resulting in gradual retention of sodium ions (20–30 mEq/wk), and this in turn leads to increased thirst. Increased thirst during gestation leads to further intake of free water and the eventual retention of 950 mEq of sodium and 7 L of water (8). This excess is widely thought to be distributed between the fetal and reproductive tissues (80%) and the maternal extracellular space (20%)(11). Interestingly, studies of limb volume in pregnancy show that edema of the lower extremities accounts for no more than 500 mL (12). Therefore, most of the retained water must be stored elsewhere.

Urinary Problems in Pregnancy

FREQUENCY

Frequency of urination is a common complaint and occurs in 46–95% of gravidas,

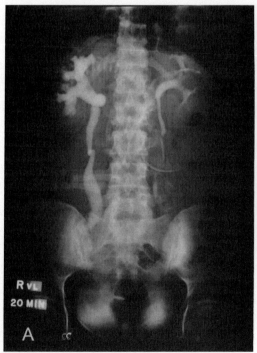 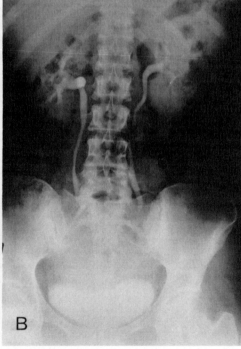

Figure 23.2.   Postpartum resolution of hydroureter. **A.** Right hydroureter above the pelvic brim at 29 weeks. **B.** Intravenous pyelogram performed 3 weeks after cesarean section shows resolution of these physiological changes.

Table 23.1. Prevalence of Lower Urinary Tract Symptoms in Pregnancy

Symptom	Prevalence (%)
Urgency	60–70
Frequency	45–95
Nocturia	55–65
Stress incontinence	30–70
Urge incontinence	20–40
Incomplete emptying	30–35

beginning in the first trimester (Table 23.1) (13). Normal nonpregnant females urinate between four and six times during the day and rarely at night. Thus, frequency is defined as voiding more than seven times during the day and more than once at night (14). Some authors describe higher incidences in primigravidas (14), whereas others show no influence of parity on frequency (4).

Frequency usually begins early in pregnancy, increases progressively in each trimester, and rapidly resolves postpartum. The postpartum incidence (10–20%) is equal to that found before pregnancy.

Bladder capacity increases in pregnancy and cannot be inferred as a cause of frequency until late in gestation when engagement of the fetal head reduces bladder capacity. The more plausible explanation for diurnal frequency is the polydipsia and polyuria of pregnancy (4). As noted above, both fluid intake and urine output rise rapidly in the first trimester and remain constant until the third trimester, when decreased sodium excretion leads to decreased output. Urinary frequency does not decrease in the third trimester, however, and this is probably due to mechanical compression of the bladder by the enlarged uterus.

NOCTURIA

The polyuria of pregnancy is in large part a nocturnal diuresis; the increase in nocturnal urine flow is double that which occurs in the daytime. Clinically evident as edema in the lower extremities, daytime fluid retention is mobilized at night when the woman reclines. Most of this nocturnal diuresis is nonosmotically obligated water. This is probably due to a reduction in renal concentrating ability in pregnancy. The mean nocturnal urine flow and solute excretion are 60–70% greater in

the first and second trimesters than before pregnancy (15). Although both urine flow and solute excretion fall somewhat in the third trimester, the incidence of nocturia continues to rise. This paradox results from the apparent decrease in functional bladder capacity of nocturic patients in the third trimester (4).

URINARY RETENTION

Although the symptoms of incomplete emptying and postvoid fullness are common, antepartum urinary retention is rare, usually associated with uterine retroversion early in the second trimester (16). Asymptomatic retroversion occurs in up to 20% of first-trimester pregnancies, with spontaneous resolution by 16 weeks most of the time. Successful manual reduction of the incarcerated uterus usually requires drainage of the bladder, adequate anesthesia, and knee-chest positioning. Presentation at term with incarceration (Fig. 23.3) has been reported and generally requires a vertical cesarean section (17, 18). Pelvic neoplasms may also cause retention by interfering with bladder neck relaxation. Cystourethrography has demonstrated that this interference resolves after the retroversion is reduced or the tumor removed (4). A similar etiology could account for the retention associated with marked uterine prolapse early in pregnancy. With both retroversion and prolapse, a Smith or Hodge pessary can serve to maintain uterine position after reduction.

Postpartum retention is far more common. After spontaneous vaginal delivery, bladder dysfunction is noted in 9–14% of patients; after forceps deliveries, this number rises to 38% (19). This retention is usually due to detrusor-sphincter dyssynergia with incomplete urethral relaxation secondary to pain and edema (4). Conversely, patients unable to void after cesarean section usually have an acontractile or underactive detrusor muscle. Kerr-Wilson and McNally (20) showed that epidural analgesia caused acute retention of greater than 850 mL after cesarean section in up to 44% of patients whose catheters were removed at the end of the operation. Tapp et al. (21) found epidurals to be associated with a significant increase in postpartum residual urine but noted spontaneous resolution in all cases by 6 weeks postpartum.

Cystometry after vaginal delivery demonstrates that 86% of patients have decreased bladder sensation and tone, which causes an increased bladder capacity (5). These changes are associated with edema and congestion of the bladder base. Most of these findings are asymptomatic and resolve spontaneously in the early postpartum period.

Significant retention requires prompt establishment of adequate drainage to avoid chronic detrusor damage. This is most easily achieved by placement of a Foley catheter for 24–72 hours. Retention due to detrusor-sphincter dyssynergia after vaginal delivery is best treated by "tincture of time," but ice to the perineum and analgesics are also helpful to relieve increased afferent sensation. Persistent retention due to detrusor hypotonia beyond the early puerperium is best treated by clean intermittent self-catheterization. Use of bethanechol or alpha blockers is usually unrewarding in these patients.

INCONTINENCE

The symptom of stress incontinence has been reported to occur in 32–85% of pregnant women (22, 23). It is usually mild and affects multiparas more often than nulliparas. Francis (22) showed an 85% prevalence in multiparas compared with a 53% prevalence in nulliparas. Nearly half of these patients noted occasional or persistent incontinence before the observed pregnancy. New onset of incontinence during pregnancy was divided equally among the trimesters. Although Francis noted no incidence in the puerperium, more recent studies note a 7% incidence. Incontinence usually increases in severity as pregnancy progresses and resolves after delivery in all but 5–14% of patients, the incidence found in multiparas before pregnancy. Viktrup et al. (23) reported that of 88 women with onset of incontinence during pregnancy, only 3 continued to lose urine 1 year postpartum. In subsequent pregnancies, these patients are at greater risk for more severe incontinence with earlier onset and persistence beyond the puerperium.

Mode of delivery has a profound impact on incontinence. Vaginal delivery can produce neurological changes in the pelvic floor, resulting in adverse effects on pudendal nerve conduction velocities, vaginal contraction strength, and urethral closure pressures. These changes are not seen after cesarean section. Presumably, these changes allow for the persistence or onset of genuine stress

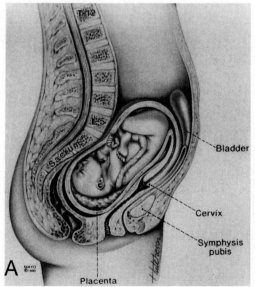

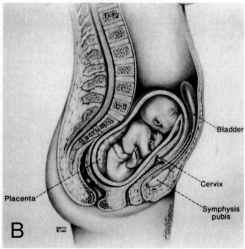

Figure 23.3. **A.** Incarcerated uterus with fetal vertex. **B.** Incarcerated uterus with fetal breech. (Reprinted from Van Winter JT, Ogburn PL, Ney JA, Hetzel DJ. Uterine incarceration during the third trimester: a rare complication of pregnancy. Mayo Clin Proc 1991; 66:608–613, with permission.)

Table 23.2. Development of Symptomatic Infection After Asymptomatic Bacteriruria

	Positive Initial Culture		Negative Initial Culture	
Author	No. of Patients	Symptomatic Infection	No. of Patients	Symptomatic Infection
Kass (1962)	95	18 (0.12%)	1,000	0 (0%)
Sleigh et al. (1964)	100	43 (43%)	100	14 (14%)
Kincaid-Smith and Bullen (1965)	55	20 (37%)	4,000	48 (1.2%)
Norden ad Kilpatrick (1965)	110	25 (23%)	105	1 (1.0%)
Whalley (1965)	179	46 (26%)	179	0 (0%)
Little (1966)	141	35 (25%)	4,735	19 (0.4%)
Brumfitt (1975)	179	55 (31%)		
Chung and Hall (1982)	212	25 (12%)	1,575	51 (3.2%)
Campbell-Brown et al. (1987)	226	1/8 (16%)	4,244	1/226 (0.4%)
Golan et al. (1989)	67	16 (24%)	1,063	17 (1.6%)
Gratacos et al. (1994)	77	2/7 (28%)	1,575	5 (0.31%)
Total	1441	333 (23%)	18,576	174 (0.94%)

incontinence in women after vaginal delivery. Whether or not this nerve damage is cumulative in multiparas is controversial. Mallett et al. (24) recently showed that absolute parity and further childbearing did not further effect pelvic floor neurophysiology. They concluded that most pudendal nerve damage occurs during the first vaginal delivery. Certainly no data exist to suggest that gravidas with prior vaginal deliveries can avoid stress incontinence or pelvic prolapse by undergoing cesarean section.

Urge incontinence is also more prevalent during and after pregnancy. The prepregnancy incidence of urge incontinence is approximately 5% and can increase to 43% by the third trimester (25). After pregnancy, the incidence remains nearly twice that noted before pregnancy.

Urodynamic evaluation of the incontinent gravida has shown, not surprisingly, that the prevalence of the symptom of stress incontinence (32%) is much higher than the diagnosis of genuine stress incontinence (7%) (25). Conversely, detrusor instability is usually present in patients complaining of urge incontinence.

URINARY TRACT INFECTIONS

Asymptomatic Bacteriuria

This pathological entity, which occurs in up to 10% of all women, whether pregnant or not, is defined as the presence of $\geq 10^5$ bacteria/mL of urine in a clean catch speci-

men from patients without symptoms of a bladder infection. The prevalence is higher in patients with lower socioeconomic status, sickle cell trait, and Lewis blood group. Race, age, and parity have no relationship to increased infection rates.

First recognized by Kass in 1960 (26), up to 40% of pregnant patients with bacteriuria will develop pyelonephritis, compared with 1% of patients without bacteriuria at the time of the initial culture. This has been consistently borne out in numerous studies showing that symptomatic infection develops in 12–43% of patients with bacteriuria during pregnancy compared with zero to 14% of patients who were abacteriuric at their initial prenatal visit (Table 23.2). Treatment of asymptomatic bacteriuria in pregnancy undisputedly reduces this risk of pyelonephritis to 5% of patients. For this reason, urine culture is recommended at the first prenatal visit. Although controversial, there also appears to be a strong link between untreated aymptomatic bacteriuria and both preterm labor and low birth weight. Metaanalysis review of 19 cohort and randomized studies found that treatment significantly reduced the risks of low birth weight and prematurity (27).

By definition, the diagnosis of asymptomatic bacteriuria is made on the basis of urine culture rather than urinalysis or dipstick tests. Attention must be given to collection and storage methods to minimize false-positive results. The most common bacteria isolated in these infections are listed in

Table 23.3. *Escherichia coli* is responsible for more than 70% of these infections, with *Klebsiella pneumoniae, Enterobacter* species, and the enterococci accounting for most of the remaining isolates.

Treatment should be based on the results of sensitivity testing. The most common oral agents are listed in Table 23.4. A 3-day course is usually sufficient. Single-dose therapy has attracted some interest, but cure rates are overall not as high (65–88%) as with more extended treatment (28). However, failure to respond to single-dose therapy may identify a high-risk group that will subsequently become reinfected 50% of the time compared with only 5% of those pregnant women who respond to single-dose therapy (29). Thus, single-dose therapy acts not only as an effective treatment with minimal side effects but also offers the advantage of being a test to identify those patients at high risk for subsequent reinfection. It is postulated that these women who fail to respond to single-dose therapy have renal bacteriuria as demonstrated by antibody-coated bacteria. This subgroup of patients might be better treated after initial therapy by low-dose antibiotic suppression rather than by surveillance.

Table 23.3. Common Bacterial Isolates in Asymptomatic Pregnant Women

Escherichia coli
Klebsiella pneumoniae
Enterobacter sp.
Enterococcus
Streptococcus sp.
Staphylococcus sp.
Proteus mirabilis
Pseudomonas aeruginosa

Enthusiasm for ampicillin has waned in recent years because of widespread resistance, reportedly up to 30% with *E. coli* and almost universal with *K. pneumoniae* (30). However, when sensitivity testing indicates, ampicillin is an excellent choice because it is inexpensive, safe, and may be used in nonallergic patients throughout pregnancy. Amoxicillin has an easier dosing schedule and may lessen side effects. The addition of clavulanic acid to amoxicillin greatly increases gram-negative coverage, making it useful in recurring or resistant infections. Cephalexin is safe throughout pregnancy, and higher-generation cephalosporins offer no further advantage against urinary tract infection. Although cross-reactivity to cephalosporins has been widely taught to occur in 8% of patients allergic to penicillins, our clinical experience suggests that this is much lower.

Nitrofurantoin is an excellent choice for initial therapy because of its safety, broad coverage of uropathogens, and high concentration in the urine. However, nausea and vomiting have been reported in up to 8% of patients. Nitrofurantoin has also rarely been associated with pulmonary hypersensitivity reactions. Nitrofurantoin can cause hemolytic anemia in patients with a deficiency in glucose-6-phosphate-dehydrogenase (G6PD). Black patients have a 10% risk for G6PD deficiency. Theoretically, nitrofurantoin should not be used in pregnant patients at term or in labor because of the risk to the neonate of hemolytic anemia, but such an effect has never been reported.

Sulfonamides, including sulfisoxazole and sulfamethoxazole, should not be used in patients near term because they displace biliru-

Table 23.4. Oral Antibiotics for Treatment of Asymptomatic Bacteriuria and Cystitis

Agent	Dose	Cost[a] ($)	Generic Available
Ampicillin	250 mg q.i.d.	5.89	Yes
Amoxicillin	250 mg t.i.d.	5.89	Yes
Amoxicillin/clavulanic acid	250 mg t.i.d.	22.09	No
Cephalexin	250 mg q.i.d.	8.59	Yes
Nitrofurantoin	50 mg q.i.d.	11.19	Yes
Nitrofurantoin monohydrate	100 mg b.i.d.	13.49	No
Sulfamethoxazole/Trimethoprim	800 mg/160 mg b.i.d.	5.89	Yes
Nalidixic acid	1000 mg q.i.d.	30.29	No

[a]Price in the Chicago area as of July 1995.

bin from binding sites on albumin in the fetus. Toxicities reported in neonates after in utero exposure to sulfonamides include severe jaundice and hemolytic anemia but, surprisingly, not kernicterus (31). Trimethoprim may interfere with folic acid metabolism and is relatively contraindicated in the first trimester of pregnancy, although many reports and trials have failed to demonstrate an increase in fetal abnormalities (31).

Nalidixic acid is safe in pregnancy but frequently causes side effects of nausea, vomiting, rash, headache, and drowsiness, limiting its usefulness. It should also not be given to patients with G6PD deficiency. Because of its limited spectrum and excellent urinary concentration, however, it can work well for patients with multiple allergies or recurrent infections.

Tetracyclines and fluoroquinolones should not be used in pregnancy. Tetracycline causes staining of fetal decidual teeth after 20 weeks gestation and has been associated with maternal hepatic toxicity. Fluoroquinolones, although very effective in nonpregnant women, can erode fetal cartilage of weight-bearing joints, causing permanent arthropathy.

After initial treatment, close follow-up with biweekly cultures is as effective as suppressive medication in preventing pyelonephritis, even though the untreated patients have a higher incidence of recurrent bacteriuria. Suppressive therapy may thus be reserved for resistant infections, patients with pyelonephritis in pregnancy, and patients for whom close follow-up may be difficult. Suppressive therapy is usually accomplished with nitrofurantoin, ampicillin, or cephalexin in a once-daily dose at bedtime.

Recurrent bacteriuria in pregnancy is associated with underlying structural disease in 40% of patients. Up to 50% of all patients with asymptomatic bacteriuria have positive fluorescent antibody tests for antibody-coated bacteria, implying renal infection (32). The fluorescent antibody test is nearly as effective as direct methods (ureteral catheterization and bladder washout techniques) in the determination of renal bacteriuria. These patients often have decreased kidney function, with mildly elevated blood urea nitrogen and serum creatinine levels. Forty-five percent have creatinine clearances of less than 100 mL/min. These abnormalities revert to normal within 6 weeks after treatment in most patients.

Long-term follow-up shows that 38% of patients with asymptomatic bacteriuria in pregnancy have bacteriuria 10–14 years later (33). Those with recurrent bacteriuria in pregnancy have a 10% incidence of chronic pyelonephritis. In subsequent pregnancies, 38% of asymptomatic bacteriuric patients have symptomatic infections (34).

Cystitis

Cystitis, or uncomplicated urinary tract infection, is a syndrome of urinary urgency, frequency, and dysuria in the absence of systemic symptoms. The incidence in pregnancy is 1–3%. Diagnosis can be made with as few as 10^2 colonies from a catheterized specimen. Only 6% of these patients have antibody-coated bacteria. Pathogens are similar to those in asymptomatic bacteriuria, with *E. coli* the most common isolate by far.

Initial antepartum screening is of limited effectiveness for predicting who will develop cystitis. Two thirds of patients who develop cystitis had negative cultures initially. This differs markedly from the rate in patients who develop pyelonephritis in pregnancy, in which only one fifth of these patients had negative cultures initially. In addition, recurrent infection after treatment is far less common in patients with cystitis (17%) than in patients with pyelonephritis (75%) or asymptomatic bacteriuria (33%).

Treatment for cystitis is identical to that used for asymptomatic bacteriuria. Success is common, and there is little risk of subsequent pyelonephritis. Only 9% of these patients will have recurrent bacteriuria. The low recurrence risk is probably due to the low incidence of renal involvement (6%) in these patients.

Pyelonephritis

Pyelonephritis complicates 1% of all pregnancies. Although pregnancy does not increase the incidence of aymptomatic bacteriuria, it does increase the risk of developing pyelonephritis. The normal dilation of the ureters and subsequent urinary stasis, as well as enhanced growth of coliform bacteria in pregnant urine, are largely responsible for this increased risk. Three quarters of kidney infections in pregnant women are predated by asymptomatic bacteriuria. Conversely, less than 5% of women whose bacteriuria is successfully treated develop pyelonephritis.

The onset of symptoms of pyelonephritis usually occurs during the second or third trimester (67%) or intra- or postpartum (27%) and rarely presents in the first trimester. The most common symptoms are listed in Table 23.5 (34). Urinalysis reveals pyuria, bacteriuria, and white cell casts. Identification of white blood cells and bacteria on a drop of unspun urine correlates well with a positive culture (35). Temporary renal dysfunction leads to an elevation in blood urea nitrogen and creatinine in 20% and decrease in creatinine clearance below 100 mL/min in 46% of patients (34). If not treated, up to 10% of women may develop septic shock and multiorgan failure. Respiratory distress with pulmonary edema occurs in 2% of cases, rarely before the third trimester (36). Unrecognized pyelonephritis has also been associated with spontaneous rupture of the urinary tract during pregnancy (37).

Pyelonephritis has been clearly associated with an increased incidence of anemia (25–60%), secondary to endotoxin-mediated hemolysis. Prospective controlled studies have not confirmed suspected associations with pregnancy-induced hypertension or low birth weight. Premature labor requiring tocolysis occurs in approximately 4% of patients with pyelonephritis, with only those patients presenting in labor being at increased risk for premature delivery. Appropriately treated patients are at low risk for preterm labor requiring tocolysis.

Treatment generally consists of hospital admission, intravenous fluid hydration, antibiotics (Table 23.6), and close observation.

Because of widespread hospital resistance to ampicillin, a first-generation cephalosporin such as cefazolin is the preferred empirical treatment, which is successful in 75% of patients. Because 95% of these patients will be afebrile in 72 hours, patients not responding by this time should have gentamicin or aztreonam added with drug levels monitored to ensure adequate therapy and prevent toxicity. A renal ultrasound or "one-shot" intravenous pyelogram should also be obtained to evaluate the possibility of urolithiasis or obstruction.

Once the patient has been afebrile for 24–48 hours, she may be changed to oral therapy for 7–14 days followed by suppressive therapy as outlined above for the duration of the pregnancy. This reduces the risk of recurrent pyelonephritis to about 5%. Surveillance with biweekly cultures is an alternative for reliable patients, but a third of these women will develop positive cultures.

Alternatively, two recent prospective randomized studies suggest that selected patients with pyelonephritis may be safely treated as outpatients. Angel et al. (38) found that oral antibiotic therapy (cephalexin) and intravenous therapy (cephalothin) were equally effective. Millar et al. (39) showed that in patients at less than 24 weeks estimated gestational age, outpatient therapy with ceftriaxone and cephalexin is safe and as effective as inpatient therapy. Patients treated as outpatients should be reliable and able to return to the hospital quickly if their condition worsens.

Follow-up studies reveal that 30–45% of women with pyelonephritis in pregnancy have radiological evidence of renal disease or anomalies (Fig. 23.4). These patients are at higher risk (40%) for developing recurrent pyelonephritis in subsequent pregnancies.

Table 23.5. Common Signs and Symptoms in Patients With Pyelonephritis

Symptom	Frequency (%)
Costovertebral tenderness	97
Fever ≥38.3° C	84
Flank pain and chills	82
Dysuria, frequency, urgency	40
Nausea, vomiting	24

Table 23.6. Intravenous Antibiotics for Treatment of Pyelonephritis in Pregnancy

Agent	Dose
Cephazolin	2 g q6h
Gentamicin	2.0 mg/kg loading dose, then 1.5 mg/kg q8h
Aztreonam	2 g q8h

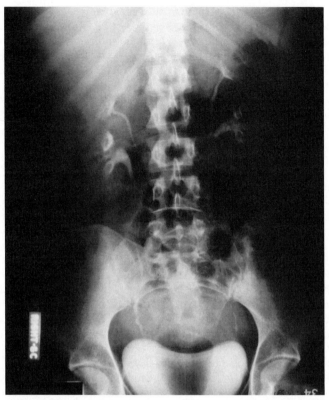

Figure 23.4. Urinary anomalies in pyelonephritis patients. Intravenous pyelogram performed 6 weeks after a pregnancy complicated by recurrent pyelone- phritis shows bifid collecting systems to the pelvic brim.

Postpartum Urinary Infection

Recurrent pyelonephritis occurs postpartum in as many as 10% of patients who have antepartum infection. Many of these infections may be iatrogenic after routine intrapartum catheterization. Bacteriuria develops twice as often in patients who are catheterized intrapartum (9.1% versus 4.7%). Indwelling catheters increase the risk of bacteriuria to nearly 25%. Catheterization should not be routinely performed.

THE URINARY TRACT DURING LABOR AND DELIVERY

Moderate amounts of urine in the bladder do not have a deleterious effect on the course of labor (40). Epidural anesthesia can eliminate the urge to void and result in overdistention of the bladder (41). For this reason, many patients with labor epidurals are subjected to continuous bladder drainage throughout labor. However, a rapid ultra- sound assessment can approximate bladder volume and reduce or eliminate the need for catheterization in most cases.

Minor trauma to the bladder during spontaneous vaginal delivery is common, with urinary retention occurring in 10–15% of all postpartum patients. Obstructed labor leading to necrosis of the anterior vaginal wall and bladder (and thus vesicovaginal fistula) has been essentially eradicated in Western countries but remains a significant problem in underdeveloped nations.

The abdominal position of the bladder during pregnancy subjects it to a higher risk of injury at laparotomy. The incidence of urinary tract injury at cesarean section is overall less than 1% (42) but increases with Pfannenstiel incision, lower segment uterine incision, prior cesarean section, prolonged second stage of labor, uterine rupture, and cesarean hysterectomy. Barclay (43) reported bladder and ureteral injury in the latter case to be 4.8% and 0.5%, respectively. Outlet forceps should confer little increased risk, but several studies document increased risk of urinary tract injury with midpelvic maneuvers such as Kielland forceps and Scanzoni rotation. Kibel et al. (44) recently reported a bladder perforation in a primigravid patient with no history of pelvic surgery. Although the laceration occurred during the vacuum-assisted delivery of a 4200-g infant, it was not detected until 3 days postpartum when the patient presented with renal failure and ascites.

Most bladder injuries involve laceration of the bladder dome, which can be easily repaired in two layers using 00 or 000 chromic or polyglactin suture. Injuries extending onto the trigone or close to the ureteral orifices demand more careful attention as ureteral reimplantation is sometimes necessary. Infant feeding tubes or umbilical artery catheters available in the delivery room can be passed retrograde to ensure patency of the ureters.

Urinary fistulas are rare and usually result from unrecognized injury at the time of operative delivery. Vesicovaginal fistula is the most common, with an incidence of 0.7% in Barclay's study. Fistula formation is classically heralded by continuous incontinence 7–14 days after injury. Patients with vesicouterine or vesicocorporeal fistulas (Fig. 23.5*A*) have cyclic hematuria as the menstrual flow empties into the bladder (menouria). Finally, the patient presenting with normal menses but loss of urine from the external cervical os may have a vesicocervical fistula (Fig. 23.5*B*).

If a fistula is identified, it should be evaluated by cystoscopy and intravenous pyelography to rule out other fistulous tracts and ureteral compromise. Drainage and decompression above the site of the fistula may result in the resolution of some small fistulae. Timing and route of surgical repair are controversial and are discussed elsewhere in the text.

VESICOURETERAL REFLUX

Vesicoureteral reflux can cause radiating flank pain with urination and occurs in up to 3.5% of pregnancies but is rarely found before the third trimester except in patients with bacteriuria, who have a 50% incidence of reflux. Many of these latter patients probably have reflux before pregnancy. In normal pregnancy, ureteral catheter studies demonstrate an increase in resting basal pressure but somewhat decreased ureteral contractility. This increase in ureteral pressure offsets a similar increase in bladder pressure until the third trimester, when detrusor pressure is often higher than 25 cm H_2O. This increase in pressure may lead to a further reduction of ureteral ejaculation of urine, with total stasis occurring at pressures above 41 cm H_2O. Pressures this high are usually only reached in the third trimester with a full bladder and predispose to reflux.

UROLITHIASIS

Urolithiasis in pregnancy is rare, with an incidence of 0.03–0.44%, a rate similar to that in the general population (Table 23.7). The higher incidences are found in the Southeast and mid-Atlantic "stone belt." Urolithiasis is twice as common in the multipara, but this may be largely due to the increase in urinary calculi with advancing age.

Pregnancy does not influence calculus disease unless nausea and vomiting prevent treatment for preexisting stones. For unknown reasons, calculus disease is four times as common in women who spontaneously abort as in pregnant and nonpregnant controls.

The onset of symptomatic urolithiasis occurs predominantly (88%) after 20 weeks gestation when ureteral dilation is prominent. The composition of these stones are the same as those found in nonpregnant patients, with the exception of an increased incidence of struvite stones ("infection stones") in pregnant patients.

The signs and symptoms of urolithiasis in pregnancy are identical to those in the nonpregnant patient. In the presence of physiological hydroureter, however, colic and hematuria are frequently absent. Stones should be suspected in any patient presenting with lateralizing flank pain and tenderness without fever. It should also be suspected in those patients with pyelonephritis who do not respond to parenteral antibiotics within 48–72 hours.

Patients with suspected urolithiasis should be evaluated with ultrasound studies.

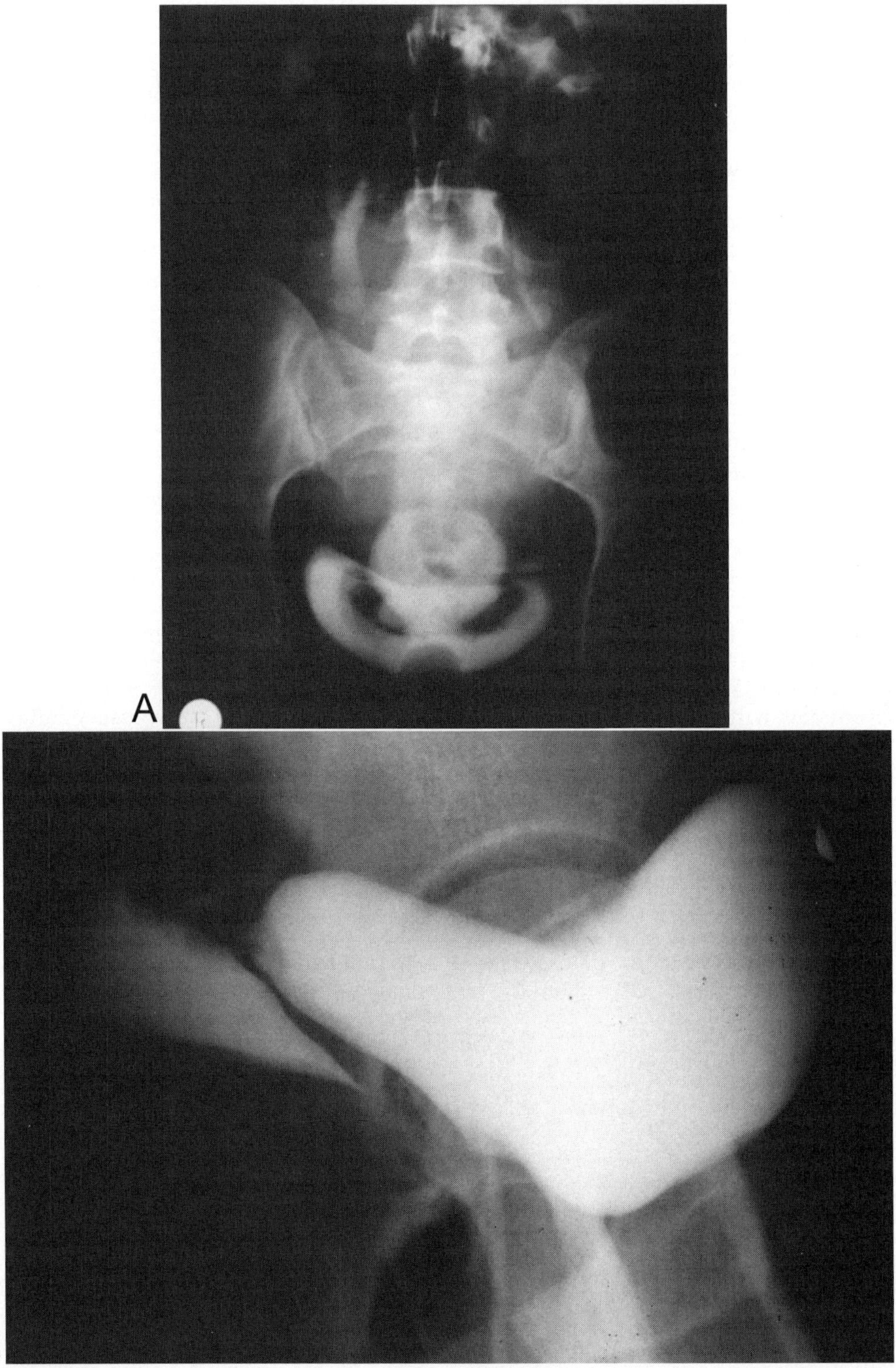

Figure 23.5. **A.** Vesicouterine fistula discovered during investigation of cyclic hematuria after cesarean section. (Courtesy of Dr. Allan Shanberg.) **B.** Lateral view of a vesicovaginal fistula masquerading as a vesicocervical fistula in a patient presenting with continuous leakage of urine 3 days after emergent cesarean section for a ruptured uterus while attempting a vaginal birth after cesarean section.

Table 23.7. Urolithiasis in Pregnancy

Author	Incidence	Spontaneous Passage	
Arnell and Getzhoff (1942)	12/9,882 (0.12%)		
Solomon (1954)	6/13,484 (0.04%)	5/6	(83%)
Byrd and Given (1963)	12[a]	3/12	(25%)
McVann (1964)	12/45,582 (0.03%)	7/12	(58%)
Simmens (1964)	9/2,037 (0.44%)	3/9	(33%)
Harris and Dunnihoo (1967)	19/11,977 (0.16%)	10/19	(53%)
Strong et al. (1978)	14/22,495 (0.06%)	11/14	(79%)
Coe et al. (1978)	20[a]	20/20	(100%)
Cumming and Taylor (1979)	13/21,277 (0.06%)	5/13	(38%)
Lattanzi and Cook (1980)	11/11,292 (0.09%)	7/11	(64%)
Total	96/138,026 (0.07%)	71/116	(61%)

[a]Not included in total incidence calculations.

Renal stones as small as 0.5 mm can sometimes be visualized with this technology (45). If this is inadequate, a one-shot intravenous pyelogram 20 minutes after dye injection may be done, followed by a 1-hour film if necessary. This results in less than 1 cGy to the fetus. A dose of 5–15 cGy in the first trimester is associated with an increased risk of congenital anomalies of 1–3%. The risk of carcinogenesis is less than 1% at doses less than 10 cGy, and the risk of leukemia in these infants is 1.5 cases per million people exposed to 1 cGy. These risks are far lower than those associated with failure to diagnose and treat urolithiasis. However, because ultrasound is safe, noninvasive, and readily available, its use before intravenous pyelography should be encouraged.

Initial treatment of urolithiasis should always be conservative. Over 60% of all stones will pass spontaneously. Stones 4 mm or less in diameter pass 80% of the time, but stones greater than 7 mm have a spontaneous passage rate of only 20% (45). For patients in whom the composition of the stone is unknown, initial therapy consists of aggressive hydration, analgesia, and bed rest. Experimental work suggests that a bolus of 250 mg of hydroxyprogesterone results in the prompt passage of stones in nonpregnant patients (46). This may be due to an acute progestational effect that simulates the hormonal milieu of pregnancy.

Where conservative management fails or complete obstruction is present, surgical intervention may be necessary. Simple procedures such as lithotripsy, cystoscopy with basket extraction, or the passage of a stent beyond the obstruction may be all that is necessary until after delivery. However, when major procedures such as ureterolithotomy, pyelolithotomy, or the very rare nephrectomy are necessary, they have been accomplished with minimal complications to either the mother or the fetus.

Determination of the exact etiology can usually be deferred until the postpartum period. When a previous etiology is known, specific therapy and aggressive hydration should be used. D-Penicillamine and all opurinol have both been used successfully and safely in pregnancy for cysteine and uric acid stones, respectively. Likewise, thiazide diuretics have been useful in curtailing calcium stone formation in hypercalciuric patients. Whenever possible, these medications should be avoided in the first trimester.

HEMATURIA

Hematuria in pregnancy is usually caused by catheterization or trauma at the time of labor and delivery. Outside of these, it is decidedly abnormal and must be investigated. Causes include urinary tract infection, calculi, trauma, urological cancer, and placenta percreta. Infection and calculus disease are discussed above. Seven percent of all pregnancies is complicated by trauma, with half occurring during the third trimester. Most of these are blunt abdominal injuries incurred in motor vehicle accidents. Although rare, the gravida with a full bladder may experience extraperitoneal rupture of the bladder with sudden blood loss and shock. The lower urinary tract is injured in 15% of pelvic fractures. Hematuria, gross or microscopic, warrants prompt investigation in the trauma setting.

Renal adenocarcinoma is the most common urological cancer of pregnancy, causing hematuria in almost half of the patients (47). A palpable abdominal mass, however, is present in most patients. Transitional cell carcinoma of the bladder has been reported in 13 patients (48), with most patients presenting with painless hematuria. Ultrasound evaluation of the urinary tract combined with cystoscopy and biopsy is usually sufficient for diagnosis. When the patient presents late in pregnancy, treatment may be delayed until after delivery. Placenta percreta is a rare condition in which the placenta penetrates the myometrium and can invade surrounding structures such as the bladder. It is most commonly associated with placenta previa and a history of prior cesarean section. In the past, diagnosis was made at the time of delivery, but antepartum diagnosis can now be made in most cases with ultrasound or magnetic resonance imaging. Cystoscopy can be a valuable adjunct. Cesarean hysterectomy and partial cystectomy are often mandated to control profuse bleeding. If the patient is not actively bleeding, the placenta may be left in situ with high ligation of the umbilical cord. The patient is then treated with antibiotics to minimize risk of infection. Methotrexate may be useful in accelerating reabsorption of the trophoblastic tissue, but a failure was recently reported (49).

PREGNANCY COMPLICATED BY PRIOR BLADDER SURGERY

Pregnancy is not contraindicated in patients having had surgery on the bladder or bladder neck. Successful outcomes have been reported in patients who have undergone continent urinary diversion, augmentation cystoplasty, and artificial urinary sphincter placement (50, 51). These patients are at high risk for urinary tract infection, and antibiotic suppression may be indicated. Most patients can deliver vaginally. For patients with previous antiincontinence surgery on the bladder neck, classic cesarean section has been recommended to minimize damage to the surgical site. The potential benefits of this procedure should be carefully weighed against the increased morbidity and necessity for future cesarean sections. Data are lacking regarding vaginal delivery after antiincontinence surgery, but a recent retrospective review found that 11 of 13 (85%) pregnant patients with an artificial urinary sphincter were able to have vaginal deliveries with no intra- or postpartum complications (51). Another report suggests that vaginal delivery is possible after pelvic floor reconstruction (52). We reevaluate patients during pregnancy to reassess their anatomic support and urodynamic parameters before deciding on mode of delivery. The patient should be an active participant in this decision.

REFERENCES

1. Iosif S, Ingemarsson I, Ulmsten U. Urodynamic studies in normal pregnancy and in puerperium. Obstet Gynecol 1980;137:696–700.
2. Tong Y, Wein AJ, Levin RM. Effects of pregnancy on adrenergic function in the rabbit urinary bladder. Neurourol Urodyn 1992;11:525–533.
3. Brown ADG. The effects of pregnancy on the lower urinary tract. Clin Obstet Gynaecol 1978;5:151–168.
4. Francis WJA. Disturbances of bladder function in relation to pregnancy. J Obstet Gynaecol Br Emp 1960;67:353–366.
5. Bennetts FA, Judd GE. Studies of the postpartum bladder. Am J Obstet Gynecol 1941;42:419–427.
6. Schulman A, Herlinger H. Urinary tract dilatation in pregnancy. Br J Radiol 1975;48:638–645.
7. Pitkin RM. Morphologic changes in pregnancy. In: Buchsbaum HJ, Schmidt JD, eds. Gynecologic and obstetric urology, 3rd ed. Philadelphia: WB Saunders Co., 1993:586.
8. Dafnis E, Sabatini S. The effect of pregnancy on renal function: physiology and pathophysiology. Am J Med Sci 1992;303:184–205.
9. Davison JA, Dunlop W. Renal hemodynamics and tubular function in normal human pregnancy. Kidney Int 1980;18:152–161.
10. Sims EAH, Krantz KE. Serial studies of renal function during pregnancy and the puerperium in normal women. J Clin Invest 1958;37:1764–1774.
11. Little B. Water and electrolyte balance during pregnancy. Anesthesiology 1965;26:400–408.
12. Hytten FE, Taggart N. Limb volumes in pregnancy. J Obstet Gynaecol Br Commonw 1967;74:663–668.
13. Cutner A, Cardozo LD, Benness CJ. Assessment of urinary symptoms in early pregnancy. Br J Obstet Gynaecol 1991;98:1283–1286.
14. Stanton SL, Kerr-Wilson R, Harris VG. The incidence of urological symptoms in normal pregnancy. Br J Obstet Gynaecol 1980;87:897–900.
15. Parboosingh J, Doig A. Studies of nocturia in normal pregnancy. J Obstet Gynaecol Br Commonw 1973;80:888–895.

16. Myers DL, Scotti RJ. Acute urinary retention and incarcerated, retroverted, gravid uterus. J Reprod Med 1995;40:487–490.
17. Jackson D, Elliot JP, Pearson M. Asymptomatic uterine retroversion at 36 weeks' gestation. Obstet Gynecol 1988;71:466–468.
18. Van Winter JT, Ogburn PL, Ney JA, Hetzel DJ. Uterine incarceration in the third trimester: a rare complication of pregnancy. Mayo Clin Proc 1991; 66:608–613.
19. Ramsay IN, Torbet TE. Incidence of abnormal voiding parameters in the immediate postpartum period. Neurourol Urodyn 1993;12:179–183.
20. Kerr-Wilson RHJ, McNally S. Bladder drainage for caesarean section under epidural analgesia. Br J Obstet Gynaecol 1986;93:28–30.
21. Tapp AJS, Meire H, Cardozo LD. The effect of epidural analgesia on post-partum voiding. Neurourol Urodyn 1987;6:235–237.
22. Francis WJA. The onset of stress incontinence. J Obstet Gynaecol Br Emp 1960;67:899–903.
23. Viktrup L, Lose G, Rolff M, Barfoed K. The symptom of stress incontinence caused by pregnancy or delivery in primiparas. Obstet Gynecol 1992;79:945–949.
24. Mallett V, Hosker G, Smith ARB, Warrell D. Pelvic floor damage and childbirth: a neurophysiologic follow up study. Neurourol Urodyn 1994;13: 357–358.
25. Cutner A, Cardozo LD, Benness CJ. Assessment of urinary symptoms in the second half of pregnancy. Int Urogynecol J 1992;3:30–32.
26. Kass EH. Bacteriuria and pyelonephritis of pregnancy. Arch Intern Med 1960;105:194–198.
27. Romero R, Oyarzun E, Mazor M, Sirtori M, Hobbins JC, Bracken M. Meta-analysis of the relationship between asymptomatic bacteriuria and preterm delivery/low birth weight. Obstet Gynecol 1989;73:576–582.
28. Vercaigne LM, Zhanel GG. Recommended treatment for urinary tract infection in pregnancy. Ann Pharmacother 1994;28:248–251.
29. Jakobi P, Neiger R, Merzbach D, Paldi E. Single-dose antimicrobial therapy in the treatment of asymptomatic bacteriuria of pregnancy. Am J Obstet Gynecol 1987;156:1148–1152.
30. Dunlow S, Duff P. Prevalence of antibiotic-resistant uropathogens in obstetric patients with acute pyelonephritis. Obstet Gynecol 1990;76: 241–244.
31. Briggs GG, Freeman RK, Yaffe SJ. Drugs in lactation and pregnancy, 4th ed. Baltimore: Williams & Wilkins, 1994:796–847.
32. Harris RE, Thomas VL, Shelokov A. Asymptomatic bacteriuria in pregnancy: antibody-coated bacteria, renal function, and intrauterine growth retardation. Am J Obstet Gynecol 1976;126: 20–25.
33. Zinner SH, Kass EH. Long-term (10 to 14 years) follow-up of bacteriuria of pregnancy. N Engl J Med 1971;285:820–824.
34. Gilstrap LC III, Cunningham FG, Whalley PJ. Acute pyelonephritis in pregnancy: an anterospective study of 656 women. Obstet Gynecol 1981;57:409–413.
35. Kunin CM. The quantitative significance of bacteria visualized in the unstained urinary sediment. N Engl J Med 1961;265:589–590.
36. Cunningham FG, Lucas MJ, Hankins GDV. Pulmonary injury complicating antepartum pyelonephritis. Am J Obstet Gynecol 1987;156: 797–807.
37. Meyers SJ, Lee RV, Munschauer RW. Dilatation and nontraumatic rupture of the urinary tract during pregnancy: a review. Obstet Gynecol 1985; 66:809–815.
38. Angel JL, O'Brien WF, Finan MA, Morales WJ, Lake M, Knuppel RA. Acute pyelonephritis of pregnancy: a prospective study of oral versus intravenous antibiotic therapy. Obstet Gynecol 1990;76:28–32.
39. Millar LK, Wing DA, Paul RH, Grimes DA. Outpatient treatment of pyelonephritis in pregnancy. Obstet Gynecol 1995;86:560–564.
40. Read JA, Miller FC, Yeh SY, Platt LD. Urinary bladder distention: effect on labor and uterine activity. Obstet Gynecol 1980;56:565–570.
41. Weil A, Reyes H, Rottenberg RD, Beguin F, Herrmann WL. Effect of lumbar epidural analgesia on lower urinary tract function in the immediate postpartum period. Br J Obstet Gynaecol 1983;90: 428–432.
42. Evrard JR, Gold EM, Cahill TF. Cesarean section: a contemporary assessment. J Reprod Med 1980; 24:147–152.
43. Barclay DL. Cesarean hysterectomy: thirty years' experience. Obstet Gynecol 1970;35:120–131.
44. Kibel AS, Staskin DR, Grigoriev VE. Intraperitoneal bladder rupture after normal vaginal delivery. J Urol 1995;153:725–727.
45. Swanson SK, Heilman RL, Eversman WG. Urinary tract stones in pregnancy. Surg Clin North Am 1995;75:123–142.
46. Perlow DL. The use of progesterone for ureteral stones: a preliminary report. J Urol 1980;124: 715–716.
47. Walker JL, Knight EL. Renal cell carcinoma in pregnancy. Cancer 1986;58:2343–2347.
48. Loughlin KR, Ng B. Bladder cancer during pregnancy. Br J Urol 1995;75:421–422.
49. Jaffe R, DuBeshter B, Sherer DM, Thompson EA, Woods JR. Failure of methotrexate treatment for term placenta percreta. Am J Obstet Gynecol 1994;171:558–559.
50. Fenn N, Barrington JW, Stephenson TP. Clam enteroplasty and pregnancy. Br J Urol 1995;75: 85–86.
51. Creagh TA, McInerney PD, Thomas PJ, Mundy AR. Pregnancy after lower urinary tract reconstruction in women. J Urol 1995;154:1323–1324.
52. Kovac SR, Cruikshank SH. Successful pregnancies and vaginal deliveries after sacrospinous uterosacral fixation in five of nineteen patients. Am J Obstet Gynecol 1993;168:1778–1786.

CHAPTER 24

Urethral Syndrome

Richard J. Scotti and Donald R. Ostergard

*Any pain within two feet of the female urethra
which does not seem to be adequately accounted
for by some definite pathology should be suspected
of being due to the urethral syndrome.
Folsom and Alexander—1934*

Introduction

The above statement (1) made in 1934 still has much relevance today, more than 50 years later. Although much progress has been made since Folsom's early pioneering work, the urethral syndrome is still one of the most perplexing topics in urogynecology today. It is considered by some to be a "wastebasket" term for urethral symptoms that do not fit into other more well-delineated diagnostic categories. The term urethral syndrome suggests a set of symptoms rather than a clearly defined clinical entity. In fact, the urethral syndrome is a disease of multiple etiologies. Causation has been variably ascribed to infection, inflammation of urethral glands, hypoestrogenism, vitamin deficiency, allergy, psychiatric disturbances, vaginal metaplasia, urethral spasm, urethral stenosis, connective tissue disease, and a host of other factors. It is no small wonder that the treatment modalities range from operative techniques to local applications of estrogen and steroids to psychotherapy.

The term urethral syndrome was originally coined by Gallagher et al. (2) in 1965. They reported that 41% of women seen in general practice who had symptoms of urinary tract infection (i.e., frequency, suprapubic discomfort, and dysuria) in fact had sterile urine.

Probably the best working definition for the urethral syndrome, as it is understood today, is that it is a *condition of lower urinary tract symptoms in the absence of obvious bladder or urethral abnormalities of other known etiologies and in the absence of significant bacterial urinary growth.* Any combination of symptoms may be present. The most common are frequency, urgency, and dysuria. Postvoid fullness, urge incontinence, apparent stress incontinence, suprapubic tenderness, dyspareunia, urinary hesitancy, incomplete bladder emptying, reduced caliber of urinary stream, general malaise, back discomfort, and many other symptoms may be present.

Many synonyms for the urethral syndrome can be found in the literature. These include aseptic urethritis, aseptic urethrotrigonitis, chronic urethritis, granular urethrotrigonitis, pseudomembranous urethrotrigonitis, senile or hypoestrogenic urethritis, senile mucosal atrophy, and irritative cystourethritis. These descriptive terms reflect the wide spectrum of cystourethroscopic findings and the myriad of postulations regarding pathophysiology. Urethral syndrome is often lumped together with interstitial cystitis. The constellation of symptoms is termed "sensory bladder disorders" or "painful bladder syndromes."

The most sober approach to the proper diagnosis and management of urethral syndrome is to attempt to isolate the etiology of urethral symptomatology in a particular individual by all means at the urogynecologist's disposal and then, as rationally as possible, to formulate a treatment plan based on probable causation. One should begin with the least complicated, least invasive treatment for the particular causative entity and proceed to more complex forms of therapy. Should uncertainty of the correct diagnosis arise during a particular treatment plan or should treatment fail, the possibility that the symptoms in fact may represent another clinical entity must be considered. Reevaluation or further testing may then be necessary.

This chapter is a review of the various pathophysiological and etiological factors in the causation of the urethral syndrome; it is also a review and update of the various methods of diagnosis and treatment. Rational approaches to therapy based on probable causation are recommended.

Embryology, Anatomy, and Physiology

The upper female urethra and trigone are formed by the upper anterior division of the urogenital sinus, whereas the lower urethra and periurethral glands and part of the vestibule are formed by the pelvic component of the lower urogenital sinus. Hence, the trigone and upper urethra are embryologically, anatomically, and physiologically related to each other. Likewise, the upper vestibule, distal urethra, and urethral and periurethral glands are similarly related (see Chapters 1 and 2).

The most extensive work describing the anatomy of the female urethra and periurethral and urethral glands in the English medical literature was done by Huffman (3). He serially sectioned the urethra and made wax reconstructions of its glands and then estimated that there are 6–21 of these ducts varying from 0.27–1.2 cm in length extending cephalad. The ducts are lined with low columnar epithelium. By mucicarmine staining techniques, he demonstrated the presence of mucus in these glands. Hutch (4)

reproduced Huffman's work from autopsy specimens and postulated that the glands in the mucosa of the urethra have a function similar to that of mucus-secreting epithelium in other parts of the body, namely, lubricating and slowing down or preventing the ascent of bacteria. This assumption had been previously made by Cox (5), who by an ingenious collection device initially designed for males by Helmholz (6) found that the upper urethra is particularly free of microorganisms, whereas the distal urethra harbors many of the organisms common to the vestibule and vagina. Both urethra and bladder probably contain antibacterial factors (7, 8).

Seddon and Bruce (9) enumerated other urethral defense mechanisms, including "urethral washout" voiding, the midurethral high-pressure zone, secretory immunoglobulin A (which reduces bacterial adherence), and paraurethral gland mucus (which traps bacteria). Mayo and Hinman (10) demonstrated in female dogs that an inoculum of bacteria above the high-pressure zone caused bacteriuria, whereas an inoculation below the zone did not. These studies all demonstrate the role the urethra plays in the defense against infection.

Between the urethra and the vagina is a layer of connective tissue that has received considerable attention in the literature, particularly by Richardson (11) and Evans (12). Richardson removed this tissue and found increased amounts of "fibroelastosis" at this site. Evans described increased amounts of hydroxyproline in patients with urethral syndrome and postulated an increased amount of collagenous tissue in this area as a cause for obstruction and urethral syndrome.

Incidence

The true incidence of urethral syndrome is unknown, but in patients referred for urinary complaints other than uncomplicated urinary tract infections, approximately 20–30% were found to have the urethral syndrome (13–16).

There are no good epidemiological studies describing the urethral syndrome, most likely because of the various differences among many authors in characterizing the syndrome itself. There do not appear to be any racial or age-related differences, although most patients are women in the reproductive years. The condition has also been reported in children and in the geriatric population (17, 18).

Evaluation and Differential Diagnosis

To diagnose urethral syndrome, one must exclude all other etiologies that can cause urinary symptoms. It is important to rule out bladder or urethral stones, bladder cancer, and tuberculosis. Tuberculosis is again on the rise, particularly in HIV-positive patients. It should be remembered that sterile pyuria can be caused by tuberculosis. Cancer of the bladder can be ruled out by bladder cytology and cystoscopy with biopsy.

Interstitial cystitis must also be ruled out because it may cause frequency, dysuria, and suprapubic discomfort with frequent small voidings. Bladder biopsy may reveal the typical lesion and may show an increase in the number of mast cells (19).

Other sources of dysuria must also be considered, including urethral diverticula, caruncle, urethral prolapse, cystocele, condyloma, herpes, and vaginitis. These may be obvious on physical examination and could cause voiding symptoms that may be suggestive of urethral syndrome.

EVALUATION

Because the diagnosis of urethral syndrome is made essentially by excluding other conditions that cause symptoms in the lower urinary tract, a fairly extensive urogynecological workup is necessary to make the diagnosis. One may therefore follow the guidelines for the triage of women with lower urinary tract symptoms outlined in Chapter 6. Urinalysis and urine culture and sensitivity are mandatory to rule out cystitis. Urethral cultures for gonorrhea, chlamydia, and ureaplasma should also be performed if acute urethritis is suspected or found.

A thorough history is essential. The urethral syndrome presents with protean manifestations. Frequency, dysuria, postvoid full-ness, and urgency are the most common symptoms. Other symptoms include bladder discomfort, incontinence, hematuria, chills and fever, dyspareunia, childhood enuresis, and tenesmus.

The history should include a urolog, which is a 24-hour diary of spontaneous micturitions. The patient is asked to document for at least one 24-hour period the time and volume of each micturition. The frequency and amount of both daytime and nighttime voidings are useful indicators of urinary tract disease. Most patients with urethral syndrome do not have significant nocturia.

A physical examination is necessary to assess anatomic abnormalities, including urethrohymenal fusion, hypospadias, urethral caruncle, cystocele, rectocele, uterine prolapse, enterocele, and other associated pelvic pathology, that may contribute to frequency, dysuria, and other symptoms. A neurological examination is necessary to rule out any nerve root damage involving the lower urinary tract.

Urethral calibration is also included in the workup because it may uncover severe degrees of urethral stenosis. Urethral calibration has no real validity without concurrent determination of urinary flow rates (20) (see "Uroflowmetry" in Chapter 6). Dynamic urethroscopy is also carried out. The urethra is examined for signs of chronic urethritis, such as exudate, redness, or inspissated glandular material. Marked pallor, atrophy, and friability suggest hypoestrogenism. The urethrovesical junction is also observed during filling, Valsalva, cough, rectal tightening, and urine holding to assess its functional competence. The urethra is carefully scrutinized for evidence of diverticula, which may present with symptomatology similar to the urethral syndrome. The trigone is examined for signs of trigonitis, granularity, or vaginal metaplasia. Because the trigone and the urethra are closely related embryologically and anatomically, signs of hypoestrogenism and chronic urethritis frequently extend to the trigone. Finally, the urethra is thoroughly massaged with a vaginal finger while the urethroscope is being withdrawn, viewing the posterior urethra during withdrawal. At this time, a thorough search is made for exudate from glandular orifices or possible diverticula.

Cystoscopy will rule out bladder pathology such as bladder diverticula, acute cystitis, interstitial cystitis, tuberculosis, radiation changes, carcinoma, or carcinoma in situ. All of these conditions may have symptoms in common with the urethral syndrome.

A cystometrogram is essential to rule out vesical instability. It should be performed in the erect position because 15–30% of persons with vesical instability will manifest it only in the standing position (see Chapter 6). Imaging radiological techniques have added little to the diagnosis of urethral syndrome (21–24). Lyon and Smith (21) described a "spinning top" appearance in young women and girls with distal urethral stenosis. Most authors report some degree of endothelial thickening in the urethra or at the bladder neck ultrasonographically (22, 24). Most imaging techniques, however, require meticulous interpretation and have not had widespread use in the diagnosis of urethral syndrome.

The urethroscope is useful for excluding other causes of symptoms, including hypoestrogenism (16, 25).

Treatment of Urethral Syndrome Based on Probable Etiology

The urethral syndrome may be caused by many different etiological factors. Therefore, many treatment modalities are in current use. The guiding principle in successful treatment is to treat the most probable cause(s) of symptoms in the individual patient after a thorough diagnostic workup is performed. Table 24.1 provides a summary of the various etiologies, pathological and urethroscopic findings, and treatment modalities.

CHRONIC URETHRITIS

Background

In 1900, Bierhoff (26) described a disease that he termed irritable bladder. His classic paper describes a condition in which the patient exhibits an "abnormal frequency of urination in the absence of pus in the urine." His cases probably included many patients with vesical instability, interstitial cystitis, and a large number of patients with urethral syndrome. He described some of the granular changes frequently seen in the trigone and urethra in patients with urethral syndrome secondary to chronic urethritis. He treated them mainly with irrigations of boric acid and/or silver nitrate.

In 1931, Folsom (27) described various changes in the urethra of women suffering from urethral syndrome. He graded these changes with respect to severity. The first phase was narrowing of the urethral lumen, followed by inflammation, engorgement, granulation, and "pin head-sized cysts." He took many biopsies that showed inflamed and inspissated glands. He postulated infection and inflammation of these glands as the cause of urethritis and recommended dilatation as a treatment of choice.

In 1935, Ormond (28) described a condition that he termed nonpurulent urethritis or granular urethritis-cystalgia, in which the patient had urinary symptoms with "no abnormal urinary findings or very minor ones." He described the changes of chronic urethrotrigonitis, which began in the urethra and spread upward to the trigone. He recommended dilatation with massage of the inflamed and inspissated periurethral glands twice weekly and local instillations of silver nitrate.

Diagnosis

Today, chronic urethritis is still considered to be caused by inflammation and/or chronic infection of periurethral and urethral glands. Various changes that have been described endoscopically take place within the urethra (27, 28). Redness and exudate are salient features. The exudate may take on a pseudomembranous appearance after a period of weeks to months. The disease progresses to granularity in the urethra and the trigone with eventual development of inflammatory fronds, polyps, and cysts (see Chapter 12, color tip page). Histologically, the urethra contains inspissated mucus and chronic inflammatory cells in the glands. There is increased vascularity and hyperplasia of the transitional epithelium.

Table 24.1. Urethral Syndrome: A Summary

Etiology	Clinical and Endoscopic Features	Histopathology	Current Recommended Treatment
Chronic urethritis	Redness, exudate, granularity, occasional inflammation, polyps, and cysts in urethra and trigone; inspissated glands	Chronic inflammatory cells; increased vascularity and hyperplasia	Urethral dilatation and massage or urethral steroids or cryotherapy
Hypoestrogenic (senile) urethritis	Pale, atrophic urethra and trigone; reddened if coexistent inflammation; postmenopausal status	Atrophic changes	Estrogen cream or suppositories
Urethral stenosis (obstruction)	Two types: Lyon's ring, constrictive band at distal urethra diagnosed with bougie, and fibroelastosis of urethrovaginal septum	Fibroelastic tissue	Breaking constrictive ring with bougie; Richardson procedure
Urethral spasm	External sphincter and/or smooth muscle spasticity diagnosed urodynamically or with selective therapeutic trials of alpha blockers and smooth muscle relaxants	None	Diazepam (skeletal muscle); alpha blockers (smooth muscle); dilatation; external meatotomy
Infection (acute urethritis)	Acute urethritis; dysuria, redness, exudative urethral mucosa; pyuria; often a negative culture	Causative organism may or may not be found; acute inflammatory cells	Specific treatment of causative agent; empirical tetracycline, erythromycin or azithromycin for all patients with pyuria
Psychogenic	Dysuria, dyspareunia, frequency, etc. (general findings of urethral syndrome)	None	Psychotherapy; supportive therapy
Allergy	Symptoms of urethral syndrome; redness	Eosinophilia, inflammation	Removing offending agents; steroid suppositories; antihistamines
Neurologic disorders	General findings of urethral syndrome; possibly low back pain	Related to neurological findings (cord compression, nerve root injury, etc.)	Treatment specific neurologic entity; injecting trigger points with local anesthetic
Trauma and noxious agents	Disruption or redness of urethral mucosa; bleeding; signs of trauma or inflammation	Evidence of injury; hemorrhage; possible acute inflammatory cells	Removing offending agents; possible prophylactic antibiotics
Anatomic variations	Urethrohymenal fusion Hypospadias	None None	Hymenoplasty Meatus transposition; neourethra

Other associated findings may be fibromuscular hyperplasia and squamous metaplasia, often with cystic degeneration (29). Pathological changes vary with the severity of the disease process and correlate well with the endoscopic appearance (30).

Treatment

Many treatments have been suggested for chronic urethritis without much control data. They are described below.

Urethral Dilatation. Dilatation is still the time-honored method for treatment and is relatively safe (Fig. 24.1). In canines, Tanagho and Lyon (31) showed that urethral dilatation causes no long-term histological or structural changes compared with urethrotomy, which causes thickening and induration of the urethral mucosa and excessive fibrous reaction involving the submucosa and the inner fibers of the muscular wall. The posttreatment incidence of urinary tract infection is less than 0.6% if prophylactic antimicrobials are given (32).

The rationale for urethral dilatation is based on the belief that dilators are rigid surgical instruments against which inspissated, inflamed, or infected urethral glands may be massaged. The exudate in these glands may be expressed in this manner. It is also thought that urethral dilatation massages the mucous membranes, stretches the submucosal tissue, and remedies strictures.

Dilatation is also thought to relieve meatal stenosis and to promote laminar flow. Because there are no significant differences in urethral caliber between affected and unaffected individuals, dilatation may act by improving drainage of congested paraurethral glands or by relieving urethral spasm. Urethral dilatation is particularly effective in those patients with chronic urethritis who also have evidence of obstructed flow.

Unfortunately, most studies on dilatation in the literature are uncontrolled or are anecdotal in nature. Antimicrobials are often given posttreatment for prophylaxis, which introduces another uncontrolled variable.

In treating recurrent cystourethritis, Kapland et al. (33) found no differences in cure rates between those patients who took medication only and patients after dilatation or internal urethrotomy. The same control data

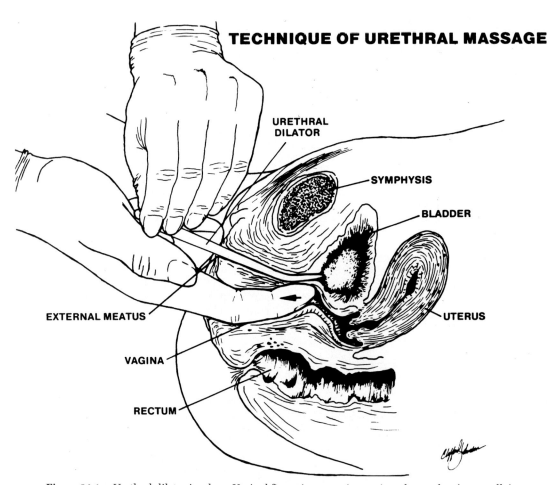

Figure 24.1.   Urethral dilator in place. Vaginal finger is massaging against the urethra (outwardly).

present in this study are not available to assess dilatation as a treatment for chronic urethritis.

Bergman et al. (34) compared urethral dilatation with tetracycline and placebo in a group of 60 patients with chronic urethral syndrome. They achieved a subjective cure, defined as an absence of symptoms at follow-up visits, in 20% of the placebo group, 50% of the tetracycline group, and 75% of the urethral dilatation group ($P >$ 0.01). This was the first prospective study using the patients as their own controls. There were no differences in other variables in the three groups of patients who were consecutively assigned to one of three treatment modalities.

Cryotherapy. Sand et al. (35) enrolled 24 women with recurrent urethral syndrome in a prospective randomized crossover study comparing dilatation and massage to cryosurgery. Short-term (6–12 month) success with a specially designed cryoprobe was 86.4%. These patients were all treated with tetracycline for 2 weeks prophylactically or had negative direct immunofluorescence testing to rule out chlamydial urethritis before admission to the study. Although their preliminary data showed some promise for this technique, long-term follow-up has been disappointing (PK Sand, personal communication, 1996).

Parkes and Boreham (36) retrospectively compared 35 cases treated with cryosurgery to 35 treated with dilatation. They showed cryosurgery to be effective in totally relieving symptoms in 18 of 35 patients compared with only 10 of 35 treated with dilatation. In a subsequent study, Boreham (37) reported his results on 111 patients followed for 3 months. Fifty-four percent of those patients were cured of their symptoms, 28% were improved, and none were made worse. Boreham also suggested that cryosurgery remissions were longer lasting than those achieved with urethral dilatation.

In recent years, cryosurgery has been all but abandoned as a method for treating chronic urethral syndrome because of the lack of long-term success and the cost and inconvenience of special instruments needed for this procedure.

Marsupialization or Unroofing (Reiser Operation). In 1968, Reiser (38) described an operation for destruction of inflamed periurethral glands that consisted of unroofing these glands with needle-point electrocautery. Using this technique, Leiter (39) treated 16 patients "refractory to all modes of therapy." Ten patients were cured, 5 improved significantly, and 1 was unchanged. Using this operation, Lewis and Griffith (40) achieved an 88% cure rate in 70 women with recurrent cystourethritis. Hedlund (41), however, treated 42 women with severe therapy-resistant chronic urethritis and found that 25 (60%) did not benefit from the operation. Currently, this operation is not widely used.

Steroids. Intraurethral steroid suppositories, topical steroid cream, and intraurethral submucosal steroid injections have been used as a treatment for chronic urethritis. In 66 women, Altman (42) injected 1 mL (10 mg) of triamcinolone acetonide along the entire length of the urethra. Eighty-seven percent of the patients who were followed (54 of the original 66) were free of symptoms from 6 months to 5 years posttreatment. Because injection is subject to individual variations in technique, we reserve the use of intraurethral steroid suppositories to patients refractory to dilatation, with variable success. Suppositories must be made by specialty pharmacists. Additionally, various sizes and shapes (FA Giglio, unpublished data and personal communication, 1996) may have to be tested to arrive at optimal urethral retention. In general, suppositories are very safe, of reasonable cost, and certainly merit consideration before attempting more invasive procedures. No well-controlled clinical trials are available for review.

Diathermy. Taylor (43) used diathermy to treat 67 females with urethral syndrome. The entire trigone and the full circumference of the upper third of the urethra were cauterized. Significant postoperative dysuria and frequency were present for several weeks. Three years posttreatment, 45% of the patients had no further attacks and 90% believed the treatment was worthwhile. Because of the severe symptomatology postoperatively, the possibility of damage to deeper structures with use of cautery, and our lack of experience with this method, we cannot recommend it presently.

Bladder Pillar Block. Ostergard (44) described the usage of local anesthesia to block the bladder pillars to carry out urethral dila-

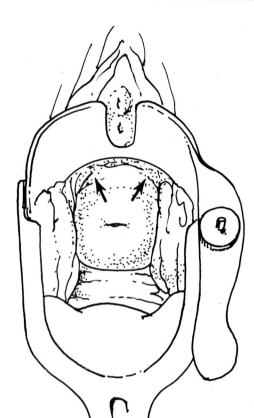

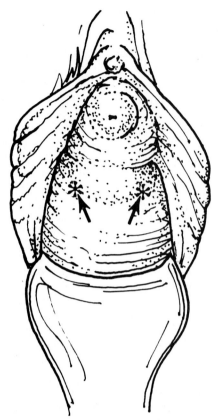

Figure 24.2. With the speculum in place, the bladder pillars are located at 10 and 2 o'clock at their attachments to the cervix (*arrows*). (From Ostergard DR. Bladder pillar block anesthesia for urethral dilatation in women. Am J Obstet Gynecol 1980;136: 187–188.)

Figure 24.3. When the uterus is absent, the urethrovesical junction is visualized and the injections are placed at 5 and 7 o'clock (*arrows*). (From Ostergard DR. Bladder pillar block anesthesia for urethral dilatation in women. Am J Obstet Gynecol 1980;136: 187–188.)

tation in women with extreme urethral pain during this procedure (Figs. 24.2 and 24.3). He has also used this technique with a long-acting anesthetic to provide relief of longer duration. There are no objective long-term outcome data for this treatment. However, it is relatively safe and carries no known risk of adverse sequelae.

Other Modalities. Other treatment modalities suggested and used for chronic urethritis are topical silver nitrate, topical phenol, and topical antibiotics. None of these are commonly used at present.

HYPOESTROGENIC (SENILE OR ATROPHIC) URETHRITIS

Background

The first report of a "vaginal-type epithelium" came from Cifuentes (45) in 1947, who saw small white patches in the distal parts of the trigone that on biopsy were found to be identical to squamous vaginal epithelium. He found these patches in many patients and ascribed no pathological significance to them. He specifically distinguished these from the exudative pseudomembranous cystitis that he and others (46, 47) had previously described.

Ney and Erlich (48) found similar slight patches and postulated estrogenic sensitivity based on the previously published work of Papanicolaou (49), who discovered squamous epithelium in the urine of pregnant women. Later, Youngblood et al. (50) took Pap smears from the urethra of postmenopausal women, both before and after estrogen administration. They found conversion of urethral epithelium from a hypoestrogenic state to a mature well-estrogenized state.

Since then, many investigators have duplicated these studies. Ingelman-Sundberg et al. (51) and Iosif et al. (52) found significant quantities of estrogen receptors in the urethra, further documenting the urethra as an estrogen-sensitive organ.

In a clinical study, Youngblood et al. (53) demonstrated marked improvement in postmenopausal urethral syndrome in women treated with nitrofurazone and diethylstilbestrol vaginal suppositories, compared with a group treated with placebo and nitrofurazone alone. Many other authors have found beneficial effects of estrogen on the urethra, including the reduction of urgency and frequency in postmenopausal women (54) and an overall improvement of atrophic changes in the urethra (55–58).

Diagnosis

Atrophic urethritis caused by relative hypoestrogenism is characterized endoscopically by a pale, somewhat stenotic, friable urethra, which may be sensitive to the touch. Hypoestrogenism is characterized histologically by atrophic epithelial lining with or without inflammation. Blood vessels are close to the surface. Vaginal and urethral cytology parallel each other in respect to estrogen effect (59). The cytological and histological effects of aging differ from person to person and may be quite variable. Estrogen, however, will reverse these changes of urogenital atrophy (59).

Treatment

The treatment for urethral syndrome secondary to hypoestrogenism is topical vaginal estrogen. If other conditions, such as obstructive flow or inflammation, are present, these should be specifically treated concurrently (e.g., dilatation). We have found that intravaginal insertion of estrogen cream is the most convenient way of administering estrogen. This may be given in the dosage of 1.25 mg of conjugated equine estrogens (one-half applicator) nightly or every other night for the first 2 weeks of treatment, followed by the same dosage twice a week for an indefinite period of time.

In a double-blind study, Youngblood et al. (53) obtained good results in 91% of postmenopausal women with urethral syndrome who used urethral suppositories containing 0.01 mg of diethylstilbestrol and nitrofurazone compared with other groups of women who used furazone suppositories and blank control suppositories. Unfortunately, these suppositories are no longer commercially available but can be prepared to order at a modest cost by a few specialty pharmacies. Vaginal cream, however, is well absorbed by the urethral tissue and is the current method of choice for treatment of urethral syndrome caused by hypoestrogenism.

Vaginal estrogens are helpful even in patients who are on oral or patch therapy. Local effects as measured by cytology are more prominent with local therapy than oral therapy (59–61). This is most likely related to the local effects of estrogen on the estrogen-sensitive urethra. Therefore, this treatment should be continued indefinitely in patients with estrogen deficiencies. Estrogen has been shown to increase blood flow to the urethra and to increase urethral tone. It acts on both smooth muscle and mucosa. Should the patient develop symptoms such as breast tenderness, alterations in dosage and timing may have to be made in either or both systemic and topical therapy.

The clinical effects of locally applied estrogen are not observable for 1–3 months (62). Conversely, when patients discontinue local estrogen therapy, they may not sense the effects of withdrawal for 1–3 months. This causes some confusion in their ability to clinically relate withdrawal of estrogen to the onset of symptoms because there is a temporal delay of several months. One must be aware of this in treating patients with topical estrogen therapy (62).

Some authors recommend urethral dilatation for hypoestrogenism on the basis that dilatation improves the integrity of the urethral mucosa. No controlled outcome data are available to substantiate the efficacy of dilatation for the hypoestrogenic urethra.

URETHRAL STENOSIS (OBSTRUCTION)

Urethral stenosis has been advanced as a cause of urethral syndrome in women. Stenosis has been described proximally and distally. Functional urethral spasm has also been reported as a cause of urethral syndrome.

Meatal Stenosis

Many articles have appeared in the literature describing meatal stenosis, both in young girls and adult women. Many of these articles have been anecdotal and without controls. In 1963, Lyon and Smith (21) described a constrictive ring of fibrous tissue situated in the distal urethra of young girls. This ring, which is usually called Lyon's ring, was identified with a *bougie à boule* and was dilated to the point of rupture, with marked improvement in urinary flow and diminution in the frequency of urinary tract infections. Later, Lyon and Tanagho (63) demonstrated radiographical evidence of this ring and also found that it consisted histologically of a collection of collagenous tissue. More recent investigators have had initial success with dilatation alone (64).

Richardson (11) and Richardson and Stonington (65) described an abundance of fibroelastic tissue in the distal urethra from biopsy specimens of young girls and women with urethral syndrome. They popularized the "Richardson technique" (11) for removing this tissue. They demonstrated marked improvement in urinary flow rates after this operation with remission of the annoying symptoms accompanying urethral syndrome in 80% of their patients.

The role of stenosis and obstruction as a cause of recurrent cystourethritis and urethral syndrome has often been questioned in the literature. Hinman (66) suggested that interruption of laminar flow of urine through the urethra causes cystourethritis. Corrière et al. (67), using technetium-labeled colloidal sulfur, showed that turbulent flow caused by urethral stenosis created backflow of urethral bacteria into the proximal urethra and bladder.

With the bougie à boule, Uehling (68) measured the mean urethral caliber of 250 women undergoing cystoscopy and found it to be 22F. He established that the mean (± SD) placed 95% of normal values between 18 and 28 F.

Hole (14) also measured the urethral caliber of two groups of women aged 17–45. One group consisted of patients without symptoms who were about to undergo minor gynecological surgery and the second group consisted of patients with symptoms of dysuria and frequency. Patients with active urinary tract infections were excluded from this study. He found that urethral caliber was similar in both groups and concluded that meatal or distal urethral caliber is highly unlikely to be a factor in producing the symptoms of dysuria and frequency. Gleason et al. (20) questioned the usefulness of bougie calibration alone as an indicator of urethral stenosis because of its lack of correlation with symptoms, trabeculation, reflux, residual urine, and urinary flow rates.

Richardson and Stonington (65) emphasized that the determination of flow rate is essential to accurately assess urethral stenosis. Farrar et al. (69), in their urodynamic evaluation of 298 females with lower urinary tract symptoms, showed that it is clearly impossible to differentiate between those females who have outlet obstructions and those who do not on the basis of symptoms alone. They concluded that "the clinical assessment of urinary stream in the female is, on the whole, unreliable, and outlet obstruction in the female can only be diagnosed by measuring urinary flow rates." We are in agreement that the flow rate is most likely a better indicator of obstruction than is calibration and should be abnormal if obstruction is postulated as a cause of urethral syndrome.

Bladder Neck Obstruction

Winsbury-White (70) was the first to describe vesical neck obstruction and surgical treatment by resection. Young (71) subsequently described hypertrophied urethral glands, urethral polyps, and a "rounded bar" of heaped-up tissue at the bladder neck, which was thought to cause urinary symptoms of hesitancy, hematuria, dysuria, and retention. He successfully treated these women with electrocautery and/or silver nitrate applications.

Treatment

Dilatation. Dilatation, as described previously, has been the main treatment for urethral syndrome based on obstructive etiology. Internal urethrotomy and urethrolysis have also been used.

Internal Urethrotomy. Internal urethrotomy was first described by Winsbury-White

(70) in 1936. McLean and Emmett (72) popularized the operation and reported an 80% cure rate in more than 700 patients. Keitzer and Allen (73) and Immergut and Gilbert (74) reported similar cure rates. The operation consists of removal of the mucosa and part of the submucosa, avoiding the muscularis at the level of the proximal urethra just distal to the vesical neck. Different operators have used urethrotomes, cautery, and punch biopsy instruments to remove or destroy varying amounts of tissue. McLean and Emmett (72) reported a 2% incidence of temporary incontinence and a 1% incidence of prolonged intermittent incontinence in their series. They ascribed their success to the fact that proximal obstructions were the causative factor of the urethral syndrome. They were unable, however, to find a relationship between preoperative urethral caliber and their results. Flow rates were not performed in their study.

Smith (75) reported "good postoperative results" in 53% of 39 adult female patients who had chronic urethritis treated with internal urethrotomy. We cannot recommend this treatment because of its potential for damage to urethral mucosa and musculature. Moreover, success rates are no better than other modalities.

Urethrolysis. Richardson (11) described a procedure for patients who had a thickened urethrovaginal septum with an obstructive flow pattern. Initially, he removed a small piece of tissue from the urethrovaginal septum. Later, he modified his operation to scoring with a scalpel and sharply teasing this tissue away from the muscularis of the urethra.

In this procedure, care is taken to incise only the fibroelastic tissue. The surgical incision is made through the vaginal mucosa up to but not including the urethral mucosa. The procedure is performed with a dilator in place to promote stabilization of the tissue.

Splatt and Weedon (76) performed this operation with similarly good results. They microscopically examined the tissue taken from this area in 50 patients and compared it with tissue removed from the urethra of 44 cadavers. They found a significant increase in fibrous tissue in the urethrovaginal septum in those patients with urethral syndrome and thus were able to advance a pathological

basis for this syndrome, thereby justifying this treatment modality.

In 105 patients, Darling and McLean (77) compared the three most commonly used surgical methods for treating the urethral syndrome: dilatation, internal urethrotomy, and urethrolysis. They reserved internal urethrotomy for patients with severe symptoms and for patients in whom dilatation had failed. They reserved urethrolysis for patients who had a thickened urethrovaginal septum. Their results were similar in all three groups (a 50% cure rate). In this paper, McLean dampened his previous enthusiasm for internal urethrotomy as a primary treatment for urethral syndrome.

URETHRAL SPASM

Background

In 1976, Raz and Smith (78) demonstrated external sphincter spasticity in females by use of urethral pressure profiles. They were able to reduce this spasticity by pudendal blocks, diazepam, or alpha-adrenergic blocking agents. Urethral dilatation had much less therapeutic value in this group of patients. The authors concluded that urethral spasticity was responsible for the urethral syndrome in this select group of patients.

Khalaf et al. (79) showed similar results in a group of female dogs to which they gave phentolamine (an alpha blocker) and d-tubocurarine (a skeletal muscle nerve-blocking agent). Urethral pressures were taken separately at the levels of both the proximal and the distal urethra of these animals and each drug was found to have selective activity on smooth muscle and skeletal muscle, respectively.

Lipsky (80) evaluated 43 women with urethral syndrome urodynamically. He found two types of obstruction. The first was seen in postmenopausal women who had a narrowed distal segment of the urethra. These women responded well to dilatation and external urethroplasty. The second type of obstruction was mainly seen in younger women. The cause was an incomplete relaxation or spasm of the external striated sphincter. Dilatation and urethroplasty did not cure all patients in this group. This study may partially explain why dilatation has variable cure rates.

Barbalias and Meares (81) described 18 women with the urethral syndrome who were studied urodynamically with synchronous video-pressure flow studies and electromyography of the external urethral sphincter. The most striking finding in this group of patients was a significantly higher than normal maximum urethral closure pressure. Some also had abnormally low urinary flow rates, instability of the intraurethral pressure at rest, incomplete funneling of the bladder neck, and distal urethral narrowing during voiding. The authors did not observe detrusor-sphincter dyssynergia or primary striated sphincter spasm. They concluded that an anatomically mediated spasm of the smooth muscle sphincter was a plausible explanation for both the urodynamic findings and for a favorable response in four patients treated with alpha blocking agents. The question remains, however, as to what caused the spasm in this group of patients: was it a primary pathology or was it a result of either acute or chronic urethritis?

Drutz et al. (82) found that a combination of Stelabid (an anticholinergic and alpha-adrenergic antagonist containing trifluoperazine hydrochloride and isopropamide iodine), antibiotics, and bladder drill markedly improved symptoms in 96% of women with the urethral syndrome. They assessed their patients urodynamically and found that 84% had detrusor sphincter dyssynergia, 8% had bladder instability, 8% had external urethral sphincter spasticity, and 1% had sensory urgency. They excluded all patients with positive urine cultures. Cystourethroscopically, urethrotrigonitis was visualized in all patients. Most had previous antibiotic therapy for lower urinary tract symptoms. After 1 month of treatment, 44 (45%) patients were cured of all symptoms, 49 (51%) were improved, 3 (3%) were unchanged, and 1 (1%) was worse. They suggest that the spasm caused by urethral syndrome is most likely due to irritation or chronic urethral inflammation rather than actual infection.

Treatment

When spasm is the cause of urethral syndrome, both smooth and skeletal muscle relaxants have been effective in relieving symptoms. Kaplan et al. (83) treated six women with urodynamic and electromyographic evidence of detrusor and/or sphincter dyssynergia caused by external sphincter spasm. All women had prolonged and intermittent urinary flow. They were given diazepam (Valium®) for 2–6 months, with slow tapering of the medication. All six women had a complete remission of symptoms.

Raz and Smith (78) report similar success with diazepam combined with phenoxybenzamine hydrochloride in progressive doses from 10–40 mg/d until an adrenolytic effect occurs. Patients treated with phenoxybenzamine must be carefully monitored for postural hypotension, tachycardia, and possible shock. Because the voluntary muscle spasm is thought to be a more prominent cause of detrusor sphincter dyssynergia, most clinicians will use diazepam alone for urethral spasm.

We recommend diazepam, 5 mg three to four times daily for 2–4 weeks. Once the cycle of urethral spasm is broken, the patient usually voids without difficulty. No long-term follow-up has been reported.

INFECTION (ACUTE URETHRITIS)

Background

Infection is thought to be the most important cause of the urethral syndrome by many investigators. Bacteria are often not retrieved from patients with urethral syndrome. This inconsistency probably relates to either the fastidiousness of the organism or the difficulty in culturing the urethra.

Cox (5) devised an instrument to selectively culture the urethra in centimeter increments. In 38 normal females, he found a 27% incidence of pathogenic bacteria (*Escherichia coli*, *Aerobacter*, *Pseudomonas*), a 15% incidence of nonpathogenic bacteria (nonhemolytic *Staphylococcus albus* and diphtheroids), and a 58% incidence of questionable pathogens (hemolytic *S. albus* and enterococcus). Only one patient had a concurrent positive urine culture (*E. coli*) in whom the same organism was isolated from the urethra. Therefore, he postulated that the noninfected state of the normal bladder was maintained by its natural resistance rather than by the lack of available pathogens.

Brooks and Maudar (84) in their series of 138 patients with urethral syndrome found that 67 (49%) patients with symptoms had significant bacteriuria and that 66% of the remaining 71 patients had insignificant bacteriuria, compared with only 9% with bacteriuria in a control group. They contended that organisms in insignificant colony counts ($\leq 10^5$ colonies/mL) probably relate to the patient's symptoms, should not be considered as contaminants, and, in fact, may be the etiological agents for their urethral symptomatology.

Findings of small numbers of bacteria in symptomatic patients may cast doubt on the original hypothesis by Kass (85) that a patient must have a colony count of 10^5 organisms/mL to have a significant infection.

O'Grady et al. (86) found a high correlation between the finding of enterobacteria in the urethra and the presence of urethral symptomatology. These investigators also found that 58% of women with urethral enterobacteria developed urinary tract infections within the ensuing 9 months. In these subjects with enterobacteria in the urine, they also found similar bacteria in the introitus. In patients without introital colonization, they found no pathogens in the urethra. They concluded that the urethral syndrome in these patients was likely due to an ascending infection.

Bruce et al. (87) recovered pathogenic bacteria from the vestibule, urethra, and vagina with significantly greater frequency in patients with urethral syndrome than in a group of controls. The bacterial flora were similar in all three areas. They suggested that the specimen taken from one region only (vestibule) would give adequate bacteriologic information.

Since 1975, many authors (88–93) have cultured *Chlamydia trachomatis* from the urethra of women with urethral symptoms. Stamm et al. (91) found chlamydial infection in 11 of 42 women with the urethral syndrome and in 1 of 35 patients with cystitis. All 42 patients with the urethral syndrome had pyuria, and 37 had coliform organisms, *S. saprophyticus* or *C. trachomatis*, in insignificant ($\leq 10^5$/mL) amounts. These cultures were obtained by suprapubic aspiration. They also found pyuria in 3 of 66 women without symptoms. The authors suggested

that the usual colony counts of $\geq 10^5$/mL may be an insensitive diagnostic indicator when applied to symptomatic lower urinary tract infection. The authors found that antibiotic therapy was effective in all patients who were culture positive and pyuria positive. Antibiotic therapy had no effect on patients without pyuria.

Paavonen and Vesterinen (90) found chlamydia to be the most common causative agent in so-called "abacterial urethritis" in Scandinavia. They concluded, as did Stamm et al. (91), that in the culture-negative specimen with pyuria, infection with chlamydia is likely to be present. They recommended antimicrobial therapy (tetracycline, doxycycline, or erythromycin).

Other authors have not found positive chlamydial cultures in patients complaining of urethral symptoms. Bump and Copeland (94), in their prospective review of 86 patients complaining of urethral syndrome, were unable to grow chlamydia in any of their subjects. Sand et al. (33) were likewise unable to culture chlamydia in their prospective study of 24 patients with urethral syndrome. More recent studies using polymerase chain reaction (PCR) techniques, enzyme immunoasssay, and direct fluorescent antibody tests found a close correlation between cervical and urethral colonization with chlamydia (95–97). These methods may increase the yield of chlamydia-positive urethral specimens in the future.

Mycoplasma organisms as a cause of apparent nongonococcal nonbacterial urethritis, particularly *Mycoplasma hominis* and *Ureaplasma urealyticum* (so called T strains), have also received attention in the literature (98–100). It is uncommon for these organisms to invade the urethra only, yet their role as infectious agents is not easily discovered because they, like chlamydia, do not grow in the usual culture medium. PCR techniques may aid in their detection in the future (101). Their role as pathogens is not well established. They respond to the tetracyclines.

Maskell et al. (102) found 82 strains of CO_2 dependent, slow growing, gram-positive organisms in the urine of 9 male and 73 female patients. All of the men and 93% of the women had urinary symptoms at the time of isolation, and 66% of the specimens showed pyuria. They suggested that these organisms may account for the urinary symptoms of some patients previously diagnosed as having urethral syndrome. Treatment with antibacterial agents rendered these patients symptom free, and the organism was no longer isolated from the urine.

Papapetropoulou and Pappas (103) also found fastidious organisms similar to those found by Maskell et al. (102). Vitoratos et al. (104) found ureaplasma, mycoplasma, and chlamydia as principal organisms in 38%, 28%, and 11%, respectively, of 135 of 237 patients with urethral symptoms.

The role of ureaplasma organisms and the causation of urethral syndrome is open to question. Bump and Copeland (94) report "no significant changes in urologic symptoms or urodynamic diagnosis between patients with a positive ureaplasma urethral culture and patients with a negative culture" in their group of 86 subjects with chronic urological complaints. This evidence may suggest that ureaplasma, although present in the urethra, may not be a significant pathogen in urethral syndrome.

Intercourse has been implicated in the transference of vestibular and vaginal bacteria into the urethra, causing acute and, later, chronic urethritis. Kent (105) postulated that the bacteria is massaged into the periurethral glands during intercourse. The urethral symptoms may be present before an infection occurs or after it has been treated successfully.

Many of the infectious causes of urethral syndrome may represent a type of acute and sometimes chronic urethritis, even though a urine culture may be persistently negative. The finding by Stamm et al. (91) that patients with urethral syndrome with pyuria, with or without bacteriuria, respond to antibiotic therapy may be presumptive evidence that these patients in fact have an ongoing urethral infection in which the usual criteria for infection are not applicable. These "culture-negative patients" probably represent a different population from those who have chronic, granular, or pseudomembranous urethrotrigonitis. Other organisms, such as *Trichomonas*, *Candida*, and human papilloma virus (HPV), have also been known to cause the urethral syndrome. PCR techniques have also been applied to detection of HPV in

the urethra (106–108). In general, good correlation has been found with the presence of HPV in the urethra when it is present in the cervix and lower genital sites. Agliano et al. (109) found a high correlation between HPV in urethral samples from patients with recurrent urethritis and cystitis. Many patients may be asymptomatic in the presence of a positive urethral specimen, so the role of HPV in the causation of symptoms, even if present in urethral specimens, is under question (107). Nonetheless, a thorough search for the typical HPV lesion should be made by urethroscopy, if lesions are present in other sites.

Diagnosis

Infection is best diagnosed by *urethral* culture or newer assays mentioned above, if available. All patients suspect for infection should have gonococcal, chlamydial, and ureaplasma cultures. Herpes cultures should be obtained if suspected. A thorough search for HPV should be carried out, particularly if there is evidence of condyloma in the lower genital tract. Urethroscopic evaluation should be performed on all patients with lower genital condyloma to rule out the presence of urethral condyloma, even if the patient is asymptomatic.

If chlamydial cultures, immune assay, direct fluorescent antibody, or PCR techniques are readily available, they may be performed before instituting therapy. Cost may play a significant role in the performance of these tests, so a therapeutic trial may be undertaken.

Treatment

If an infectious etiology is determined, specific agents should be used. In patients treated with nitrofurazone urethral applications, Youngblood (110) reported a 90% remission of frequency, a 75% decrease in dysuria, a 58% decrease of urgency, and a 55% relief of difficulty initiating or passing urine. Unfortunately, this mode of treatment is no longer available commercially. Should other obvious infectious agents, including *Candida*, *Trichomonas*, or condyloma, be the cause of urethral symptomatology, they should be specifically treated.

Because chlamydia as a cause of chronic and acute urethritis has received such widespread attention, a 2-week trial of doxycycline, erythromycin, or tetracycline may be attempted in patients not responding to other treatment modalities. The newer macrolide antibiotics (e.g., azithromycin) may also be tried. A therapeutic trial of one of these agents for the patient and her sexual partner(s) is cost effective and may avoid more expensive complicated methods of treatment.

PSYCHOGENIC

Background

Bierhoff (26) was the first to coin the term "bladder neurosis." Many of his patients with urgency and frequency may have had undiagnosed unstable bladder or interstitial cystitis; most of them, however, by his own description, seemed to meet the criteria for urethral syndrome. A number of these patients may have had apparent psychogenic causes for their symptoms.

Zufall (111), in his series of 190 women with the urethral syndrome, suggested that the condition is mainly psychic in origin, because he failed to document any objective findings on physical examination, urinalysis, studies of residual urine, pyelography, or cystoscopy. Carson et al. (112) studied 160 patients with urethral syndrome by use of urinalysis, urine culture, cystoscopy, excretory urography, and the Minnesota Multiphasic Personality Inventory (MMPI). Only the MMPI revealed any significant positive findings, revealing "evidence for conversion or psychophysiological etiology." More recently, using questionnaires and laboratory analysis, others reported no association of the urethral syndrome with increased psychiatric morbidity (113, 114).

Diagnosis

Various psychological tests may be used, such as an MMPI or a more simple visual analog scale, to ascertain the degree of psychiatric symptoms either causing or attributable to urethral syndrome.

That patients affected with lower urinary tract symptoms have a definite psychological component has been recorded since ancient times. An old Chinese proverb states that "the bladder is the mirror of the soul." There is no doubt that patients suffering with urethral syndrome are very distressed by their recurrent symptoms and are in need of emotional support. In many cases, however, their psychiatric disorder results from situational stress brought on by their distressing urinary symptoms.

Treatment

Supportive therapy is most helpful in all patients with urethral syndrome, regardless of the etiology. Understanding and patience are paramount in managing patients with chronic and recurrent lower urinary tract symptomatology. Many of these patients with urethral syndrome have been treated by several physicians and often are labeled as hypochondriacs. Patients who have no other obvious etiology and who have failed other treatment measures may respond to several psychotherapeutic measures. Hypnosis, desensitization drills, and guided visual imagery may be used for allaying symptoms in this group of patients.

ALLERGY

Background

Kindall and Nickels (115) first suggested allergy as a cause of symptoms in the urinary tract. They described two cases of renal colic with edema and redness in the bladder without pyuria. Both patients responded to epinephrine. Bladder biopsies showed eosinophilia and mononuclear cell infiltration. Other authors (116, 117) described dysuria or frequency in patients with sterile urine and allergic sensitivities. Many of these patients had eosinophilia in their bladder biopsies. The symptoms disappeared with avoidance of the suspected allergens. In our experience, allergy is a rare cause of urethral symptoms.

Treatment

Treatment of the urethral syndrome caused by allergy is based on antihistamine therapy and the avoidance of known allergens.

NEUROLOGICAL DISORDERS

Background

Hoyt (118) reported four cases of urethrotrigonitis caused by reflex pain from spinal injuries or neurological abnormalities. This pain was found along bladder and urethral nerve roots. With local injections of anesthetic in dermatomes supplying these same areas (the so-called trigger zones), he was able temporarily and, in some cases, permanently to reverse the urethral symptoms. Trigger zones were previously reported by Travell and Rinzler (119) in 1946, when they were able to relieve cardiac pain by injecting zones of marked hyperesthesia in the skin and tissue of the chest wall. More recently, Slocumb (120) and Mercer and Slocumb (121) reported a 91% improvement rate injecting trigger points in patients with urethral syndrome. They coined the term pelvic hyperpathia syndrome to describe a multiplicity of complaints referred to the urethra and other pelvic areas in their group of patients. Petersén and Franksson (122) reported 23 patients with urethrotrigonitis. Nerve lesions were found from S1 and S5 in 20 of these patients. The authors experimentally injected local anesthetics into intradural spinal nerve roots in these patients, with resultant relief of symptoms.

Nerve root damage is a frequent cause of bladder symptoms, both hypertonic and hypotonic. How frequently nerve root irritation causes urethrotrigonitis and urethral syndrome is unknown, but neurological disease must be considered in the differential diagnosis of urethral syndrome. Conditions such as spinal stenosis and back injury are known causes of both bladder and urethral symptoms.

Schmidt (123) reported urodynamic evidence for external sphincter spasm in most patients with urethral syndrome. He postulated spastic behavior in the external sphincter as a cause for urethral syndrome and gave urodynamic evidence for his postulation. He demonstrated that these patients respond to neurostimulation of S3 or S4, further corroborating his theory that urethral spasm, transmitted through these nerve roots, is responsible for the condition. He reported excellent response to needle electric stimulation of the S3 and S4 foramina. This study may lend some credence to Drutz's theory (82) that urethral spasm, mediated perhaps through motor nerves, may be the common final expression of all urethral irritants, including infection, and that spasm may be the principal cause of symptoms in the urethra.

Treatment

Treatment is aimed at treating the specific neurological disorder. Injection of trigger points, as suggested by Mercer and Slocumb (121) and Petersén and Franksson (122) may be attempted.

TRAUMA AND NOXIOUS AGENTS

Background

Trauma has often been cited as a cause of acute and chronic urethritis. "Honeymoon cystitis" is a well-known clinical entity. There is often a very clearcut association between the onset of urethritis and the time of first intercourse or the time of increased frequency or intensity of intercourse. Bran et al. (124) found a higher percentage of organisms in the urine after gentle massage of the urethra. These organisms were in most cases identical to those at the external meatus. Most of these organisms, however, disappeared in 48 hours.

Instrumentation, bubble baths, excessive vaginal douches, perineal sprays, and tampon insertion (125–129) have been shown to be associated with urethritis.

Treatment

Noxious agents, bubble baths, irritating tampons, and offending chemical substances, including deodorant soap, should be avoided if they are suspect as the cause of urethral syndrome.

ANATOMIC VARIATIONS

Background

Anatomic variations such as urethrohymenal fusion, hypospadias, urethral caruncle, or urethral prolapse may predispose patients to acute urethritis (62) with later development of chronic urethritis. In these conditions, the urothelium may become inflamed or infected because of its close proximity to the vaginal microflora or as a result of sexual activity.

Treatment

If urethrohymenal fusion or hypospadias is present and causing urethral syndrome or recurrent urinary tract infections, a hymenoplasty or definitive surgical treatments of hypospadias, urethral prolapse, or caruncle should be undertaken (130).

Hymenoplasty for urethrohymenal fusion consists of incising transversely across the hymen about 1 cm lateral to the urethral meatus bilaterally and then reapproximating the tissue in a longitudinal plane, thereby separating the hymen (and vestibule) from the urethra. The exact cure rate with use of this procedure is unknown. Hypospadias can be treated by urethral meatus transposition (130) or, in severe cases, by the creation of a neourethra using vaginal tissue or pedicle flaps (131–133).

The treatment for urethral caruncle is cautery, although most caruncles are asymptomatic and need no treatment. Surgical excision is the treatment for urethral prolapse.

OTHERS

Deficiencies in vitamins A, C, and D have also been implicated in urethral syndrome, but no substantial documentation is available. Treatment is vitamin supplementation.

What's Ahead— Solving the Riddle

In an attempt to piece together the puzzle of the urethral syndrome, several questions still remain unanswered. How does one scientifically measure the endpoint of cure or improvement of urethral syndrome since the only measure of cure is the patient's subjective response? What is the spontaneous remission rate of the urethral syndrome? What effect would massage alone without dilatation have on chronic urethritis? What effect would the use of urethral suppositories with massage have on the cure of urethral syndrome? These questions and many others still must be answered before we solve the riddle of the urethral syndrome.

Summary

The urethral syndrome is an elusive disease that defies easy categorization and is therefore difficult to treat. It is a confusing disorder with multiple etiologies. Almost any treatment method will help about one half of patients. Cystoscopy alone, for example, has been shown to reduce symptoms in most patients suffering from urethral syndrome.

Dilatation remains the treatment of choice for chronic urethritis by virtue of its widespread usage and long-term record of safety. Estrogen should be used empirically in a patient who is peri- or postmenopausal, whether or not she has convincing evidence of local hypoestrogenism. These patients often respond to estrogen, and it should be used liberally if there are no contraindications to its use. It is also advisable to begin one therapy at a time to scientifically evaluate the response to individual treatment modalities. Antibiotics can be used empirically in patients suspect for infection.

In conclusion, the urethral syndrome is difficult to diagnose and difficult to treat, but if the clinician makes a reasonable search for the etiology and begins to separate out the various possible etiologies by careful diagnostic evaluation and careful observation of the patient's complaints and response (or nonresponse) to therapy, a rational approach to treatment based on probable causation can be successful.

REFERENCES

1. Folsom AI, Alexander JC. Referred pain from the female urethra. J Urol 1934;31:731–739.
2. Gallagher DJ, Montgomerie JZ, North JD. Acute infections of the urinary tract and the urethral syndrome in general practice. Br Med J 1965; 543:622–626.
3. Huffman JW. The detailed anatomy of the paraurethral ducts in the adult human female. Am J Obstet Gynecol 1948;55:86–101.
4. Hutch JA. The role of urethral mucus in the bladder defense mechanism. J Urol 1970;103: 165–167.
5. Cox CE. The urethra and its relationship to urinary tract infection: the flora of the normal female urethra. South Med J 1966;59:621–626.

6. Helmholz HF Sr. Determination of the bacterial content of the urethra: a new method, with results of a study of 82 men. J Urol 1950;64: 158–166.

7. Cox CE, Hinman F Jr. Factors in resistance to infection in the bladder. In: Kass EH, ed. Progress in pyelonephritis. Philadelphia: Davis, 1965:563.

8. Kaye D. Antibacterial activity of human urine. J Clin Invest 1968;47:2374–2390.

9. Seddon JM, Bruce AW. Cystourethritis. Urology 1978;11:1–10.

10. Mayo ME, Hinman F. Role of mid-urethral high pressure zone in spontaneous bacterial ascent. J Urol 1973;109:268–272.

11. Richardson FH. External urethroplasty in women: technique and clinical evaluation. J Urol 1969;101:719–723.

12. Evans AT. Etiology of urethral syndrome: preliminary report. J Urol 1971;105:245–250.

13. Dans PE, Klaus B. Dysuria in women. Johns Hopkins Med J 1976;138:13–18.

14. Hole R. The calibre of the adult female urethra. Br J Urol 1972;44:68–70.

15. Seng M, Cochrane WJ, Mack FG. The vesical neck syndrome in women of middle age. Can Med Assoc J 1949;60:39–44.

16. Scotti RJ, Ostergard DR, Guillaume AA, Kohatsu KE. Predictive value of urethroscopy as compared to urodynamics in the diagnosis of genuine stress incontinence. J Reprod Med 1990;35: 772–776.

17. Smith PJ. The management of the urethral syndrome. Br J Hosp Med 1979;22:578–587.

18. Tait J, Peddie BA, Bailey RR, et al. Urethral syndrome (abacterial cystitis)—search for a pathogen. Br J Urol 1985;57:522–526.

19. Larsen S, Thompson SA, Hald T, et al. Mast cells in interstitial cystitis. Br J Urol 1982;54: 283–286.

20. Gleason DM, Bottaccini MR, Lattimer JK. What does the bougie à boule calibrate? J Urol 1969; 101:114–116.

21. Lyon RP, Smith DR. Distal urethral stenosis. J Urol 1963;89:414–421.

22. Jackson EA. Urethral syndrome in women. Radiology 1976;119:287–291.

23. Shopfner CE. Roentgen evaluation of distal urethral obstruction. Radiology 1967;88:222–231.

24. Sugaya K, Nishizawa O, Noto H, et al. Vesical ultrasonography and internal examination of female patients with urethral syndrome. Jpn J Urol 1992;83:1094–1100.

25. Scotti RJ, Ostergard DR. Predictive value of urethroscopy in genuine stress incontinence and vesical instability. Int Urogynecol J 1993;4: 255–258.

26. Bierhoff F. On the so-called "irritable bladder" in the female. Am J Med Sci 1900;120: 670–695.

27. Folsom AI. The female urethra: a clinical and pathologic study. JAMA 1931;97:1345–1351.

28. Ormond JK. Non-purulent urethritis in women. "Granular urethritis—cystalgia." J Urol 1935; 33:483–497.

29. Powell EM, Wattenberg CA. Treatment of urethritis in the female: with a clinical and pathological study. J Urol 1954;72:392–399.

30. Powell NB, Powell EB. The female urethra: a clinico-pathological study. J Urol 1949;61: 557–570.

31. Tanagho EA, Lyon RP. Urethral dilatation versus internal urethrotomy. J Urol 1971;105:242–244.

32. Fujita K, Matsushima H, Nakano M, Kaneko M, Munakata A. Prophylactic oral antibiotics in urethral instrumentation. Jpn J Urol 1994;85: 802–805.

33. Kapland GW, Sammons TA, King LR. A blind comparison of dilatation, urethrotomy and medication alone in the treatment of urinary tract infection in girls. J Urol 1973;109: 917–919.

34. Bergman A, Karram M, Bhatia NN. Urethral syndrome. A comparison of different treatment modalities. J Reprod Med 1989;34:157–160.

35. Sand PK, Bowen LW, Ostergard DR, Bent A, Panganiban R. Cryosurgery versus dilation and massage for the treatment of recurrent urethral syndrome. J Reprod Med 1989;34:499–504.

36. Parkes AC, Boreham P. Cryosurgery for the urethral syndrome: preliminary communication. J R Soc Med 1980;73:428–430.

37. Boreham P. Cryosurgery for the urethral syndrome. J R Soc Med 1984;77:111–113.

38. Rieser C. A new method of treatment of inflammatory lesions of the female urethra. JAMA 1968;204:378–384.

39. Leiter E. Management of recurrent cystourethritis in women. Urology 1973;1:111–113.

40. Lewis EL, Griffith TH. Recurring cystourethritis in women: is an effective therapy available? J Urol 1973;110:544–545.

41. Hedlund PO. Experience of the Rieser operation for chronic female urethritis. A follow-up study of 42 cases. Scand J Urol Nephrol 1979;13: 217–219.

42. Altman BL. Treatment of urethral syndrome with triamcinolone acetonide. J Urol 1976;116: 583–584.

43. Taylor JS. Diathermy to the trigone and urethra in the management of the female urethral syndrome. Br J Urol 1977;49:407–409.

44. Ostergard DR. Bladder pillar block anesthesia for urethral dilatation in women. Am J Obstet Gynecol 1980;136:187–188.

45. Cifuentes L. Epithelium of vaginal type in the female trigone: The clinical problem of trigonitis. J Urol 1947;57:1028–1037.

46. Orr L. Chronic pseudomembranous trigonitis. South Med J 1933;26:359–361.

47. Ryall EC. Pseudo-membranous trigonitis. Br J Urol 1929;1:254–257.

48. Ney C, Erlich JC. Squamous epithelium in the trigone of the human female urinary bladder. With a note on cystoscopic observations during estrogen therapy. J Urol 1955;73:809–819.

49. Papanicolaou GN. Diagnosis of pregnancy by cytologic criteria in catheterized urine. Proc Soc Exp Biol Med 1948;67:247–249.

50. Youngblood VH, Tomlin EM, Williams JO, Kim-

melstiel P. Exfoliative cytology of the senile female urethra. J Urol 1958;79:110–113.

51. Ingelman-Sundberg A, Rosen J, Gustafsson SA, Carlstrom K. Cystosol estrogen receptors in the urogenital tissues in stress-incontinent women. Acta Obstet Gynaecol Scand 1981;60:585–586.

52. Iosif CS, Batra S, Ek A, Astedt B. Estrogen receptors in the human female lower urinary tract. Am J Obstet Gynecol 1981;141:817–820.

53. Youngblood VH, Tomlin EM, Davis JB. Senile urethritis in women. J Urol 1957;78:150–152.

54. Ishigooka M, Hashimoto T, Tomaru M, Nakada T, Mitobe K. Effect of hormonal replacement therapy in postmenopausal women with chronic irritative voiding symptoms. Int Urogynecol J 1994;5:208–211.

55. Burton G, Cardozo LD, Abdalla H, Kirkland A, Studd JW. The hormonal effects on the lower urinary tract in 282 women with premature ovarian failure. Neurourol Urodyn 1991;10:318–319.

56. Batra S, Bjellin L, Sjögren C, Iosif S, Widmark E. Increases in blood flow of the female rabbit urethra following low dose estrogens. J Urol 1986;136:1360–1362.

57. Batra S, Iosif CS. Female urethra: a target for estrogen action. J Urol 1983;129:418–420.

58. Longhurst PA, Kauer J, Leggett RE, Levin RM. The influence of ovariectomy and estradiol replacement on urinary bladder function in rats. J Urol 1992;148:915–919.

59. Smith P. Age changes in the female urethra. Br J Urol 1972;44:667–676.

60. Mandel FP, Geola FL, Meldrum DR, et al. Biological effects of various doses of vaginally administered conjugated equine estrogens in postmenopausal women. J Clin Endocrinol Metab 1983;57:133–139.

61. Koloszar S, Kovacs L. Treatment of climacteric urogenital disorders with an estriol-containing ointment. Orvosi Hetilap 1995;136:343–345.

62. Scotti RJ. Urethral syndrome: non-infectious etiology. Infect Surg 1989;8:178–181.

63. Lyon RP, Tanagho EA. Distal urethral stenosis in little girls. J Urol 1965;93:379–388.

64. Holubar J, Ungar V, Gal P. Urethral dilation in the treatment of urinary tract infections in girls. Ceskoslovenska Pediatrie 1991;46:408–400.

65. Richardson FH, Stonington OG. Urethrolysis and external urethroplasty in the female. Surg Clin North Am 1969;49:1201–1208.

66. Hinman F Jr. Mechanisms for the entry of bacteria and the establishment of urinary infection in female children. J Urol 1966;96:546–550.

67. Corrière JN Jr, McClure JM III, Lipschultz LI. Contamination of bladder urine by urethral particles during voiding: urethrovesical reflux. J Urol 1972;107:399–401.

68. Uehling DT. The normal caliber of the adult female urethra. J Urol 1978;120:176–177.

69. Farrar DJ, Whiteside CG, Osborne JL, Turner-Warwick RT. A urodynamic analysis of micturition symptoms in the female. Surg Gynecol Obstet 1975;141:875–881.

70. Winsbury-White HP. Two cases of retention of urine in women. Lancet 1936;1:1008–1009.

71. Young HH. The pathology and treatment of obstructions at the vesical neck in women. JAMA 1940;115:2133–2136.

72. McLean P, Emmett JL. Internal urethrotomy in women for recurrent infection and chronic urethritis. J Urol 1969;101:724–728.

73. Keitzer WA, Allen JS. Operative treatment of chronic cystitis by urethrotomy: 10 years of experience. J Urol 1970;103:429–431.

74. Immergut MA, Gilbert EC. The clinical response of women to internal urethrotomy. J Urol 1973;109:90–91.

75. Smith GI. Internal urethrotomy for recurrent or chronic urethritis. Clinical experience in 40 women. Urology 1973;2:144–147.

76. Splatt AJ, Weedon D. The urethral syndrome: morphological studies. Br J Urol 1981;53:263–265.

77. Darling MR, McLean PA. The female urethral syndrome: a comparison of three different methods of treatment. Ir Med J 1977;70:338–339.

78. Raz S, Smith RB. External sphincter spasticity syndrome in female patients. J Urol 1976;115:443–446.

79. Khalaf IM, Toppercer A, Elhilali MM. Urethral pressure changes in reflex micturition. Invest Urol 1979;17:141–145.

80. Lipsky H. Urodynamic assessment of women with urethral syndrome. Urologe A 1976;15:207–212.

81. Barbalias GA, Meares EM Jr. Female urethral syndrome: clinical and urodynamic perspectives. Urology 1984;23:208–212.

82. Drutz HP, Mainprize TZ, Tremblay P, Baker KR. Detrusor sphincter dyssynergia, detrusor instability, and urethral syndrome: role of treatment with a combined anticholinergic and alpha blocking agent, bladder drill and antibiotics. Int Urogynecol J 1991;2:10–15.

83. Kaplan WE, Firlit CF, Schoenberg HW. The female urethral syndrome: external sphincter spasm as etiology. J Urol 1980;124:48–49.

84. Brooks D, Maudar A. Pathogenesis of the urethral syndrome in women and its diagnosis in general practice. Lancet 1972;2:893–898.

85. Kass EH. Chemotherapeutic and antibiotic drugs in the management of infections of the urinary tract. Am J Med 1965;18:764.

86. O'Grady FW, Mcherry MA, Richards B, Cattell WR, O'Farrell SM. Introital enterobacteria, urinary infection, and the urethral syndrome. Lancet 1970;2:1208–1210.

87. Bruce AW, Chadwick P, Hassan A, VanCott GF. Recurrent urethritis in women. Can Med Assoc J 1973;108:973–976.

88. Holmes KK, Handsfield HH, Wang SP, et al. Etiology of nongonococcal urethritis. N Engl J Med 1975;292:1199–1205.

89. Johannisson G, Lowhagen GB, Lycke E. Genital *Chlamydia trachomatis* infection in women. Obstet Gynecol 1980;56:671–675.

90. Paavonen J, Vesterinen E. *Chlamydia trachoma-*

tis in cervicitis and urethritis in women. Scand J Infect Dis Suppl 1982;32:45–54.

91. Stamm WE, Wagner KF, Amsel R, et al. Causes of the acute urethral syndrome in women. N Engl J Med 1980;303:409–415.

92. Tait IA, Rees E, Jameson RM. Urethral syndrome associated with chlamydial infection of the urethra and cervix. Br J Urol 1978;50:425.

93. Morris RE, Legault J, Baker C. Prevalence of isolated urethral asymptomatic *Chlamydia trachomatis* infection in the absence of cervical infection on incarcerated adolescent girls. Sex Transm Dis 1993;20:198–200.

94. Bump RC, Copeland WE Jr. Urethral isolation of the genital mycoplasmas and *Chlamydia trachomatis* in women with chronic urologic complaints. Am J Obstet Gynecol 1985;152:38–41.

95. Sellors JW, Mahony JB, Jang D, et al. Comparison of cervical, urethral, and urine specimens for the detection of *Chlamydia trachomatis* in women. J Infect Dis 1991;164:205–208.

96. Naher H, Drzonek H, Wolf J, von Knebel Doeberitz M, Petzoldt D. Detection of *C trachomatis* in urogenital specimens by polymerase chain reaction. Genitourin Med 1991;67:211–214.

97. Hay PE, Thomas BJ, Horner PJ, MacLeod E, Tenton AM, Taylor-Robinson D. *Chlamydia trachomatis* in women: the more you look, the more you find. Genitourin Med 1994;70:97–100.

98. Kaufman RE, Wiesner PJ. Nonspecific urethritis [abstract]. N Engl J Med 1974;291:1175–1177.

99. Taylor-Robinson D, McCormack WM. The genital mycoplasmas (first of two parts) [abstract]. N Engl J Med 1980;302:1003–1010.

100. Taylor-Robinson D, McCormack WM. The genital mycoplasmas (second of two parts). N Engl J Med 1980;302:1063–1067.

101. Blanchard A, Hamrick W, Duffy L, Baldus K, Cassell GH. Use of the polymerase chain reaction for detection of *Mycoplasma fermentans* and *Mycoplasma genitalium* in the urogenital tract and amniotic fluid. Clin Infect Dis 1993; 17(Suppl 1):S272–S279.

102. Maskell R, Pead L, Allen J. The puzzle of "urethral syndrome": a possible answer? Lancet 1979;1:1058–1059.

103. Papapetropoulou M, Pappas A. The acute urethral syndrome in routine practice. J Infect 1987;14:113–118.

104. Vitoratos N, Gregoriou O, Papadias C, Liapis A, Zourlas PA. Sexually transmitted diseases in women with urethral syndrome. Int J Gynaecol Obstet 1988;27:177–180.

105. Kent S. Urinary tract problems in women are linked to sexual activity. Geriatrics 1975;30: 145–146.

106. Rymark P, Forslund O, Hansson BG, Lindholm K. Genital HPV infection not a local but a regional infection: experience from a female teenage group. Genitourin Med 1993;69:18–22.

107. van Doornum GJ, Hooykaas C, Juffermans LH, et al. Prevalence of human papillomavirus infections among heterosexual men and women with multiple sexual partners. J Med Virol 1992;37: 13–21.

108. Allen PM, Davis GD, Bowen LW, et al. The female urethral syndrome is rarely associated with human papillomavirus infection types 6/11, 16, 18, 31, 33. Int Urogynecol J 1995;6: 195–197.

109. Agliano AM, Gazzaniga P, Cervigni M, et al. Detection of human papillomavirus type 16 DNA sequences in paraffin-embedded tissues from the female urinary tract. Urol Int 1994;52: 208–212.

110. Youngblood VH. Nitrofurazone in the treatment of nonspecific urethritis in females. J Urol 1953; 70:926–929.

111. Zufall R. Treatment of the urethral syndrome in women. JAMA 1963;184:894–895.

112. Carson CC, Segura JW, Osborne DM. Evaluation and treatment of the female urethral syndrome. J Urol 1980;124:609–610.

113. Sumners D, Kelsey M, Chait I. Psychological aspects of lower urinary tract infections in women. BMJ 1992;304:17–19.

114. Nazareth I, King MB. The urethral syndrome: a controlled evaluation. J Psychosom Res 1993; 37:737–743.

115. Kindall L, Nickels TT. Allergy of the pelvic urinary tract in the female: A preliminary report. J Urol 1949;61:222–232.

116. Frensilli FJ, Sacher EC, Keegan CT. Eosinophilic cystitis: observations on etiology. J Urol 1972; 107:595–596.

117. Powell NB, Powell EB, Thomas OC, Queng JT, McGovern JP. Allergy of the lower urinary tract. J Urol 1972;107:631–634.

118. Hoyt HS. Segmental nerve lesions as a cause of the trigonitis syndrome. Stanford Med Bull 1953;2:61.

119. Travell J, Rinzler SH. Relief of cardiac pain by local block of somatic trigger areas. Proc Soc Exp Biol Med 1946;63:480.

120. Slocumb JC. Neurological factors in chronic pelvic pain: trigger points and the abdominal pelvic pain syndrome. Am J Obstet Gynecol 1984;149:536–543.

121. Mercer LJ, Slocumb JC. The pelvic hyperpathia syndrome: a urethral syndrome variant. Presented at the Gynecologic Urology Society Annual Scientific Meeting, Florida, October 1–3, 1984.

122. Petersén I, Franksson C. Urethro-trigonitis and spinal nerve root lesions. Acta Obstet Gynaecol Scand 1955;34:399–411.

123. Schmidt RA. The urethral syndrome. Urol Clin North Am 1985;12:349–354.

124. Bran JL, Levison ME, Kaye D. Entrance of bacteria into the female urinary bladder. N Engl J Med 1972;286:626–629.

125. Marshall S. The effect of bubble bath on the urinary tract. J Urol 1965;93:112.

126. Pieterse HF. Various concepts in the aetiology of recurrent urinary tract infections in girls. 3. S Afr Med J 1974;48:123–127.

127. Pieterse HF. Various concepts in the aetiology of recurrent urinary tract infections in girls. II. S Afr Med J 1974;48:82–86.

128. Pieterse HF. Various concepts in the aetiology of

recurrent urinary tract infections in girls. S Afr Med J 1974;48:41–42.

129. Simmons RJ. Acute vulvovaginitis caused by soap products. Obstet Gynecol 1955;6:447–448.

130. Van Bogaert LJ. Surgical repair of hypospadias in women with symptoms of urethral syndrome. J Urol 1992;147:1263–1264.

131. Mitchell ME, Hensle TW, Crooks KK. Urethral reconstruction in the young female using a perineal pedicle flap. J Pediatr Surg 1982;17:687–694.

132. Hendren WH. Construction of female urethra from vaginal wall and a perineal flap. J Urol 1980;123:657–664.

133. King LR, Wendel RM. A new application for transvaginal plication in the treatment of girls with total urinary incontinence due to epispadias or hypospadias. J Urol 1969;102:278–282.

CHAPTER 25

Urethral Diverticula

Jack R. Robertson

The first successful repair of a urethral diverticulum was described by Hey in 1805 (1). Hunner (2) reported three urethral diverticula in female patients and commented on the apparent rareness of the condition. In 1953, Novak (3) stated, "This is a relatively rare condition and no gynecologist will see more than a few in a lifetime." A few years later, Davis and Cain (4) and then Tratner developed catheters with double balloons (C.R. Bard, Covington, GA) (Fig. 25.1). The two balloons effectively isolate the urethra between an intravesical balloon and a sliding or wedge-shaped balloon that tamponades the external meatus. This allows the introduction of radiopaque dye into the urethra to outline urethral diverticula (Figs. 25.2 and 25.3). This new diagnostic technique revealed 50 diverticula in 1 year, more than in the entire previous history of Johns Hopkins Hospital. Before 1950, only a little over 100 cases were found in the medical records of Johns Hopkins, the Mayo Clinic, and the Cleveland Clinic combined.

Incidence

Incidence figures are infrequently reported. A recent study showed that 5% of patients in a urogynecology clinic had diverticula, and a second study of patients before radiation for carcinoma of the cervix revealed a frequency of 4.7%.

Etiology

A classic study by Huffman in 1984 (5) gave a detailed description of paraurethral ducts and periurethral glands. It is postulated that diverticula develop secondary to obstruction of the duct between the urethra and the paraurethral gland. This may lead to abscess formation and rupture back into the urethra. Stones may develop, but carcinoma is infrequent.

Clinical Symptoms

The clinical symptoms of urethral diverticula are common to other maladies of the lower urinary tract (Table 25.1). None are diagnostic, and the classic symptoms of post-micturition dribbling and expression of pus are frequently absent. Any patient with chronic lower urinary tract symptoms unresponsive to conventional therapy should be suspected of having a urethral diverticulum. Dysuria and difficulty in voiding after intercourse are common complaints. Some patients have symptoms.

Symptoms of urethral diverticula are produced on a mechanical basis and are of great variety. Symptoms may be present for many years because diagnosis is usually delayed. Wide-mouthed diverticula with good drainage are asymptomatic unless they become infected. A small closed-off diverticulum may produce severe pain and yet be difficult to diagnose.

Classic Physical Findings

The classic physical findings are a palpable suburethral mass and expression of pus from a tender urethra. However, urethral palpation is neglected. Fantl (personal communica-

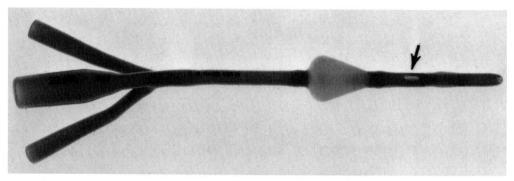

Figure 25.1. The Tratner catheter. This three-lumen catheter has two balloons that isolate the urethra. Radiopaque dye then enters the urethra through the port indicated by the arrow.

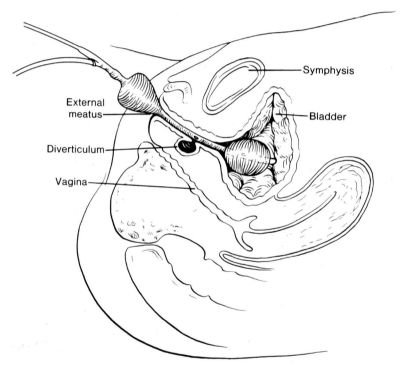

Figure 25.2. The placement of the Tratner catheter. Isolation of the urethra between the balloons allows positive pressure urethrography.

tion) reported 100 urological charts and found that the male urethra was palpated in 75% of cases. He reviewed 100 gynecological charts and found a 20% incidence of urethral palpation.

Diverticula are easier to palpate with a sound in the urethra. A soft cushion may be palpated in 50% of patients. However, in the author's experience, 50% of known diverticula cannot be outlined while palpating the urethra with the examining finger. If pus is expressed, a diverticulum must be ruled out.

However, pus may be expressed from an infected Skene's gland. Unfortunately, the patient may have no physical findings.

Location of Diverticular Orifices

The anatomy of the urethra reveals the presence of a large number of periurethral glands entering the posterior urethra, with the largest of these glands emptying into the distal urethra (see Chapter 1). The location of urethral diverticular orifices parallels the site of entry of these glands into the urethra, with more than half opening into the middle third of the urethra.

Diagnosis

In the author's experience, 50% of patients with urethral diverticula have more than one. It is not uncommon to see as many as three. Urethral diverticula may be diagnosed with a voiding cystogram. If the diagnosis of a urethral diverticulum is made with a voiding cystogram, urethroscopy may reveal two or

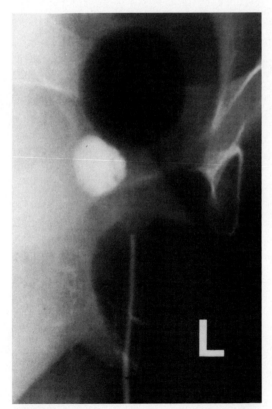

Figure 25.3. Radiographic view of urethral diverticulum utilizing a Tratner catheter. Note the air-filled balloons, which are part of the triple-lumen system of the Tratner catheter. The contrast material is injected into the third lumen and exits into the urethra. The diverticulum is seen filled with contrast material after completion of the procedure (courtesy of A.E. Bent, M.D.).

more diverticula hidden behind the larger diverticulum filled with dye.

Radiographic Diagnostic Procedures

Two radiographic diagnostic procedures in common use are voiding cystourethrography and positive pressure urethrography. The voiding radiograph depends on the chance filling of the diverticulum during the study. Its accuracy is about 65%. Positive pressure urethrography with use of either the Tratner or the Davis catheter is comparable with urethroscopy for accuracy (Fig. 25.3). The accuracy with either method is 90%.

Kohorn and Glickman (6) recently described three aids for the diagnosis and management of urethral diverticula. In the first, double-balloon urethrography technique is modified. Diluted contrast medium is used to inflate the intravesical and external balloons, so that improved delineation of the anatomy of the diverticular pockets is obtained with undiluted contrast medium. Second, an angiographic catheter is placed in the most distal pouch, using a fluoroscope for a guide. The purpose is to identify and irrigate with antibiotic solution the nondraining pouches of the compound diverticula. Third, a 7F Foley catheter balloon is then placed in the thin-walled and friable diverticular pouches to facilitate dissection.

Table 25.1.   Clinical Symptoms of Urethral Diverticula

Asymptomatic
Dysuria
Frequency
Urgency
Hematuria
Dyspareunia
Vaginal mass
Postmicturition dribbling
Recurrent cystitis
Pain
Incontinence
Urinary retention
Nocturia

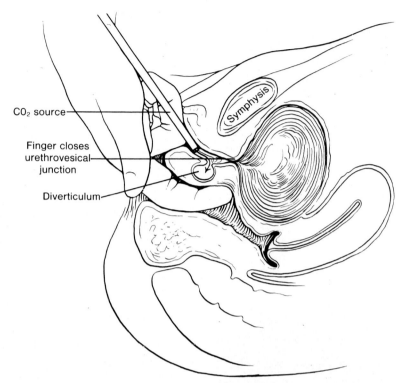

CO₂ source

Finger closes
urethrovesical
junction

Diverticulum

Symphysis

Figure 25.4. The technique of urethra distention with CO_2. Occlusion of the urethrovesical junction with the finger allows distention of the urethra and visualization of diverticular orifices.

Urethroscopic Diagnostic Procedures

Urethroscopy is essential to diagnose urethral diverticula. The technique of urethroscopy for diverticula begins with the placement of 200 mL of carbon dioxide into the bladder. Two fingers in the vagina push the vesical neck up against the symphysis to trap the gas in the urethra (Fig. 25.4). Under direct vision, urethral massage reveals the presence of pus or urine exuding from the diverticular orifice.

Urodynamic Evaluation

Urodynamic assessment of the urethra aids in the selection of the proper operative procedure for treatment of the diverticulum. The most important urodynamic technique is the urethral closure pressure profile and its relationship to the diverticular orifice

(Fig. 25.5). If the opening of the diverticulum into the urethra is distal to the peak urethral closure pressure, the Spence procedure (7) is the operation of choice. If the diverticular orifice is proximal to the area of peak closure pressure, direct dissection of the diverticulum with closure of the urethra in layers is required.

If a Spence procedure is done and the diverticular orifice is not distal to peak closure pressure, genuine stress incontinence will result because of disruption of the muscular sphincteric mechanism of the urethra.

Reid et al. (8) and Bhatia et al. (9) reported the role of urodynamics in detecting the association of urethral diverticula and incontinence. A postoperative complication of incontinence may be more distressing to the patient than the symptoms from her diverticulum.

A prophylactic urethropexy is accomplished when preoperative genuine stress incontinence is documented and/or if intraoperative profilometry shows a significant reduction in urethral closure pressure post-urethral diverticulectomy. Intraoperative profilometry is accomplished after induction of anesthesia and repeated after diverticulectomy.

Leach and Bavendam (10) reported that none of eight women who had only a urethral diverticulectomy (because their preoperative urethroscopic evaluation showed no genuine stress incontinence or urethral hypermobility) had postoperative urinary incontinence. However, when the preoperative endoscopic evaluation demonstrated genuine stress incontinence, poor urethral support, or a large proximal diverticulum, a simultaneous transvaginal needle suspension prevented postoperative incontinence in 21 of 22 patients.

Surgical Repair

The standard operative approach for urethral diverticula is through the vagina. Two procedures are in use. The actual choice of the surgical method depends on the location of the diverticular orifice in relation to the site of peak urethral closure pressure. As previously stated, if the orifice is proximal to this area, direct dissection of the diverticulum is necessary. Dissection is difficult because of the normal anatomic fusion of the urethra to the anterior vaginal wall, the associated infection, and the tendency of the diverticulum to partially surround the urethra or extend up under the base of the bladder. No cleavage planes exist, and a

tedious time-consuming operation results. Basic principles of fistula surgery prevail, with adequate dissection and closure in layers with minimal tension.

Normal saline solution is injected submucosally for hemostasis. A half-moon incision is made in the anterior vaginal wall about 0.5 cm below the urethral meatus. A vaginal flap is developed over the diverticulum, and it is reflected inferiorly. A transverse incision is made in the periurethral tissue; this tissue is reflected superiorly and inferiorly to expose the diverticulum.

The diverticulum is monitored endoscopically. The size of the diverticular orifice, the condition of the tissue, and the presence of other diverticula are noted.

The diverticulum is opened from the vaginal side. The cavity is inspected with the endoscope. If peridiverticulitis is found, a partial ablation is indicated, and the friable mucosa is not separated from the vaginal mucosa and fascia. Sharp dissection is required to separate the sac from the vagina and floor of the urethra. Care must be taken to preserve the mucosa of the urethral floor.

The urethral defect is closed with interrupted sutures of 3-0 catgut, inverting the edges. A second row of mattress sutures approximates the periurethral fascia over the primary sutures. The vaginal flap is trimmed and approximated with interrupted catgut sutures.

The procedure begins with the vaginal incision and exposure of the entire area oc-

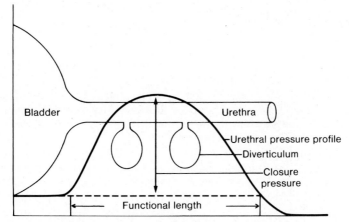

Figure 25.5. The urethral closure pressure profile with superimposed diverticular orifices proximal and distal to peak closure pressure.

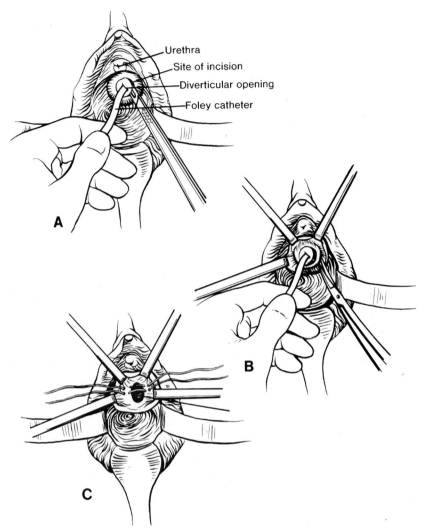

Figure 25.6. Total excision of urethral diverticulum. **A.** The vaginal incision and exposure of the diverticulum for direct dissection with placement of a Foley catheter for traction. **B.** Gradual dissection of the diverticulum frees it from its attachment to the urethra. **C.** Interrupted sutures close the urethra and the base of the diverticulum. (Redrawn from Urologic Surgery, edited by J.F. Glenn. Hagerstown, MD: Harper & Row, 1975.)

cupied by the diverticulum (Fig. 25.6A). At this point, it may be helpful to enter the diverticulum and place a Foley catheter for traction (Fig. 25.6B). Tedious sharp dissection continues until the entire diverticulum is free from all surrounding attachments and the connection to the urethra is definitively identified (Fig. 25.6B). The division of the urethral attachment completes the removal of the diverticulum, and closure of the urethra follows (Fig. 25.6C).

An alternative technique for closure involves the creation of two vaginal flaps, one of which is denuded of its vaginal epithelial covering (Fig. 25.7A). Placement of the denuded flap between the dissection site and the full thickness of the vaginal wall allows a layered closure without tension (Fig. 25.7B).

Another technique recently reported by Mizrahi (11) describes transvaginal periurethral injection of polytetrafluoroethylene (Polytef®) in the treatment of the urethral diverticula. After the injection, the diverticulum is collapsed. Bovine collagen is still experimental but could be substituted for the Polytef®. Polytef® has been shown to migrate to the lungs and brain in animal studies.

The Spence Procedure

When the diverticular ostium is distal to the peak urethral closure pressure, the Spence procedure is the operation of choice. This is an operation designed to marsupialize the diverticulum. The endoscope is used to locate the diverticulum, and a Kelly clamp is placed on the anterior vaginal wall opposite the diverticular orifice. One blade of the scissors is placed in the urethra and the other in the vagina (Fig. 25.8*A*). The scissors divide the intervening septum between the floor of the urethra and the vagina to complete the marsupialization (Fig. 25.8*B*). After the edges are trimmed, a running locking suture along the edges ensures hemostasis (Fig. 25.8*C*). The operation is performed in 30 minutes in an outpatient facility. A vaginal pack is not used nor is a catheter inserted. Catheteriza-

tion is not necessary, and the patients go home a few hours after the procedure. Subsequent granulation creates the appearance of a large meatotomy.

SURGICAL RESULTS OF THE SPENCE PROCEDURE

In two reported series, genuine stress incontinence followed the Spence procedure in 1 of 30 and 1 of 26 patients, respectively. Both patients with failures responded to vaginal estrogen application with cure of the incontinence. By comparison, direct excision of urethral diverticula has a complication rate approaching 20%. These complications are primarily urethrovaginal fistulae, urethral strictures, and urinary incontinence.

Partial Ablation Technique

The vaginal mucosa is dissected free, leaving the diverticulum intact in this method

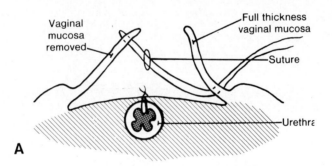

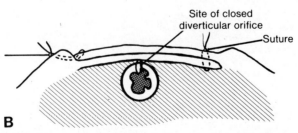

Figure 25.7. The vaginal flap technique for closure over the urethral defect. **A.** After one side of the freed vaginal flaps is denuded, the denuded flap is sutured underneath the intact full-thickness flap (**B**). (Re-

drawn from Judd GE, Marshall JR. Repair of urethral diverticulum or vesicovaginal fistula by vaginal flap technique. Obstet Gynecol 1976;47:627–629.)

devised by Tancer et al. (12) (Fig. 25.9*A*). The sac is entered longitudinally. The urethral opening is identified and the easily accessible portion of the sac is excised (Fig. 25.9*B*). An effort is made not to enucleate the sac at its neck. The opening is closed side to side with 3-0 chromic catgut (Fig. 25.9*C*). A second layer of sutures is placed, imbricating the previous urethral defect. The remainder of the diverticular wall is closed in a double-breasted fashion. The vaginal mucosa is closed.

The average hospital stay is 6 days. Urinary incontinence, fistula formation, or recurrence did not occur in Tancer et al.'s series. The pathology of peridiverticulitis as well as the site and extent of the lesion is taken into account with partial ablation.

After surgery, the bladder is filled with 300 mL saline and a suprapubic catheter is inserted. Suprapubic bladder drainage avoids injury to the suture line from an indwelling urethral catheter or from complications resulting from intermittent catheterization.

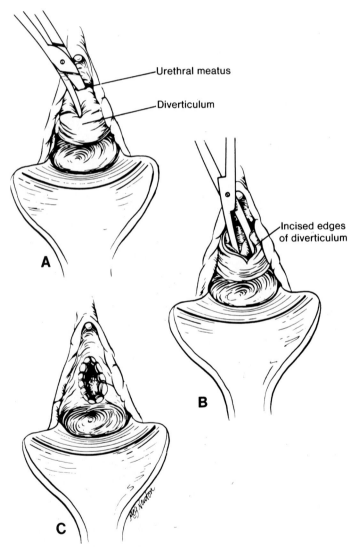

Figure 25.8. The Spence procedure for marsupialization of urethral diverticula. The scissors enter the diverticulum (**A**) and incise the full thickness of the urethrovaginal diverticulum septum (**B**). **C.** A running locking suture around the incised edges secures hemostasis.

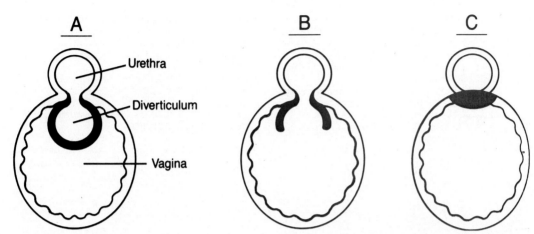

Figure 25.9.   Partial ablation. If the ostium is small and the periurethral tissue not inflamed, do a standard enucleation (**A**), but if peridiverticular and urethral inflammation is present, do a partial ablation

(**B**). Close the urethral opening without compromising the urethral floor (**C**). (Reproduced from Sanz L. Gynecologic surgery. Oradell, NJ: Medical Economics Company, Inc. Copyright 1988. All rights reserved.)

COMPLICATIONS

The rate of complications is 17%, using the standard technique. Urethral strictures result from removal of too much urethral mucosa. Treatment is by gradual dilation. Fistulae occur in about 5%. Antibiotic control of infection reduces fistula occurrence. If the fistula is located distal to the continence zone and is symptomatic, it may be corrected by a Spence procedure.

Summary

Diverticular symptoms and physical findings mimic many other lower urinary tract abnormalities. Urethroscopic examination may reveal the presence of one or more diverticula. It is helpful to combine urethroscopic, radiological, and urodynamic evaluations to select the correct operative procedure. If the diverticular orifice is distal to the area of peak urethral pressure, the Spence marsupialization operation is the procedure of choice; otherwise, direct dissection and removal is indicated.

REFERENCES

1. Hey W. Practical observations in surgery. Philadelphia: Humphreys, 1805.

2. Hunner GL. Calculus formation in a urethral diverticulum in women: report of three cases. Urol Cutan Rev 1938;42:336–341.
3. Novak R. Editorial comment. Obstet Gynecol Surv 1953;8:422–424.
4. Davis HJ, Cain LG. Positive pressure urethrography: a new diagnostic method. J Urol 1956;75:753–757.
5. Huffman JW. Detailed anatomy of the paraurethral ducts in adult human female. Am J Obstet Gynecol 1948;55:86–101.
6. Kohorn E, Glickman M. Technical aids in the investigation and management of urethral diverticula in the female. Urology 1992;50:322–325.
7. Spence HM, Duckett JW. Diverticulum of the female urethra: clinical aspects and presentation of a single operative technique for care. J Urol 1970;104:432–437.
8. Reid RE, Gill B, Laor E, et al. Role of urodynamics in management of urethral diverticulum in females. Urology 1986;28:342–346.
9. Bhatia NN, McCarthy TA, Ostergard DR. Urethral pressure profiles in women with urethral diverticulae. Am J Obstet Gynecol 1981;58:375–378.
10. Leach GE, Bavendam TG. Female urethral diverticula. Urology 1987;30:407–415.
11. Mizrahi S. Transvaginal periurethral injection of polytetrafluoroethylene (Polytef®) in the treatment of urethral diverticula. Br J Urol 1988;62:280.
12. Tancer ML, Moopan MMU, Pierre-Louis C, et al. Suburethral diverticulum: treatment by partial ablation. Obstet Gynecol 1983;62:511.

SUGGESTED READINGS

Andersen MJF. The incidence of diverticula in the female urethra. J Urol 1967;98:96–98.
Cook EN, Pool TL. Urethral diverticulum in the female. J Urol 1949;62:495–497.

Hirschorn RC. A new surgical technique for removal of urethral diverticula in the female patient. J Urol 1964;92:206–209.

Hyams JA, Hyams NM. New operative procedure for treatment of diverticulum of the female urethra. Urol Cutan Rev 1939;43:573–577.

Judd GE, Marshall JR. Repair of urethral diverticulum or vesicovaginal fistula by vaginal flap technique. Obstet Gynecol 1976;47:627–629.

Lichtman AS, Robertson JR. Suburethral diverticula treated by marsupialization. Obstet Gynecol 1976; 47:203–206.

Moore TD. Diverticulum of the female urethra: improved technique of surgical excision. J Urol 1952; 68:611–616.

Robertson JR. Genitourinary problems in women. Springfield, IL: Charles C. Thomas, 1978: 65–80.

Young HH. Diverticulum of female urethra. South Med J 1938;31:1043–1057.

CHAPTER 26

Vesicovaginal Fistula: Vaginal Repair

Jack R. Robertson

Vesicovaginal fistulae are uncommon. However, they are the most common postsurgical fistula between the lower urinary tract and the genitalia. Most are secondary to hysterectomy; obstetrical fistulae are now uncommon except in Third World countries. They are repairable through the vagina because of their location at the apex of the vaginal vault. The fistula lies just anterior to the site of the posthysterectomy scar, and its border abuts the scar. On the intravesical side, the fistula is usually just above and occasionally extends into the trigone. At times, the ureteral orifice is seen at the border of the fistula. This location decreases the need for the previous technique of direct dissection and closure of the fistulous tract. The much simpler Latzko (1) technique (partial colpocleisis) is preferred for posthysterectomy vesicovaginal fistulae.

Diagnosis and Preoperative Evaluation

If the patient has had previous irradiation, the possibility of a tiny vesicovaginal fistula must always be considered. It may occur years later. The details of working up a patient with a vesicovaginal fistula are important, because the best chance for a cure rests in the hands of the first surgeon. Chances of a successful closure decrease with each attempt. The following are standard methods of evaluation:

1. Methylene blue, sterile milk, or water and air (flat tire test);
2. Indigo carmine test;
3. Cystoscopy;
4. Intravenous pyelogram;
5. Retrograde pyelogram.

Endoscopy is essential in the preoperative evaluation of patients with vesicovaginal fistula. The patient is placed in the knee-chest position as originally described by Marion Sims (2). It is not necessary to reposition for cystoscopy. A Sims' speculum is inserted into the vagina to retract the rectum. Either a rigid or flexible endoscope is introduced through the urethra into the bladder. Carbon dioxide is used for insufflation; structures are seen more clearly through a gas medium. The fistula is easily observed just above the interureteric ridge, and the location and function of both ureteral orifices are observed. The pliability of the bladder wall is observed by manipulating the vaginal aspect of the fistulous tract.

The endoscope is removed, and the vaginal aspect of the fistula is observed. If a flexible scope is used, it can usually be maneuvered through the fistulous tract to view the edges and the vaginal aspect of the fistula. Since 1975, I have coupled a television camera to the endoscope. This allows a truly objective evaluation of the fistula's readiness for closure. The fistula should be closed whenever the endoscopic view shows that it is clean. No two fistulae or patients are the same.

Suprapubic repair may be extraperitoneal or transperitoneal. Either approach requires

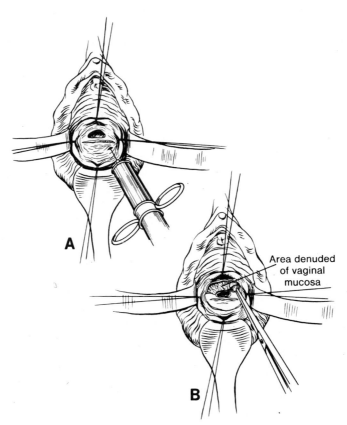

Figure 26.1. The Latzko procedure. **A.** The fistulous site after application of four traction sutures showing typical location of fistula and the injection of a hemostatic solution. **B.** The vaginal mucosa around the fistula is removed.

excision of the tract and mobilization of the bladder from the underlying vagina. This may require ureteral catheterization or, occasionally, a ureteral neocystostomy, both of which cause patient discomfort and prolong hospitalization. If suprapubic repair fails, the fistula is larger than it was originally.

With the Latzko procedure, ureteral integrity is never threatened, even if the ureteral orifice is near the fistula's edge. The patient is free of dressings, catheters, and drains. She is ambulated the day of surgery without discomfort and is discharged in a few days. The surgery is close to 100% effective. If failure occurs, the fistula is no larger than the original lesion.

There have been no controlled randomized studies of alternative treatments of genitourinary fistulae; therefore, the most effective method of management is debatable. The low morbidity, short hospital stay, and success rate make the Latzko procedure the treatment of choice for posthysterectomy vesicovaginal fistula repair.

Postoperative care is simple, and discomfort is minimal. Bladder drainage may be discontinued in 24 hours. After discharge, the patient continues a high-fiber diet and stool softeners and avoids Valsalva maneuvers. Nothing is to enter the vagina until her postoperative examination at 6 weeks.

Preoperative Cortisone

The use of cortisone preoperatively remains controversial, but I have used this technique for 30 years. The usual dose is 100 mg of cortisone three times a day, which allows repair of the fistula within 10 days to 2 weeks of injury in about 75% of cases. It is important to recognize whether or not the tissues are pliable and noninflamed before surgery. Endoscopic evaluation with the urethroscope aids in this critical determination. If infection remains, surgery is delayed. If cortisone is used, the removal of the suprapubic catheter should be delayed 7–10 days because cortisone may possibly delay healing.

Latzko Partial Colpocleisis Procedure

The Latzko technique for vesicovaginal fistula repair by the vaginal route is a relatively new and simple surgical technique. Its success does not depend on the basic principles of fistula repair, because excision of the fistulous tract, extensive mobilization of the bladder and vagina, and layered closure are not part of the procedure. There is little disturbance of the fistulous site itself, and the repair depends only on the viability of surrounding vaginal mucosa and submucosa. Therefore, the procedure lends itself to early use, thus avoiding the traditional waiting period of 4–6 months.

Figures 26.1 and 26.2 illustrate the procedure. The typical location of the fistula is just anterior to the vaginal cuff line of incision. All small acute fistulae should have 10–14 days of catheter drainage; they may close spontaneously.

A Foley catheter is inserted through the fistula, and the bulb is inflated. This gives excellent traction and simplifies exposure. Placement of four traction sutures and injection with a dilute epinephrine solution or normal saline solution facilitate the dissection of the vaginal wall (Fig. 26.1*A*). Denudation of an elliptical portion of the vaginal wall at least 2.5 cm beyond the tract in all directions follows (Fig. 26.1*B*). Closure in three layers with 3-0 absorbable suture completes the procedure (Fig. 26.2, *A* and *B*). The

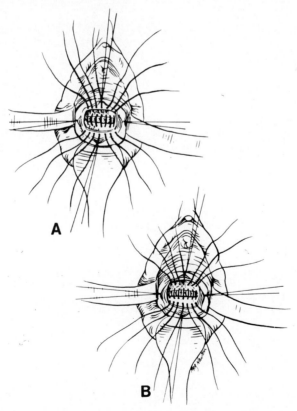

Figure 26.2. The Latzko closure. **A.** The submucosa is closed in layers with interrupted sutures. **B.** The vaginal wall is similarly closed.

posterior vaginal wall now becomes the posterior vesical wall and eventually reepithelializes with transitional epithelium. Postoperatively, a suprapubic catheter provides adequate drainage and is left in place for 24 hours, although many surgeons recommend bladder drainage for 7–14 days.

I never insert a ureteral catheter when using the Latzko procedure. If the ureteral orifice is at the edge of the fistula, the ureter is turned into the bladder by this operation. I have never seen ureteral encroachment.

Postoperative Care

Postoperative care is important; the patient has minimal discomfort, requiring only simple analgesia. She is ambulated within 24 hours. Stool softeners are started on the first postoperative day. The patient is discharged 3 or 4 days after surgery, after having a normal bowel action. The patient is encouraged to eat a high-fiber diet, to continue stool softeners, and to avoid Valsalva maneuvers. Sexual intercourse should not be resumed until 3 months postsurgery.

REFERENCES

1. Latzko W. Postoperative vesicovaginal fistulas: genesis and therapy. Am J Surg 1942;58:211–228.
2. Sims JM. On the treatment of vesico-vaginal fistula. Am J Med Sci 1852;23:59–82.

SUGGESTED READINGS

Collins CG, Pent D, Jones FB. Results of early repair of vesicovaginal fistula with preliminary cortisone treatment. Am J Obstet Gynecol 1960;80:1005–1012.
Diaz-Ball FL, Moore CA. A diagnostic aid for vesicovaginal fistula. J Urol 1969;102:424–426.
Graham JB. Vaginal fistulas following radiotherapy. Surg Gynecol Obstet 1965;120:1019–1030.
Robertson JR. Genitourinary problems in women. Springfield, IL: Charles C. Thomas, 1978:81–91.

CHAPTER 27

Vesicovaginal and Ureterovaginal Fistulae[a]

Raymond A. Lee

Given a sufficient surgical experience, injury to the urinary tract with the potential for developing a fistula can and does occur in the very best of hands. The resultant constant, malodorous, unimpeded leakage of urine is one of the most devastating complications for the patient and her surgeon. Although it is impossible to determine accurately the frequency of genitourinary fistula, it is currently recognized that most fistulae in the United States result from gynecological surgery. Surgical treatment of benign conditions accounted for more than 80% of the vesicovaginal fistulae in our recent series (1); "simple" total abdominal hysterectomy was the causative procedure in 70% of the patients. Frequently, the referring physician commented that the operation had been "simple" and uncomplicated, and this dreaded complication first occurred after many years of surgical experience. Possibly, there is a greater degree of apprehension and concern with the more difficult dissections of disease conditions and so the surgeon dissects more carefully and identifies the adjacent contiguous structures, thus avoiding the injury or at least promoting recognition and prompt repair of any injury that does occur.

Responsible Conditions and Operations

URETHROVAGINAL FISTULA

In a review from our institution reported in 1988, 53 patients were seen for a urethrovagi-

nal fistula; 10 of these patients had a separate vesicovaginal fistula. Diverticulum of the urethra was the most common preceding condition (13 patients) leading to urethrovaginal fistula. Vaginal surgery for stress incontinence (11 patients) and cystocele (8 patients) were the next most common circumstances leading to fistula formation. Treatment of seven patients with carcinoma of the cervix and one each with carcinoma of the endometrium and ovary led to urethral fistulas. In the rest of the patients, we could not establish the indication for operation.

VESICOVAGINAL FISTULA

Eighty percent of vesicovaginal fistulae occur after treatment of benign gynecological conditions, mainly uterine fibroids, menometrorrhagia, uterine prolapse, carcinoma in situ, or endometriosis. Approximately 10% of vesicovaginal fistulae follow obstetric procedures such as forceps rotation, cesarean section, or cesarean/hysterectomy. Just over 5% occur after treatment of malignant disease of the cervix, uterus, or ovaries. In over 85% of cases, the vesicovaginal fistulae follow abdominal or vaginal hysterectomy. Radiation therapy for various malignancies accounts for less than 5% of the fistulas.

URETEROVAGINAL FISTULA

Treatment for benign conditions is responsible for 90% of ureterovaginal fistulae; these conditions include menometrorrhagia, uter-

---

[a]Copyright 1989 Mayo Foundation.

ine fibroids, pelvic relaxation, or endo-metriosis. Again, total abdominal hysterec-tomy is responsible for more than 90% of the cases leading to ureterovaginal fistula. Ob-stetric injuries and radiation rarely lead to the formation of a ureterovaginal fistula.

Diagnosis

The first evidence of a urinary fistula is often the onset of leakage of watery fluid from the vagina. Various causes for the develop-ment of a fistula after operation include (*a*) an unrecognized gross injury to the urinary tract, (*b*) the inadvertent placement of a su-ture through the wall of the bladder or ureter, (*c*) necrosis of the urinary tract with associ-ated hematoma or infection, or (*d*) any com-bination of these. The cause, to a large extent, determines how rapidly the fistula develops and how soon its presence becomes clini-cally evident. Likewise, the cause influences how early the presence of a fistula is sus-pected and how easily the diagnosis is made. Other factors that influence when the fistula first becomes evident are the origin and loca-tion of the fistula and the method of catheter drainage used postoperatively.

URETHROVAGINAL FISTULA

The onset of vaginal leakage of watery fluid, the first evidence of urinary fistula, was related to the site of the fistula. Other factors that may influence the time of recognition are (*a*) unrecognized gross injury to the urinary tract (onset is usually immediate), (*b*) unrec-ognized suture through the wall of the ure-thra, (*c*) necrosis of the urinary tract with associated hematoma or infection, or (*d*) any combination of these.

In the Mayo Clinic study, patients with ure-throvaginal fistula after forceps delivery or trauma had leakage immediately or within the first 24 hours (two patients). If a urethral catheter was in place temporarily (such as af-ter anterior repair or diverticulectomy), cath-eter removal was followed promptly by the leakage (6 of 10 patients with anterior repair). In six other patients who required repeat catheterization for urinary retention, leakage developed 7–20 days postoperatively.

Patients with diverticulectomy had leak-age when the catheter was removed (3–7 days; four patients). Six initially continent patients had leakage 7–14 days postopera-tively. Onset of leakage was undetermined in three patients. Patients who underwent ra-diation therapy first noted the leakage 14–33 days after cessation of therapy (for the cases in which this information was recorded—four of six patients).

VESICOVAGINAL FISTULA

Immediate leakage after operation prob-ably results from unrecognized perforation or laceration of the bladder. In our cases of vesicovaginal fistulae, leakage occurred within the first 10 days in 70% and within the first 20 days in 90%. When the fistula follows childbirth with forceps delivery, leakage fre-quently occurs within the first 24 hours.

URETEROVAGINAL FISTULA

A ureterovaginal fistula may take several days or even weeks to progress through a period of necrosis, uroma formation, and eventual dissection through a "previously closed" vaginal suture line. There frequently is an associated period of increased tempera-ture of varying degree, usually with associ-ated unilateral tenderness of the costoverte-bral angle followed by the passage of urine that enters the vagina through a small com-munication with the ureter. Spontaneous cessation of leakage of urine from the vagina may represent spontaneous healing with re-establishment of a ureteral lumen. More likely, it may be an ominous sign of complete obstruction of the ureter from scar formation that, if left untreated, would result in loss of the kidney. Only when an intravenous pyelo-gram demonstrates a normal kidney with an intact ureter can the cessation of urine drain-age be safely considered to represent correc-tion of the fistula.

Management

URETHROVAGINAL FISTULA

Depending on its location, a simple ure-throvaginal fistula may not cause symptoms

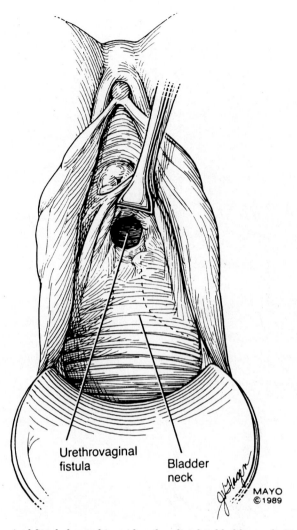

Figure 27.1.   Urethrovaginal fistula located in midurethra distal to bladder neck. (From Lee RA. Atlas of gynecologic surgery. Philadelphia: WB Saunders, 1992. By permission of Mayo Foundation.)

and may not require surgical repair. However, most urethrovaginal fistulas are associated with some leakage, and operative repair is required. The reconstruction is relatively simple, and yet success depends on meticulous attention to details during each phase of the operation.

Technique of Vaginal Repair

In Figure 27.1, the broken line indicates the junction of the urethra and the bladder neck, and the urethrovaginal fistula is located at the junction of the lower and middle thirds of the urethra. The vertical incision is made in the anterior vaginal wall, extending up and around the margins of the urethral defect (Fig. 27.2*A*). The vaginal mucosa is separated from the underlying cervicopubic fascia laterally, back to the descending pubic ramus (Fig. 27.2*B*). Infrequently, mobilization is continued laterally into the retropubic space and posteriorly to align with the entire trigone and lower segment of the base of the bladder and proximal portions of the urethra. Sufficient mobilization is required to provide a tension-free closure of the reconstructed urethra. The edges of the wall of

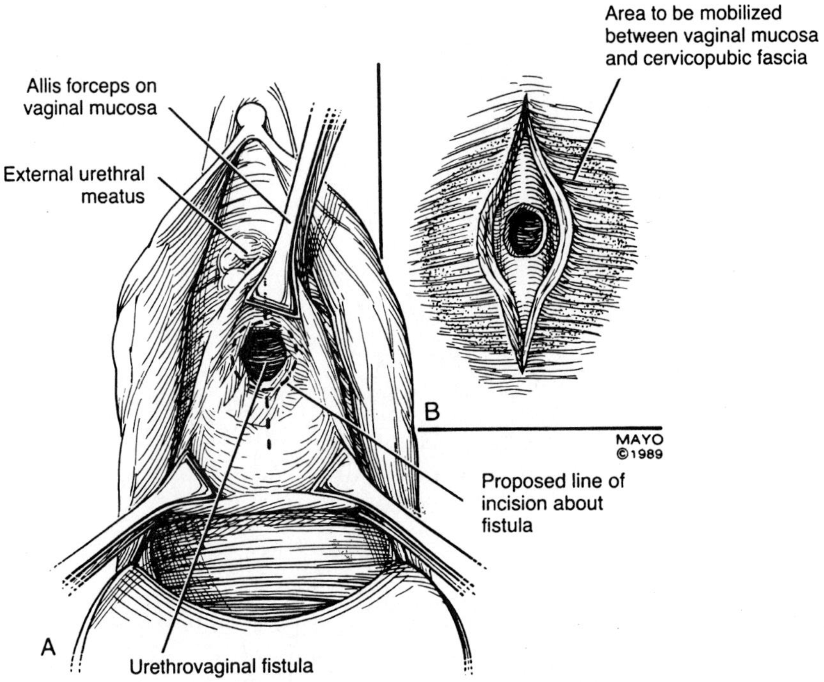

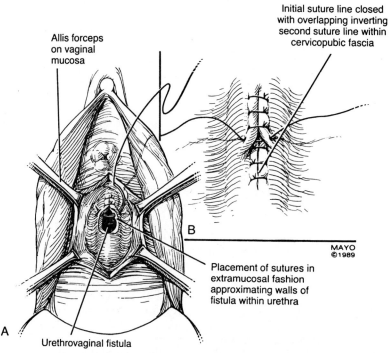

Figure 27.2. **A.** Proposed incision about fistulous opening. **B.** Area to be mobilized after excising scarred fistulous tract. (From Lee RA. Atlas of gynecologic surgery. Philadelphia: WB Saunders, 1992. By permission of Mayo Foundation.)

Figure 27.3. **A.** Closure of fistula with placement of interrupted sutures in an extramucosal position. **B.** Second suture line reinforcing inverted original suture line. (From Lee RA. Atlas of gynecologic surgery. Philadelphia: WB Saunders, 1992. By permission of Mayo Foundation.)

the urethra are accurately approximated with interrupted fine (4-0) delayed absorbable sutures placed in an extramucosal position (Fig. 27.3*A*). The initial suture line is inverted with a second suture line that incorporates the adjacent cervicopubic fascia and picks up a portion of the underlying tissue to obliterate dead space and aid in complete hemostasis (Fig. 27.3*B*). The vaginal suture line is approximated with interrupted 4-0 delayed absorbable sutures (Fig. 27.4).

In patients who have a linear urethrovaginal fistula (loss of a major portion of the floor of the urethra), urethral reconstruction may be more difficult, and urinary continence, even in what appears to be a well-constructed urethral tube, may not be predictable. The basic principles of the repair are the same as those for simple urethrovaginal fistula, as outlined above. Operative repair of the linear loss of the floor of the urethra is reviewed elsewhere and is beyond the scope of this discussion (2).

VESICOVAGINAL FISTULA

In recent years, different opinions have developed regarding the appropriate timing of fistula repair. In 1960, Collins et al. (3) suggested early repair and reported the preoperative use of cortisone to effect "resolution of the inflammatory reaction" around a vesicovaginal fistula. Of 15 fistulae operated on within 8 weeks (most within 4 weeks) of discovery, 13 were repaired successfully, all transvaginally. In 1971, Collins et al. (4) reported a 72% success rate in 29 patients treated with the same approach and medications, all within 2 weeks of discovery of the fistula. In 1979, Persky et al. (5) reported results of early repair (at 1–10 weeks) in seven patients; they used the suprapubic transvesical approach in all but one. They placed the peritoneum and omentum as an intervening layer between the bladder and vaginal repair, and the procedure was successful in all patients.

It is impossible for us to determine the cause of operative failure in patients referred after one or several unsuccessful operative attempts to correct their fistulae. In many patients, operations that were unsuccessful in correcting the fistula were performed very

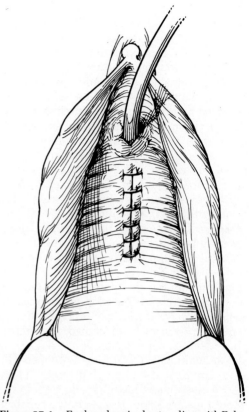

Figure 27.4. Enclosed vaginal suture line with Foley catheter in place. (From Lee RA. Atlas of gynecologic surgery. Philadelphia: WB Saunders, 1992. By permission of Mayo Foundation.)

early (at 10–15 days), and this timing is believed to be a contributing factor to the failure of the repair.

With or without preoperative steroid preparation, the presence of resolving suture material, edema, and inflammation with microabscess and macroabscess formation should have an adverse effect on the overall success rate of primary repair. In addition, preliminary catheter drainage of the urethra or bladder (or "splinting" of a ureter) for 15–30 days may provide spontaneous healing in a significant number of patients with fistulae. Thus, the need for an early operation that some advocate is avoided. In the usual postoperative (nonradiated) patient with a vesicovaginal fistula, waiting about 8–12 weeks after the formation of a fistula (or after a failed repair) ensures that the tissues will have a good blood supply and minimal edema and infection. There is little evidence of previous suture material, and cleavage planes are readily identifiable during dissection. These characteristics will permit wide mobilization and adequate dissection to allow accurate approximation of the tissues without tension to the suture lines.

Nevertheless, we are certain that there are specific fistulae that may be successfully managed by early operation (such as obstetric laceration and some of the fistulae diagnosed in the few hours after operation). Case selection is most important and is based on the type and difficulty of the causative operation and on the disease for which the original procedure was performed. Patients with pelvic inflammatory disease, abscess, malignancy, or postradiation problems are poor risks. In addition, the general physical condition of the patient should be the same consideration for early intervention. Sometimes the patient responds to news of her condition with apprehension, depression, or anger and is prompted to request or even demand immediate surgical correction. The physician must not allow these emotional factors to influence the treatment plan, even though the patient may not be easily convinced that additional time should elapse before the operative repair is undertaken.

Another area of controversy is the route of repair. Many fistulae can be repaired successfully via a vaginal, abdominal, or transvesical approach. In a specific circumstance, any of these approaches may provide a singular advantage, and on occasion, it may be necessary to incorporate all or a combination of these approaches for a successful outcome. Surgical experience with a significant number of fistula will soon indicate to the surgeon (regardless of specialty) that to manage the diverse types of genitourinary fistulae successfully, one must be familiar and adept with all approaches, as well as with various techniques.

From the patient's standpoint, the vaginal approach is easier, safer, and the most comfortable. The size or number of fistulae or a history of previous operative repair does not necessarily obviate the vaginal approach. The usual fistula resulting from an operation is located low in the bladder just above the interureteric ridge and generally lends itself to a vaginal repair, which is discussed elsewhere in this text.

Technique of Abdominal Repair

VESICOVAGINAL FISTULA

Since the work of Sims (6) more than a century ago, the surgical principles have been well established, and surprisingly little change has occurred in the modern era. More than 80% of repairs will be performed vaginally; specific indications for an abdominal repair are the presence of a large vesicovaginal fistula in proximity to the ureter and the difficulty of adequate exposure with the vaginal route even with use of the Schuchardt incision. When an abdominal approach is chosen (because of the proximity of the ureter or an adherent segment of bowel), we prefer the transperitoneal approach, which permits mobilization of the base of the bladder and ureter (usually with an indwelling ureteral catheter) so that an accurate and safe repair can be accomplished under good visibility.

Regardless of the approach chosen, the basic fundamentals of a successful repair remain the same: wide mobilization of the tissues surrounding the fistulous tract with excision of the scarred epithelialized fistulous tract (Fig. 27.5), a layered closure with extramucosal approximation by fine absorbable sutures free of tension (Fig. 27.6), and a second and third layer of inverting sutures within the wall of the bladder with a layered closure of the vaginal wall (Fig. 27.7), which again should be tension-free with excellent hemostasis. Careful attention should be given to obliteration of dead space to minimize potential infection. When possible, the peritoneum from the back and dome of the bladder is sutured between the suture lines, closing the bladder and vagina (Fig. 27.8). In the radiated patient, the omentum is freed from the right side of the transverse colon and fixed in place with fine interrupted absorbable sutures, separating the suture lines of the vagina and the bladder (Fig. 27.9).

Postoperative Management

To be successful, fistula repair of the bladder requires sound surgical judgment during

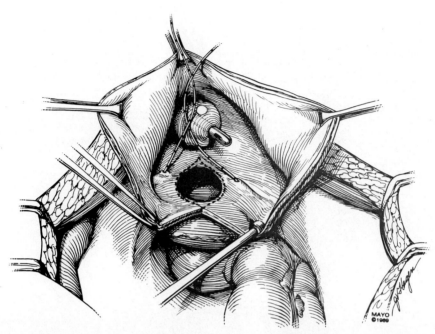

Figure 27.5. Bladder opened with outline of area to be resected before placement of initial suture line. (From Lee RA. Atlas of gynecologic surgery. Philadel- phia: WB Saunders, 1992. By permission of Mayo Foundation.)

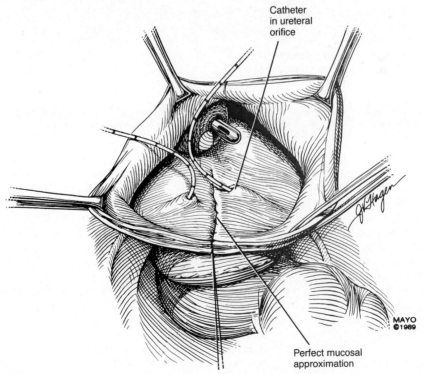

Catheter
in ureteral
orifice

Perfect mucosal
approximation

Figure 27.6. Extramucosal approximation by su- tures resulting in perfect approximation of bladder mucosa. (From Lee RA. Atlas of gynecologic surgery. Philadelphia: WB Saunders, 1992. By permission of Mayo Foundation.)

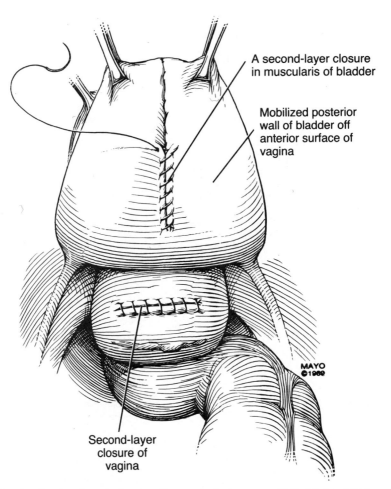

A second-layer closure in muscularis of bladder

Mobilized posterior wall of bladder off anterior surface of vagina

Second-layer closure of vagina

MAYO ©1989

Figure 27.7. Previously closed vaginal suture line separated from second layer of inverting suture within wall of bladder. (From Lee RA. Atlas of gyne-cologic surgery. Philadelphia: WB Saunders, 1992. By permission of Mayo Foundation.)

the operation and the postoperative period. Any tension or manipulation of the suture line must be avoided; competent bladder drainage with a large-caliber catheter, ure-thrally, suprapubically, or both, is manda-tory. Overdistention of the bladder due to obstructing blood or mucus can be prevented by hourly charting of the urine output and appropriate use of irrigation. Repeated ure-thral catheterization may disrupt a well-closed bladder repair and should be avoided. Some surgeons have recommended early re-moval of the urethral catheter for treatment of simple vesicovaginal fistula. Although this may be acceptable for some patients, we are unable to predict with certainty for which patients this is appropriate. As a result, we

customarily provide catheter drainage for at least 7 days and in radiated patients for several weeks. To minimize infection, appro-priate urinary specimens for culture are ob-tained, and antibiotics are administered.

URETEROVAGINAL FISTULA

When a ureteral injury is suspected, excre-tory urography is done. It is unusual for a ureterovaginal fistula to exist without some degree of radiographically identifiable ob-struction of the upper urinary tract; therefore, its presence can be excluded in most cases by demonstrating a normal upper tract on intra-venous urography. Conversely, ureteral in-volvement should always be suspected

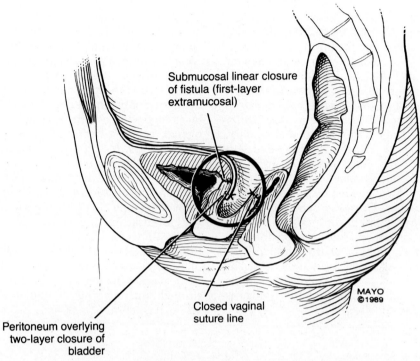

Submucosal linear closure
of fistula (first-layer
extramucosal)

Closed vaginal
suture line

Peritoneum overlying
two-layer closure of
bladder

Figure 27.8.   Peritoneum from dome of bladder sutured between closed vagina and bladder wall. (From Lee RA. Atlas of gynecologic surgery. Philadelphia: WB Saunders, 1992. By permission of Mayo Foundation.)

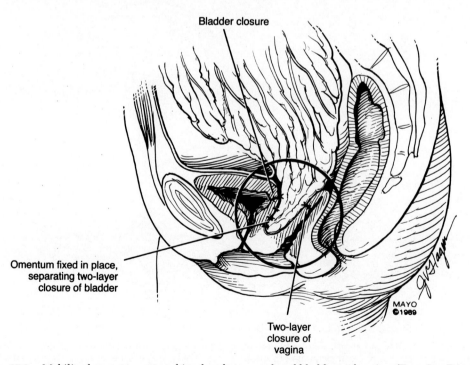

Bladder closure

Omentum fixed in place,
separating two-layer
closure of bladder

Two-layer
closure of
vagina

Figure 27.9.   Mobilized omentum sutured in place between closed bladder and vagina. (From Lee RA. Atlas of gynecologic surgery. Philadelphia: WB Saunders, 1992. By permission of Mayo Foundation.)

whenever an upper tract is shown to be partially obstructed in association with a urinary tract fistula. Once identified, an attempt should be made to introduce a guidewire and retention ureteral catheter (double J catheter), which will serve as a drain and stent. Initially, a retrograde technique should be used, and if a catheter can be negotiated through the blocked area, further therapy may not be required. If necessary, percutaneous nephrostomy can be done with the patient under local anesthesia or in the radiography department using fluoroscopy as a guide to localize the position and size of the renal pelvis. Once the needle is within the renal pelvis, a Silastic ureteral catheter can be passed to relieve the tension and preserve the function of the kidney. This permits the surgeon to delay ureteral repair until the patient is a better surgical candidate and the overall condition of the tissues is considered optimal.

The choice of the operative repair is determined by the location of the injury to the ureter and its relationship to the bladder. Ureterovaginal fistulae that occur after gynecological procedures usually result from injuries close to the bladder. For these, we prefer to use an open technique or ureteroneocystostomy. The end of the proximal ureter is incised in a vertical fashion in the six o'clock position for a distance of approximately 5 mm. A 4-0 polyglycolic acid suture is inserted through the angle of this incision. A finger is inserted inside the open bladder to tent up the bladder wall and indicate the most accessible area on the posterior lateral wall for insertion of the ureter. A 1-cm opening is dissected directly through the full thickness of the bladder by a spreading action of the dissecting scissors. A curved forceps is then passed inside the bladder and out through the opening in the bladder wall where it grasps the previously placed suture;

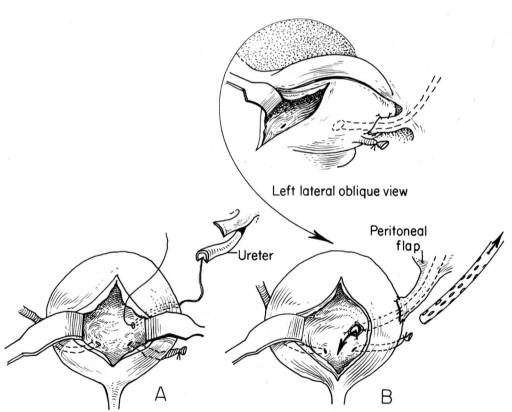

Figure 27.10. **A.** Traction suture delivering ureter through wall of bladder. **B.** Open cystotomy through which ureter is fixed to bladder mucosa. (From Symmonds RE. Ureteral injuries associated with gynecologic surgery: prevention and management. Clin Obstet Gynecol 1976;19:623–644. By permission of Harper & Row, Publishers.)

traction on the suture delivers the ureter into the bladder (Fig. 27.10*A*). From inside the bladder, five or six interrupted 4-0 polyglycolic acid sutures are used to anastomose the full thickness of the spatulated ureter to near full thickness of the bladder in a mucosa-to-mucosa approximation. Three or four interrupted sutures of the same material are placed (Fig. 27.10*B*) in the peritoneum, incorporating the peritoneum of the ureter to the muscularis and serosa of the bladder. This reinforces the repair and reduces any potential tension on the mucosal approximation. I prefer to then pass a self-retaining ureteral catheter with its most proximal end lodged in the renal pelvis and its distal end free within the bladder. This is generally left in place for 10–14 days. The bladder is drained with a suprapubic Foley catheter that is brought out through an anterior cystotomy, which is then closed with two layers of running 3-0 polyglycolic acid suture. Appropriate suction drainage and reperitonealization are accomplished in the customary fashion.

Bladder Extension

Occasionally, a ureteral fistula will be so high that it is necessary to free the bladder from the back of the symphysis pubis and either sidewall to bridge this gap without tension on the anastomosis. This permits a ureteroneocystostomy to be accomplished as far as the bifurcation of the iliac vessels on either side. Any tension on the anastomosis is relieved by stretching and fixing the upper lateral portion of the bladder wall to the iliopsoas fascia with several interrupted 2-0 polyglycolic acid sutures (Fig. 27.11).

Bladder Flap

If the above-described technique does not permit the bladder to reach the ureter free of tension, then one must consider construction of a tube of the bladder flap to bridge the defect. Methods to accomplish this have been reported by Boari (7). An obliquely placed flap is outlined on the outside of the bladder. This must be widely based superiorly (Fig. 27.12, *A* and *B*), and when care is taken to

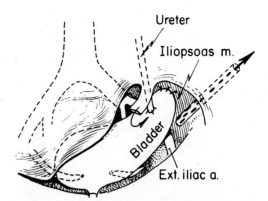

Figure 27.11. Mobilized bladder fixed to iliopsoas muscle. (From Symmonds RE. Ureteral injuries associated with gynecologic surgery: prevention and management. Clin Obstet Gynecol 1976;19:623–644. By permission of Harper & Row, Publishers.)

avoid making the flap too narrow distally, its blood supply should be excellent. Generally, an end-to-side mucosa-to-mucosa approximation can be accomplished as previously described for ureteroneocystostomy (Fig. 27.12*C*). The anastomosis is done under direct vision before the long linear defect of the anterior bladder wall produced by the creation of the tube is closed (Fig. 27.12*D*). When a peritoneal flap has been preserved along with the upper end of the ureter, this flap can be brought down well over the anterior cystotomy incision and fixed in a position so that it will additionally relieve any tension on the anastomosis.

Other equally important techniques, such as ureteroureterostomy or transureteroureterostomy, are excellent. Each has specific indications, and on occasion they are the preferred route of repair. A description of these techniques is beyond the scope of this discussion.

In all of these anastomoses, we prefer the use of a simple ureteral catheter that is passed up to the renal pelvis and down into the bladder. The catheter is left in place for an appropriate time. Drainage of the anastomotic site is essential. A large extraperitoneal suction tube is inserted and left in place for about 10 days, or longer if there is any urinary leakage. An excretory urogram is obtained between 2 and 3 weeks after the operation and every 3 months thereafter during the first year to be certain that delayed stricture does not occur.

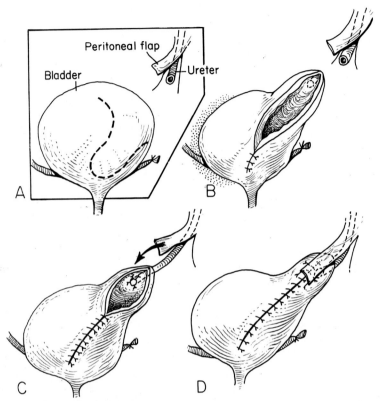

Figure 27.12. Modified Boari technique for construction of tube from bladder flap to bridge a ureteral defect. (From Symmonds RE. Ureteral injuries associated with gynecologic surgery: prevention and management. Clin Obstet Gynecol 1976;19:623–644. By permission of Harper & Row, Publishers.)

Summary

Gynecological surgery is responsible for most of the genitourinary fistulae that occur. The "easy" operation (the simple abdominal hysterectomy), and not the technically difficult operations for conditions such as pelvic inflammatory disease, endometriosis, or carcinoma, is responsible for most of these fistulae. Once a genitourinary fistula is identified, sound surgical judgment is required to choose the proper time and route of repair. Meticulous technique, approximation of tissues without tension, good hemostasis, and avoidance of infection are mandatory. The repair can be simple, but each step must be performed carefully to ensure a satisfactory outcome.

Ureteral fistulae resulting from gynecological procedures usually lend themselves to a ureteroneocystostomy. However, alternative techniques may be required and should be applied on an individual basis. Close observation and sound judgment by the operating surgeon are required during the postoperative convalescence.

REFERENCES

1. Lee RA, Symmonds RE, Williams TJ. Current status of genitourinary fistula. Obstet Gynecol 1988; 72:313–319.
2. Lee RA. Atlas of gynecologic surgery. Philadelphia: WB Saunders, 1992.
3. Collins CG, Pent D, Jones FB. Results of early repair of vesicovaginal fistula with preliminary cortisone treatment. Am J Obstet Gynecol 1960;80:1005–1009.
4. Collins CG, Collins JH, Harrison BR, Nicholls RA, Hoffman ES, Krupp PJ. Early repair of vesicovaginal fistula. Am J Obstet Gynecol 1971;111: 524–526.
5. Persky L, Herman G, Guerrier K. Nondelay in vesicovaginal fistula repair. Urology 1979;13:273–275.
6. Sims JM. On the treatment of vesico-vaginal fistula. Am J Med Sci 1852;23:59–82.
7. Boari A. Contributo sperimentale alla plastica dell'uretere. Atti Accad Sci Ferrara 1894;68: 149–154.

CHAPTER 28

Lower Urinary Tract Infection

Mickey M. Karram

Introduction

Urinary tract infections in women produce significant health problems. They are among the most common infections dealt with by primary care physicians. Although rarely followed by severe sequelae, they sometimes lead to acute pyelonephritis and bacteremia and become a major cause of morbidity and time lost from work. The health care expenditures necessitated by the diagnosis, antimicrobial treatment, and subsequent management of women with urinary tract infections has been estimated to exceed one billion dollars annually (1).

The proper management of these patients, although often simple, has recently been challenged by several occurrences: (a) the introduction of new antimicrobial agents, (b) the advent of single-dose therapy, (c) the recognition of additional lower urinary tract pathogens such as *Staphylococcus saprophyticus* and *Chlamydia trachomatis*, (d) the realization that many women with symptomatic cystitis may have less than 10^5 organisms/mL in urine cultures; and (e) the understanding that certain patients with infection-like symptoms will be termed urethral syndrome because they have no apparent cause for their symptoms.

Prevalence

Approximately 5 million cases of acute cystitis occur annually in the United States,

resulting in an estimated 6 million office visits (2). Urinary tract infections are much more prevalent among women than men (ratio of 8:1). This is probably secondary to an anatomically short urethra in proximity to a large bacterial reservoir within the introital tract and along the vaginal vestibule (3).

The incidence of urinary tract infections rises with age. At 1 year of age, there is an approximate 1–2% incidence of bacteriuria in females; pathology directly correlates with these infections. As many as 50% of patients will show abnormalities on intravenous pyelogram (IVP), that is, scarring and either ipsilateral reflux or some obstructive disease (4, 5). After 1 year of age, the infection rate decreases to approximately 1% and continues to decrease until puberty. The incidence of urological pathology associated with these infections also continues to decrease progressively. With the introduction of sexual activity and pregnancy, the incidence starts to rise and continues to progressively increase with age. Between the ages of 15 and 24, the prevalence of bacteriuria is about 2–3% and increases to about 10% at the age of 60, 20% after the age of 65, and 25–50% after the age of 80 (Fig. 28.1) (6).

Approximately 2% of all patients admitted to a hospital acquire a urinary tract infection during their stay, which accounts for 500,000 hospital-acquired urinary tract infections per year. One percent (5000) of these infections become life threatening. Instrumentation or catheterization of the urinary tract is a precipitating factor in at least 80% of these nosocomial infections (7, 8).

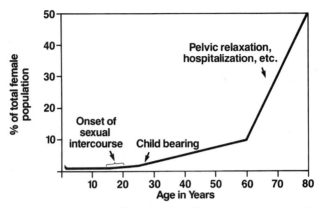

Figure 28.1. Prevalence of bacteriuria in females as a function of age.

Definitions

Before discussing urinary tract infection, an understanding of generally accepted definitions is essential because the commonly used terminology can, at times, be confusing.

Cystitis indicates inflammation of the bladder whether used as a histological, bacteriological, cystoscopic, or clinical description. Most commonly, it produces symptoms of urinary frequency and dysuria. Bacterial cystitis needs to be differentiated from nonbacterial cystitis (i.e., radiation, interstitial, and so on).

Urethritis refers to inflammation of the urethra and usually requires an adjective for modification (i.e., Chlamydial, nonspecific, and so on). In the female, symptoms of urethritis are impossible to distinguish from those of cystitis.

Trigonitis is inflammation or localized hyperemia of the trigone. This term is commonly used to describe the normal cobblestone or granular appearance of the trigone and floor of the vesical neck. The failure to recognize that this epithelium is part of the normal embryological development plus the lack of experience in cystoscopic examinations of normal women without bladder symptoms are probably responsible for the terms trigonitis and granular urethral trigonitis.

Bacteriuria implies the presence of bacteria in the bladder urine and not contaminants that have been added to a sterile bladder urine. The term includes both renal and bladder bacteria. Symptomatic bacteriuria can have as few as 10^2 colony-forming units

(cfu)/mL, whereas asymptomatic bacteriuria requires the growth of $\geq 10^5$ cfu.

Urethral syndrome is a poorly defined syndrome of frequency, urgency, dysuria, suprapubic discomfort, and voiding difficulties in the absence of any organic pathology. This term needs clarification, and it should not be used to describe urine with bacteria counts of less than 10^5 organisms/mL or Chlamydial infection of the urethra or a hypoestrogenic urethra. When we use the term urethral syndrome, we have ruled out detrusor and urethral dysfunction as well as any lower urinary tract infection. Thus, it is basically a "wastebasket" diagnosis of lower urinary tract symptomatology without any discernable pathology (9, 10).

Pathogenesis

The pathogenesis of urinary tract infection in the female has been postulated to involve three primary mechanisms, namely hematogenous or lymphatic spread or ascending extension of organisms directly from the rectum (Fig. 28.2). Retrograde (ascending) infection is the most widely accepted mechanism and appears to be important in the management of infections. Hematogenous dissemination is the principal route by which staphylococcus organisms seed the kidney. This leads to pyelonephritis and may possibly be an important route for *Escherichia coli* in patients who do not have vesicoureteral reflux.

The normal female urinary tract is remarkably resistant to infection. Although certain risk factors for developing urinary tract infections have been identified (Table 28.1), it remains unclear why certain women are more prone to infection. Susceptibility probably also depends on the inoculum size, the virulence properties of the invading microorganism, and, most importantly, the status of the defense mechanisms of the host. These host mechanisms are found in the urine, the vagina, and throughout the female urinary tract.

The enterobacteriaceae are responsible for approximately 80% of bacteriuria in urinary tract infections. *E. coli* accounts for approximately 80% of the community-acquired infections; other organisms are responsible for a disproportionate number of infections considering their frequency in stool flora. *Klebsiella* species cause about 5% of infections, whereas *Enterobacter* and *Proteus* species each cause approximately 2% of infections outside the hospital (11). *Serratia marcescens* and *Pseudomonas aeruginosa* are almost always hospital acquired and are due to omission of infection control practices, usually after urethral catheterization or manipulation. Although anaerobes are present in abundance in the feces of normal individuals, they are rarely the cause of urinary tract

infection. The oxygen tension in the urine probably prevents their growth and persistence within the urinary tract. *Staphylococcus saprophyticus* is the second most common pathogen isolated from young women with acute cystitis and accounts for approximately 10% of these cases (9, 10, 12–16). *Staphylococcus epidermidis* is a frequent cause of nosocomial urinary tract infection in catheterized patients and is frequently resistant to antibacterial agents (17). Other gram-positive organisms, including the group B and group D *streptococcus,* cause 1–2% of urinary tract infections.

Host Defense Mechanisms

URINE

Urine has certain defense mechanisms against infection. The most important inhibitory factors include a very high or low osmolality, a high urea concentration, a high organic acid concentration, and a low pH. A very dilute urine, as well as urine with a high osmolality, especially when associated with a low pH, will inhibit bacterial growth by inhibiting phagocytosis and decreasing the reactivity of complement. In general, anaerobic bacteria and other fastidious organisms

Hematogenous ▮▶
- Rare
- Descending
- Large bacterial inoculum
- Virulent organisms

◀ **Lymphatics**
- Very rare
- From bowel

Ascending ⬆
- Most common
- Proximity of bacterial reservoir
- Short urethra
- Catheterization and instrumentation

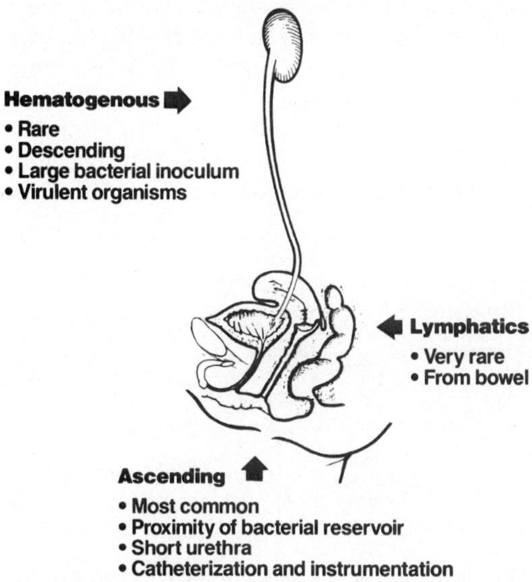

Figure 28.2. Pathways of bacterial entry into the urinary tract.

Table 28.1. Known Risk Factors for Urinary Tract Infection

Advanced age
Inefficient bladder emptying
  Pelvic relaxation
    Large cystocele with high residuals
    Uterovaginal prolapse resulting in
      obstructive voiding
  Neurogenic bladder, i.e., diabetes, multiple
    sclerosis, spinal cord injury, etc.
  Drugs with anticholinergic effects
Decreased functional ability
  Dementia
  Cardiovascular accidents
  Fecal incontinence
  Neurological deficits
Nosocomial infections
  Indwelling catheters
  Hospitalized patients
Physiological changes
  Decreases vaginal glycogen and increased
    vaginal pH in women

that make up most of the urethral flora will not multiply in urine. However, urine usually supports growth of nonfastidious bacteria (18, 19).

VAGINAL, PERIURETHRAL, AND PERINEAL COLONIZATION

There is accumulating evidence that the antibacterial defense mechanisms of the vaginal walls and periurethral area are important in preventing the progression of microorganisms from the rectum to the bladder. Normally, this area is colonized by gram-positive bacteria, lactobacillus, and diphtheroid (organisms that grow very poorly in urine and do not cause urinary tract infections). A number of studies have shown that females with recurrent cystitis will first colonize their vaginal introitus and periurethral area with enterobacteria before the onset of the symptoms of cystitis and will then be at risk for infection until this colonization reverses to a normal situation (3, 18, 20). Acidity of vaginal secretions may contribute to vaginal resistance to coliform bacteria. In premenopausal females, the vaginal pH is usually near 4.0. This low acidic pH prohibits the growth of organisms such as *E. coli* but promotes the growth of the normally present organisms (e.g., lactobacillus) that will interfere with the growth of uropathogens (21, 22). High vaginal pH seems to be associated with the growth of enterobacteria (23).

NORMAL PERIODIC VOIDING

Periodic voiding is one of the most important known bladder defense mechanisms. One study noted the introduction of 10 million bacteria into normal male bladders failed to establish infection because the organisms were rapidly cleared by voiding, diluting with fresh urine, and voiding again (24). Voiding displaces infected urine with sterile urine and flushes out bacteria attached to desquamated uroepithelial cells.

PREVENTION OF BACTERIAL ADHERENCE

The ability of an organism to bind to the epithelial cell has been shown to correlate with its ability to infect the urinary tract. The ascending loop of Henle secretes Tamm-

Horsfall protein, which is a uromucoid, rich in mannose. This protein may inhibit bacterial adherence and trap bacteria in the urine, allowing them to be flushed from the urinary tract (25). Also, the presence of urinary immunoglobulin and the lining of the bladder with a glycosaminoglycan may be important factors in the blocking of bacterial adherence. The reduction of glycosaminoglycan probably plays a role in recurrent cystitis (26, 27).

Host Susceptibility Factors

BACTERIAL ADHERENCE

Adherence of microorganisms to mucosal cells is considered to be a prerequisite to colonization and infection (28). As previously mentioned, when these organisms enter the urethra and bladder in most women, they do not adhere and are easily washed away. In persons who are susceptible to urinary tract infections, the organisms will quickly lock into the defective epithelial cells. The fecal flora is almost invariably the source of the infecting organisms. *E. coli* is the major pathogen, although *S. epidermidis,* enterococcus, *Klebsiella,* and *Proteus* can sometimes be identified (Fig. 28.3). The interaction of the mucosal and bacterial cells is probably dependent on both receptors on the mucosa and some type of attachment mechanism used by the bacteria. *E. coli* has been shown to possess surface organelles that mediate attachment to specific host receptors. These structures are called pili and can be present in large numbers on the microbial cell. Two types that appear to be important in urinary infections have been identified. Type

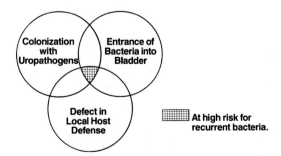

Figure 28.3. Factors determining host risk and susceptibility to bacterial cystitis in normal females with anatomically normal urinary tracts.

I pili seek mannose as a receptor and are isolated from individuals with cystitis. They tend to bind with a low affinity, and their presence is not correlated highly with pathogenicity. Type II pili are mannose-negative or "p pili" and adhere to the P blood group. *E. coli* strains possessing p fimbriae are more virulent and more likely to cause pyelonephritis than strains without them (29–31).

Schaeffer et al. (32) studied the adherence of *E. coli* to vaginal epithelial cells in control subjects and in women who had experienced at least three urinary tract infections in the past year. He found adherence to be greater in the study patients than in the controls. The vaginal cells of those receiving a sustained course of antimicrobial showed less adherence than the vaginal cells of patients who were not on antibiotics. If the antibiotics were discontinued, adherence returned, and reinfection usually occurred (32). In another study, Schaeffer et al. (33) noted that adherence tended to be higher during the early estrogen-dependent phase of the menstrual cycle.

Furthermore, high-risk women with recurrent urinary tract infections may be more genetically prone to recurrent infection because they have a higher prevalence of the human leukocyte antigen-A3 subtype than do women who have never had urinary tract infections (34). Recent work also suggests that women of blood group B or AB who are nonsecretors of blood group substances have a significantly higher risk of developing infections compared with women of other blood groups (35).

Thus, these genetic differences at the cellular level seem to influence bacterial adherence and make certain women more prone to urinary tract infections. These differences also influence the anatomic level of the infections.

SEXUAL INTERCOURSE

In women, sexual intercourse appears to be a major determinant for bacterial entry into the bladder. Prospective studies have shown that many urinary tract infections develop the day after sexual intercourse (36). Both the frequency and recency of sexual intercourse increase the risk of urinary tract infection. It has been shown that women who have engaged in sexual intercourse within the prior 48 hours have a risk of infection 60 times greater than women who have not (36). This appears to occur through inoculation of periurethral bacteria into the bladder during active intercourse. Women who have not colonized their vaginal and periurethral areas with coliform bacteria will have introduction of normal vaginal flora (e.g., lactobacillus, diphtheroid, or *S. epidermidis*), which will not produce infection and are rapidly cleared with voiding. However, in the colonized women, the pathogenic organisms, such as *E. coli,* will infect the bladder.

Another commonly overlooked factor is the use of diaphragms. A number of studies have confirmed that diaphragm users are at increased risk of urinary tract infection even after statistically controlling for sexual activity and history of previous urinary tract infection (37, 38). The mechanism is unknown; it is believed that it may be related to urethral obstruction caused by the diaphragm (39, 40). Also, diaphragm users have reduced vaginal colonization with lactobacillus, but coliform are isolated three times more often than in women using other contraceptive methods (38).

SYSTEMIC FACTORS

Diabetics are prone to develop neurogenic bladder dysfunction and severe vascular disease, both of which can predispose to urinary tract infections. Other genetic problems that are commonly associated with urinary tract infections are gouty nephropathy, sickle cell trait, and cystic renal disease.

It must be understood that the explanations mentioned for the pathogenesis of urinary tract infections only apply to those females who have normal urinary tracts. Bacteria in the presence of obstructions, stones, or a neurogenic bladder does not need to have special invasive properties other than the ability to grow in urine.

Clinical Presentation

The signs and symptoms of urinary tract infection in females can be diverse. It is helpful to distinguish lower urinary tract infection (cystitis) from upper tract infection (pyelonephritis) to aid in the selection of proper antimicrobial therapy and to plan appropriate follow-up.

Cystitis and associated urethral irritation are usually manifested by lower urinary tract irritative symptoms in the form of dysuria, frequency of small amounts of urine, urgency, nocturia, suprapubic discomfort, and low backache and flank pain. Occasionally, there may be mild incontinence and hematuria at the end of voiding. Rarely, the urine will be grossly bloody. Systemic symptoms in the form of fever, chills, and so on are usually absent in lower urinary tract infections.

Upper urinary tract infections involving the renal pelvis, calyces, and parenchyma will commonly present with fever, chills, malaise, and, occasionally (especially in elderly patients), nausea and vomiting. Costovertebral angle tenderness and flank pain are usually present. There will be colicky pain if acute pyelonephritis is complicated by either a renal calculus or a sloughed renal papilla secondary to diabetic or analgesic nephropathy.

Diagnosis of Bacteriuria

Before performing any tests to document the presence or absence of pathogenic bacteria in the urine, the method of urinary collection must be considered. Considerable care must be taken in the collection of urine from ambulatory females. Kass (41, 42) published results demonstrating that one whole voided urine specimen with a colony count of greater than 10^5 cfu/mL has only an 80% chance of representing true infection. Three specimens increased the odds to 95% (41, 42). Even when intelligent educated patients are given clear detailed instructions for collection of urine, errors can occur. Certain patients, because of physical disability or obesity, are simply unable to obtain a clean voided specimen without assistance. When necessary to avoid these limitations, specimens can be obtained via urethral catheterization, the patient can lie in the lithotomy position on an examining table and void

after the perineum is cleaned with soap and water while the nurse collects a midstream specimen, or bladder urine can be aspirated suprapubically (43). Although urethral catheterization is the most time-honored method, it should be kept in mind that catheterization is not without risks. Reports have noted that catheter-induced infection rates range from 1% in young healthy females to as high as 20% in hospitalized females (44, 45).

URINE MICROSCOPY

Microscopic analysis of urine is an easy and valuable method of evaluating women with symptoms of urinary tract infection. A thorough microscopic examination of an uncentrifuged sample of urine can detect the presence of significant bacteria, leukocytes, and red blood cells. If infection with greater than 10^4 cfu/mL is present, the finding of one or more bacteria on a Gram stain specimen of urine correlates highly with the presence of urinary tract infection, having a sensitivity of 80% and a specificity of 90% with a positive predictive value of approximately 85% (46). Thus, a Gram stain of the urine is useful in detecting abundant bacteriuria but is of little help in infection with colony counts of less than 10^4 cfu/mL.

Fresh unspun urine should also be quantitatively assessed with a hemocytometer for the number of white blood cells. The hemocytometer is positioned on the microscope stage. The number of leukocytes is counted in each of nine large squares, divided by 9 and multiplied by 10 to yield the number of white blood cells per milliliter. Pyuria is defined as greater than 10 leukocytes/mL. Pyuria is present in nearly all women with acute urinary tract infection. Studies note the presence of pyuria to be 80–95% sensitive (even when bacteria counts are less than 10^4) and 50–75% specific for the presence of urinary tract infection. It is also of value to ascertain whether red blood cells are present or to perform a urine dipstick for blood. Microscopic hematuria can be found in about 50% of women with acute urinary tract infection and is rarely present in patients who have dysuria due to other causes (47, 48).

OFFICE URINE KITS

If expertise for office microscopy is not available or feasible, it is reasonable to substitute a rapid diagnostic test for bacteriuria, pyuria, and hematuria, although, in general, these lead to less accurate results than microscopy. The most common rapid detection test is the nitrite test. This test depends on the conversion of urinary nitrate to nitrite by bacterial action. Numerous test kits are available (N-Multisticks, N-Multisticks C, N-Multisticks-SG from the Ames Division of Miles Laboratory; Chemstrip 9 and Chemstrip LN from Boehringer Mannheim Diagnostics; and Kyotest 8 Fe from Kyoto Diagnostics) (49). The test is often integrated with a test for esterase that suggests the presence of pyuria by a substrate color change caused by the esterase found in leukocytes. The sensitivity of these tests is directly related to the bacterial counts. Wu et al. (50) showed a sensitivity of only 22% in infections with 10^4 to 10^5 cfu/mL versus 60% for those with greater than 10^5 cfu/mL. The test should be performed on concentrated first-morning voided specimens. It has been suggested that false-negative results are more likely if the test is used as a sampling technique at other times during the day (51). False-negative results can also occur in infections due to enterococci because they do not convert nitrate to nitrite and also in the presence of certain dyes such as bilirubin, methylene blue, or phenazopyridine that may interfere with the interpretation of the test (52, 53). Some believe that these are good screening tests for asymptomatic bacteriuria (51–53), whereas others believe that the high false-negative rate limits their value (50).

Other rapid detection tests, such as filter methods (e.g., Back-T-Screen, Marion Laboratories, Inc., Kansas City, MO), concentrate a specific quantity of urinary sediment on a filter of controlled pore size. One milliliter of urine is mixed with 3 mL of a diluent containing glacial acetic acid and other ingredients that dissolve crystals and increase adherence of bacteria and leukocytes. The diluted mixture is then passed through the filter and rinsed with a diluent. A safranin dye is then used to stain the bacteria and leukocytes, and a decolorizer is added to remove excess dye. Resulting colors are compared with a reference to quantitate the presence of bacteria and leukocytes. The sensitivity of these tests for urine infected with 10^4 to 10^5 cfu/mL is from 34% to 65%. As the number of organisms increases to greater than 10^5, the sensitivity also increases to 79–85%. The specificity of this test at lower bacterial counts is approximately 75% (50, 54). The main advantage of these tests is a more reliable detection of smaller numbers of bacteria at the expense of lower specificity (55). The test is believed by some to be a good screening method because it detects both bacteria and pyuria.

URINE CULTURE

In the patient who has clinical signs of acute lower urinary tract infection and is noted to have pyuria, bacteriuria, or hematuria on one of the previously mentioned office tests, it is reasonable to initiate antibiotic therapy without obtaining a urine culture. However, if one of the screening techniques is deemed inappropriate or inconclusive or the patient has recurrent infection that has not been subjectively relieved with previous antibiotics or if signs and symptoms are consistent with upper urinary tract infection, then a bacterial culture and sensitivity should be performed. The traditional approach to the interpretation of a urinary culture has been that there must be growth of greater than or equal to 10^5 cfu/mL to consider it positive. This criterion is based on studies demonstrating that the finding of greater than 10^5 cfu/mL on two consecutive urine cultures distinguishes women with asymptomatic bacteriuria or pyelonephritis from those with contaminated specimens (41, 42, 46). The use of this cutoff, however, has two limitations for the clinician who treats these patients. First, 20–24% of women with symptomatic urinary infections will present with less than 10^5 bacteria/mL of urine (43, 56–58). This is probably secondary to a slow doubling time of bacteria in urine combined with frequent bladder emptying from persistent irritation. A study by Stamm and associates (59) proposed that the best diagnostic criterion for culture detection in young symptomatic women is 10^2 cfu/mL, not 10^5 cfu/mL. The second limitation of the 10^5 cutoff is one of overdiagnosis. In the original studies by Kass (41, 42, 60), a single culture of $\geq 10^5$ cfu/mL had a 20% chance of representing contamination. Because patients who are susceptible to infection will often carry large numbers of pathogenic bacteria on the perineum, contamination of an otherwise sterile urine can at times occur. For this reason, care in the collection of the urine specimen must again be emphasized.

Although methods of obtaining cultures in the office are available, most clinicians use commercial laboratories. One should be familiar with the individual laboratory policy of reporting culture results. Some laboratories report any culture of less than 10^5 cfu/mL as negative and often report only the predominant organism in mixed cultures.

Sensitivity testing is also usually obtained via commercial laboratory even though office tests have been described. The disadvantages of sensitivity testing include the time involved, which is typically 24–48 hours; the absence of control of processing by the referring physician; and the relatively high cost.

Cystourethroscopy

Indications for endoscopic evaluation in females with urinary tract infection has been a controversial issue. Fowler and Pulaski (61) reported on 74 cystoscopies performed in women with two or more previous infections and noted the only abnormality that altered treatment was the presence of a urethral diverticulum in three cases. Engel et al. (62) reviewed 153 women who had undergone cystoscopy for urinary tract infection. Although abnormalities were noted in 62% of the cases, 84% of these abnormalities were inflammatory in nature and presumably secondary to prior infection. Only one abnormality, a colovesical fistula, had an effect on treatment (62). Cystoscopy under local anesthesia has basically no risk and occasionally will reveal findings useful in subsequent patient management. Therefore, it should be considered in patients with recurrent or persistent urinary tract infection or asymptomatic hematuria.

Radiological Studies

Although it has long been believed that urinary tract infection constitutes one of the important indications for urography, the use of routine IVPs in women with otherwise uncomplicated infection has recently been challenged. The minimal (1–2%) yield of the IVP makes it an inefficient and expensive method of identifying underlying disease (61–66). The cost of detecting a single significant and treatable urological disorder has been estimated at 9 thousand dollars (66). However, the IVP is a valuable diagnostic test when properly indicated. In the author's opinion, the indications for obtaining an IVP for urinary tract infection are (*a*) a history of previous upper urinary tract infection; (*b*) a history of childhood urinary tract infections; (*c*) history of recurrent infections caused by the same organism, particularly if the organism is urea-splitting, such as *Proteus mirabilis*, because this is frequently associated with infected stones (Fig. 28.4); (*d*) all cases of infection associated with painless hematuria; (*e*) women with a history of stones or obstruction; and (*f*) patients that have bacterial evidence of rapid recurrence, suggesting bacterial persistence or the presence of an enterovesical fistula.

A voiding cystourethrogram or a double-balloon catheter study should be performed if a urethral diverticulum is thought to be contributing to recurrent infections. Signs and symptoms of urethral diverticulum include leakage of urine and the finding of pus or pain on palpation and massage of the urethra.

Urodynamic Studies

Urodynamic studies involving a range of procedures from a simple cystometrogram and flow studies to complicated video-urodynamic studies are sometimes useful to demonstrate abnormal contraction and emptying of the bladder. A vicious cycle of repeated lower urinary tract infections can lead to an obstructed voiding pattern, with high residuals resulting from spasm of the external striated urethral sphincter secondary to infection or to the pain of the acute cystitis

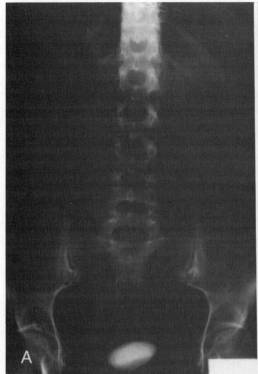
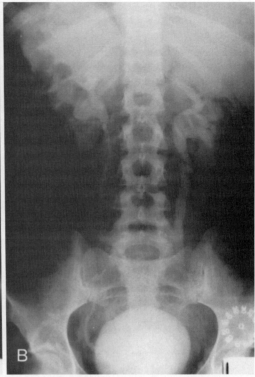
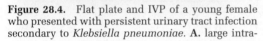

Figure 28.4. Flat plate and IVP of a young female who presented with persistent urinary tract infection secondary to *Klebsiella pneumoniae*. **A.** large intra- vesical bladder calculi. **B.** Bilateral hydronephrosis and hydroureter.

(67). These tests can prove helpful in patients with recurrent urinary tract infection who have neurological disease or a history of pelvic or spinal surgery.

Differential Diagnosis

In women whose history or laboratory findings are not consistent with urinary tract infection, other causes of their lower urinary tract symptoms must be considered.

Vaginitis is a major cause of lower urinary tract symptoms, with *Trichomonas* and *Candida* being the most commonly implicated organisms. Nonspecific urethritis is a term that has been used by some to describe patients with dysuria secondary to what is believed to be an inflamed urethra. Several organisms have been proposed as potential pathogens in such cases. These have included *Chlamydia trachomatis*, lactobacilli, *Staphylococcus saprophyticus*, corynebacte- ria, as well as other fastidious organisms such as *Ureaplasma urealyticum,* and *Mycoplasma hominis.* However, data to substantiate correlation between clinical symptoms and the presence of these organisms are lacking (68, 69). Trauma related to intercourse or other activities may also produce symptoms of urinary tract infection. Unfortunately, many of these patients are unnecessarily treated with repetitive courses of antibiotics. Dysuria is also a common presenting symptom in sexually transmitted diseases, particularly *C. trachomatis* and, less commonly, herpes simplex virus or *Neisseria gonorrhoeae.*

Some patients can distinguish internal from external dysuria. Discomfort that is centered inside the body is more commonly associated with urinary tract infection or urethritis due to *C. trachomatis*; pain that starts when the urine flows across the perineum is more commonly associated with vaginitis or herpetic infection. Frequency, urgency, and voiding small amounts of urine are common in urinary tract infection and in sexually transmitted diseases and rare in vaginitis. Virtually all women with acute symptomatic urinary tract infection have pyuria and about half will have microscopic hematuria. Pyuria can also exist in patients with urethritis secondary to sexually transmitted diseases. It is not present in vaginitis. Hematuria is not a feature of either sexually transmitted diseases or vaginitis; therefore, its presence is a strong clue toward the diagnosis of cystitis. Postmenopausal females may have dysuria secondary to desiccation of the urethra and the vaginal mucosa caused by estrogen deficiency (70). A group of women exists who are not estrogen deficient and who complain of persistent lower urinary tract symptoms despite negative urine, vaginal, and urethral cultures. The term *urethral syndrome* (68–71) has been introduced to describe these patients, and a full discussion of this condition is presented elsewhere. A suggested approach to the evaluation and management of women with dysuria is shown in Figure 28.5.

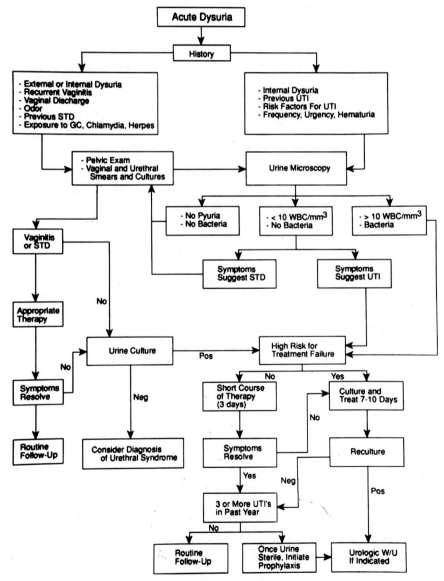

Figure 28.5. Algorithm for diagnosis and management of females presenting with acute dysuria.

Management of Lower Urinary Tract Infection

General measures, such as rest and hydration, should always be emphasized in women with urinary tract infection. Hydration will dilute bacterial counts and, perhaps, destroy cell wall-deficient bacterial strains. Acidification of the urine is only helpful in recurrent infections and in patients taking methenamine compounds, which demonstrate maximal antibacterial activity at a pH of 5.5 or less. Urinary analgesic agents such as phenazopyridine hydrochloride (Pyridium) help relieve pain and burning on urination. If prescribed, they should be used for only 2–3 days along with a specific antibacterial agent. It has also been noted that the ingestion of cranberry juice may be protective against the development of cystitis by inhibiting bacterial adherence (72).

With regard to the therapeutic management of this condition, certain factors should be kept in mind. Because the fecal flora is the reservoir for most of the organisms causing the infection, a drug that has little or no effect on these microbes should ideally be prescribed. The reason to avoid altering these bacteria is because 20% of females with simple cystitis will have a recurrence shortly after stopping medication. A drug can alter bacteria in the bowel by either passing through the gastrointestinal tract without being absorbed or by having a high serum level. It is also important that a drug maintain a low serum level to avoid disrupting the flora in other parts of the body, such as the vagina. If a drug appropriately matched to bacterial sensitivity causes a yeast vaginitis, the subsequent therapy for the vaginitis will increase patient morbidity and raise the cost of therapy. In addition, the vaginitis set up by the antibiotic could lead to a vaginitis-cystitis circle that may be difficult to treat. These therapeutic goals should be kept in mind when treating these infections because there are many misconceptions about commonly prescribed antibiotics. For example, ampicillin and tetracycline are both frequently prescribed for simple cystitis, despite the fact that they have an incidence of yeast vaginitis that may approach 25% and

70–80%, respectively, because both drugs are excreted in the fecal stream unchanged and will have a stool level three times the urine level (73–76). Nitrofurantoin, on the other hand, has excellent activity against *E. coli* and has no significant serum level. It has a 19-minute serum half-life and is metabolized in every tissue in the body, resulting in no significant changes in fecal or vaginal flora, which is why no increase in bacterial resistance to nitrofurantoin is seen after 30 years of use in the United States (75–80). The most common sulfonamide preparation used in the management of urinary tract infection is the combination of trimethoprim with sulfamethoxazole (TMP-SMX, Bactrim, Septra). These drugs have become very popular in the management of urinary tract infections because of their broad range of activity against uropathogens, low incidence of adverse effects, twice-daily dosage, and infrequent occurrence of bacterial resistance. However, these agents have been shown to have a moderate effect on bowel and vaginal wall flora (81, 82).

A group of synthetic quinoline derivatives, which are related chemically to nalidixic acid, has recently been introduced as antibacterial agents for urinary tract infections. Derivatives include norfloxacin (Noroxin), ciprofloxacin, enoxacin, ofloxacin, pefloxacin, and amifloxacin. These agents are more active than nalidixic acid against gram-negative urinary tract pathogens (e.g., *E. coli*). In addition, they have an expanded antibacterial spectrum that includes *Pseudomonas aeruginosa* and gram-positive bacteria (e.g., staphylococci, enterococci). All of these agents are administered orally, and parenteral formulations are available for some (e.g., ciprofloxacin). Adverse effects have been infrequent; however, their cost limits their routine use. Because they have no advantage over more standard agents (e.g., nitrofurantoin, TMP-SMX) for uncomplicated infections, they should be reserved for use in patients with resistant infections or as an alternative to parenteral antibiotics in certain complicated infections and cases of pyelonephritis (83–89). Unfortunately, their attractiveness has lead to widespread use, making ciprofloxacin the fourth most commonly prescribed antibiotic in the United States. This overuse has been accompanied by an in-

Table 28.2. Dosage and Toxicity of Antibiotics Commonly Used in the Treatment of Urinary Tract Infections

Drug	Oral Dose and Frequency	Minor Toxicity	Major Toxicity
TMP-SMX	1 tab bid	Allergic	Serious skin reactions, blood dyscrasia
Nitrofurantoin	50–100 mg q6–8h	Gastrointestinal upset	Peripheral neuropathy, pneumonitis
Ampicillin	250–500 mg q6h	Allergic candidal overgrowth	Allergic reactions, pseudomembranous colitis
Tetracyclines	250–500 mg q6h	Gastrointestinal upset, skin rash, candidal overgrowth	Hepatic dysfunction, nephrotoxicity
Cephalexin	250–500 mg q6h	Allergic	Hepatic dysfunction
Norfloxacin	400 mg q12h	Nausea, vomiting, diarrhea, abdominal pain, skin rash	Convulsions, psychoses, joint damage

Table 28.3. Spectrum of Antimicrobial Activity Against Common Lower Urinary Tract Pathogens

Organisms	TMP-SMX	Nitrofurantoin	Ampicillin	Tetracycline	Cephalexin	Carbenicillin	Gentamicin	Norfloxacin
Escherichia coli	++	++	++	±	++	++	++	++
Pseudomonas	–	–	–	–	–	++	++	++
Klebsiella	++	±	–	±	++	–	++	++
Proteus	++	–	++	–	++	++	++	++
Enterobacter	++	–	–	–	–	++	++	++
Enterococcus	–	±	++	++	±	–	–	++
Staphylococcus	–	±	++	+	++	++	+	++
Serratia marcescens	+	–	–	–	–	–	++	++

++, Excellent; +, good; ±, occasionally effective; –, resistant.

crease in bacterial resistance; already, strains of *E. coli* are resistant to ciprofloxacin.

Listed in Tables 28.2 and 28.3 are the dosage, toxicity, and spectrum of antimicrobial activity of some of the commonly prescribed oral antibiotics.

ASYMPTOMATIC BACTERIURIA IN PATIENTS WITHOUT CATHETERS

By definition, asymptomatic bacteriuria is the recovery of $\geq 10^5$ cfu/mL of a single bacterial species in at least two consecutive clean-voided urine specimens in the absence of clinical symptoms (41). Little is known about the natural history of untreated bacteriuria in women because most are treated once the diagnosis is made. Two studies have, however, compared antibiotic treatment with placebo in women with asymp-

tomatic bacteriuria. They noted that 60–80% of these patients will spontaneously clear their infection whether they are treated or receive placebo (90, 91). Although the long-term effects of asymptomatic bacteriuria are not completely known, there seems to be no association with renal scarring, hypertension, or progressive renal azotemia.

Screening for asymptomatic bacteriuria has little apparent value in adults, with two exceptions: before urological surgery and during pregnancy. Postoperative complications, including bacteremia, are reduced by recognizing and treating asymptomatic bacteriuria before urologic surgery (92). All pregnant women should be screened for bacteriuria in the first trimester and should be treated if bacteriuria is present to reduce their markedly increased risk of acute pyelonephritis and the accompanying risks of prematurity and low birth weight in their infants (93, 94).

To date, there is no definite advantage to treating asymptomatic bacteriuria in the non-pregnant female. There are, however, recent studies that have shown a significant assoc-iation between asymptomatic urinary tract infection and overall mortality (95, 96). Whether this mortality is a false-positive re-sult or the bacteriuria is serving as a marker for a chronic disease that was the actual cause of death needs to be confirmed by further studies.

FIRST INFECTIONS OR INFREQUENT REINFECTIONS

Many treatment regimens have been re-ported for initial therapy of simple cystitis, ranging from one dose to 2 or more weeks of medication. The longer treatment regimens were instituted in an attempt to prevent the relapse rate that occurs in about 20% of patients treated for cystitis. Almost all of these relapses are attributable to the coloni-zation of the vaginal walls and urethra with gram-negative bacteria that have continued to grow on the perineum or reappeared when the drug was stopped. It does not indicate that the prescribed drug has failed to eradi-cate the bacteriuria.

There are numerous studies in the litera-ture evaluating single-dose therapy in the management of acute uncomplicated cystitis (97–106). When single-dose therapy was compared with 10 days of TMP-SMX, there was a significantly higher treatment failure rate with single-dose therapy (106). Further concern has been raised that single-dose re-gimes are less likely to be effective in treat-ment of infections when an unrecognized complicating factor is present, such as preg-nancy, diabetes, or an anatomic or functional abnormality of the urinary tract. Single-dose therapy has also been noted to be suboptimal in the treatment of occult upper urinary tract infection (107).

A plethora of studies has been conducted in recent years to define the optimal antimi-crobial agent and length of treatment for uncomplicated cystitis in women. With most antimicrobial agents, 3-day regimes appear optimal, with efficacy comparable with 7-day regimes but with fewer side effects and lower cost. Nitrofurantoin, cefadroxil, amoxicillin,

and TMP-SMX have been shown to be effec-tive in 3-day regimes, either in open trials or in comparative trials with longer regimes. A recent prospective randomized trial com-pared these four antimicrobial agents in a 3-day regime in young women with acute cystitis (108). The findings demonstrated that a 3-day regime of twice daily TMP-SMX was more effective than 3 days of nitrofurantoin, cefadroxil, or amoxicillin. Moreover, TMP-SMX was the least expensive of the four regimes, mainly because compared with the other regimes, patients were less likely to have to return for evaluation of persistent or recurrent urinary tract infection or for yeast vaginitis (108). We thus favor the use of TMP-SMX as our first-line agent for empiri-cal treatment of acute uncomplicated cystitis in women.

Alternate regimes that can be used in women who have a history of intolerance to TMP-SMX are nitrofurantoin 100 mg four times daily or TMP 100 mg twice daily. We try to avoid the use of amoxicillin or first-generation cephalosporin because we have experienced a relatively high failure rate with these agents in our clinic. Single-dose therapy or a short course of therapy should only be considered in patients who are at very low risk for treatment failures. Thus, patients (*a*) with systemic diseases such as diabetes mellitus, (*b*) who have a history of acute pyelonephritis, (*c*) who have a his-tory of a treatment failure in the last 6 months, (*d*) who have a history of childhood urinary tract infections, or (*e*) with known structural abnormalities of the urinary tract should be given a longer 7- to 10-day course of therapy.

For patients with acute simple cystitis who have complete resolution of their symptoms, it is not necessary to perform any routine posttreatment urinary assessment. However, in those patients whose urinary symptoms persist beyond the 3 days of therapy, a urine culture and sensitivity should be obtained. Persistence of symptoms should suggest the possibility that either the initial diagnosis of urinary tract infection was in error or that the patient's infection is secondary to a resistant organism that was present from the onset of therapy or has developed during initial therapy. In cases of resistance, a 7- to 10-day course of a sensitive antibiotic should then be prescribed.

RECURRENT INFECTIONS

Approximately 75% of all women who experience a urinary tract infection will subsequently experience less than one infection per year (109). However, the other 25% of women will develop reinfections at a rate of almost three infections per year. These women comprise 50% of all women presenting with acute urinary tract infections (109–112).

Once the urine has been sterilized by appropriate antimicrobial therapy, the pattern of culture-documented reinfection or recurrence is very helpful in the subsequent management of these patients (Fig. 28.6). It can also be used to classify patients with different infectious etiologies to identify those who may be at increased risk or require further urological evaluation. The most common type of recurrence is a reinfection by bacteria different from the initially infecting strain. Even though the infections may be caused by the same species (e.g., *E. coli*), the organisms can usually be differentiated on the basis of colonial morphology and antimicrobial sensitivities. These infections are almost invariably due to a recurrent ascending infection from the vaginal introital area. It has been shown that the same strain can exist in the introital area for many months and cause multiple reinfections. Sexual intercourse and occult urinary tract abnormalities may also facilitate reinfection and must always be considered in these patients.

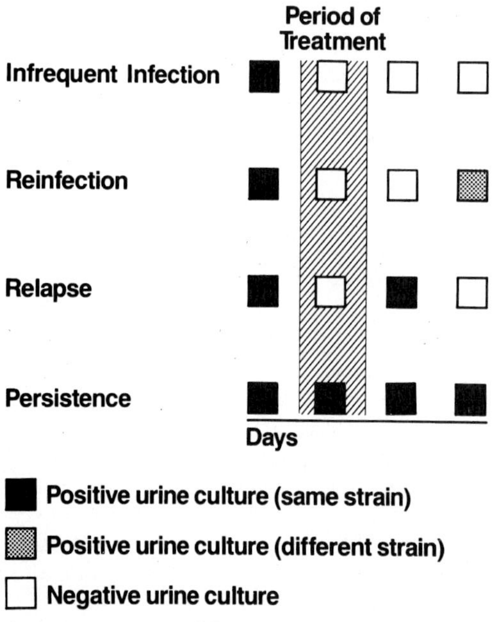

Relapsing infection from an upper urinary tract source of an infected stone should be suspected if the same organism is repeatedly isolated 7–10 days after treatment with an antimicrobial agent to which the organism is sensitive. In many of these patients, one cannot obtain sterile urine, and thus these are termed bacterial persistence. Causes of these are listed in Table 28.4. Endoscopic and radiographic evaluations must be selectively performed in cases of relapse or persistence of infection.

The goal of the management of reinfected urine is to achieve sterile urine; this is the basis for subsequent successful use of antimicrobial agents. To successfully eradicate urinary tract infections, antimicrobial agents should be administered in sufficient doses to exceed by a wide margin the minimal concentration required to inhibit growth. Lower dosages lead to the selection of resistant organisms from the original population in about 10% of the cases and complicates the treatment of these already difficult patients.

Recurrent cystitis should be documented by culture at least once and then managed by one of three strategies: continuous prophylaxis, postcoital prophylaxis, or therapy initiated by the patient (self-start therapy). Continuous prophylaxis has been shown to be highly cost effective and is recommended as the initial form of therapy in women who have frequent reinfections (113, 114). Its success depends on using the minimal dosage of an antimicrobial agent that has minimal or no adverse effect on the fecal flora. Once the urine has been completely sterilized by a full-dose course of therapy, nightly therapy is

Figure 28.6. Natural history of urinary tract infection.

Table 28.4. Correctable Urinary Tract Abnormalities Causing Persistent Bacteriuria

Urethral diverticulum
Infected stone
Significant anterior vaginal wall relaxation
Papillary necrosis
Foreign body
Duplicated or ectopic ureter
Atrophic pyelonephritis (unilateral)
Medullary sponge kidney

Table 28.5. Oral Antimicrobial Agents Useful for Prophylactic Prevention of Recurrent Urinary Tract Infections

Agent	Dosage
Nitrofurantoin	100 mg
Cephalexin	250 mg
TMP-SMX*	1 tablet
Cinoxacin	250–500 mg

*Each regular tablet contains 80 mg trimethoprim and 400 mg sulfamethoxazole.

begun with one of many different drugs (Table 28.5). Nitrofurantoin (113) 100 mg or cephalexin (114) 250 mg have been shown to be effective therapy. These drugs do not cause resistance in the fecal flora; however, vaginal colonization with sensitive bacteria does continue. Their efficacy depends on nightly bactericidal activity in the bladder urine against sensitive reinfecting organisms. The efficacy of cephalexin is dependent on use of a minimal dosage. If it is given four times a day in full dosages, it gives rise to resistant strains. When it is given in a dose of 250 mg nightly, it does not. TMP-SMX (115) is active, not only because of bactericidal activity against urinary bacteria but also because TMP diffuses into the vaginal fluid at a concentration bactericidal to most urinary pathogens (116). Low-dose TMP-SMX or TMP alone causes resistance in about 10% of rectal cultures (115). Most of these patients will continue to maintain sterile urine while on prophylactic therapy, although breakthrough infections may infrequently occur and should be treated with full-dose sensitive antimicrobial therapy. We empirically continue the prophylactic therapy for approximately 6 months and, at that time, follow the patient off therapy with frequent cultures. Approximately 30% of women will have a spontaneous remission for at least the following 6 months (112). Unfortunately, a remission does not necessarily reflect a complete cure. If reinfection occurs, it must be managed by reinstitution of low-dose nightly prophylaxis.

Self-start intermittent therapy can be an alternative to continuous prophylactic therapy in patients with recurrent urinary tract infections. When this regimen is used, the patient is given a dip-slide device and instructed to perform a urine culture when she has symptoms consistent with a recur-

rent urinary tract infection. She then empirically starts a 3-day course of full-dose antimicrobial therapy, usually with one of the previously mentioned antibiotics. Full-dose nitrofurantoin, cinoxacin, or norfloxacin are excellent choices. Norfloxacin seems to be an ideal drug for self-start therapy. It has a broader spectrum of activity than any other oral agent and is comparable with or better than most available parenteral antimicrobial agents. In addition, it has activity against multiple resistant bacteria, and bacteria exposed to this agent have a low rate of spontaneous mutation to resistant organisms. In a multicenter comparative study of over 350 patients with urinary tract infections, the percentage of strains susceptible to norfloxacin was 99%. This was significantly greater than the percentage of strains susceptible to TMP-SMX, which was approximately 90%. Also, the percentage of bacteriological cures was significantly higher with the norfloxacin (than TMP-SMX), and side effects were minimal (117).

If a patient's history suggests that reinfections are preceded by intercourse, she may take a single antimicrobial tablet before or after intercourse (118). Vosti (119) first demonstrated that nitrofurantoin given after coitus prevented recurrent urinary tract infection. More recently, Pfau et al. (120) showed that TMP-SMX, nalidixic acid, nitrofurantoin, and sulfonamide were all effective in preventing recurrent urinary tract infections when given to young sexually active women whose infections occurred postcoitally. If feasible, a woman who has recurrent urinary tract infections and uses a diaphragm as her mode of contraception should consider another method. If she is unable or unwilling to change to another method, she should be closely questioned about symptoms of urinary obstruction occurring with the diaphragm in place. If such symptoms occur, it should be ascertained if the fit of the diaphragm is too large. Women in this category of intercourse-related infection should also be advised to void as promptly as possible after intercourse. Postmenopausal women may also have frequent reinfections. These infections are sometimes attributable to residual urine after voiding, which is often associated with pelvic organ prolapse. In addition, the lack of estrogen causes marked changes in the vaginal microflora, including loss of bacilli and increased colonization by *E. coli* (121). Antimicrobial prophylaxis or topically applied estrogen cream are alternative preventive measures in such women.

COMPLICATED INFECTIONS

Complicated urinary tract infections occur in patients with functionally, metabolically, or anatomically abnormal urinary tracts or are caused by pathogens that are resistant to antibiotics. The clinical spectrum can range from mild cystitis to life-threatening urosepsis. In addition, there may be long periods of asymptomatic bacteriuria. Urine cultures therefore must be obtained in patients suspected of having complicated infection to identify the infecting pathogen and perform susceptibility testing. The wide variety of underlying conditions and diverse spectrum of possible etiologic agents make generalizing about antimicrobial therapy difficult. For empirical therapy in patients with mild to moderate illness who can be treated as outpatients, the fluoroquinolones provide a broad spectrum of antimicrobial activity covering most expected pathogens and achieve high levels in the urine. At least 10–14 days of therapy is usually necessary. Pseudomonas and enterococcal infections are especially difficult to treat and may warrant more prolonged therapy. Without correction of the underlying anatomic, functional, or metabolic defect, infection often recurs. For this reason, a urine culture should be repeated 1–2 weeks after the completion of therapy.

CATHETER-ASSOCIATED INFECTION

Catheter-associated urinary tract infection is the most common hospital-associated infection and is the most frequent source of bacteremia in hospitalized patients (122). One recent study showed a threefold increase in mortality in these patients (123). The mechanism through which bacteriuria is related to mortality is uncertain. Risk factors of catheter-associated infection are advanced age, female sex, and an increasing degree of underlying illness (124). The pathogenesis of catheter-associated urinary infection has not been studied as well as urinary tract infection of noncatheterized patients. Points of bacte-

Table 28.6. Prevention of Bladder Infection in Elderly Long-Term Catheterized Patients

Monitor urine level in bag every 4 h; exchange catheter if cessation of flow for 4 h
Fluid intake of 1.5 L/d
Avoid catheter manipulations
Exchange catheter if infection is suspected
Exchange catheter every 8–12 wk

rial entry, however, have been well defined and include introduction of bacteria residing in the urethra into the bladder at the time of catheterization, subsequent entry of bacteria colonizing the urethra meatus along the mucus sheath external to the catheter, and ascent of bacteria within the catheter lumen itself. The relative proportion of infections occurring through these different routes of entry have not been clearly defined. Recent prospective studies demonstrated that organisms causing infection in catheterized patients can be identified in the urethral or rectal flora 2–4 days before the onset of bacteriuria in 70% of women (125). Until more is known about the pathogenesis of nosocomial bacteriuria, the bulk of preventive efforts should continue to focus on aseptic care of the urinary catheter (126) (Table 28.6). There has been no demonstrable efficacy of local antimicrobial ointments applied to the meatal junction despite the apparent association of meatal colonization with subsequent infection (127, 128). The use of antimicrobial irrigants has also been ineffective in reducing the prevalence of bacteriuria (129). Although systemic antimicrobial agents reduce the occurrence of bacteriuria for the first few days of catheterization, their use cannot be widely recommended at this time because the benefit accrued, that is, reduction of asymptomatic bacteriuria, may not be worth the cost and attendant risk of development of resistant microorganisms (130).

The diagnosis and management of these urinary tract infections in elderly nursing home patients with long-term catheterization (greater than 3 months) can present a challenge. All patients with indwelling catheters for any length of time will develop bacteria in their urine (Fig. 28.7). However, as long as the catheter system is a closed functioning system and the patient is asymptomatic with no local or systemic symptoms or signs, there is no advantage to empirical systemic antibiotics. On the other hand, 10% of elderly patients with indwelling catheters will develop bacteremia and gram-negative septicemia, a serious disease with a 20–50% mortality. These patients must be promptly identified because they require hospitalization and vigorous systemic antibiotic therapy. A traumatic event consisting of ob-struction, manipulation, or removal of an inflated indwelling bladder catheter often precedes the onset of urosepsis. In addition to antibiotic therapy, it is essential to estab-lish free flow of urine for the catheterized patient with acute urosepsis. The complica-tions of concomitant bacteremia (shock, adult respiratory distress syndrome, dis-seminated intravascular coagulation, and gastric hemorrhage) must be readily recog-

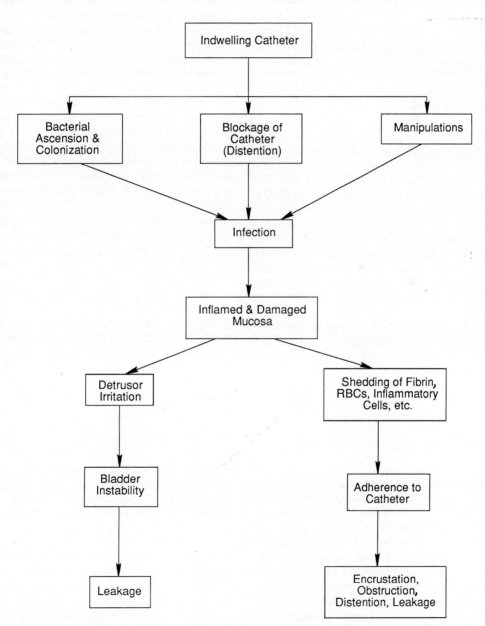

Figure 28.7. Pathogenesis of infection and clinical picture of females with long-term indwelling catheters.

64666486464644

nized and managed appropriately. Certain measures can be taken to prevent these life-threatening complications in patients with chronic indwelling catheters (Table 28.6). Catheters should be checked every 4 hours by experienced personnel to ensure proper drainage and no formation of any encrustation within the tubing of the catheter, and indwelling catheters should be changed every 8–12 weeks, depending on whether they are silicon- or Teflon-coated catheters.

Lower Urinary Tract Instrumentation

Whether patients undergoing lower urinary tract instrumentation for diagnostic or therapeutic purposes need prophylactic antibiotics is, currently, an unresolved issue. A recent prospective double-blind placebo-controlled study did note that when patients underwent urodynamic evaluations, endoscopic evaluations of the lower urinary tract, or urethral dilatations, patients receiving placebo had a significantly higher infection rate that those receiving either one dose of cefadroxil or three doses of nitrofurantoin (131). For this reason, we have adopted the policy of routine prophylaxis after patients undergo lower urinary tract instrumentation. In patients undergoing intermittent catheterization, bacteriuria may be reduced by bladder irrigation with a solution of neomycin or polymyxin or by oral methenamine, nitrofurantoin, or TMP-SMX prophylaxis (132).

Acute Pyelonephritis

Pyelonephritis is defined as inflammation of the kidney and renal pelvis, even though the diagnosis is based on clinical findings. Patients with acute pyelonephritis have chills, fever, and unilateral or bilateral costovertebral angle tenderness. These upper tract signs are often accompanied by dysuria, increased urinary frequency, and urgency. The urine is usually cloudy and malodorous, and in very rare cases, acute renal failure may be present.

Urine analysis notes the urinary sediment to show increased white cells, white blood cell casts, and red blood cells. Bacteria rods or chains of cocci are also often seen. Urine cultures grow various amounts of bacteria. Systemic blood tests may show polymorphonuclear leukocytosis, increased erythrocyte sedimentation rate, elevated C-reactive protein, and elevated creatinine if renal failure is present. The most common bacteria to cause acute pyelonephritis are those of the Enterobacteriaceae family. These include *E. coli* and species of *Klebsiella*, *Proteus*, *Enterobacter*, *Pseudomonas*, *Serratia*, and *Citrobacter*.

Only recently, the radiological findings characteristic of acute pyelonephritis have been emphasized. It has previously been thought that intravenous urogram in these patients were normal; however, in 24–28% of patients with acute pyelonephritis, abnormal urograms have been attributed to the acute disease (133, 134). Findings on intravenous urogram in patients with acute pyelonephritis have included renal enlargement, impaired contrast excretion, nonobstructive dilatation of the urinary collecting system, cortical striations in the nephrogram, and ureteral striations. Although renal ultrasound is useful to show renal size in most infected kidneys, no findings are seen on ultrasound that are not seen on the urogram. Contrast-enhanced CT are very sensitive for detection of renal enlargement, attenuated parenchyma, and compressed collecting systems characteristic of acute pyelonephritis. CTs, however, are not indicated unless the diagnosis cannot be established on urogram or renal ultrasound or if the patient does not respond to therapy.

The treatment of acute pyelonephritis should be subdivided into three categories: patients who have mild symptoms and do not warrant hospitalization; patients who are ill enough to warrant hospitalization for parenteral antibiotics; and infection associated with hospitalization, catheterization, urological surgery, or urinary tract abnormalities. For patients needing parenteral therapy, ampicillin and aminoglycoside have proven efficacy and offer effectiveness against most of the Enterobacteriaceae, *Pseudomonas*, and other gram-negative bacilli. In nonhospital-acquired infections, a third-generation cephalosporin is an

effective alternative. Both oral fluoroquinolones and TMP-SMX have proven to be
efficacious in those receiving outpatient
therapy. It is important that the patient understand that fever and flank pain may persist for several days after the initiation of
successful antimicrobial therapy. However,
if symptoms persist beyond this time, the
possibility of underlying renal or urinary
tract abnormalities should be considered
and radiological investigation with either
ultrasound, urography, or CT should be performed. The duration of therapy for acute
pyelonephritis should be 14 days (135). Repeat urine culture should be performed 5–7
days after initiation of therapy and 4–6
weeks after discontinuation of antimicrobial
therapy to ensure that the urinary tract remains free of infection. Between 10% and
30% of individuals with acute pyelonephritis relapse after a 14-day course of therapy.
Individuals who relapse usually are cured
by a second 14-day course of therapy, but
occasionally a 6-week course of therapy is
necessary.

REFERENCES

1. Fihn SD. Urinary tract infections in primary care obstetrics and gynecology. Clin Obstet Gynecol 1988;31:1003–1016.
2. National Center for Health Statistics. Ambula-tory medical care rendered in physicians offices. United States 1975. Adv Data 1977;12:1–8.
3. Cox LE, Lacy SS, Hinman F. The urethra and its relationship to urinary tract infection. II. The urethral flora of the female with recurrent uri-nary tract infection. J Urol 1968;99:632–638.
4. Winberg J, Anderson HJ, Bergstrom T, et al. Epidemiology of symptomatic urinary tract in-fection in childhood. Acta Paediatra Scand 1974;252(Suppl):3–21.
5. Rolleston GL, Shannon FT, Utley WLF. Relation-ship of infantile vesico-ureteric reflux to renal damage. Br Med J 1970;1:460–464.
6. Mulholland SG. Controversies in management of urinary tract infection. Urology 1986;27(Suppl):3–8.
7. Mayer TR. UTI in the elderly: how to select treatment. Geriatrics 1980;35:67–73.
8. Turck M, Stamm W. Nosocomial infection of the urinary tract. Am J Med 1981;70:651–659.
9. Maskell R. Importance of coagulase-negative Staphylococci as pathogens in the urinary tract. Lancet 1974;1:1155–1159.
10. Scllin M, Cooke DI, Gillespie WA, Sylvester DGH, Anderson JD. Micrococcal urinary tract infections in young women. Lancet 1975;2:570–575.
11. Cunha B. Urinary tract infections. I. Pathophysi-ology and diagnostic approach. Postgrad Med 1981;70:141–158.
12. Hovelius B. Urinary tract infections caused by *Staphylococcus saprophyticus* recurrences and complications. J Urol 1979;122:645–650.
13. Marrie T, Kwan C, Noble M, et al. *Staphylococ-cus saprophyticus* as a cause of urinary tract infections. J Clin Microbiol 1982;6:427–432.
14. Bailey RR. Significance of coagulase-negative Staphylococcus in urine. J Infect Dis 1973;127:179–183.
15. Wallmark G, Arremark I, Telander B. *Staphylo-coccus saprophyticus*: a frequent cause of acute urinary tract infection among female outpa-tients. J Infect Dis 1978;138:791–794.
16. Lewis JF, Brake SR, Anderson DJ, Vredeveld GD. Urinary tract infection due to coagulase-negative Staphylococcus. Am J Clin Pathol 1982;77:736–742.
17. Nicolle LE, Hoban SA, Harding GKM. Charac-terization of coagulase-negative Staphylococci from urinary isolates. J Clin Microbiol 1983;17:267–271.
18. Bryant RE, Sutcliffe MC, McGee FE. Human polymorphonuclear leukocyte function in urine. Yale J Biol Med 1973;46:113.
19. Kaye D. Antibacterial activity of human urine. J Clin Invest 1968;47:2374.
20. Stamey TA. Urinary tract infections in women. In: Stamey TA, ed. Pathogenesis and treatment of urinary tract infections. Baltimore: Williams and Wilkins, 1980:122–209.
21. Eden CS, Eriksson B, Hanson LA. Adhesion of *Escherichia coli* to human uroepithelial cells in vitro. Infect Immun 1977;18:767–773.
22. Stamey TA, Timothy MM. Studies of introital colonizations in women with recurrent urinary infections. I. The role of vaginal pH. J Urol 1975;114:261–265.
23. Parsons DL, Schmidt JD. Control of recurrent lower urinary tract infections in the postmeno-pausal women. J Urol 1982;128:1224.
24. Cox CE, Hinman F. Experiments with induced bacteriuria, vesical emptying and bacterial growth on the mechanism of bladder defense to infection. J Urol 1961;86:739.
25. Orskov I, Ferencz A, Orskov F. Tamm-Horsfall protein or uromucoid is the normal urinary slime that traps type I fimbriated *Escherichia coli*. Lancet 1980;1:887–893.
26. Parsons CL. Prevention of urinary tract infection by the exogenous glycosaminoglycan sodium pentosan polysulfate. J Urol 1982;127:167–173.
27. Parsons CL, Greenspan C, Moore SW, et al. Role of surface mucin in primary antibacterial de-fense of bladder. Urology 1977;9:48–52.
28. Reid G, Sobol JD. Bacterial adherence in the pathogenesis of urinary tract infection: a review. Rev Infect Dis 1987;9:470–487.
29. Kallonius G, Mollby R, Svenson SB, et al. The P^k antigen as receptor for the haemagglutinin of pyelonephritic *Escherichia coli*. FEMS Micro-biol Lett 1980;7:297.
30. Vaisanen V, Elo J, Tallgreen LG, et al. Mannose-resistant haemagglutination and P antigen rec-ognition are characteristic of *Escherichia coli*

causing primary pyelonephritis. Lancet 1981;2: 1366–1371.

31. Iwahi T, Abe Y, Nakao M, Imada A, Tsuchiya K. Rule of type I fimbriae in the pathogenesis of ascending urinary tract infection induced by *Escherichia coli* in mice. Infect Immun 1983;39: 307–314.

32. Schaeffer AJ, Jones JM, Dunn JK. Association of in vitro *Escherichia coli* adherence to vaginal and buccal epithelial cells with susceptibility of women to recurrent urinary tract infections. N Engl J Med 1981;304:1062–1066.

33. Schaeffer AJ, Amundsen SK, Schmidt LN. Adherence of *Escherichia coli* to human urinary tract epithelial cells. Infect Immunol 1979;24: 753–757.

34. Schaeffer AJ, Radvany RM, Chmiel JS. Human leukocyte antigens in women with recurrent urinary tract infections. J Infect Dis 1983;148: 604–610.

35. Kinane DF, Blackwell CC, Brettle RP, et al. ABO blood group, secretor state and susceptibility to recurrent urinary tract infection in women. Br Med J 1982;285:7–11.

36. Nicolle LE, Harding GKM, Preiksaitis J, Ronald AR. The association of urinary tract infection with sexual intercourse. J Infect Dis 1982;146: 579–584.

37. Strom BL, Collins M, West SL, et al. Sexual activity, contraceptive use, and other risk factors for symptomatic and asymptomatic bacteriuria. Ann Intern Med 1987;107:816–823.

38. Fihn SD, Latham RH, Roberts P, et al. Association between diaphragm use and urinary tract infection. JAMA 1985;253:240–244.

39. Foxman B, Frerichs RR. Epidemiology of urinary tract infection. I. Diaphragm use and sexual intercourse. Am J Public Health 1985;75:1308–1315.

40. Fihn SD, Johnson L, Pinkstaff C, Stamm WE. Diaphragm use and urinary tract infection. Analysis of urodynamic and microbiologic factors. J Urol 1986;136:853–856.

41. Kass EH. Asymptomatic infections of the urinary tract. Trans Assoc Am Physicians 1956; 69:56.

42. Kass EH. Bacteriuria and diagnosis of infections of the urinary tract. Arch Intern Med 1967;100: 709–714.

43. Stamey TA, Govan DE, Palmer JM. The localization and treatment of urinary tract infections: the role of bactericidal urine levels as opposed to serum levels. Medicine 1965;44:1–8.

44. Turck M, Goffe B, Petersdorf RG. The urethral catheter and urinary tract infection. J Urol 1962; 88:834–837.

45. Thiel G, Spuhler O. Urinary tract infection by catheter and the so-called infectious (episomal) resistance. Schweiz Med Wochenschr 1965;95: 1155.

46. Fihn SD, Stamm WE. Management of women with acute dysuria. In: Rund D, Wolcott BW, eds. Emergency medicine annual. Connecticut: Appleton-Century-Crofts, 1983;2:225.

47. Stamm WE. Measurement of pyuria and its relation to bacteriuria. Am J Med 1983;75:53.

48. Johnson JR, Stamm WE. Diagnosis and treatment of acute urinary tract infection. Infect Dis Clin North Am 1987;1:773–779.

49. Free AH, Free HM. Urinalysis: its proper role in the physician's office. Clin Lab Med 1986;6: 253–259.

50. Wu TC, Williams EC, Koo SY, et al. Evaluation of three bacteriuria screening methods in a clinical research hospital. J Clin Microbiol 1985;21: 796–814.

51. Kunin CM. Detection, prevention and management of urinary tract infection, 4th ed. Philadelphia: Lea and Febiger, 1987:195–234.

52. Schaeffer AJ. The office laboratory. Urol Clin North Am 1980;7:29–58.

53. Reid G. The office microbiology laboratory. Urol Clin North Am 1986;13:569–576.

54. Bixler-Forell E, Bertram MA, Bruckner DA. Clinical evaluation of three rapid methods for the detection of significant bacteriuria. J Clin Microbiol 1985;22:62–68.

55. Needham CA. Rapid detection methods in microbiology: are they right for your office? Med Clin North Am 1987;71:591–605.

56. Kraft JK, Stamey TA. The natural history of symptomatic recurrent bacteriuria in women. Medicine 1977;56:55–61.

57. Mabeck CE. Studies in urinary tract infections. I. The diagnosis of bacteriuria in women. Acta Med Scand 1969;186:35–41.

58. Kunz HH, Sieberth HG, Freiberg J, et al. Zur Bedeutung der Blasenpunktion fur den sicheren Nachweis einer Bacteriurie. Dtsch Med Wochenschr 1975;100:2252.

59. Stamm WE, Counts GW, Running KR, et al. Diagnosis of coliform infection in acutely dysuric women. N Engl J Med 1982;307:463–467.

60. Kass EH. The role of asymptomatic bacteriuria in the pathogenesis of pyelonephritis. In: Quinn EL, Kass EH, eds. Biology of pyelonephritis. Boston: Little, Brown, 1960:399.

61. Fowler JE Jr, Pulaski T. Excretory urography, cystography, and cystoscopy in the evaluation of women with urinary tract infection. N Engl J Med 1981;304:462–468.

62. Engel G, Schaeffer AJ, Grayhack JT, et al. The role of excretory urography and cystoscopy in the evaluation and management of women with recurrent urinary tract infection. J Urol 1980; 123:190–198.

63. DeLange HE, Jones B. Unnecessary intravenous urography in young women with recurrent urinary tract infections. Clin Radiol 1983;34: 551–556.

64. Fair WR, McClennan BL, Jost RG. Are excretory urograms necessary in evaluating women with urinary tract infections? J Urol 1979; 121:313.

65. Mogensen P, Hansen LK. Do intravenous urography and cystoscopy provide important information in otherwise healthy women with recurrent urinary tract infection? Br J Urol 1983; 55:261.

66. Newhouse JH, Rhea JT, Murphy RX, et al. Yield of screening urography in young women with urinary tract infection. Urol Radiol 1982;4:187.

67. Tanagho EA, Miller ER, Lyon HP, Fisher R. Spastic striated external sphincter and urinary tract infection in girls. Br J Urol 1971;43:69.

68. Gallagher DJ, Montgomerie JZ, North JD. Acute infections of the urinary tract and the urethral syndrome in general practice. Br Med J 1965; 1:622.

69. Gillespie WA, Henderson EP, Linton KB, et al. Microbiology of the urethral (frequency and dysuria) syndrome. A controlled study with 5 year review. Br J Urol 1989;64:270–274.

70. Bergman A, Karram MM, Bhatia NN. Urethral syndrome: a comparison of different treatment modalities. J Reprod Med 1989;34:157–160.

71. Stamm WE, Running K, McKevitt M, et al. Treatment of acute urethral syndrome. N Engl J Med 1981;304:956–960.

72. Sobota AE. Inhibition of bacterial adherence by cranberry juice: potential use for the treatment of urinary tract infections. J Urol 1984;131: 1013–1017.

73. Kunin CM, Finland M. Clinical pharmacology of the tetracycline antibiotics. Clin Pharmacol Ther 1961;2:51.

74. Francke EL, Neu HC. Chloramphenicol and tetracyclines. Med Clin North Am 1987;71: 1155–1168.

75. Parsons CL. Urinary tract infections in the female patient. Urol Clin North Am 1985;12: 355–361.

76. Reed MD, Blumer JL. Urologic pharmacology in the office setting. Urol Clin North Am 1988;15: 737–751.

77. Conklin JD. The pharmacokinetics of nitrofurantoin and its related bioavailability. Antimicrob Agents Chemother 1978;25:233–237.

78. Mayrer AR, Andriole VT. Urinary tract antiseptics. Med Clin North Am 1982;66:199–216.

79. Hoener B, Patterson SE. Nitrofurantoin disposition. Clin Pharmacol Ther 1981;29:808–815.

80. Kalowski S, Rudford N, Kincaid-Smith P. Crystalline and macrocrystalline nitrofurantoin in the treatment of urinary tract infection. N Engl J Med 1974;290:385–389.

81. Reed MD, Besunder JB, Blumer JL. Sulfonamides. In: Koren G, Prober CG, Gold R, eds. Antimicrobial therapy in infants and children. New York: Marcel Dekker, 1988:153–172.

82. Weinstein L, Madoff MA, Samet CM. The sulfonamides. N Engl J Med 1960;263:793–801.

83. Hooper DC, Wolfson JS. The fluoroquinolones: pharmacology, clinical uses and toxicities in humans. Antimicrob Agents Chemother 1985; 28:716–722.

84. Neu HC. Quinolones: a new class of antimicrobial agents with wide potential uses. Med Clin North Am 1988;72:623–636.

85. Wise R, Griggs D, Andrews JM. Pharmokinetics of the quinolones in volunteers: a proposed dosing schedule. Rev Infect Dis 1988;10(Suppl 1):S83–S89.

86. Wolfson JS, Hooper DC. The fluoroquinolones: structures, mechanisms of action and resistance, and spectra of activity in vitro. Antimicrob Agents Chemother 1985;28:581–590.

87. Childs SJ, Goldstein EJ. Ciprofloxacin as treatment for genitourinary tract infection. J Urol 1989;141:1–5.

88. Goldstein EJ, Alpert ML, Najem A. Norfloxacin in the treatment of complicated and uncomplicated urinary tract infections: a comparative multicenter trial. Am J Med 1987;82:65–69.

89. Lee C, Ronald AN. Norfloxacin: its potential in clinical practice. Am J Med 1987;82:27–34.

90. Guttmann D. Follow-up of urinary tract infection in domiciliary patients. In: Brumfitt W, Asscher AW, eds. Urinary tract infection. London: Oxford University Press, 1973:62.

91. Mabeck CE. Treatment of uncomplicated urinary tract infection in non-pregnant women. Postgrad Med 1972;48:69–81.

92. Zhanel GG, Handing GRM, Guay DRP. Asymptomatic bacteriuria: which patients should be treated? Arch Intern Med 1990;150:1389–1396.

93. Andreole VT, Patterson TF. Epidemiology, natural history, and management of urinary tract infections in pregnancy. Med Clin North Am 1991;75:359–373.

94. Kass EH, Platt R. Urinary tract and genital mycoplasmal infection. In: Wald NJ, ed. Antenatal and neonatal screening, 1st ed. New York: Oxford University Press, 1984:345–357.

95. Platt R. Adverse consequences of acute urinary tract infections in adults. Am J Med 1987; 82(Suppl 6B):47–52.

96. Evans DA, Kass EH, Hennekens CH, et al. Bacteriuria and subsequent mortality in women. Lancet 1982;1:156–161.

97. Fihn SD. Single-dose antimicrobial therapy for urinary tract infections: "less is more?" or "reductio ad absurdum?" J Gen Intern Med 1986;1: 62–65.

98. Brumfitt W, Faiers MC, Franklin INS. The treatment of urinary infection by means of a single dose of cephaloxidine. Postgrad Med 1970;46: 65–72.

99. Buckwold FJ, Ludwid P, Godfrey KM, et al. Therapy for acute cystitis in adult women: randomized comparison of single-dose sulfasoxazole vs trimethoprim-sulfamethoxazole. JAMA 1982;247:1839–1843.

100. Rubin RH, Fang LST, Jones SR, et al. Single-dose amoxicillin therapy for urinary tract infection. JAMA 1980;244:561–564.

101. Greenberg RN, Sanders CV, Lewis AC, et al. Single-dose cefaclor therapy of urinary tract infection: evaluation of antibody-coated bacteria test and C-reactive protein assay as predictors of cure. Am J Med 1981;71:841–847.

102. Bailey RR, Abbott GD. Treatment of urinary tract infection with a single dose of amoxicillin. Nephron 1977;18:316–321.

103. Ireland D, Tacchi D, Bint AJ. Effect of single-dose prophylactic cotrimoxazole on the incidence of gynaecological postoperative urinary tract infection. Br J Obstet Gynaecol 1982;89:578–585.

104. Tolkoff-Rubin NE, Weber D, Fang LST, et al. Single dose therapy with trimetho-prim-sulfamethoxazole for urinary tract infection in women. Rev Infect Dis 1982;4:443–447.

105. Fang LST, Tolkoff-Rubin NE, Rubin RH. Efficacy of single-dose and conventional amoxicillin

therapy in urinary tract infection localized by the antibody-coated bacteria technic. N Engl J Med 1978;298:413–418.

106. Fihn SD, Johnson C, Roberts PL, Running K, Stamm WE. Trimethoprim-sulfamethoxazole for acute dysuria in women: a double-blind, randomized trial of single-dose versus 10-day treatment. Ann Intern Med 1988;108:350–357.

107. Ronald AR, Boutros P, Mourtada H. Bacteriuria localization and response to single-dose therapy in women. JAMA 1976;235:1854–1858.

108. Hooten TM, Winter C, Tiu F, Stamm WE. Randomized comparative trial and cost analysis of 3-day antimicrobial regiments for treatment of acute cystitis in women. JAMA 1995;273: 41–45.

109. Wathne B, Hovelius B, Mardh PA. Causes of frequency and dysuria in women. Scand J Infect Dis 1987;19:223.

110. Kraft JK, Stamey TA. The natural history of symptomatic recurrent bacteriuria in women. Medicine 1977;56:55–64.

111. Stamm WE, McKevitt M, Counts GW, et al. Is antimicrobial prophylaxis of urinary tract infections cost effective? Ann Intern Med 1981;94: 251–256.

112. Nicolle LE, Ronald AR. Recurrent urinary tract infections in adult women. Infect Dis Clin North Am 1987;1:793–814.

113. Stamey TA, Condy M, Mihara G. Prophylactic efficacy of nitrofurantoin macrocrystals and trimethoprim-sulfamethoxazole in urinary infections: biologic effects on the vaginal and rectal flora. N Engl J Med 1977;296:780–788.

114. Martinez FC, Kindrachuk RW, Thomas E, et al. Effect of prophylactic low dose cephalexin on fecal and vaginal bacteria. J Urol 1985;133: 994–998.

115. Stamm WE, Counts GW, McKevitt M, et al. Urinary prophylaxis with trimethoprim and trimethoprim-sulfamethoxazole: efficacy, influence on the natural history of recurrent bacteriuria, and cost control. Rev Infect Dis 1982;4: 450–461.

116. Stamey TA, Condy M. The diffusion and concentration of trimethoprim in human vaginal fluid. J Infect Dis 1975;131:261–268.

117. Sabbaj J, Hoagland VL, Shih WJ. Multiclinic comparative study of norfloxacin and trimethoprim-sulfamethoxazole for treatment of urinary tract infections. Antimicrob Agents Chemother 1985;27:297–302.

118. Wong ES, McKevitt M, Running K, et al. Management of recurrent urinary tract infections with patient–administered single-dose therapy. Ann Intern Med 1985;102:302–309.

119. Vosti KL. Recurrent urinary tract infections: prevention by prophylactic antibiotics after sexual intercourse. JAMA 1975;231:934–938.

120. Pfau A, Sacks T, Englestein D. Recurrent urinary tract infections in premenopausal women: pro-

phylaxis based on an understanding of the pathogenesis. J Urol 1983;129:1152–1160.

121. Raz R, Stamm WE. A controlled trial of intra-vaginal estriol in postmenopausal women with recurrent urinary tract infections. N Engl J Med 1993;320:753–756.

122. Kreger DE, Creven DE, Carling PC, McCabe WA. Gram negative bacteremia. III. Reassessment of etiology, epidemiology and ecology in 612 patients. Am J Med 1980;68:332–338.

123. Platt R, Polk BF, Murdock B, Rosner B. Mortality associated with nosocomial urinary tract infection. N Engl J Med 1982;307:736–745.

124. Garibaldi RA, Burke JP, Dickman ML, Smith CB. Factors predisposing to bacteriuria during indwelling urethral catheterization. N Engl J Med 1974;291:215–221.

125. Garibaldi RA, Burke JP, Britt MR, Miller WA, Smith CB. Meatal colonization and catheter-associated bacteriuria. N Engl J Med 1980;303: 316–321.

126. Wong ES, Hooton TM. Guidelines to prevention of catheter-associated urinary tract infection. Infect Control 1980;2:125–136.

127. Burke JP, Jacobson JA, Garibaldi RA, Conti MT, Alling DW. Evaluation of daily meatal care with poly-antibiotic ointment in prevention of urinary catheter-associated bacteriuria. J Urol 1983;129:331–334.

128. Burke JP, Garibaldi RA, Britt MR, Jacobson JA, Conti MT, Alling DW. Prevention of catheter-associated urinary tract infections. Am J Med 1981;70:655–661.

129. Warren JW, Platt R, Thomas RJ, Rosner B, Kass EH. Antibiotic irrigation and catheter-associated urinary tract infections. N Engl J Med 1978;299:570–576.

130. Britt MR, Garibaldi RA, Miller WA, Helertson RM, Burke JP. Antimicrobial prophylaxis for catheter-associated bacteriuria. Antimicrob Agent Chemother 1977;11:240–246.

131. Bhatia NN, Bergman A. Role of antibiotic prophylaxis following instrumentation of the lower urinary tract. In: Proceedings of the International Continence Society. London: International Continence Society, 1985:301.

132. Kuhlemeier K, Stover SL, Lloyd LK. Prophylactic antibacterial therapy for preventing urinary tract infections in spinal cord injury patients. J Urol 1985;134:514–518.

133. Little PJ, McPherson DR, Wardener HE. The appearance of the intravenous pyelogram during and after pyelonephritis. Lancet 1965;1: 1186–1190.

134. Silver TM, Kass EM, Thornburg JR, et al. The radiological spectrum of acute pyelonephritis in adults and adolescents. Radiology 1976;118: 65–69.

135. Ronald AR. Optimal duration of treatment for kidney infection. Ann Intern Med 1987;106: 467–468.

CHAPTER 29

Interstitial Cystitis

C. Lowell Parsons

Introduction

Interstitial cystitis (IC) is a clinical syndrome composed of significant urinary urgency, frequency, and/or pain in the absence of any other definable cause. In most patients, onset is gradual with an insidious progression. The question could be posed "what is the diagnosis for an individual in an early phase of IC?" To define this syndrome, it is important to consider this fact, especially since the early (mild) phase of this problem may be known by many names, such as chronic bacterial cystitis, urethral syndrome, trigonitis, urgency-frequency syndrome, or pseudomembranous trigonitis. All these descriptions reduce to one common problem, urinary urgency, frequency, and/or pain in the absence of bacterial infection (or other definable pathology). Most patients may belong to the same disease process but represent different phases (early versus late). The milder form of disease may be present in perhaps 50% of individuals who are initially diagnosed as having recurrent urinary tract infection but who, in fact, will have negative cultures (1). These are the people whose symptoms persist despite antibiotic therapy. Most will resolve spontaneously after several weeks or months and go undiagnosed because they represent no major clinical problem (or the person will learn to "live with their symptoms"). These individuals would not be diagnosed with IC but, in fact, are likely to have it.

There are many misconceptions concerning IC because it is a diagnosis of exclusion. Confusion exists as to what an abnormal voiding pattern is, what cystometrogram findings should be present, what a normal bladder capacity under anesthesia is, what a Hunner's ulcer looks like, whether or not glomerulations exist, and what pathological changes are found. We review these problems to clarify what changes are present and actually represent the pathological processes known to be associated with IC to better understand the diagnosis and therapy.

Definition

The definition of IC has been changing significantly in recent years secondary to the marked interest in studying this disease. In 1987, a group of interested researchers met at the National Institutes of Health to establish clinical criteria for characterizing the IC syndrome patient for research studies (2). Although these were not meant to be diagnostic criteria for IC, they represented the first attempt to quantify some of the changes. In fact, most researchers have become much more liberal in their definition of the disease. Although these were criteria meant to be used to study IC, it was well accepted by the group that they represented only a portion of the patients (perhaps one third or less) because many people with the IC syndrome do not have all the published parameters of IC. For example, it was stated that the symptoms had to be present more than 12 months or the patient needed to have glomerulations on cystoscopy, and neither criterion is important.

The sine qua non of the definition of IC is that the patient has significant urinary urgency, frequency, and/or bladder pain sufficient to be an iatrogenic stimulus. Upon clinical evaluation, these patients should have no other definable pathology such as urinary infections, carcinoma, radiation, or medication-induced cystitis. It may well be that this syndrome encompasses a number of different etiologies but with a bladder insult that ultimately results in urinary frequency and urgency that is essentially its only clinical response to noxious stimuli. This expansion of the definition is controversial, but as clinical and epidemiological data accumulate, it is steadily becoming accepted. In this review of IC, this more liberal definition is used.

An important purpose for using a broad definition of the syndrome is that IC is underdiagnosed. Many patients with milder forms could readily benefit from therapy if the diagnosis is considered. Treatment may be withheld if the physician reserves the diagnosis of IC for the more severe and "classic" symptoms.

Incidence/Epidemiology

Although IC was first identified in 1907 by Nitze (3), few epidemiological studies have been reported. In a Finnish study of 103 people with IC, Oravisto (4) estimated an annual incidence of 1.2 cases per 100,000 and a prevalence of about 10–11 per 100,000.

The incidence in the United States has been estimated from two sources. Held et al. (5) estimated about 44,000 cases in the United States; the author's estimate extrapolated from San Diego County is placed at 40–60,000. Held et al. also estimated a worst case scenario in the United States at 450,000.

DEMOGRAPHIC FACTORS

The studies mentioned above reveal several risk factors. Sex is a risk factor, with a female-to-male ratio of about 9:1 (5–8) in all reports. Age is also a risk factor, with incidence generally limited to those over 18 years of age but some reported cases in younger people (9–12). Median age of diagnosis is between 40 and 46 in most series, with disease appearing several years earlier (5, 6, 13). Race and ethnicity appear to be a risk factor, occur-

ring mostly in caucasians (14–16) but also reported in African-Americans (17).

In a review of 300 cases at the University of California, San Diego, it was also observed that those without diabetes (no diabetes seen) seem to be at a greater risk (13). Finally, a 400% increased incidence was seen in Jewish people. All these findings are similar to those seen in inflammatory bowel diseases (6, 18–23).

Pathogenesis

IMMUNE SYSTEM

Since the original description of the "elusive ulcer" of Hunner approximately 75 years ago, there has been slow progress in defining the etiology of this disorder (24, 25). Many etiologies have been suggested, including lymphatic, chronic infection, neurological, psychological, autoimmune disorders, and vasculitis (26–34). Most of the proposed etiologies are hypothetical, with little data to define the role of these mechanisms. Oravisto (33) suggested mild increases in antinuclear antibodies in approximately 50% of patients with IC. More recently, Ochs et al. (35) also found mild elevation of antinuclear antibodies, which may represent an effect of chronic injury rather than a primary immune activity. Currently, there is little to suggest the immune system as a major etiological factor in most cases, but perhaps it is important in some subsets or in disease progression.

EPITHELIAL LEAK

One major theory of the etiology of IC is that there is a defective bladder epithelium with loss of the "blood-urine" barrier resulting in a leaky membrane (36–38). An epithelium permeable to small molecules could then explain many of the symptoms associated with the complex. Chronic leak of small solutes such as potassium could actually induce sensory nerves to depolarize, resulting in urgency-frequency (39–41). This concept is attractive, particularly because most patients do not have any significant signs of inflammatory responses in their bladder muscle or urine, and no more than one third of patients has mast cells to explain the sensory/urgency induced from their degranulation (32, 42–44).

An epithelial leak could be secondary to problems such as vascular defects, mast cells, defective mucus, or urinary factors. There have been some limited data to support the concept that such a leak existed (36, 38). Regarding the morphological data, a subsequent study was unable to confirm the initial electron microscopic observations that both normals and IC patients (three) had similar findings in their tight junctions relative to ruthenium red penetration. However, a controlled study in 56 patients provided data to support the hypothesis that the bladder surface in patients with IC may indeed leak solutes (37). These investigators subsequently reported a more sensitive assay to detect an epithelial leak. In their patient population, approximately 70% of patients with IC have a "leaky epithelium," whereas 30% do not. They suggested that those who do not leak have some other problem, such as neurological abnormality (e.g., neurogenic inflammation). They further emphasized that these findings support the concept of several etiologies of urgency-frequency syndrome.

GLYCOSAMINOGLYCANS: THE BLOOD-URINE BARRIER

Control of epithelial permeability in the bladder has long been believed to be due to tight junctions unique to the bladder epithelium, the hydrophobic bilipid membrane, and ion pumps (36, 45–51). However, recent studies provided data to suggest that the bladder surface proteoglycans or glycosaminoglycans (GAG) may actually be another critical component of the mechanism by which the epithelium maintains a barrier between the bladder wall and urine, the so-called "blood-urine" barrier (37, 39, 40).

Surface proteoglycans (GAG, mucus) appear to have multiple roles in the bladder, including antiadherence and regulation of transepithelial solute movement (40, 52–54). The cell's external surface GAG are capable of preventing the adherence of bacteria, crystals, proteins, and ions, a function that is lost when this layer is removed with a dilute acid or detergent (55) but restored when GAG is replaced by exogenous polysaccharides such as heparin or pentosanpolysulfate (PPS) (52, 56, 57). GAG prevents solute movement by tightly binding water, which acts as a physical barrier to molecular movement (Fig. 29.1).

Highly charged cationic amines, on the other hand, have a high affinity for sulfated polysaccharides and will displace the water bound to the oxygen groups (58–60). It has been demonstrated both in animal and human models that protamine sulfate will inactivate native cell surface polysaccharides and result in increased epithelial permeability and induce symptoms of urgency and frequency (39, 40). The impermeability to urea in normal individuals increases from 5% to 25%. In these studies, the increased permeability in normal human subjects resulted in urgency, frequency, and bladder pain, symptoms that were reversed with a subsequent treatment with heparin. Because damage to the transitional cell mucus can be reversed by

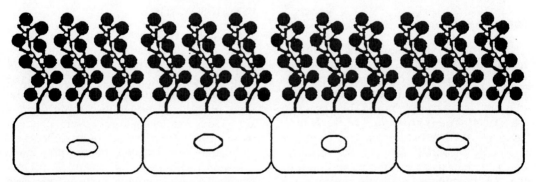

Figure 29.1. The concept of a biofilm layer at the bladder surface is schematically shown and demonstrates the location of the trapped water at the surface. Circles represent bound water and the wavy lines the protein backbone.

the addition of GAG such as heparin or PPS, it opens new possibilities for therapeutic roles for these agents (39, 40).

Based on these concepts, Parsons and colleagues (61–63) proposed that the surface polysaccharide is functionally defective (not absent) in patients with IC. The cause for the deficiency could include diminished density or thickness of material, reduced sulfation of the polysaccharides, or the presence of a compound such as a urinary quaternary amine. Based on these studies, sulfated polysaccharides were examined for treatment in IC and are discussed under Therapy.

INFECTION

From the time the disease was defined by Hunner, infection has been implicated as a possible etiological factor for IC, especially because infection induces the same symptoms. Studies, however, to document bacterial infection in IC have been unsuccessful. No clearcut evidence to date exists to suggest bacteria, fungi, or virus plays a role (28, 64, 65), and of course the disease is defined in part by having sterile urine by conventional cultures.

More recently, Lowentritt et al. (66) used cultures of bladder biopsies to grow fastidious forms of bacteria and the polymerase chain reaction (PCR) technique. A well-conserved bacterial gene has been used for PCR (16S rRNA) studies and may have some promise as a tool to find fastidious bacteria causing an infection similar to peptic ulcer where bacteria interferes with the function of gastric mucus.

INFLAMMATION

Controversy exists concerning the role of mast cells in IC. Mast cells have been reported by a number of investigators to be present in IC biopsies, whereas others believe they are also present in non-IC bladders (32, 34, 43, 44). The central point of the controversy is whether or not mast cells play a causative, secondary, or no role. Causative here is defined as degranulating and producing the symptoms or, on the other hand, representing a response to whatever is causing IC (e.g., an epithelial leak) and becoming

a type of defense mechanism that may ultimately be part of the problem.

There have been attempts at quantitating mast cells (granulated and degranulated) both in the mucosa and in the subepithelial tissues (67–69) to better understand what may be occurring in the bladder wall. Degranulation of mast cells in an animal model causes a significant epithelial leak (70, 71). Although not yet resolved, the presence of mast cells in one third of patients may result in degranulation and symptom aggravation. Control of this degranulation (even though the cells may be a defense mechanism) may be helpful therapy, especially in allergic or atopic patients, and is discussed later.

The role of inflammation and inflammatory mediators in IC is not known. Traditionally, the concept that inflammation is present in IC is probably not the case in most patients. Several points can be made that support the notion that inflammation plays little role in IC. First, on biopsy specimens, almost no inflammation is seen. Second, no systemic signs are found (e.g., no leucocytosis) (72). And finally, no inflammatory mediators are found in the urine of over 90% of these patients (73). Also against the role of inflammation, patients with IC do not suffer from other generalized inflammatory problems such as collagen vascular diseases (26, 31). Additionally, steroids and nonsteroidal anti-inflammatory agents are ineffective in controlling IC pain, whereas narcotics will relieve it. On the other hand, there may be significant interplay between mast and inflammatory cells (their mediators) that is yet to be determined in subsets of patients.

PSYCHOSOMATIC

IC has been suggested to be of psychosomatic origin, but this is not substantiated by any clinical data. Most patients (especially with chronic pain) are secondarily affected by their disease and as a result may show signs of mild or moderate chronic depression. Those suffering from severe nocturia will exhibit even more profound depression and agitation due to sleep deprivation. Early researchers reported that essentially no one has ever been cured of IC by psychotherapy (27). This is certainly true in the author's experience. Treating depression can improve overall sense of well-being for a patient and help them cope with their disease, but it will not cure the IC or reduce the number of their daily voids. It is true that acute emotional stress will flare IC symptoms and stress reduction will improve them, but the patient will continue to have IC. The physician should emphasize to the patient that IC is not a psychological disorder.

Pathology

One of the main diagnostic problems with IC is the lack of pathological findings readily identified and quantified. Various nonspecific descriptions have been proposed, but unfortunately there is nothing pathognomonic of IC in bladder biopsy specimens. In addition, in reported studies, biopsies are usually obtained after a hydrodistention that causes severe artifacts such as edema and hemorrhage. The mast cell controversy has already been reviewed; approximately one third of these patients have increased mast cell infiltration of their bladder wall and mucosa, significance unknown. Light microscopy generally reveals a urothelium that is thinned, readily detached, and nearly absent in many areas.

Unlike the normal six- or seven-layer-thick epithelium, the mucosa is frequently only two to four cell layers thick. These changes are consistent with a dysfunctional epithelium (37). A generalized pancystitis (64, 74–76) with infiltration of the lamina propria by mononuclear and chronic inflammatory cells is seen. However, these changes are also consistent with the effects of hydrodilation.

The ulcer originally described by Hunner (24, 25) is not a true ulcer because the epithelium over it is usually intact. Instead, it is a reddish patch that appears quite similar to carcinoma in situ. When present, it is best seen clinically with little to observe pathologically. These ulcers are rare (6–8% of patients) and represent a late or severe manifestation of disease seen in "end-stage bladders" (13).

The distribution of collagen within the bladder wall is controversial (77). One hypothesis suggests that as the disorder progresses, a fibrotic small end-stage type bladder develops. There is little or no data to support this theory. The author believes this to be untrue and, instead, believes that an epithelial leak and frequent low volume voiding leads to a thinned epithelium with atrophic muscle bundles resulting in a small bladder. Furthermore, the only scarring present in the bladder wall is probably iatrogenic, stemming from prior biopsies because many of these patients undergo multiple biopsies over years (77). This is exemplified by the study of Johansson and Fall (77), who biopsied scar sites (shown in their illustrations) and found fibrosis but normal appearing areas showed no fibrosis. As the entire bladder shrinks from frequent low volume voiding, this scar tissue takes on a disproportionate and artifactual enlarged total volume of the bladder wall. In the author's experience (over 500 biopsies), scarring, in fact, is not identified when biopsies are obtained from an area of the bladder not previously biopsied.

Although cell surface mucus (GAG) appears to be physiologically dysfunctional, its anatomic presence is hard to quantify. Studies have conflicted on the presence or absence of this layer. Morphological quantification of this material is not reliable, but recent advances (78, 79) may help provide a marker for this disease. Both believe the surface GAG or its associated proteoglycans may be altered in IC.

The main point relative to biopsy is that IC cannot be diagnosed by it. There is no way to rule in or out this disorder by pathological examination of bladder tissue. Some of the changes as mentioned above, however, do support the diagnosis. Although it is rare that these patients are confused with those having carcinoma in situ of the bladder, the biopsy may be necessary to rule out cancer. A combination of cytological evaluation of the urine and bladder washings plus the biopsy may be necessary to exclude malignancy. If cystoscopy is normal, cytologies are sufficient.

Signs and Symptoms

The primary symptom of IC is the presence of abnormal sensory urgency. From sensory urgency derives urinary frequency. In addition, most patients have associated bladder pain. A recent study (13) showed that of the patients presenting with IC, approximately 15% have little to no bladder pain, whereas 85% present with significant pain. It is important to determine whether or not the pain is of bladder origin. To do this, ask the patient if the pain (despite being constantly present) worsens as the bladder fills with urine and improves (not disappears) with voiding. Bladder pain of IC is experienced suprapubically, in the perineum, vaginally, or in the low back or medial aspect of the thighs (27). Two thirds of patients do not experience dysuria.

Nocturia is variable, but in general, 90% of the patients complains of voiding at least one to two times per night (13). Nocturia increases with the severity and duration of the disease. The average patient voids approximately 16 times per day; a minimum for diagnostic purposes is 8 voids per day (2). The average voided volume is 106 mL (Table 29.1).

Between 85% and 90% of individuals with IC are female. Of those who are sexually active, most (75%) complain of exacerbation of the symptom complex associated with sexual intercourse (13). It is likely that any woman regularly taking antibiotics after sexual intercourse does not have recurrent cystitis but rather IC. Symptoms usually flare for 2–3 days and then subside, corresponding to the usual length of antibiotic therapy. The increase in symptoms may be felt during sexual activity, immediately after, or within 24 hours. In addition, most women who are still menstruating will complain of a flare of symptoms just before or at the time of the menstrual cycle (13, 27).

The typical age of diagnosis in IC is between 40 and 46 years with an average duration of symptoms for 3–4 years (13, 27).

Evaluation

The physician struggles to establish a diagnosis of IC primarily because no objective "blood test" exists. Evaluation of large numbers of patients with the urgency-frequency syndrome reveals historical and clinical findings that help establish the diagnosis.

In August 1987, a group of investigators and patients interested in IC met at the National Institutes of Health and defined the National Institute of Diabetes and Digestive and Kidney Diseases (NIDDKD) criteria to establish the diagnosis for research purposes (2). These criteria are a practical attempt to quantitate findings in IC. In part, they were based on a study reported by Parsons (13) where the symptoms of over 200 IC patients were measured and analyzed. From Parsons' data, each variable was examined; the point that included 90% of the patients was the number taken for the NIDDKD criteria. For example, 90% of IC patients were found to void at least one to two times at night, complained of eight or more voidings during the day, and had moderate urinary urgency, but the presence of bladder pain was optional. Nocturia is not necessary to establish a diagnosis. The data upon which these criteria were based are reported in Table 29.2. It is important to note that these criteria were developed to provide uniform findings for researchers investigating IC. They were never meant to be a gold standard for diagnosis. Patients meeting this criteria have advanced disease. There are many patients with IC (perhaps most) who do not meet these criteria but have the disease and will benefit from therapy.

VOIDING FREQUENCY

Assessment of voiding frequency is quite useful and can be determined from a 3-day voiding log where each voiding is measured and recorded. From such data it was found that the average patient voids 16 times per day with a capacity of 106 mL (Table 29.1). The voiding profile is a useful method to

Table 29.1. Voiding Profiles of 250 Patients With Interstitial Cystitis

	Number of Voidings (per day)	Voided Volumes (mL)	Nocturia
Average	15.6	121	4.7
90% Confidence limit[a]	9	175	1.5
Range	7–45	26–325	0–13

[a]90% of patients had at least this level.

Table 29.2. Urinary Symptoms

	Values
Nocturia	
Mean	4.7
90% cutoff level[a]	1.5 (1–2 voidings)
Range	0–13
1–2	41 (18%)
2–4	90 (90%)
4.5–8	63 (28%)
Daytime frequency	
Mean	16.0
90% cutoff level	7
Range	5.5–40
Urgency	
Mild	8 (3.5%)
Moderate	63 (28%)
Moderate-Severe	35 (15.5%)
Severe	119 (53%)
Pain	
None	41 (18%)
Mild	16 (7%)
Moderate	82 (36%)
Severe	86 (39%)

Symptoms reported in 225 patients. Included are frequency distributions for symptom severity.
[a]Present in 90% of patients.

Table 29.3. Changes Associated With Duration of Interstitial Cystitis

	Average at 1 Year[a]	Average at >7 Years[b]
Number of patients	34	42
Voidings	15.2	17.3
Voided volume (mL)	128	105
Anesthetic capacity (mL)	711	518

[a]Represents patients with 1 year of symptoms.
[b]Represents patients with >7 years of symptoms.

establish not only the diagnosis of IC but also subsequently to create and evaluate the success of a therapeutic plan during follow-up care. As might be anticipated, patients with a longer disease history have a smaller functional bladder capacity as reflected in the average voided volume and number of daily voidings (Table 29.3).

Duration of symptoms helps to define patients with IC requiring therapy from those with a milder urgency-frequency syndrome. Because response to treatment takes time, the presence of continuous symptoms for at least 6 months helps distinguish those patients who need therapy from the milder problems that resolve spontaneously.

PHYSICAL EXAMINATION

There is one important part of the examination that helps to confirm the diagnosis of IC. On physical examination, over 95% of patients complains of a tender bladder base during the pelvic examination. Their discomfort is easily elicited by palpation of the anterior vaginal wall and the bladder.

Urine analysis on voided specimens is not useful in these patients because their low voided volumes make midstream collection impossible. One sees primarily vaginal secretions unless a catheterized specimen is obtained. A catheterized specimen examined under the microscope should show no bacteria and most show no red or white blood cells. Urine should be sent for cytological evaluation to rule out the possibility of carcinoma. In the absence of hematuria, cytology alone in the female is sufficient to rule out carcinoma.

URINARY MARKERS

A number of studies attempted to identify a possible urinary marker for IC. A variety of inflammatory factors have been examined, including interleukins, but no real differences between most IC patients and normals have been found (81). There is increased output of kallikrein in the urine (82), especially those with prominent pain as a symptom.

Urinary GAG excretion seems to be reduced overall in the IC population as does a glycoprotein called GP51 (83, 84). Metaloproteases are also increased in the IC population and have a potential as a marker for IC (85).

Although it is possible that some of these markers may be beneficial in understanding the pathogenesis of IC and also as a marker of the disease, it is not yet clear as to what their usefulness will be.

Urodynamics

The cystometrogram (CMG) is a valuable study to perform in patients with this syndrome in that a normal CMG essentially excludes the diagnosis of clinically significant IC. Because all patients complain of significant urinary urgency, this can usually be documented with cystometry. If gas is used, patients experience a sensation of significant urgency at less than 125 mL, and with water, <150 mL (water is recommended as more reliable). If this portion of the CMG is normal, they probably do not have IC or only a mild form. In 75 patients with CMGs reported by Parsons (13), the average bladder capacity was 220 mL with over 90% of patients having a volume of less than 350 mL (Table 29.4). However, there is an important caveat relative to maximum bladder capacity. A small group of patients with significant IC will develop detrusor myopathy (about 5%) (13, 86). Individuals with this complication have large atonic bladders with little muscle present. They have moderate to severe sensory urgency, large bladder capacities (>1000 mL), and usually carry residual urine (>100 mL). Detrusor function is poor or absent. Because most patients are females, they are able to void but primarily with a Valsalva maneuver. This subgroup represents approximately 5% (Table 29.4) of patients with IC (13). Males with detrusor myopathy may require a program of intermittent catheterization as part of their treatment.

POTASSIUM TEST

A simple method has been devised by Parsons (the Parsons test) to measure epithelial permeability. The test is based on the hypothesis that if one places a solution of KCl into a normal bladder, it provokes no symptoms of urgency or pain. On the other hand, if placed into a bladder with an impaired mechanism to maintain the impermeable epithelium, then the potassium diffuses across the transitional cells to stimulate sensory nerves and cause urgency or pain.

To perform the test, two solutions are placed into a bladder for 5 minutes. Solution 1 is sterile water and solution 2 contains 400 mEq/L of KCl. The volume used is 40 mL to reduce stimulation due to volume.

After instilling the solution for 5 minutes, the patient is asked about their symptoms on a scale of 0–5 (Table 29.5). If the patient does not respond to water and states the KCl solution is causing their symptoms to increase (2 or better), this is considered a positive test. In a recent study, 70% of patients (58) had provocation of symptoms, whereas only 4% (1 of 22) of normals responded. It is a useful test to separate epithe-

Table 29.4. Results of Cystometrograms in 200 Patients With Interstitial Cystitis

	Values
Average capacity	242 mL ± 110
90% cutoff level	<350 mL
Postvoid residual >50 mL	12/200 (6%)
Number with increased sensory urgency[a]	192/200 (96%)
Patients with uninhibited contractions	11/200 (5.5%)
Detrusor myopathy	8/200[b](4%)

Average capacities and 90% cutoff levels are listed. Patients with uninhibited contractions did not respond to anticholinergic therapy.
[a]Patients with urgency at <100 mL. All had urgency at <125 mL.
[b]Detrusor myopathy is described by Holm-Bentzen.[86]
All patients suspected had cystometrograms demonstrating increased sensory urgency, postvoid residuals >50 mL, and poor detrusor contractions. Detrusor volumes were >750 mL.

Table 29.5. Grading Scale for Symptoms

	None	Mild		Moderate		Severe
Pain	0	1	2	3	4	5

	None	Mild		Moderate		Severe
Urgency	0	1	2	3	4	5

Questions
1. Which solution is worse? ____ Solution 1 ____ Solution 2 ____ Neither
2. Is the difference between solutions
   ____ None ____ Mild ____ Moderate ____ Severe

NOTE: Each subject was told to consider their symptoms at the start as baseline of 0. When a solution was added, they were asked if it provoked symptoms (pain or urgency) on a scale of 0–5.

lial leakers from nonleakers and to detect an abnormal permeability barrier.

CYSTOSCOPIC EVALUATION

Cystoscopic evaluation of the bladder under anesthesia is both a diagnostic and therapeutic maneuver but is more useful for therapy because absence of findings does not exclude the diagnosis. Examination under local anesthesia is to be discouraged because it offers little help in diagnosis (except to exclude carcinoma) and causes the patient severe discomfort. It is recommended that when IC is suspected and a cystoscopy is necessary (e.g., hematuria is present in a male over 40), then it should be performed under anesthesia.

The cystoscopy under anesthesia is performed in a manner to both diagnose and treat. The diagnosis depends on discovering one of two findings, a Hunner's ulcer, or the presence of glomerulations or petechial hemorrhages. However, not all patients show these changes, so absence does not exclude the diagnosis.

Cystoscopy

The cystoscopy should be performed in two phases. Phase one is the initial inspection. Here the physician should obtain specimens for cytology and urine for regular and tuberculosis culture (optional because it is almost never diagnosed). Visual examination of the bladder may reveal a true Hunner's ulcer (patch). The patch is velvety red and present in only 8% of patients (13) and is very similar in appearance to carcinoma in situ. However, it is not actually a true ulcer. A biopsy should not be performed at this part of the cystoscopy. Prior biopsy site scars, frequently mistaken for ulcers, may also be seen (77). Bladders with IC appear to heal poorly, and biopsy scars are frequently large but are recognized by the spoke wheel growth of neovascularity that radiate from the central scarred portion. These scars frequently tear and bleed after distention and account for most so-called epithelial disruptions. Parsons (13) reported as many as 75% of ulcers described at previous cystoscopy by other urologists to actually be biopsy site scars.

The second phase of the cystoscopic procedure is the hydrodistention to demonstrate glomerulations, which will also induce a disease remission in 60% of patients. Hydrodistention is performed by filling the bladder slowly up to 80–100 cm H_2O pressure maximum. The urethra of the female should be manually compressed over the cystoscope to prevent leakage of fluid or else adequate distention for therapy will not be achieved. After several minutes, the bladder is emptied. The last part of the effluent is usually bloody if glomerulations (petechial hemorrhage) or ulcers are present. When the bladder is reexamined, the glomerulations should be demonstrated. They are diffusely located around the bladder, at least 10–20 per field of vision. Hemorrhages on the trigone or posterior bladder wall are irrelevant and do not constitute a positive finding because they represent cystoscope trauma. Hemorrhages probably represent abnormal and fragile microvasculature but are by no means pathognomonic for IC and their absence does not exclude the diagnosis.

What constitutes an abnormal bladder capacity under anesthesia is surprising to many physicians. A normal female bladder holds well over 1000 mL, whereas the IC bladder usually holds less than 850 mL (13). The average anesthetic capacity for IC patients is between 550 and 650 mL (Fig. 29.2). Patients with a longer history of symptoms have smaller bladder capacities, suggesting the disease is slowly progressive (13). This is also supported by the fact that patients with Hunner's ulcers have the worst symptoms and also have the smallest bladder capacities and the greatest epithelial leaks (13, 37).

BIOPSY

The last part of the cystoscopic procedure should be the biopsy. One should *never* biopsy before hydrodistention because the bladder could tear at the biopsy site, leading to a significant bladder rupture. If one is using a caustic agent for therapy, *never* biopsy before the solution is placed in the bladder. Should the solution extravasate through the biopsy site, severe tissue damage may occur.

The biopsy itself is not diagnostic for IC but can rule out other diseases such as carcinoma in situ. The findings on pathological exami-

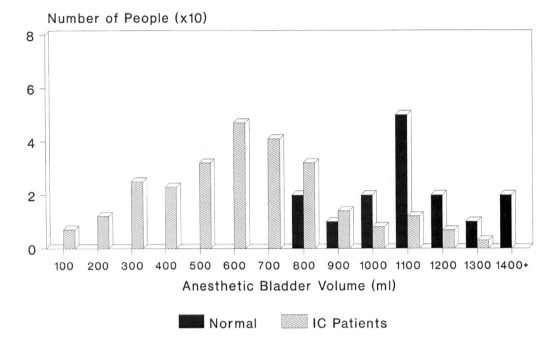

Number of People (x10)

Anesthetic Bladder Volume (ml)

■ Normal ▨ IC Patients

Avg Normal = 1115 ml, N=15   Avg IC = 575 ml, N=270

Figure 29.2. Normal bladder capacities for 270 IC patients were measured under anesthesia, and for purposes of presentation each unit of the ordinate represents 10 people. Fifteen normals, females being treated for stress incontinence, were also measured.

nation include the presence of mast cells (demonstrated by toluidine blue staining) (67, 69), inflammatory cells, and a thinned mucosa. A normal biopsy does not exclude IC and should not be used in diagnosis.

Although diagnosis of IC depends in part on abnormal cystoscopic findings, one cannot arbitrarily rule out the disease purely by the endoscopic findings. There are many patients who have IC without such findings who benefit from therapy. The physician needs to be aware of the fact that this disease complex is still primarily manifested by significant urinary urgency or frequency and perhaps few or no other findings other than negative tests.

Therapy

Few advances had been made in therapy for IC until recently. Most medications were used empirically, and all were studied without controls. Drugs used for IC included anticholinergics, antihistamines, analgesics, and antiinflammatories. Future drug efficacy studies should include controls to demonstrate whether therapy is active but are unlikely to be performed for readily available medications. Traditional and newer therapies that should aid the physician treating IC are reviewed.

When discussing therapy with an individual who has IC, it is important for the physician to emphasize that for symptoms present for more than 1 year, no particular therapy is likely to be curative. Although he or she may have a significant remission of symptoms, in all probability, relapse will eventually occur. If patients are prepared for this eventuality, they are much less distressed when symptoms return and cope better with their disease. The physician-patient relationship is strengthened in terms of credibility if this area is addressed before treatment. Patients readily accept this explanation and overall appear to cope better with their problem when they have a realistic outlook.

ANTIDEPRESSANT THERAPY

Chronic pain and sleep loss cause depression; thus, it is valuable to place most IC patients on antidepressant medications. Tricyclic antidepressants have several beneficial modes of action. They cause side effects of drowsiness (aids sleep), increase pain thresholds, and elevate the mood. If tricyclic antidepressants are used, start with low doses (25 mg amitriptyline 1 hour before bedtime) and warn patients they will be tired (for 12–15 h/d) for the first 2–3 weeks of therapy. Once they become tolerant to this side effect, increase slowly, if needed, to a larger dose. Amitriptyline, or imipramine (87), can be prescribed in doses beginning at 25 mg (or even 10 mg) 1 hour before bedtime. If fluoxetine (Prozac®) is selected, use 20 mg/d and increase if needed to 40 mg. Sertraline (Zoloft) is another well-tolerated antidepressant used in a dose of 50 mg/d and may be increased to 100 mg if needed.

Antidepressant therapy is an important adjunct to treatment. It does not cure IC, but patients function much better with their disabling symptoms if not depressed. In essence, they "feel better" even if they still void 20 times per day. Antidepressants may not cure IC, but surprisingly, many will improve dramatically only with this therapy, especially those with a negative potassium test (normal epithelium), which suggests these patients may have a type of "neurogenic inflammation."

HYDRODISTENTION OF THE BLADDER UNDER ANESTHESIA

The report by Bumpus in 1930 (88) of bladder hydrodistention improving the symptoms of IC resulted in this procedure becoming a mainstay of therapy. Few would question the activity of hydrodistention in ameliorating the symptoms in 60% of IC patients. The procedure must be performed under anesthesia because the dilation causes pain. The procedure for hydrodistention has been described under diagnosis. Pressure dilatation of the bladder using a syringe is not recommended because it can result in bladder rupture; a maximum of 80–100 cm H_2O pressure is best to use.

The mechanism by which hydrodistention improves symptoms is unknown; several theories have been postulated. Neuropraxis induced by mechanical trauma may occur in some individuals. Few patients awaken with decreased pain, which would support the neuropraxis concept. Rather, most (80%) awaken from anesthesia with significantly worse pain that slowly improves over 2–3 weeks. This pain usually requires narcotic analgesia until remission occurs. We believe most patients' symptoms are exacerbated by hydrodistention because of epithelial damage by mechanical trauma. The disruption in the integrity of the mucosal cells increases the epithelial leak, causing symptoms to flare. Healing may occur over the next several weeks, which correlates with the time of clinical remission. Perhaps the epithelium regenerates and for a period of time is "healthy" and impermeable. Then, whatever events initiate the disease continue and relapse occurs.

Remission may persist between 4 and 12 months, and hydrodistention may be repeated as needed. If no remission is obtained, repeat the dilation at least two more times because frequently in our experience, patients respond to a subsequent dilation. In general, most patients obtain less beneficial effects as the procedure is repeated.

DIMETHYLSULFOXIDE

Dimethylsulfoxide (DMSO) was approved for use in IC in 1977 (89). Although no controlled clinical trials were ever conducted with DMSO, it does appear to induce remission in 34–40% of the patients. The difficulty with DMSO is that it may induce an excellent remission in the first one to three cycles of therapy, but as an individual relapses and requires subsequent treatment, progressive resistance to its beneficial effects is seen in most patients.

For treatment, 50 mL of 50% DMSO is instilled into the bladder for 10–15 minutes. Longer periods are unnecessary because DMSO rapidly exerts its effect. Instillations are performed on an outpatient basis or patients can be taught to perform it themselves. The author recommends that patients receive six to eight weekly treatments to determine whether a therapeutic response is achieved. If the patient has moderate or worse symptoms, continue the therapy for an additional 4–6 months once every other week. Remember, once DMSO therapy is stopped, the patient is likely to become resistant to its use. Many patients experience a flare of symptoms when DMSO is placed into the bladder. This phenomenon may be related to DMSO's ability to destroy the surface epithelial cells in a detergent-like effect (in a sense it works similarly to distention) (41, 90). Nonetheless, DMSO may be very effective at treating these patients. Should the patient experience pain with DMSO, it is recommended that he or she receive intravesically 10 mL of 2% viscous xylocaine jelly 15 minutes before placing DMSO. If this is not successful, then use an injectable narcotic before the intravesical instillation. The flare of symptoms associated with DMSO usually disappears over 24 hours. As these patients receive subsequent treatments, the pain tends to diminish.

Patients may also receive indefinite therapy using DMSO. As originally reported by Stewart et al. (89), patients used DMSO weekly for several years without problems. DMSO has been associated with cataracts in animals; however, this complication has not been reported in humans. If your patient is on chronic therapy, it is recommended that he or she have a slit lamp evaluation at perhaps 6-month intervals.

ANTIHISTAMINES

Antihistamines have been tried in IC but without controlled studies. Antihistamines were chosen because of the possible role of mast cells (74, 75, 91, 92). In the author's experience, antihistamines are very useful in the management of IC in patients with allergies (pollen, food, sinusitis). In fact, atopic individuals may not respond to other therapies (e.g., DMSO) unless their mast cells are inhibited. Theoharides (93) recommended the chronic use of hydroxyzine (Atarax®, Vistaril®) at doses of 25–50 mg daily. This medication is believed to work best if used for at least 2–3 months. Chronic use stabilizes mast cells and reduces allergic symptoms. We have likewise found hydroxyzine to be the best antihistamine to use and very effective at suppressing the seasonal flares of IC. Like amitriptyline, it is a tricyclic compound and results in a tiring effect that will dis-

appear after 2–3 weeks of use. The patient should be warned of this effect and encouraged to stay on the drug.

ANTIINFLAMMATORIES

Because of the assumption that inflammation plays a role in this disorder, patients have received both steroidal and nonsteroidal drugs. Badenoch (94) found significant improvement in 19 of 25 patients treated with prednisone. However, all were treated after hydrodistention under anesthesia that may have been responsible for most of the benefit. In this author's experience, neither steroidal nor nonsteroidal analgesics work to ameliorate the symptoms of this complex. As with most drugs, clinical trials have not been conducted on the efficacy of these compounds in IC. Perhaps the lack of effect on inflammation-suppressing agents further suggests the immune system is not usually involved in causing symptoms in IC.

INTRAVESICAL SILVER NITRATE

Intravesical silver nitrate was first reported in 1926 by Dodson (95). Pool (96) fashioned a treatment regimen in which bladder irrigations were begun under anesthesia with a 1:5000 concentration. This was followed subsequently by gradually increasing the concentrations on a daily basis, ultimately using a 1% solution. Again, this was done in an uncontrolled setting on patients who had dilatation of the bladder under anesthesia. Pool reported good results in 89% of patients. Other uncontrolled studies reported that this compound is helpful, but it is not very widely used today. One caution in the use of silver nitrate: never instill into the bladder after biopsy. If there is a perforation and this solution is placed into the bladder, intra- and extraperitoneal extravasation could occur, resulting in major tissue damage. Silver nitrate activity is probably related to its ability to injure surface epithelial cells (similar to distention, DMSO) inducing new production of umbrella cells and their mucus.

INTRAVESICAL SODIUM OXYCHLOROSENE (CLORPACTIN WCS-90®)

Clorpactin is a highly reactive chemical compound that is a modified derivative of

hypochlorous acid in a buffered base. Its
activity is dependent on the liberation of
hypochlorous acid and its resulting oxidiz-
ing effects and detergency (97). Wishard et
al. (97), who treated 20 patients with five
weekly instillations of 0.2% Clorpactin
WCS-90 under local anesthesia, reported
improvement in 14 of 20 patients, and
follow-up was brief. Messing and Stamey
(8), treating 38 patients with 0.4% Clorpactin, reported significant improvement in
72%. Ureteral reflux is a contraindication to
the use of Clorpactin. It is recommended
that the compound usually be used under
anesthesia. Chlorpactin also causes a pain
flare before its beneficial effects occur, suggesting a similar activity as distention,
DMSO, and silver nitrate.

HEPARIN

Heparin, when given by injection, has
been reported to alleviate the symptoms of
IC (98). Again, this was not in a controlled
study. Chronic systemic heparin therapy
cannot be used in most individuals because
it results in osteoporosis in 100% of patients
who use it for 26 weeks. In the author's
experience, intravesical heparin has significant activity in approximately 50% of patients. Here too the data were obtained in an
uncontrolled investigation. Previous controlled studies (examining the activity of
pentosanpolysulfate) by the author demonstrated a placebo effect in IC patients of
approximately 20%. Assuming a similar rate
for the heparin study, the 50% activity of
heparin may be real (62). The technique uses
10,000 units of heparin in 10 mL of sterile
water. The patient is instructed in self-
administration at home. Initially, this solution is instilled intravesically five to seven
times per week. This treatment can be carried on indefinitely. It takes 3–6 months to
see improvements. The best improvements
are noted after 1–2 years. Long-term therapy
is recommended for patients with moderate
or worse disease who respond to its use.
However, once the patient shows improvement, they can be slowly tapered to three
times per week. Serum prothrombin time,
partial thromboplastin time, and platelets
are monitored for the first 3 weeks after
therapy begins to rule out the formation of
an unusual antibody to heparin. After 3

weeks, if no problems are found, these blood
studies are no longer necessary. Heparin is
not absorbed across the bladder mucosa so
it is safe to use indefinitely.

PPS

Parsons and colleagues (61–63) first reported PPS as active at ameliorating the
symptoms of IC. Because PPS (Elmiron®) is
a highly charged anionic sulfated polysaccharide, theoretically it may augment the
bladder surface defense mechanism or de-
toxify in urine agents that have a capacity to
attack the bladder surface (e.g., quaternary
amines or other highly charged cations). In
a controlled clinical study, 42% of patients
had their symptoms controlled versus 20%
for placebo (62). This has been borne out in
several subsequent studies, including a five-
center trial where 28% of patients versus
13% on placebo improved (63) and in a
seven-center study of 150 patients where
there was a 32% patient improvement versus 15% on placebo (99). Additionally, an
English-Danish study also found a significant reduction of pain in patients on drug
compared with placebo (44). Elmiron® is not
currently approved for use in the United
States but may be available soon and one
could check its status with the manufacturer
Baker-Norton, Inc. in Miami, Florida. It is
used in an oral dose of 100 mg three times
per day but may be increased to 400–600
mg/d. In patients with moderate disease, it
appears to have about 40–50% activity. In
the controlled clinical trials that were done
on patients with severe disease, its activity
was lower. Continued use of Elmiron® for
several years leads to long-term disease control in most of the drug responders. Response to therapy is first seen after 6–10
weeks but may take 6–9 months to work.
Patients do better after 6–12 months of
therapy.

SURGERY

Approximately 3% of patients presenting
with IC to the University of California, San
Diego, Medical Center have ultimately undergone some type of surgery for disease that
is severe and refractory to all treatment. The
question is the type of surgery to be performed.

CYSTOLYSIS

Attempts at surgical ablation of the bladder innervation by cystolysis are to be discouraged because most patients will fail this and develop a neurogenic bladder with significant urinary pain as the nerves regenerate.

BLADDER AUGMENTATION

A concept exists that these patients have small bladders and thus void frequently. Actually the reverse is true. They have sensory urgency, void frequently, and subsequently develop a small bladder. Hence, attempts to augment the bladder with a patch of bowel are likely to fail. Patients will then have a capacity that is large, have more difficulty emptying (usually requiring intermittent catheterization), but still retain all their sensory urgency and pain (100). Almost all reports of successful therapy have subsequently been recanted by the authors performing this surgery.

URINARY DIVERSION ALONE

There are no controlled studies evaluating diversion alone, but studies suggest it is not effective (101). In counseling, one should tell patients that diversion alone may not be sufficient to control their pain and they may subsequently require a cystectomy. The patient can then decide whether or not they want a risk of more than one surgery.

CYSTECTOMY AND DIVERSION

This is the mainstay of therapy for patients with "end-stage bladder." Before contemplating major therapy, several caveats are offered. First, the patient should have failed all above conservative treatment. Second, the clinician should be sure that the pelvic pain is from the bladder. The pain should be increased when the patient holds her urine and somewhat relieved by voiding. A CMG should be performed to be sure that filling the bladder causes pain. If these conditions are met, then in our experience 95% of patients will be relieved of their pain (Table 29.6). We performed 16 continent diversions for IC and four patients developed pouch pain (after 2–3 years). All 16 patients are at least 5 years

Table 29.6. Surgery for Interstitial Cystitis[a]

Treatment	Persistent Pain	No Pain
Cystectomy	1/25	24/25 (96%)

[a]Twenty-five patients underwent cystectomy for interstitial cystitis at University of California, San Diego. After 6 months, only one patient had persistent pelvic pain. That patient did not have "classic bladder pain" that increases with bladder filling but rather pelvic pain unrelated to voiding.

status after diversion. It would appear that most do not develop pouch pain. The pouch pain has been controlled with chronic instillation of 10,000 units of heparin placed into the pouch after each catheterization.

BLADDER TRAINING

Whatever therapy is successful at alleviating the pain and sensory urgency of IC, the individual afflicted with the chronic form of the disease will have a small capacity bladder that is in part based on sensory urgency and in part on frequent low volume voiding, a type of disuse atrophy. The author discovered that in several controlled clinical trials, even with good remission of pain and urgency, there is almost no change in urinary frequency over a 12-week period. This issue must be addressed to obtain a functional recovery of the bladder. Persistent urinary frequency from a small bladder can be reversed after therapy has controlled urgency and pain. This is accomplished by training the patients to undergo a program of progressively holding their urine to increase their bladder capacity (102). A urological nurse can direct this therapy. To begin this treatment, obtain a 3-day voiding profile from the patient (to include time of voiding and a measurement of volume). Determine the average time interval between voids and gradually increase this interval monthly. For example, if the patient voids every hour, it is recommended that he or she attempt to void every 1.25 hours and at the end of 1 month increase that to 1.5 hours. The patient should never progress too quickly because he or she will become discouraged and drop out. It takes 3–5 months of this protocol to see results. At the end of 3–4 months, the bladder capacity will increase approximately two and one half times with a corresponding reduction in urgency and the number of voidings per day (102).

We also discovered that in patients who have minimal or no pain associated with their urinary frequency, bladder training may be the only therapy required to improve them and in fact the only therapy that is effective. For more details concerning the use of this protocol, the reader is referred elsewhere (102).

Summary

IC is a syndrome in a state of rapid change regarding the understanding of the pathogenesis and the development of therapy due to a significant increase in research activity. These investigations will help the clinician quantitate the symptoms and clinical findings to better diagnose the syndrome and will simultaneously lead to improved treatment strategies which will result in symptom reduction (hydrodistention, DMSO, Elmiron®, heparin, or hydroxyzine). In addition, bladder training methods can further rehabilitate the patient with the IC bladder. As reviewed herein, perhaps 75–85% of patients with moderate to severe IC can experience significant remission with conservative therapy and avoid the need for extirpative surgery.

REFERENCES

1. Hamilton-Miller JMT. The urethral syndrome and its management. J Antimicrob Chemother 1994;33(Suppl A):63–73.
2. Gillenwater JY, Wein AJ. Summary of the National Institute of Arthritis, Diabetes, Digestive and Kidney diseases workshop on interstitial cystitis, National Institutes of Health. Bethesda, Maryland, August 28–29, 1987. J Urol 1988;140:203–206.
3. Nitze M. Lerbuch der Kystoscopie: Ihre Technik und Klinische Bedeuting. Berlin: JE Bergman, 1907:410.
4. Oravisto KJ. Epidemiology of interstitial cystitis. 1. In: Hanno PM, Staskin DR, Krane RJ et al, eds. Interstitial cystitis. London: Springer-Verlag, 1990:25–28.
5. Held PJ, Hanno PM, Pauly MV, et al. Epidemiology of interstitial cystitis. 2. In: Hanno PM, Staskin DR, Krane RJ, et al. Interstitial cystitis. London: Springer-Verlag, 1990:29–48.
6. Oravisto KJ. Epidemiology of interstitial cystitis. Ann Chir Gynaecol Fenn 1975;64:75–77.
7. Walsh A. Interstitial cystitis. In: Harrison JH, Gittes RF, Perlmutter AD, et al., eds. Campbell's urology, 4th ed. Philadelphia: WB Saunders, 1978.
8. Messing EM, Stamey TA. Interstitial cystitis: early diagnosis, pathology, and treatment. Urology 1978;12:381–392.
9. Farkas A, Waisman J, Goodwin WE. Interstitial cystitis in adolescent girls. J Urol 1977;118:837–839.
10. Bowers JE, Lattimer JK. Interstitial cystitis. Surg Gynecol Obstet 1957;105:313.
11. McDonald HP, Upchurch WE, Artime M. Bladder dysfunction in children caused by interstitial cystitis. J Urol 1958;80:354.
12. Lapides J. Observations on interstitial cystitis. Urology 1975;5:610–611.
13. Parsons CL. Interstitial cystitis: clinical manifestations and diagnostic criteria in over 200 cases. Neurourol Urodyn 1990;9:241–250.
14. Pool TL. Interstitial cystitis: clinical considerations and treatment. Clin Obstet Gynecol 1967;10:185–191.
15. De Juana CP, Everett JC. Interstitial cystitis: experience and review of recent literature. Urology 1977;10:325–329.
16. Hanno P, Wein A. Interstitial cystitis, parts I and II. Baltimore: American Urological Association, Update Series 1987:19.
17. Smith BH, Dehner LP. Chronic ulcerating interstitial cystitis (Hunner's ulcer). Arch Pathol 1972;93:76–81.
18. Bures J, Fixa B, Komarkova O, et al. Nonsmoking: a feature of ulcerative colitis. Br Med J 1982;285:440.
19. Calkins B, Lilienfeld AM, Mendeloff AI, Garland C, Monk M, Garland FC. Smoking factors in ulcerative colitis and Crohn's disease in Baltimore. Am J Epidemiol 1984;122:498.
20. Cope GF, Heatley RV, Kelleher J, Lee PN. Cigarette smoking and inflammatory bowel disease: a review. Human Toxicol 1987;6:189–193.
21. Paulley JW. Ulcerative colitis: a study of 173 cases. Gastroenterology 1950;16:566.
22. National Center for Health Statistics. Health and nutrition examination survey, cycle II, 1976–1980. Washington DC: Government Printing Office, 1985.
23. Lilienfeld AM, Lilienfeld DE. Foundations of epidemiology, 2nd ed. New York: Oxford, 1980.
24. Hunner GL. A rare type of bladder ulcer in women. Report of cases. Boston Med Surg J 1915;172:660–664.
25. Hunner GL. Elusive ulcer of the bladder: further notes on a rare type of bladder ulcer with a report of 25 cases. Am J Obstet 1918;78:374.
26. Oravisto KJ, Alfthan OS, Jokinen EJ. Interstitial cystitis. Clinical and immunological findings. Scand J Urol Nephrol 1970;4:37–42.
27. Hand JR. Interstitial cystitis, a report of 223 cases. J Urol 1949;61:291.
28. Hanash KA, Pool TL. Interstitial and hemorrhagic cystitis: viral, bacterial and fungal studies. J Urol 1970;104:705–706.
29. Oravisto KJ, Alfthan OS. Treatment of interstitial cystitis with immunosuppression and chloroquine derivatives. Eur Urol 1976;2:82–84.

30. Gordon HL, Rosen RD, Hersh EM, Yium JJ. Immunologic aspects of interstitial cystitis. J Urol 1973;109:228–233.

31. Silk MR. Bladder antibodies in interstitial cystitis. J Urol 1970;103:307–309.

32. Holm-Bentzen M, Lose G. Pathology and pathogenesis of interstitial cystitis. Urology 1987;29(4 Suppl):8–13.

33. Oravisto KJ. Interstitial cystitis as an autoimmune disease. A review. Eur Urol 1990;6:10–13.

34. Weaver RG, Dougherty TF, Natoli C. Recent concepts of interstitial cystitis. J Urol 1963; 89:377.

35. Ochs RL, Stein TW Jr, Peebles CL, Gittes RF, Tan EM. Autoantibodies in interstitial cystitis. J Urol 1994;151:587–592.

36. Eldrup J, Thorup J, Nielsen SL, Hald T, Hainau B. Permeability and ultrastructure of human bladder epithelium. Br J Urol 1983;55:488–492.

37. Parsons CL, Lilly JD, Stein P. Epithelial dysfunction in non-bacterial cystitis (interstitial cystitis). J Urol 1991;145:732–735.

38. Völter D, Weisswange V, Ziegler H, Schubert GE. Die xenon-exhalationsmessung im rahmen der diagnostik von hernblasenerkrankungen. Urologe 1975;14:38–40.

39. Lilly JD, Parsons CL. Bladder surface glycosaminoglycans: a human epithelial permeability barrier. Surg Gynecol Obstet 1990;171:493–496.

40. Parsons CL, Boychuk D, Jones S, Hurst R, Callahan H. Bladder surface glycosaminoglycans: an epithelial permeability barrier. J Urol 1990;143: 139–142.

41. Hohlbrugger G, Lentsch P. Intravesical ions, osmolality and pH influence the volume pressure response in the normal rat bladder, and this is more pronounced after DMSO exposure. Eur Urol 1985;11:127–130.

42. Lynes WL, Flynn SD, Shortliffe LD, et al. Mast cell involvement in interstitial cystitis. J Urol 1987;138:746–752.

43. Hanno P, Levin RM, Monson FC, et al. Diagnosis of interstitial cystitis. J Urol 1990;143:278–281.

44. Holm-Bentzen M, Jacobsen F, Nerstrom B, et al. Painful bladder disease: clinical and pathoanatomical differences in 115 patients. J Urol 1987; 138:500–502.

45. Englund SE. Observation on the migration of some labeled substances between the urinary bladder and blood in rabbits. Acta Radiol 1956; 135(Suppl):9–13.

46. Kerr WK, Barkin M, D'Aloisio J, Merczyk Z. Observations on the movement of ions and water across the wall of the human bladder and ureter. J Urol 1963;89:812–819.

47. Lewis SA, Diamond JM. Active sodium transport by mammalian urinary bladder. Nature 1975;253:747–748.

48. Fellows GJ, Marshall DH. The permeability of human bladder epithelium to water and sodium. Invest Urol 1972;9:339–344.

49. Hicks RM. The permeability of rat transitional epithelium. J Cell Biol 1966;28:21–31.

50. Hicks RM, Ketterer B, Warren RC. The ultrastructure and chemistry of the luminal plasma membrane of the mammalian urinary bladder: a structure with low permeability to water and ions. Phil Trans R Soc Lond B 1974;268:23–38.

51. Staehelin LA, Chlapowski FJ, Bonneville MA. Luminal plasma membrane of the urinary bladder. J Cell Biol 1972;53:73–91.

52. Parsons CL, Stauffer C, Schmidt J. Bladder surface glycosaminoglycans: an efficient mechanism of environmental adaptation. Science 1980;208:605–607.

53. Parsons CL, Greenspan C, Mulholland SG. The primary antibacterial defense mechanism of the bladder. Invest Urol 1975;13:72–76.

54. Parsons CL, Greenspan C, Moore SW, Mulholland SG. Role of surface mucin in primary antibacterial defense of bladder. Urology 1979; 9:48–52.

55. Gill WB, Jones KW, Ruggiero KJ. Protective effects of heparin and other sulfated glycosaminoglycans on crystal adhesion to urothelium. J Urol 1982;127:152–154.

56. Hanno PM, Parsons CL, Shrom SH, Fritz R, Mulholland SG. The protective effect of heparin in experimental bladder infection. J Surg Res 1978;25:324–329.

57. Parsons CL, Mulholland S, Anwar H. Antibacterial activity of bladder surface mucin duplicated by exogenous glycosaminoglycan (heparin). Infect Immun 1979;24:552–557.

58. Menter JM, Hurst RE, Nakamura N, West SS. Thermodynamics of mucopolysaccharide-dye binding. III. Thermodynamic and cooperatively parameters of acridine orange-heparin system. Biopolymers 1979;18:493–505.

59. Hurst RE, Rhodes SW, Adamson PB, Parsons CL, Roy JB. Functional and structural characteristics of the glycosaminoglycans of the bladder luminal surface. J Urol 1987;138:433–437.

60. Bekturov EA, Bakauova KH, eds. Synthetic water-soluble polymers in solution, New York: Hüthig and Wepf, Verlag, 1986:38–54.

61. Parsons CL, Schmidt JD, Pollen J. Successful treatment of interstitial cystitis with sodium pentosanpolysulfate. J Urol 1983;130:51–53.

62. Parsons CL, Mulholland SG. Successful therapy of interstitial cystitis with pentosanpolysulfate. J Urol 1987;138:513–516.

63. Mulholland SG, Hanno P, Parsons CL, Sant GR, Staskin DR. Pentosan polysulfate sodium for therapy of interstitial cystitis: a double-blind placebo-controlled clinical study. Urology 1990;35:552–558.

64. Fall M, Johansson SL, Vahlne A. A clinicopathological and virological study of interstitial cystitis. J Urol 1985;133:771–773.

65. Hedelin HH, Märdh PA, Bronson JE, Fall M, Miller BR, Pettersson KG. Mycoplasma hominis and interstitial cystitis. Sex Transm Dis 1983; 10:327.

66. Lowentritt JE, Kawahara K, Human LG, Hellstrom WJ, Domingue GJ. Bacterial infection in prostatadynia. J Urol 1995;154:1378–1381.

67. Theoharides TC, Sant GR. Bladder mast cell activation in interstitial cystitis. Semin Urol 1991;9:74–87.

68. Lynes WL, Flynn SD, Shortliffe LD, et al. Mast cell involvement in interstitial cystitis. J Urol 1987;138:746–752.
69. Larsen S, Thompson SA, Hald T, et al. Mast cells in interstitial cystitis. Br J Urol 1982;54: 283–286.
70. Bjorling DE, Saban MR, Zine MJ, et al. In vitro passive sensitization of guinea pig, rhesus monkey and human bladders as a model of noninfectious cystitis. J Urol 1994;152:1603.
71. Saban R, Christensen M, Keith I, et al. Experimental model for the study of bladder mast cell degranulation and smooth muscle contraction. Semin Urol 1991;9:88–101.
72. MacDermott JP, Miller CH, Levy N, Stone AR. Cellular immunity in interstitial cystitis. J Urol 1991;145:274–278.
73. Felsen D, Frye S, Bavendam T, Trimble L, Vaughan ED Jr. Interleukin-6 activity in the urine of interstitial cystitis (IC) patients. J Urol 1992;147:460A.
74. Larsen S, Thompson SA, Hald T, et al. Mast cells in interstitial cystitis. Br J Urol 1982;54:283.
75. Smith B, Dehner LP. Chronic ulcerating interstitial cystitis. A study of 28 cases. Arch Pathol 1972;93:76.
76. Jacobo E, Stamler FW, Culp DA. Interstitial cystitis followed by total cystectomy. Urology 1974;3:481.
77. Johansson SL, Fall M. Clinical features and spectrum of light microscopic changes in interstitial cystitis. J Urol 1990;143:1118–1124.
78. Dixon JS, Holm-Bentzen M, Gilpin CJ, et al. Electron microscopic investigation of the bladder urothelium and glycocalyx in patients with interstitial cystitis. J Urol 1986;135:621–625.
79. Cornish J, Nickel JC, Vanderwee M, Costerton JW. Ultrastructural visualiation of human bladder mucous. Urol Res 1990;18:263–266.
80. Burford HE, Burford CE. Hunner ulcer of the bladder: a report of 187 cases. J Urol 1958;79: 952–955.
81. Felsen D, Frye S, Trimble LA, et al. Inflammatory mediator profile in urine and bladder wash fluid of patients with interstitial cystitis. J Urol 1994; 152:355–361.
82. Zuraw BL, Sugimoto S, Parsons CL, Hugli T, Lotz M, Koziol J. Activation of urinary kallikrein in patients with interstitial cystitis. J Urol 1994; 152:874–878.
83. Hurst RE, Rhodes SW, Adamson PB, Parsons CL, Roy JB. Functional and structural characteristics of the glycosaminoglycans of the bladder lumenal surface. J Urol 1987;138:433–437.
84. Moldwin RM, Shupp-Byrne D, Callahan HJ, Mulholland SG. The presence of an antibacterial glycoprotein in a spectrum of transitional gel carcinomas. J Urol 1992;148:154–157.
85. O'Hara SM, Marley GM, Stein P, Parsons CL, Veltri RW, Howard E. Investigation of matrix metalloproteinases (MMPs) as new biomarkers for detection and monitoring of patients with interstitial cystitis syndrome. J Urol 1995;153: 290A.
86. Holm-Bentzen M, Larsen S, Hainau B, Hald T. Non-obstructive detrusor myopathy in a group of patients with chronic bacterial cystitis. Scand J Urol Nephrol 1985;19:21.
87. Hanno PM, Buehler J, Wein AJ. Use of amitriptyline in the treatment of interstitial cystitis. J Urol 1989;141:846–848.
88. Bumpus HC. Interstitial cystitis. Med Clin North Am 1930;13:1495.
89. Stewart BH, Persky L, Kiser WS. The use of dimethylsulfoxide (DMSO) in the treatment of interstitial cystitis. J Urol 1968;98,671.
90. Hohlbrugger G, Lentsch P, Pfaller K, Madersbacher H. Permeability characteristics of the rat urinary bladder in experimental cystitis and after overdistention. Urologia Int 1985;40: 211–216.
91. Bohne AW, Hodson JM, Rebuck JW, Reinhard RE. An abnormal leukocyte response in interstitial cystitis. J Urol 1962;88:387.
92. Simmons JL. Interstitial cystitis: an explanation for the beneficial effect of an antihistamine. J Urol 1961;85:149.
93. Theoharides T. Hydroxyzine in the treatment of interstitial cystitis. Urol Clin North Am 1994;21: 113–119.
94. Badenoch AW. Chronic interstitial cystitis. Br J Urol 1971;43:718.
95. Dodson AI. Hunner's ulcer of the bladder: a report of 10 cases. Virginia Med Monthly 1926; 53:305.
96. Pool TL. Interstitial cystitis: clinical considerations and treatment. Clin Obstet Gynecol 1967; 10:185.
97. Wishard WN, Nourse MH, Mertz JHO. Use of clorpactin WCS90 for relief of symptoms due to interstitial cystitis. J Urol 1957;77:420.
98. Lose G, Frandsen B, Hojensgard JC, et al. Chronic interstitial cystitis: increased levels of eosinophil cationic protein in serum and urine and an ameliorating effect of subcutaneous heparin. Scand J Urol Nephrol 1983;17:159.
99. Parsons CL, Benson G, Childs SJ, Hanno P, Sant GR, Webster G. A quantitatively controlled method to study prospectively interstitial cystitis and demonstrate the efficacy of pentosanpolysulfate. J Urol 1993;150:845–848.
100. Nielsen KK, Kromann-Andersen B, Steven K, Hald T. Failure of combined supratrigonal cystectomy and Mainz ileocecocystoplasty in intractable interstitial cystitis: is histology and mast cell count a reliable predictor for the outcome of surgery? J Urol 1990;144:255–258.
101. Eigner EG, Freiha FS. The fate of the remaining bladder following supravesical diversion. J Urol 1990;144:31–33.
102. Parsons CL, Koprowski P. Interstitial cystitis: successful management by a pattern of increasing urinary voiding interval. Urology 1991;37: 207–212.

CHAPTER 30

Overflow Incontinence

Michelle M. Germain and Donald R. Ostergard

Overflow incontinence, as defined by the International Continence Society (ICS), is "any involuntary loss of urine associated with over-distension of the bladder" (1). Traditionally, overflow incontinence has been associated with urinary retention and large bladder volumes that result from outflow obstruction or impaired detrusor activity. The original definition of overflow incontinence, used by the ICS in 1976, was "involuntary loss of urine when the intravesical pressure exceeds the maximal urethral pressure due to elevation of intravesical pressure, associated with bladder distension but in the absence of detrusor activity" (2). Using this definition, decreased bladder compliance, which causes increased intravesical pressure with increasing bladder volume, and low urethral pressure can be considered in the etiology of overflow incontinence.

It is difficult to determine the true incidence of overflow incontinence because of variation in study populations and definitions. Gender differences are also difficult to determine, but a higher incidence of overflow incontinence due to urinary retention and urethral obstruction occurs in men. The literature on overflow incontinence is sparse, especially concerning female incontinence. This may be because the true clinical problem is urinary retention and its associated morbid sequelae and not the incontinence (3).

Symptoms

Patients with overflow incontinence have a variety of urinary symptoms. They may report urine loss without awareness, intermittent dribbling of urine, or constant wetness. They may describe a slow and intermittent urine stream, difficulty initiating voiding, and needing to strain or use suprapubic pressure to void. In some cases, these women may report symptoms consistent with stress incontinence and urine loss with position change. These patients often report frequent urinary tract infections, presumably secondary to large residual urine volumes. In cases of decreased bladder compliance, these women may report large-volume urine loss and symptoms of urinary urgency associated with urine loss.

It is important to remember, however, that history alone may not be an accurate tool in determining the etiology of incontinence (4). Urinary symptoms of voiding difficulty were not found to be a reliable guide to the final urodynamic diagnosis or to the severity of the voiding dysfunction (5). These researchers reported that the most valuable symptoms for the prediction of voiding dysfunction are poor urinary stream, incomplete bladder emptying, straining to void, and nocturia.

Evaluation

For any patient complaining of urinary incontinence, a thorough history and physical examination, with a neurological examination, 24-hour voiding diary, urinalysis and urine culture, and measurement of the postvoid residual urine volume are essential. Complaints of constantly feeling wet and of urine loss without awareness suggest the presence of a fistula or an ectopic ureter, which is located beyond the urethral continence mechanism, and therefore cystourethroscopy is necessary. In addition, evaluation of bladder capacity and bladder wall compliance, with multichannel urodynamic equipment and electromyography, are essential. Voiding function should also be investigated, whether by uroflowmetry, pressure voiding studies, or voiding cystourethrography. Finally, because urinary retention, decreased bladder compliance, and increased vesical pressure can result in reflux, imaging of the kidneys and ureters to rule out hydronephrosis, either by ultrasound or intravenous pyelography, is important. In most cases, overflow incontinence indicates an underlying major pathology, and thus once the diagnosis is made, careful investigation for the etiology is imperative.

Etiology

The normal act of micturition involves urethral relaxation followed by detrusor contraction; this is centrally controlled in the pontine and sacral micturition centers. Impaired bladder emptying may occur as a result of defective functioning in the central or peripheral nervous systems or in the lower urinary tract.

A firm definition of elevated postvoid residual urine volume has not been universally accepted. A postvoid residual urine volume less than or equal to 50 mL is considered normal, whereas a residual urine volume above 200 mL is unquestionably abnormal and consistent with urinary retention. However, it is the significance of volumes between 50 and 199 mL that is debated (6).

In women, urinary retention is the major cause of overflow incontinence; there are both acute and chronic causes of urinary retention. If the acute causes are not promptly resolved, more permanent damage can result, presumably because the detrusor muscle, or the parasympathetic ganglia in the bladder wall, becomes compromised. We discuss the various conditions that can lead to urinary retention, as outlined in Table 30.1. Additionally, however, we present the newer concept that altered bladder compliance and sphincter function can result in overflow incontinence.

Table 30.1. Causes of Overflow Incontinence

Urinary retention
  Iatrogenic
    Surgery
    Obstetric trauma
  Infectious
  Neurological
    Cerebral cortical lesions
    Spinal cord trauma
    Nerve root damage
    Demyelinating diseases
    Peripheral neuropathy
  Anatomic urethral obstruction
    Extrinsic compression
    Urethral sphincter
  Pharmacological
  Psychiatric disorders
Decreased bladder compliance
Urethral sphincter dysfunction

IATROGENIC

Postoperative and postpartum patients account for the major proportion of women with acute urinary retention. This phenomenon may result from bladder trauma and edema secondary to surgery or obstetric delivery, epidural anesthesia, pelvic nerve stretching or trauma, pelvic hematoma, or episiotomy pain and abdominal incision pain, especially for patients who void mainly by Valsalva maneuver.

Long-standing urinary retention due to prior antiincontinence surgery, especially retropubic urethral suspension, is a rare but troubling complication. Although retropubic urethropexy has the highest long-term success rates, the incidence of voiding dysfunction is reportedly as high as 20% (7). It is critical in all antiincontinence procedures to avoid overcorrection of the urethrovesical junction. Women identified preoperatively with abnormal voiding mechanisms are at high risk of postoperative voiding difficulties (8). Most women with postoperative urinary retention improve with time and adequate bladder drainage.

INFECTIOUS

Severe dysuria, either because of urethritis or cystitis, can be associated with acute urinary retention. Infection and inflammation of the bladder and urethra may interfere with the normal micturition reflex. Acute urinary retention may also occur in women with primary anogenital herpes simplex virus infections (9). This may be secondary to pain (10) or pelvic neuritis involving the bladder (11). Herpes zoster has also been implicated in urinary retention, presumably as a result of invasion of the sacral spinal ganglia by the virus (12).

NEUROLOGICAL DISEASE

Neurological disease is one of the most common causes of urinary retention in women, with multiple sclerosis being the most common condition (5). In fact, impaired bladder emptying may be the first indication of neurological disease.

The duration of a detrusor contraction is controlled by efferent fibers from the brainstem to the sacral micturition center. In cases of herniated lumbosacral disk disease, lesions of the sacral spinal cord or nerve roots, and "spinal shock" secondary to trauma, both motor and sensory control of the bladder are lost. Nontraumatic conditions include spinal cord tumors, vascular disease, and demyelinating diseases, like multiple sclerosis. Patients with interruption of this pathway have high-volume high-compliance bladders and are more prone to overflow incontinence. In time, however, if the lesion is above the sacral micturition center, detrusor hyperreflexia may develop and can be associated with detrusor sphincter dyssynergia and incomplete emptying.

The pudendal nerve provides the circuitry for coordination of detrusor and urethral muscular activity during voiding. In addition to spinal cord lesions noted above, diseases that result in peripheral neuropathy, such as diabetes, hypothyroidism, alcoholism, uremia, tabes dorsalis secondary to syphilis, and collagen vascular disease, can destroy this function. Patients with these diseases may have detrusor sphincter dyssynergia and obstructive voiding symptoms or uninhibited urethral relaxation.

ANATOMIC URETHRAL OBSTRUCTION

Bladder neck obstruction is an uncommon cause of urinary retention and overflow incontinence in women. However, there have been reports of pelvic tumors, both benign leiomyomata and malignant neoplasms, that compressed and obstructed the urethra. Additionally, vaginal mesonephric or paramesonephric remnant cysts have been reported to cause obstruction (13). An entrapped, retroverted, gravid or nongravid uterus (14), uterine prolapse, or a severe cystocele can result in urethral kinking and obstruction. There has also been a report of bladder neck obstruction due to circular smooth muscle hypertrophy, although the underlying etiology of this was not addressed (15). Chronic inflammation can result in urethral stricture, as can prior urethral surgery for diverticula or fistula repair.

PHARMACOLOGICAL AGENTS

There are a number of medications for cardiovascular, neurological, psychological, and allergic disorders that can affect voiding function. In addition to causing urinary retention, these agents have been associated with frequency, hesitancy, and irritative bladder symptoms. These include anticholinergic agents, anticonvulsants, phenothiazines, ganglionic blockers, antidepressants and alpha-adrenergic agonists. In patients with underlying voiding disorders, these drugs can lead to significant urinary retention.

Finally, there are a number of chemotherapeutic agents that can cause peripheral neuropathy, thus resulting in impaired bladder function. These include vincristine and cisplatin.

PSYCHIATRIC DISORDERS

Urinary retention resulting from psychiatric disorders is difficult to diagnose and should be considered a diagnosis of exclusion. It can be seen with conversion disorders, hysteria, and depression, to name a few. Voiding dysfunction is thought to result from subconscious inhibition, by the central nervous system, of normal detrusor and urethral function. However, psychotropic drugs, such as tricyclic antidepressants, must be excluded as a contributing factor (5).

BLADDER AND URETHRAL DYSFUNCTION

Injury to the bladder wall, either as a result of radiation therapy, surgery, or inflammation, can result in a small-volume low-compliance bladder. Decreased bladder compliance places the upper urinary tract at high risk secondary to vesicoureteral reflux and chronic pyelonephritis; this may subsequently lead to renal failure (16). The loss of bladder wall compliance results in an increase in intravesical pressure with increased volume, although the bladder volume may not be excessive. Eventually, the intravesical pressure exceeds the intraurethral pressure, and urinary incontinence results (3). In women with urethral sphincter deficiency, non-stress-related pressure equalization incontinence can occur at lower bladder volumes because intravesical pressure exceeds resting urethral pressure at smaller bladder volumes (VL Handa, unpublished data, 1995).

Treatment

ACUTE URINARY RETENTION

In patients presenting with acute urinary retention, the immediate treatment should be bladder drainage. Because of the risk of bladder hemorrhage with rapid bladder drainage, after draining the first 500–750 mL to relieve immediate discomfort, the remainder of the volume should be drained at a rate of 250 mL/h. Continuous drainage may be necessary for a number of days or weeks. Antibiotic therapy is not necessary unless there is a documented urinary tract infection.

CHRONIC URINARY RETENTION

In cases of chronic urinary retention, intervention is essential if the patient has recurrent urinary tract infections or evidence of upper tract disease. Additionally, patients with irritative bladder symptoms and/or urinary incontinence may seek medical evaluation and request medical intervention to relieve these symptoms.

Long-term management of patients with urinary retention should be directed at preventing renal damage and correcting the underlying cause of urinary retention. All urinary tract infections should be treated before initiating a diagnostic evaluation and proceeding with other therapy for urinary retention. More specific therapeutic interventions

Table 30.2.   Treatment of Overflow Incontinence

Urinary retention
  Acute retention
    Bladder drainage
    Antibiotic therapy
  Chronic retention
    Pharmacological agents
    Intermittent self-catheterization
    Behavioral modification
    Surgical intervention
Detrusor/sphincter dysfunction
  Pharmacological agents
  Behavioral modification

are outlined in Table 30.2 and discussed in the following sections.

Pharmacological Therapy

Most studies with pharmacological agents are uncontrolled, and there are contradictory results reported about their efficacy (17). In patients with detrusor areflexia, there are two drug categories that can be used. Acetylcholine agonists are promoted as detrusor contractility enhancers. Unfortunately, they really only increase detrusor tone, and therefore they have been used with mixed results. Alpha-adrenergic blocking agents, in combination with cholinergic agonists, decrease outlet resistance (18).

For women with detrusor hyperreflexia, the goal is to obtain a sustained and coordinated detrusor contraction at the time of desired micturition and to decrease outlet resistance in the presence of detrusor sphincter dyssynergia. However, this goal has not been achieved. Parasympathomimetic drugs have been used, including anticholinergics, smooth muscle relaxants, calcium channel blockers, and beta-adrenergic agonists. These drugs have been used with limited success, most likely because they do not increase the strength of detrusor contractions but merely increase the resting tone of the detrusor muscle (19). Tricyclic antidepressants may also be used, although these do have alpha-agonist properties and thus may increase urethral tone. However, in patients with decreased bladder compliance and/or urethral sphincter dysfunction, tricyclic antidepressants are the drug of first choice. In cases of detrusor sphincter dyssynergia, skeletal sphincter spasm is most commonly seen with detrusor hyperreflexia. Diazepam can be used in these patients to decrease outlet resistance. Prazosin hydrochloride and phenoxybenzamine, which are alpha-adrenergic blocking agents, can also be used to decrease the contractility of the smooth muscle component of the sphincter.

Intermittent Self-Catheterization

Continuous bladder catheter drainage is best avoided in cases of urinary retention, because of the high complication rate from infections, ulcerations, calculi, and bladder spasms. Over the long term, permanent drainage can result in a small-volume low-compliance bladder, with subsequent upper urinary tract damage (20). Intermittent catheterization is a much less morbid treatment intervention and is an acceptable option for women with sufficient mobility and manual dexterity. The rate of cystitis is low and can be controlled by antibiotic prophylaxis.

Behavior Modification

Patients with urinary retention can use a number of simple techniques to decrease the likelihood of elevated residual urine volume. The patient should be instructed to void in the sitting position, not in the squatting position, because this posture does not facilitate adequate relaxation of the pelvic floor. Patients should be educated about normal voiding and instructed to relax the muscles of the pelvic floor. Because constipation can lead to bladder dysfunction, every attempt should be made to prevent this. Finally, the double voiding technique requires two episodes of micturition a few minutes apart.

In patients with hypotonic bladders, timed voiding is a very useful maneuver to decrease the likelihood of incontinence. The patients are instructed to void on a preset schedule regardless of their bladder sensation. This schedule is usually every 2–3 hours depending on their frequency of incontinent episodes. This concept of scheduled voiding can also be used in patients who have overflow incontinence due to decreased bladder compliance and low urethral pressure. With this technique, the bladder volume is never allowed to reach the volume at which bladder

pressure exceeds urethral pressure, and thus incontinence is avoided.

Finally, in patients with detrusor areflexia, application of manual pressure over the bladder, with or without Valsalva maneuver, can facilitate bladder emptying. However, some clinicians do not advocate this technique because of the possibility of vesicoureteral reflux (20) with increased detrusor pressure.

Surgical Intervention

In cases of detrusor areflexia, there are two therapeutic options. Although still under study, reduction cystoplasty has been used in some patients with excessively large bladders. With progressive upper tract disease, presumably because of vesicoureteral reflux, urinary diversion has been used.

Conversely, patients with detrusor hyperreflexia may be treated with a number of surgical procedures, such as peripheral bladder denervation, selected sacral nerve resection, and augmentation cystoplasty, if more conservative options have failed. These procedures have not been widely studied, however.

REFERENCES

1. Abrams P, Blaivas JG, Stanton SL, Andersen JT. The standardization of terminology of lower urinary tract function recommended by the International Continence Society. Int Urogynecol J 1990; 1:45–58.
2. Bates P, Bradley WE, Glen E, et al. First report on the standardisation of terminology of lower urinary tract function. Br J Urol 1976;48:39–42.
3. Richardson DA. Overflow incontinence and urinary retention. Clin Obstet Gynecol 1990;33: 378–381.
4. Jensen JK, Nielsen FR, Ostergard DR. The role of patient history in the diagnosis of urinary incontinence. Obstet Gynecol 1994;83:904–910.
5. Dwyer PL, Desmedt E. Impaired bladder emptying in women. Aust NZ J Obstet Gynecol 1994; 34:73–78.
6. Urinary Incontinence Guideline Panel. Urinary incontinence in adults. Clinical Practice Guideline. Rockville, MD: U.S. Department of Health and Human Services. AHCPR Publication No. 92-0038. March 1992.
7. Lose G, Jorgensen L, Mortensen SO, et al. Voiding difficulties after colposuspension. Obstet Gynecol 1987;69:33–38.
8. Bhatia NN, Bergman A. Use of preoperative uroflowmetry and simultaneous urethrocystometry for predicting risk of prolonged postoperative bladder drainage. Urology 1986;28:440–445.

9. Caplan LR, Kleeman FJ, Berg FS. Urinary retention probably secondary to herpes genitalis. N Engl J Med 1977;297:920–921.

10. Person DA, Kaufman RH, Gardner HL, et al. Herpesvirus type 2 in genitourinary tract infections. Am J Obstet Gynecol 1973;116:993–995.

11. Greenstein A, Matzkin H, Kaver I, Braf Z. Acute urinary retention in herpes genitalis infection: urodynamic evaluation. Urology 1988;31: 453–456.

12. Patel BR, Rivner MH. Herpes zoster causing acute urinary retention. South Med J 1988;81:929–930.

13. Muram D, Jerkins GR. Urinary retention secondary to a Gartner's duct cyst. Obstet Gynecol 1988;72:510–511.

14. Nelson MS. Acute urinary retention secondary to an incarcerated gravid uterus. Am J Emerg Med 1986;4:321–322.

15. Diokno AC, Hollander JB, Bennett CJ. Bladder neck obstruction in women: a real entity. J Urol 1984;132:294–298.

16. McGuire EJ. Editorial: Bladder compliance. J Urol 1994;151:965–966.

17. Finkbeiner AE. Is bethanechol chloride clinically effective in promoting bladder emptying? A literature review. J Urol 1985;134:443–449.

18. Tammela T. Prevention of prolonged voiding problems after unexpected postoperative urinary retention: a comparison of phenoxybenzamine and carbachol. J Urol 1986;136:1254–1257.

19. Wein AJ. Pharmacologic treatment of incontinence. J Am Geriatr Soc 1990;38:317–325.

20. Madersbacher H. The various types of neurogenic bladder dysfunction: an update of current therapeutic concepts. Paraplegia 1990;28:217–229.

CHAPTER 31

The Mind-Bladder Syndrome

Charles B. Stone and Stanley A. Brosman

Syndromes of lower urinary tract dysfunction in women are complex phenomena with multiple etiologies that may include psychological factors. Psychological contributions to symptom production may be quite significant, even crucial, in some patients with frequency-urgency-pain syndrome, incontinence associated with bladder instability, or some instances of retention. On the other hand, significant psychiatric problems may occur because of the psychological effects on patients experiencing symptoms of organic disease such as urethral diverticula, stress urinary incontinence, or interstitial cystitis. Profound psychosocial distress and disability usually accompany chronic urinary incontinence from any cause. In patients with interstitial cystitis, the frequency-urinary-pain syndrome that occurs in the natural history of the disease may be psychologically devastating.

Review of Urogynecological Literature

The significance of voiding dysfunction associated with psychological causes may have been appreciated but was rarely discussed in the literature before 1963. In 1900, Bierhoff (1) described the irritable bladder syndrome or bladder neurosis. Apparently, he regarded the etiology of this syndrome as almost always organic rather than psychogenic. He noted that a phlegmatic woman describes her pain as "only a little discomfort," whereas the neurasthenic type may magnify this into unbearable discomfort or "stabbing, cutting pains."

In 1962, Smith (2) reported his experience with psychosomatic "cystitis." He found little in the literature about the influence of the psyche on urinary function, although physicians have known of such influence since ancient times. He quoted a Chinese proverb, "The bladder is the mirror of the soul." Smith condemned empirical organic therapy, including any form of manipulative or operative treatment, because it convinced the patient erroneously of serious organic disease. He emphasized that psychotherapy was the definitive treatment because, in addition to their urinary symptoms, these patients had psychosexual difficulties with deep and basic psychological problems.

In 1963, Zufall (3) reported that in 8 years he had treated 190 women with urethral syndrome, manifested by frequency, dysuria, and pain in the back, flanks, or abdomen. In diagnostic studies, including pyelograms and cystoscopies, he found no consistent pathology. With any form of treatment, he noted that about one third of his patients improved for more than 12 weeks. He also noted a history of dyspareunia in only nine patients. He regarded his patients as suffering from psychoneurosis with hysterical somatization of emotional problems.

Bors and Comarr (4) stated that psychic causes account for the symptom of frequency in 10% of women with this complaint. Accompanying psychogenic bladder dysfunction are various autonomic complaints, such as headache, nausea, and constipation; these women refer associated pain to the suprapubic region, lower abdomen, urethra, or vagina.

In 1963, Hodgkinson et al. (5), pioneers in urogynecology, introduced the term dyssynergic detrusor dysfunction. They calculated the incidence of detrusor dyssynergia as 8.7% in a series of 735 patients with deficient urinary control. They commented that, on the basis of medical custom, the term neurogenic was as acceptable as dyssynergic. They emphasized that extreme detrusor dysfunction may develop in the apparently normal woman. In their terminology, "apparently normal" seems to imply the absence of positive neurological or gynecological findings but avoids taking psychogenic factors into account. In responding to discussions of their paper, Hodgkinson described a patient who was operated on five times for stress incontinence and was apparently never cured. Finally, direct urethrocystometry showed a voluntary voiding pattern. He considered her to have psychogenic incontinence associated with difficulties relating to her husband, a chronic alcoholic, who remained sympathetic and relatively sober only so long as she had urinary difficulties. Hodgkinson then pointed out that she used her incontinence to keep her husband from drinking. Thus, he implicitly acknowledged a psychogenic factor, that is, the secondary gain to the patient from her symptoms.

In 1975, Green (6) reported detrusor dyssynergia as the second most common cause of urinary incontinence in women. He reported that the management of these patients with bladder instability was frequently difficult, and the results of treatment were unpredictable and often unsatisfactory.

Jeffcoate and Francis (7) and Frewen (8–10) emphasized psychosocial factors in reviewing the etiology of functional types of urinary incontinence. Frewen found that the doctor-patient relationship cannot be overemphasized both with regard to mutual understanding and the development of an aura of sustained optimism. In follow-up of 50 patients treated with bladder drill for urge incontinence, he found a subjective cure rate of 86%. Twelve of 50 patients had a history of emotional disturbances since childhood.

Marshall and Judd (11) found psychiatric consultation helpful in a number of cases in which lower urinary tract symptoms proved to be a component of an unrecognized emotional disturbance, usually depression.

Fantl (12) reported that over 90% of women with bladder instability appear to have no other recognizable pathology. This disorder of unknown etiology is the second most common cause of urinary incontinence in women. Fantl emphasized the need to avoid unsuccessful surgery. As a pioneer in the use of bladder drill, he found the essential subjective elements of the protocol to be positive reinforcement and reward, feeling of accomplishment, reassurance of expected success, and continuous encouragement.

In their comprehensive review of the literature on urethral syndrome, Scotti and Ostergard (13) reported that patients who have no other obvious cause and in whom other treatment measures have failed may respond to several psychotherapeutic measures, including hypnosis, desensitization drills, and guided visual imagery.

The problem of chronic urinary incontinence in geriatric practice was addressed in a National Institutes of Health Consensus Development Conference in 1988 (14). The conclusions developed included the statement that urinary incontinence leads to stigmatization and social isolation.

Weber et al. (15) found women with prolapse and urinary incontinence do not differ from continent women without prolapse in measures of sexual function. Increasing age was the only significant factor for worsening sexual function.

Lagro-Janssen et al. (16) evaluated 110 women aged 20–65 with urinary incontinence. The reported consequences of incontinence included low self-esteem, changing lifestyle to avoid potentially embarrassing situations, and, most importantly, fear of odor was mentioned as the worst effect in 40% of cases. They found a significant relationship between the objective severity of the incontinence and its psychosocial impact. In particular, the fear of odor was of the utmost importance.

Review of Psychiatric Literature

Some types of lower urinary tract dysfunction in women, such as chronic incontinence associated with bladder instability or frequency-urgency-pain syndrome without urological findings, are common psychosomatic disorders. The basic emotional problem in these patients is shame. It is shame that influences patients to keep the problem a secret, to delay seeking treatment, and sensitizes patients to the attitudes of health-care providers. The emotional and behavioral effects of shame are related to its intensity and the coping capability of those afflicted with it. Depression in female patients with lower urinary tract dysfunction is usually one of the manifestations of shame. Therefore, in addition to treating symptoms of depression, it is useful to address the underlying shame.

Although here we focus our attention and discussion on women, the same statements can be applied to men who have similar problems related to their lower urinary tract.

In 1905, Freud (17) wrote that children concern themselves with the problem of what sexual intercourse consists of, and they usually seek a solution to the mystery in some common activity concerned with the function of urination or defecation. Urination particularly appeals to their developing sense of logic because it is a function of the phallus that is known to them. Also, Freud thought that the urinary apparatus served temporarily in the place of the as yet undeveloped sexual apparatus to satisfy the child's curiosity. In 1908, Freud (18) described the sexual instinct of humans as highly complex, with important contributions to sexual excitation furnished by stimulation of certain specifically designated areas of the body, including genitals, mouth, anus, and urethra, which therefore are designated "erotogenic zones."

In 1941, Menninger (19) found that urination may at times express both erotic and aggressive elements of the personality. In some cases, he regarded urination as having a sexual masturbatory meaning. He thought that either frequency or retention on a psychogenic basis expressed self-punitive tendencies, which the individual used to attempt to atone for guilt over sexual thoughts or activities.

Wahl and Golden (20) offered the hypothesis that urinary symptoms in adults may at times represent somatization of repressed wishes to reexperience infantile pleasure in urination that is no longer acceptable to adults. Repression of this early infantile wish

might account for the symptom of retention. They found with remarkable regularity that patients with urinary retention had repressed genital sexual conflicts. Genitals were considered taboo, and the individual invested the act of urination with forbidden, sensual, erotic feelings. Also, the wish for catheterization had sexual meaning, that of vicarious sexual gratification. They found that their patients used their symptoms to permit avoidance of sexual relations, to provide an opportunity to be dependent, or to serve as acceptable punishment for the patient's neurotic guilt feelings.

Nesbitt et al (21) found that women with psychogenic urinary retention struggled within themselves with the need to control angry, hostile, or aggressive impulses. Repressed conflict over aggressive impulses may take the form of a bodily symptom such as urinary retention.

Larson et al. (22) reported 37 cases of psychogenic urinary retention. Each patient had psychosomatic symptoms in other organ systems, predominantly headaches, low back pain, and a variety of gastrointestinal symptoms. They evaluated 25 patients psychiatrically and found 17 to be neurotic and 8 psychotic. Of the 17 neurotics, they diagnosed conversion hysteria in 12 and neurotic depression in 3. Of the eight psychotics, five were schizophrenic and three psychotically depressed.

Yazmajian (23) reported the psychoanalytic treatment of three adult patients, all toilet trained before the age of 2 years and never enuretic, in whom excessive functional urination took the place of weeping, crying, or sobbing. Each patient went through a prolonged period in early childhood when he or she wept, cried, or sobbed bitterly because of the mother's withdrawal of love and attention. Weeping released feelings of abandonment coupled with rage and a sense of absolute helplessness that was the affective tone that dominated this phase of their lives. As an adult, one patient found that whenever she was inclined to weep, the impulse to urinate supervened to restore emotional detachment. When aware of this, the patient wept briefly, and while shedding tears, the impulse to urinate disappeared.

In 1949, Straub et al. (24) reported what is probably the first experimental psychiatric study of both women and men patients with either urinary urgency and frequency or retention. They found bladder hyperfunction and frequency commonly associated with a reaction of anxiety and resentment accompanying conflict. Bladder hypofunction with urinary retention usually accompanied emotional repression and a general reaction of withdrawal and a sense of being overwhelmed. In some patients, the two patterns of disturbance alternated. In the authors' opinion, such patients dealt differently from time to time with conflict situations. They found an association of tension, anxiety, and comparatively aggressive behavior with vesical hyperfunction and an association of either blandness or dejection and nonaggressive behavior with vesical hypofunction. They concluded that recognition of psychosomatic phenomena involving the bladder depends on positive identification of situational conflicts that correlate with bladder disturbance. Their findings of bladder hypofunction with urinary retention in patients who were repressed, emotionally withdrawn, and overwhelmed are entirely compatible with our own clinical experience in noting transient urinary retention in elderly women receiving psychiatric treatment for chronic severe depression. We also found that these same patients at times complain of urgency and frequency when their mental status changes from predominantly depressive withdrawal to agitated anxiety.

In 1977, Chertok et al. (25) reported on both clinical aspects and the evolution of etiological concepts of the frequency-urgency-pain syndrome. They reviewed the German and French literature published in the past century. As early as 1859, Briquet attributed the occurrence of urgency, frequency, and pain in women to the somatization of emotional conflict. In 1911, Dejerine and Gauckler advanced etiological thought by maintaining that the disturbance of micturition and urogenital pain derived from disorders of sexuality. These authors found that about 20% of women attending a urological clinic in a Paris hospital had frequency-urgency-pain syndrome. The usual definition of disturbance of micturition and vesical pain may be too restrictive because the pain frequently involves not only the bladder area but the entire pelvic region as well. They retrospec-

tively studied the records of 55 women patients seen from 1952 to 1970. Eighteen of these patients suffered solely from pain, either vesical, urethral, or genital; 19 patients had both dysuria and pain. Sixty-three percent complained of pain in other areas, such as headaches, heaviness of the stomach, heartburn, or polysystemic complaints. In 40%, there were complaints of anxiety, depression, or phobias. The most significant line of inquiry was the patients' verbalization of their symptoms. In some, there were thinly disguised sexual or pregnancy fantasies. The age of onset was 36–50 years. Most were married, but many had no sexual activity. They reported variable results with psychotherapy, although some had "veritable therapeutic miracle cure" after one interview.

In 1977, Hafner et al. (26) reported a psychiatric study of women with urgency and urgency incontinence in the absence of organic structural bladder and urethral abnormality. They wanted to determine the extent to which these symptoms yielded to psychological and behavioral treatments. Those patients who appeared most disturbed had symptoms that were often bizarre or atypical, with pain in areas other than the bladder as a common feature. Most had grossly disturbed interpersonal relationships, had recently lost a close relative, or had a history of repeated bereavement.

In 1977, Rees and Farhoumand (27) reported the psychiatric assessment of 50 women randomly selected from among patients being evaluated for recurrent cystitis. Thirty percent had a history of anxiety disorder and/or depression antedating the onset of urinary symptoms. In 24%, the psychiatric manifestations were in reaction to or resulting from the urological disorder. Only 25% were free of psychiatric symptoms at all times.

In a psychiatric study of 20 patients with chronic urinary incontinence previously reported by Stone and Judd (28), all had severe situational stress, 19 had chronic depression, and 12 had functional symptomatology in other organ systems, namely, headaches, backaches, and gastrointestinal symptoms. Although this small group of patients mostly suffered from incontinence due to unstable bladder, the psychological effects of incontinence from any cause are very profound.

Discussion

Difficult management problems often occur with patients whose symptoms are partially psychogenic in origin and with patients whose emotional distress is a result of their physical urological disorders. We encountered the expression that the bladder is "the mirror of the soul." Why should there be a connection between the mind and the bladder? The explanation comes from the pervasiveness of feelings, especially shame, that occur with lower urinary tract dysfunction. This is not a natural or physiologic process, but one that is learned during early childhood.

Tomkins (29) described nine innate emotions, separated into two groups, positive and negative. Positive emotions include interest or excitement, enjoyment or joy, and surprise or startle. The six negative emotions include distress or anguish, fear or terror, shame or humiliation, dissmell, disgust, and anger or rage. He considered as a classic shame scene a mother ridiculing her child as a "baby" on the occasion of urinary wetting. The child feels the loss of love and respect from the mother, the provocation of too much attention and control from her, and also turning away in disgust and dissmell. The child has not only done something "wrong" as immoral but also as incompetent. Also evoked in the child may be anger at the impatient mother and distress at the loss of what had been mutually enjoyed. Such a scene implies a variety of violations of values: "urinary leakage is wrong," "urinary leakage is ugly," "you promised to control yourself," "you have no skill," and it is all "shameful." The concept that urine is dirty and smells bad is drilled into the minds of these children.

Although Tomkins was describing a classic shame scene in early childhood, his formulations also apply at the emotional level to adult women with lower urinary tract dysfunction. The psychological explanation for this is that urinary dysfunction in adults tends to have emotionally regressive effects. Thus, shame scenes in childhood may be reexperienced emotionally in adults, especially when urinary incontinence occurs.

In the management of these problems, patients expect the primary physician to provide all the necessary treatment and do not wish to be referred to psychiatrists. For treatment to be most effective, the physician is responsible for developing a "working alliance" with the patient. This concept describes the patient's regard for the physician as an ally in a mutual working relationship rather than as a formidable frightening authority figure (30). Development of a satisfactory working alliance enhances the patient's conscious and rational willingness to overcome her illness and sense of helplessness, stimulates her conscious rational desire to cooperate, and maximizes her potential ability to follow the physician's instructions. According to Greenson (31), the psychological process that makes this possible is the patient's identification with the physician's approach to understanding the patient. That is, the patient needs to realize that the physician is interested in her as a person who is ill rather than impersonally as a case of a disease.

For the patient to be as comfortable as possible in seeking treatment and for the sake of encouraging compliance with treatment, it is essential that physicians and their staff maintain sympathetic empathic attitudes. Specifically, in relating to these patients who are burdened with shame, what must absolutely be avoided is any light-hearted, superficial, or, above all, any joking references to the patient's urinary symptoms and the predicament she is in.

What can the physician do to develop the working alliance? For the urogynecologist, this can be accomplished with a brief interview, which has the practical advantage of being psychologically diagnostic and therapeutic. The diagnostic aspect consists of talking with the patient to find out how self-conscious, embarrassed, or ashamed she is. The physician should inquire about life situational problems, chronic depression, and whether she has functional symptoms in other organ systems characteristic of anxiety disorders or emotional conflict. Such an interview takes only a few minutes and useful questions include the following: Does she get satisfaction from everyday activities? Are there difficulties in her closest relationships, such as with her husband, immediate family members, relatives, co-workers, or employers? The focus is on present life situations. It is not necessary to delve deeply into the past or developmental history, except for one question about childhood enuresis. Specifically, this line of inquiry is aimed at finding out how well the patient coped with situational problems just preceding the onset of urinary symptoms. To the patient, her distress in her current life is real and as much a source of disability as the "real" genitourinary pathology for which the physician searches to explain her symptoms. When treating a patient with chronic complicated situational problems, the physician is certainly not expected to solve all the patient's life problems. It is a valuable service to offer a sympathetic ear plus useful objective advice about any part of the problem.

Chronic depression is readily recognizable, even though the patient may maintain a facade of smiling cheerfulness on certain important occasions, such as a visit to her physician. The so-called "smiling depression" is chronic. The chronic patient cannot remember specifically when the depression began nor can she spontaneously connect it with any happening in her life. She usually relates abandonment of whatever her life goals may have been. An ominous but useful finding in psychiatric history-taking is that the patient as a girl did not have any life goals or specific ambition for her future. Such history usually indicates a patient who had serious problems with the development of her self-image in early childhood. As an adult, she tends to welcome invalidism. Usually, she believes herself miserably trapped with no hope of extricating herself, often from her home situation and marriage, and she sadly accepts her fate, but in ill health. Some patients with chronic incontinence tend to feel too indisposed to participate in sex. The chronically depressed patient feels like crying, but embarrassment prevents it. She prefers to be alone to cry, and when she cries, she is not sure of just exactly what she is crying about and characteristically does not get much relief from crying.

Another area of inquiry concerns the presence of functional symptoms in other organ systems. To elicit these symptoms, it is often useful to ask the patient if she ever feels nervous in any part of her body. The physician often discovers that the patient has never before attempted to verbalize her bodily feelings. The process of verbalization

of feelings is helpful because the patient immediately changes perceptions of vague physical uneasiness into secondary process, that is, logical language. This process in itself may reduce anxiety and lead to prevention of anxiety through understanding of the emotional significance of physical sensations or symptoms. The usual alternative to this type of discussion is the prescribing of minor tranquilizers, but this approach may perpetuate the patient's feelings of helplessness to prevent symptom recurrence.

The type and extent of pain, which is a prominent clinical feature in many women patients with mind-bladder syndrome, is often etiologically related to emotional problems. On the basis of the clinical experience in gynecological psychiatry, we regard women patients with chronic painful voiding dysfunction as psychiatrically similar to those with chronic pelvic pain. Chronic lower urinary tract pain is a clinical variant or subgroup of chronic pelvic pain. Chertok et al. (25) stated that the present nomenclature is too restrictive; the patient has pain not only in the vesical area but frequently throughout the entire pelvic region as well.

Friederich (32) states that is it is possible for pain to be a completely psychic experience based on unconscious memories or fantasies. She theorizes that in the sexual sphere, if a patient felt guilty as a child about expressing sexual feelings, then as a woman she may develop pain in situations of sexual arousal. Another basis for pain is loss—actual, threatened, or fantasized. Identifying with the lost person through pain is an unconsciously determined way of continuing a relationship in the patient's mind and of emotionally holding on to the lost person. Pain is more likely if the patient had ambivalent feelings with strong anger and guilt feelings about the lost person. The pain in this sense keeps the lost one present inside the mind of the patient and helps diminish the intense grief that may threaten to overwhelm the patient.

Psychotropic Drug Therapy

The use of minor tranquilizing or antidepressant drugs involves serious therapeutic

Table 31.1. Psychotropic Drug Therapy

Drug	Indication	Daily Dose (mg)	Side Effects
Buspirone	Anxiety	30–60	Nausea Dizziness Anxiety
Clonazepam	Anxiety	0.5–2.0	Sedation Incoordination

Tricyclics
  Desipramine
  Amitriptyline
	Depression	100–300	Sedation
			Weight gain
			Orthostatic hypotension
			Anticholinergic effect

Nortriptyline		50–150	Age over 40: EKG changes, tachycardia

dilemmas in these patients (Table 31.1). Minor tranquilizers assist in the management of anxiety and mild degrees of depression. Most of the minor tranquilizers are benzodiazepines, a class of drugs associated with chemical dependency in vulnerable patients who take these medications on a regular daily basis. Prolonged use leads to loss of the initial benefit and results in habituation to the drug. The patients under consideration here all have chronic subjective distress associated with chronic situational problems and are not likely to be satisfied with only a few days' use of minor tranquilizers. The likelihood of developing chemical dependency correlates with personality traits of dependency, either clearly evident passive dependency or more subtle unsatisfied dependency needs in active vigorous people. In geriatric patients, especially in those with even slight memory impairment or cognitive loss associated with aging brain dysfunction, there is a tendency to develop slurred speech and varying degrees of confusion as side effects of benzodiazepines. This is usually dose related, occurring in elderly patients who exceed a maintenance dose in the mistaken hope that larger doses will help them to feel better. In psychiatric practice, the original benzodiazepine, diazepam, is no longer in use because of its cumulative effect with repeated daily doses. Some of the more rapidly excreted benzodiazepines, such as lorazepam, alprazolam, and triazolam, have been accorded a secondary place in psychiatric practice because of the significant risk of dependency developing with extended use. Probably the best benzodiazepine for prolonged use in

treatment of anxiety is clonazepam, which may be effective in a single daily dose of 0.5–2.0 mg.

Buspirone, a nonbenzodiazepine antianxiety drug, has become known as useful in some patients. Its advantage is the absence of potential for inducing chemical dependency. For treatment of significant degrees of depression, the tricyclic drugs, especially imipramine, desipramine, and nortriptyline, are well established for these patients. Tricyclics do not cause chemical dependency but have other limitations. Even small daily doses have been associated with significant weight gain. The physician prescribing a tricyclic drug for depression should remember that overdose of these drugs in suicide attempts are likely to be fatal due to heart block and ventricular arrhythmias. The therapeutic dosage range is narrow. The usual minimum therapeutic dose is 50–100 mg daily, with generally accepted maximum dose of 300 mg daily, although patients usually do not tolerate these higher levels because of uncomfortable side effects such as orthostatic hypotension, dry mouth, constipation, and drowsiness. Currently, in psychiatric practice the tricyclics have been relegated to a secondary role since the introduction of newer generations of antidepressant drugs. Selective serotonin reuptake inhibitors (SSRIs) are widely used, including fluoxetine, sertraline, paroxetine, and fluvoxamine. However, in urogynecological practice, tricyclics continue to be the drugs of choice, whereas the role of SSRIs has not been established.

Chronic lower tract urinary dysfunction,

regardless of its cause, can produce profoundly devastating mental and emotional effects that emanate from feelings of shame. Effective management of these patients is enhanced by understanding the significance of the mind-bladder syndrome.

REFERENCES

1. Bierhoff F. On the so-called "irritable bladder" in the female. Am J Med Sci 1900;120:670.
2. Smith DR. Psychosomatic "cystitis." J Urol 1962; 82:359.
3. Zufall R. Treatment of the urethral syndrome in women. JAMA 1963;184:138.
4. Bors E, Comarr AE. Neurological urology. Baltimore: University Park Press, 1971:120–121.
5. Hodgkinson CP, Ayers MA, Drukker BH. Dyssynergic detrusor dysfunction in the apparently normal female. Am J Obstet Gynecol 1963;87:717.
6. Green TH Jr. Urinary stress incontinence: differential diagnosis, pathophysiology, and management. Am J Obstet Gynecol 1975;122:368–400.
7. Jeffcoate TNA, Francis WJ. Urgency incontinence in the female. Am J Obstet Gynecol 1966;94: 604–618.
8. Frewen WK. Urgency incontinence. J Obstet Gynaecol Br Commonw 1972;79:77–79.
9. Frewen WK. A reassessment of bladder training in detrusor dysfunction in the female. Br J Urol 1982;54:372–373.
10. Frewen WK. The significance of the psychosomatic factor in urge incontinence. Br J Urol 1984;58:330.
11. Marshall JR, Judd GE. Guide for the management of women with symptoms arising in the lower urinary tract. Clin Obstet Gynecol 1976;19: 247–258.
12. Fantl JA. Urinary incontinence due to detrusor instability. Clin Obstet Gynecol 1984;27: 474–489.
13. Scotti RJ, Ostergard DR. The urethral syndrome. Clin Obstet Gynecol 1984;27:515–529.
14. Urinary incontinence in adults. Consensus Development Conference, Bethesda, MD: National Institutes of Health, 1988;7.
15. Weber AM, Walters MD, Schover LR, Mitchinson A. Sexual function of women with uterovaginal prolapse and urinary incontinence. Obstet Gynecol 1995;85:483–487.
16. Lagro-Janssen T, Smits A, Van Weel C. Urinary incontinence in women and the effects on their lives. Scand J Primary Health Care 1992;3: 211–216.
17. Freud S. Three essays on the theory of sexuality. In: Standard edition of the complete psychological works of Sigmund Freud. London: Hogarth Press, 1963;7:190.
18. Freud S. Character and anal erotism. In: Standard edition of the complete psychological works of Sigmund Freud. London: Hogarth Press, 1963; 9:131.
19. Menninger KA. Some observations on the psychological factors in urination and genitourinary affections. Psychoanal Rev 1941;28:117.
20. Wahl CW, Golden JS. Psychogenic urinary retention. In: Wahl CW, ed. New dimensions in psychosomatic medicine. Boston: Little Brown, 1964:313–335.
21. Nesbitt RE Jr, Hollender MH, Feldman PM, Glazer JA, Hayes RC, Ferro PL. Psychogenic urinary retention. Int Psychiatry Clin 1965;2:561.
22. Larson JW, Swenson WM, Utz DC, Steinhilber RM. Psychogenic urinary retention in women. JAMA 1963;184:697.
23. Yazmajian RV. Pathological urination and weeping. Psychoanal Quart 1966;35:40.
24. Straub LR, Ripley HS, Wolf S. Disturbances of bladder function associated with emotional states. JAMA 1949;141:1139.
25. Chertok L, Bourguignon O, Guillon F, Aboulker P. Urethral syndrome in the female (irritable bladder): the expression of fantasies about the urogenital area. Psychosom Med 1977;39:1–10.
26. Hafner RJ, Stanton SL, Guy J. A psychiatric study of women with urgency and urgency incontinence. Br J Urol 1977;49:211–214.
27. Rees DLP, Farhoumand N. Psychiatric aspects of recurrent cystitis in women. Br J Urol 1977; 49:651.
28. Stone CB, Judd GE. Psychogenic aspects of urinary incontinence in women. Clin Obstet Gynecol 1978;21:807.
29. Tomkins S. Shame. In: Nathanson DL, ed. Chapter in the many faces of shame. New York: Guilford Press, 1987:133–161.
30. Greenson RR. The working alliance and transference neurosis. Psychoanal Q 1965;34:155.
31. Greenson RR. The technique and practice of psychoanalysis. New York: International Universities Press, 1967:192–193.
32. Friederich MA. Psychological aspects of chronic pelvic pain. Clin Obstet Gynecol 1976;19:399.

CHAPTER 32

Geriatric Urogynecology

Alfred E. Bent and Mary T. McLennan

Introduction

The prevalence of urinary incontinence increases with age. Community dwelling elderly have a 15–30% prevalence of incontinence. Rates are higher with nursing home patients, with estimates of 50% or greater (1).

Although health care costs continue to be a major concern (2, 3), incontinence also has a profound psychological and physical effect on an individual's lifestyle. Reports of interference with social contacts and activity range from 8 to 52% (4). Norton et al. (5) reported that 40% of incontinent women avoided sexual activity and that 76% of patients attending a urodynamic clinic believed their mental health was affected. McCauley et al. (6) noted that 20% of women found life intolerable. Incontinence does not appear to predict or contribute to mortality (7).

Studies indicate that fewer than 40% of patients report urine loss to physicians (8–11). Burgio et al. (12) showed that the reporting of incontinence was associated with severity as measured by frequency and volume of accidents, the extent to which it restricted activities and affected mood, and the use of protection. The reason for this poor reporting is unclear. In a study of community dwelling people 65 years and older, Branch et al. (8) reported that 58% of respondents perceived urine loss as a normal consequence of aging. Of equal concern is the fact that physicians may not be asking this age group about incontinence and may be reluctant to institute treatment or refer those reporting incontinence (13). Urinary incontinence is also cited as a major reason for institutionalizing elderly family members (14, 15).

Agencies interested in geriatric incontinence include the National Institute on Aging, Veterans' Administration, Help for Incontinent People, the Simon Foundation, and the National Institutes of Health. Although urinary incontinence may comprise a large portion of urinary difficulties in the elderly, there are a number of other lower urinary tract disorders and problems that also have an impact on the health care system.

Effect of Aging on the Lower Urinary Tract

Changes with aging may directly affect lower urinary structure, neurological control of micturition, pattern of urine production, and the physical ability to perform the task associated with voiding. Physiological aging is associated with reduced tissue repair, decreased elastic tissue, increased fatty infiltration, cellular atrophy, nerve degeneration, and a reduction of smooth muscle tone. These changes cause alterations in the supports of the pelvic organs (16). There is an associated estrogen deficiency leading to decreased connective tissue, thinning of vaginal and urethral epithelium, decreased urethral submucosal vascularity, and decreased cellular glycogen in the vagina. The latter change results in a decreased lactic acid production by Doderlein's bacilli and an increase in vaginal pH. The presence of lactobacilli and the maintenance of a low pH may directly protect the vagina from colonization with uropathogens. Some lactobacilli produce hydrogen peroxide that prevents colonization. *Escherichia coli* rarely colonizes at a pH less than 4.5 (17).

These effects plus impaired emptying secondary to altered neural pathways, altered immune response, and thin atrophic epithelium may increase the incidence of urinary tract infections. In one study of 123 postmenopausal patients with urethral syndrome, distal urethral smears for cytohormonal status showed 15 normals, 85 with a decline in estrogen activity, and 23 atrophic or without estrogen effect (18). The structural response may be atrophy and shortening of the vagina, receding of the urethral meatus, and alteration of pelvic supports. In youth, the urethra has numerous submucosal venous plexuses with valve-like folds that hold large amounts of blood. With age, the valves diminish in size, the veins become less flexible, and vessel walls thicken. Urethral pressure decrease is observed with aging. The clinical response includes an increased incidence of genuine stress incontinence (GSI) from a combination of thinned urethral urothelium, decreased urethral pressure, impaired submucosal vascular plexus with secondary alteration of the pressure transmission to the proximal urethra during stress, and poor anatomic support at the urethrovesical junction or bladder neck. Detrusor instability (DI) may result from altered neural pathways and nerve conduction changes, leading to a hyperexcitable micturition reflex. Urethral syndrome may result from altered urethral sensitivity caused by a thin urothelial lining, an altered trigone, and impaired submucosal vascularity.

Bladder changes include increased permeability of the endothelium (undetermined significance) and collagenous and smooth muscle changes in the submucosa that may alter compliance and muscle function (19). There appears to be a reduction in nerve axons with advancing age (20). Postmortem studies reveal trabeculation and loss of supporting elasticity that lead to the formation of cellules and diverticula (21). The trabeculation may be due to hypertrophic changes with a thin bladder wall and accentuation of

muscle bundles. Unstable bladder and bladder outlet obstruction may also cause these changes. The incidence of transitional cell carcinoma increases with age and is discussed later. The trigone has an embryological origin similar to the urethra and is also estrogen dependent. Atrophic changes may cause a red irritated trigone. Age-related changes in glomerular filtration rate, renal blood flow, and renal tubular function result in the loss of concentrating ability of the kidneys (22). Because of these physiological changes, the resultant volume may account for the diurnal increased frequency (23, 24). Medical conditions have an effect on the voiding pattern, and these include diabetes with polyuria, cardiac and vascular disease with mobilization of peripheral edema when resting supine, and the use of diuretics.

Age-associated factors have direct and indirect effects on lower urinary tract function. Cognitive and sensory impairment obscures the need for voiding (25). Griffiths et al. (26) found that the presence of urge incontinence was strongly associated with decreased perfusion of the cortex and midbrain. Immobility results in difficulty in using the toilet, which may in turn cause incontinence (25). Central nervous system disorders that are common in the elderly (e.g., stroke, dementia, or Parkinson's disease) are associated with a high incidence of DI. Cancer growth or vascular impairment may have generalized and local effects on the bladder and the urethra. Drug use may have direct bladder and urethral effects. Asymptomatic bacteriuria increases with age and leads to an increase in symptomatic infection (27, 28).

Symptoms and Diagnoses

In a series of 100 ambulatory postmenopausal patients with urinary tract complaints, the following frequency of symptoms was identified: urgency, 65%; urge incontinence, 58%; nocturia, 57%; stress incontinence, 52%; frequency, 49%; postvoid fullness, 36%; and dysuria, 17%. The diagnoses in these patients are shown in Table 32.1 (29).

In Brussels, a survey of 1299 community dwelling women, of whom 858 were postmenopausal, showed an incontinence rate of

26.4%: stress incontinence, 5.1%; urge incontinence, 4.5%; mixed incontinence, 13%; unknown incontinence, 3.8%; urgency, 14.9%; frequency, 19.6%; and nocturia, 17.6%. A comparison of symptoms with premenopausal women in the same community is shown in Table 32.2 (11).

Table 32.1. Diagnoses in 100 Postmenopausal Patients with Lower Urinary Tract Complaints

	n
Hypoestrogenism	41
Urethral syndrome	38
Genuine stress incontinence	33
Detrusor instability	24
Pelvic relaxation	11
Distal urethral stenosis	10
Radiation changes	5
Unstable urethra	4
Urinary tract infections	3
Rigid urethra	3
Other	27
Total	199

In a 1994 survey of 2884 noninstitutionalized ambulatory patients aged 65–80, 1104 (28.4%) reported incontinence in the previous year. Of the female responders, 38% reported incontinence. Less than one half (37.6%) of incontinent responders had ever told their physicians (12). Similarly, in a study of 364 community dwelling adults with a mean age of 75, 41% reported incontinence in a home interview. Most patients did not receive treatment or referral for their problem (13).

A review of those patients referred for urodynamic assessment showed a steady increase in the percent of patients with GSI into the menopausal years. There was a gradual increase in DI with age ranging from 16% at 16–25 years to 45% over 75 years (DI and mixed) (Table 32.3) (30).

A study of 133 incontinent frail female elderly recruited from seven nursing homes in central Pennsylvania revealed 41% with a normal cystometrogram; 38% with DI; 16%

Table 32.2. Other Genitourinary Symptoms in Premenopausal and Postmenopausal Women

	Premenopausal (%)	Postmenopausal (%)
Urgency[a, b]	8.7	14.9
Frequency >6/d	17.1	19.6
Nocturia >1/night	7.9	17.6
Dysuria	6.2	5.1
Cystitis in past year	12.7	10.1
Vaginal pain	11.0	10.1
Vaginal itching[b]	32.7	23.2
Discharge[b]	58.3	22.5
Sexually active[b]	86.8	50.7
Dyspareunia[b, c]	6.2	16.1

[a]Defined as the ability to withhold urine for no longer than 5 min.
[b]$p < 0.05$.
[c]Among the sexually active women.
From Rekers H, Drodendijk AC, Valkenburg HA, Riphagen S. The menopause, urinary incontinence, and other symptoms of the genito-urinary tract. Maturitas 1992; 15:101–111.

Table 32.3. Age-Related Referrals for Urodynamic Investigations and Urodynamic Diagnoses Applied

	16–25 y	26–35 y	36–45 y	46–55 y	56–65 y	66–75 y	≥76 y	Total
Genuine stress incontinence	11 (17)	142 (40)	418 (52)	407 (55)	236 (49)	148 (48)	39 (46)	1401
Detrusor instability	3 (5)	64 (18)	98 (12)	93 (13)	67 (14)	50 (16)	13 (15)	388
Mixed	7 (11)	5 (4)	89 (11)	101 (14)	81 (17)	55 (18)	25 (30)	373
Hypersensitive	0	23 (6)	19 (2)	12 (2)	13 (3)	5 (2)	0	72
Normal	44 (67)	113 (32)	184 (23)	127 (16)	83 (17)	53 (16)	7 (9)	611
Total	65	357	808	740	480	311	84	2845

From Keane DP, Eckford SD, Shepherd AM, Abrams P. Referral patterns and diagnoses in women attending a urodynamic unit. Br Med J 1992; 305:1437–1438.

with stress incontinence; 5% with postvoid residuals greater than 500 mL, suggesting overflow type incontinence; and 60% with some fecal incontinence. Half showed severe cognitive impairment, and 63% were totally dependent (10). One hundred thirty-five stroke patients were followed for 1 year, and urinary incontinence developed in 51% within that year. Most cleared within weeks, and at 1 year, the continued incontinence rate was only 15% (31). In nursing home situations, incontinence may not be recognized by physicians when diapers and bladder conditioning are used. The three most common precipitating factors for urinary incontinence are cerebrovascular disease, immobility, and mental confusion. The more common urogynecological diagnoses in all elderly patients over 65 are DI, GSI, and mixed incontinence (29, 32, 33) (Tables 32.4 and 32.5).

Diagnostic Methods

Geriatric patients presenting with lower urinary tract disorders, including incontinence, require initial history and physical

Table 32.4. Classification of Incontinence

DI
GSI
Mixed incontinence
Bypass of continence mechanism (fistula, diverticulum)
Overflow incontinence
Functional (mobility, sensation)
Iatrogenic (drugs)

Table 32.5. Frequency and Type of Urinary Incontinence in Elderly Females

	Frequency (%)
Institutionalized elderly	
DI	27–61
GSI	21
Mixed	4
Underactive detrusor	8
Outlet obstruction	4
Noninstitutionalized elderly	
DI	27–46
GSI	46
Mixed incontinence	19
Other causes	8

examination similar to any other age group (Table 32.6). The history taking may be aided by previous completion of a detailed questionnaire by the patient, a relative, or a caregiver. A completed 24-hour voiding diary gives objective data on frequency of micturition, functional cystometric capacity, number of incontinent episodes, associated symptoms, and fluid balance. The chief complaint and history of the presenting problem are first ascertained, followed by a series of specific questions. If incontinence is present, whether it is associated with stress or urge or is spontaneous, intermittent, continuous, or nocturnal should be ascertained. Other questions should refer to irritative symptoms such as frequency, urgency, urge incontinence, nocturia, or dysuria and problems with bladder emptying such as hesitancy, a weak stream, and postvoid fullness. Associated factors include fluid intake and number and types of pads used if incontinent. Past urinary tract problems, prior surgeries of any type, and current and past treatment for urinary disorders are then discussed. General questions need to be posed regarding ambulatory capacity, mental status, community potential, medical problems, and neurological symptoms. A specific record of medications is important. Drugs that may affect the lower urinary tract include antihypertensives, antidepressants, antipsychotics, hypnotics, caffeine, muscle relaxants, antihistamines, diuretics, and hormones (34). In a study of 84 incontinent nursing home females, 70% of the 454 drugs taken by the residents had the potential to cause incontinence (35). Finally, other specific gynecological questions are addressed, including vaginal bleeding, sexual function, vaginal symptoms, menopausal symptoms, hormone replacement therapy, and symptoms of pelvic relaxation, such as pressure, bulge, or a sensation of fullness in the vagina.

Table 32.6. Simplified Evaluation for Office or Institutionalized Elderly

History and physical examination
Mobility and toilet access
Review of medication
Urolog record
Residual urine
Urinalysis and culture
Simplified cystometrogram

Although history is important, it does not establish the diagnosis. Jensen et al. (36) in a recent analysis of the literature showed that reliance on history alone to demonstrate GSI resulted in a misdiagnosis in 25% of cases. Patient history is an inaccurate predictor of DI and mixed incontinence in that the symptoms of urge incontinence lead to a misdiagnosis in 45% of cases (36). In a geriatric population, Ouslander et al. (37) demonstrated that symptoms of severe urgency and urge incontinence were less than 75% sensitive and 80% specific in identifying patients whose final diagnosis was DI.

The physical examination should be careful and complete because associated conditions in the elderly have a major impact on lower urinary tract function. Ambulatory capacity and mental status are assessed, and a general examination is completed. The finding of a high proportion of "normal cystometrograms" in Yu and colleagues's study (10, 25) of elderly incontinent in long-term care facilities suggests that mental and physical disability are important causes of incontinence or a significant aggravating factor (38). The specific neurological examination assesses cortical, suprasacral, and sacral cord function "S2–4" and includes lower extremity reflexes, sensation, bulbocavernosus reflex, anal wink, and sphincter tone. The vagina is examined with Graves' or Sims' specula to assess atrophy, urethrovesical junction mobility, and pelvic relaxation. Bimanual rectovaginal examination is then completed, during which time the ability to perform a Kegel squeeze can be assessed and fecal impaction excluded.

A number of simple evaluations can be performed to confirm and rule out common disorders. The patient is asked to void before assessment. Passage of a 14–16 French catheter allows collection of urine for microscopy ± culture and measurement of the postvoid residual (normally less than 100 mL). At this stage, a simple cystometrogram can be performed. With the patient supine, a bulb syringe is attached to the catheter and room temperature sterile water is added in 50-mL increments. The syringe is held so the 50 mL mark is approximately 15 cm above the symphysis (Fig. 32.1). The water meniscus is observed, and DI is strongly suspected if the column rises or leakage occurs around

the catheter in the absence of abdominal straining as indicated by a hand placed on the patient's abdomen. The first sensation to void and maximum cystometric capacity can also be assessed. A number of studies have demonstrated good correlation between this simple cystometry and multichannel studies. Ouslander et al. (37) and Fonda et al. (39) found simple bedside cystometry 75% and 88% sensitive, respectively, and 75% specific for the diagnosis of DI compared with multichannel studies in the geriatric population. The catheter may then be removed and a "standing stress test" done to assess for the presence of stress incontinence. In a group of 167 women age 60 and over, the provocative stress test had a sensitivity of 39.5% but, more importantly, a specificity of 98.5% in the detection of stress incontinence (40). These simple procedures are inexpensive, easy, and well tolerated and provide information for management decisions.

Complex urodynamic studies should be reserved for those in whom prior screening studies are normal, those who are not responding to initial conservative therapy, or those in whom one is contemplating operative intervention.

Cystoscopy is performed to rule out bladder cancer, interstitial cystitis, chronic cystitis, foreign body, calculi, and trabeculation. In women, bladder cancer is the eighth most common cause of cancer, accounting for 4% of all cancers and 3% of all cancer deaths. Ninety percent of transitional cell cancer occurs after the age of 50, with a fourfold increase associated with cigarette smoking. It is 2.7 times more common in men (41). When bladder cancer is present, gross or microscopic hematuria and bladder irritability are the most common presenting symptoms (42). Microscopic examination of a freshly voided specimen may help elucidate the origin of the hematuria. Erythrocytes of glomerular and tubulointerstitial disease are typically disfigured (dysmorphic), whereas nonglomerular are mostly undamaged circular and occasionally "ghosts" (lost their hemoglobin). Approximately 3% of normal individuals will excrete more than three red blood cells per high-power field (41). Cytological examination of urinary marker proteins and urine sediment analysis plus routine urinalysis

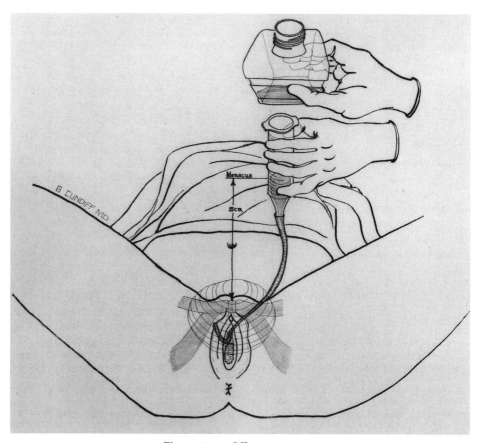

Figure 32.1. Office cystogram.

(Urocon) can help differentiate between hematuria of glomerular, tubulointerstitial urethral neoplasia, or postrenal origin. The initial diagnostic approach to asymptomatic hematuria should include cystoscopy and renal ultrasound or intravenous pyelogram. The latter will detect the rare, small, and nonobstructive renal pelvis or ureteral tumors that would be missed by ultrasound. Whether this extensive an investigation is warranted has been challenged, as Bard (43) found no cases of cancer in 177 women with asymptomatic microhematuria followed for 10 years and Mohr et al. (44) found 1 case in 353 women followed for 3 years. The evidence suggests that if these initial tests are negative, repeat investigations for microscopic hematuria are not necessary unless the patient develops gross hematuria, recurrent urinary tract infections, or changes in voiding characteristics (45). The use of urine cytology should be limited to high risk groups (e.g., previous radiation therapy for cervical cancer, exposure to aromatic amines,

long-term catheter patients, previous treatment with cyclophosphamide). Well-differentiated tumors often shed minimally, and the cells may appear to be normal. Even high-grade tumors have a false-negative cytology of 20%. First voided specimens should not be used because cells degenerate when urine remains in the bladder for prolonged periods. Saline bladder washings are more accurate (41).

Urethroscopy allows functional assessment of the urethrovesical junction during coughing and straining and "hold" maneuvers and observation for atrophic urethral changes, urethral diverticulum, ureters, and trigone. A reddened granular trigone may indicate minimal estrogen effect associated with menopause. Changes may not correlate with symptoms. A white membrane with distinct margins extending over the trigone and toward the ureteric orifices confirms the different embryologic origin of these organs from the bladder. This white membrane is squamous metaplasia, and a biopsy, if done, generally shows stratified squamous epithelium (46).

Intravenous pyelogram is indicated for suspected upper tract abnormalities, renal calculi, urinary sepsis not clearing with repeated therapy, or unexpected hematuria.

If the patient is referred for acute incontinence, the mnemonic "DRIP" devised by Ouslander (47), can be used to cover the potential causes of delirium; restricted mobility and retention; infection, inflammation, and impaction (fecal); and pharmaceutical and polyuria.

How far to pursue evaluation of urinary complaints in the elderly is controversial. All patients merit at least an initial evaluation. Even minor improvement may make a significant change in the quality of life and/or ease the burden on caregivers. The common geriatric urodynamic diagnoses are shown (Table 32.7).

Hypoestrogenism

The genitourinary indications for estrogen replacement include atrophic vaginitis, irritative urethral symptoms such as dysuria and urinary frequency (urethral syndrome), recurrent urinary tract infections, and GSI (48). Atrophic vaginitis includes symptoms of vaginal dryness, burning, itching, dyspareunia, discharge, and bleeding. The vaginal use of 0.3 mg of conjugated estrogen daily for 4 weeks has been shown to provide effective relief from atrophic vaginitis (49). Recently, a lower dose of 0.3 mg three times weekly was shown to provide both subjective relief and objective improvement in vaginal cytology (50). The endometrial effects of vaginal estrogen must be considered because estradiol is detectable in the serum in a small percentage of patients. Endometrial biopsy assessments

Table 32.7. Common Diagnoses in Geriatric Urogynecology

DI
GSI
Combined GSI and DI
Overflow incontinence
Recurrent urinary tract infections
Urethral syndrome
Pelvic relaxation
Estrogen deficiency

have shown proliferation, although to date there have been no published cases of endometrial cancer (50, 51). Therefore, contraindications to topical estrogen are the same as those for oral therapy. No protective effect on bone or heart has been demonstrated from vaginal estrogen therapy.

Hypoestrogenism probably affects the sensory threshold of the urinary tract in elderly patients, leading to a decreased volume and time to first sensation (52, 53). Studies have shown no effect on urethral function or DI, but diurnal frequency and nocturia were significantly reduced (53). Volume at first sensation and maximum cystometric capacity were increased (52–54). Estrogen therapy can improve irritative symptoms of the urethral syndrome. It also has a beneficial effect for the lower urinary tract by altering the sensory threshold, thereby subjectively improving symptoms such as urgency, frequency, and a sense of incomplete emptying (53).

Vaginal estrogen is associated with a significant decrease in vaginal pH, an increase in vaginal colonization with lactobacillus, and a decrease in the rate of colonization with enterobacteriaceae. These effects make it useful in the prevention of recurrent urinary tract infections (17).

There is an estrogen-mediated effect that increases the sensitivity of alpha-adrenergic stimulation in the urethral smooth muscle (55) and its response to alpha-adrenergic medications. Oral or vaginal estrogen plus phenylpropanolamine have proven beneficial in the treatment of stress incontinence (56, 57).

The efficacy of estrogen alone in the management of incontinence is difficult to assess. Fantl et al. (58) concluded that estrogen use provided subjective improvement with an average of 64% over placebo. A few studies provide data on objective improvement with only one of three randomized controlled trials showing a significant decrease in urine loss (58).

Urethral Syndrome

The diagnosis and treatment of urethral syndrome have already been discussed elsewhere in the text. In the elderly, many symptoms are directly due to estrogen deficiency.

A 24-hour voiding diary may show a daytime frequency of every 15–30 minutes but only two to three episodes of voiding each night. Although bladder capacity may be somewhat reduced in these patients, they are generally able to hold several times the volume of their voided amount. These patients do not complain of incontinence but frequently have been treated for recurrent urinary tract infections without appropriate documentation. Vaginal estrogen therapy in the dose of one quarter of an applicator (1 g) at night for 2 weeks or three times a week for 6 weeks followed by maintenance therapy once or twice per week has been recommended. The local effects of estrogen therapy, in addition to those already described, include urothelial proliferation, improved vascularity of the submucosa, and connective and elastic tissue growth. As with younger patients, treatment response may be seen from bladder retraining drills, low-dose antibacterials, antispasmodics, antiinflammatories, muscle relaxants, amitriptyline, and urethral dilation with or without periurethral steroids.

Pelvic Relaxation

Symptomatic pelvic relaxation (cystocele, enterocele, rectocele, uterine prolapse, vault prolapse) may present with a bulge, pressure feeling, or a visible lump. Interference with the lower urinary tract may include obstructive voiding, frank incontinence, or potential incontinence. There is evidence that denervation of the pelvic floor may be a factor in both GSI and genital tract prolapse (59, 60). The mechanism of continence or obstructive voiding in patients with severe cystocele, procidentia, or vault prolapse is related to the posterior-superior visceral descent with increased intraabdominal pressure, causing mechanical obstruction of the less mobile urethra. Relatively minor symptoms of pelvic pressure and irritative voiding may be initially managed by adjustment of fluid intake, including caffeine restriction, administration of vaginal estrogen, pelvic floor exercises, and a high-fiber intake for the control of constipation (61). Residual symptoms may be managed by insertion of a pessary, along with maintenance vaginal estrogen therapy.

The expected beneficial effects from the pessary include reduction in the pelvic relaxation, cure of the vaginal bulge and pressure symptoms, and relief of obstructive voiding. The undesirable effects include expulsion of the pessary, absence of symptom improvement, and the development of urinary incontinence.

Several types of pessaries are effective, including the ring with or without a diaphragm, inflatable, cube, Gehrung, or Gelhorn. Most patients prefer a ring diaphragm pessary because of the ease of maintenance and use. However, a large introitus may hold only the inflatable type or a suction type, such as a cube or Gelhorn. The office should be equipped with several sizes and types. Ideally, the pessary should be removed overnight and cleaned weekly or biweekly. Vaginal estrogen cream should be inserted twice per week to maintain a healthy mucosal lining. Douches are not generally recommended, but a Betadine or other douche may be used once weekly, especially if the patient wears the pessary for longer than one week at a time. The use of twice weekly Trimo-san vaginal jelly may help to destroy the odor caused by bacteria.

Failure to control symptoms by conservative measures may lead to surgical repair. Standard vaginal surgery may be used for all defects with a few precautionary steps. The patient who is sexually active or desires to retain the capacity for intercourse must not have an obliterative procedure performed (i.e., LeFort repair or colpocleisis). When performing a hysterectomy for prolapse, the cul-de-sac must be obliterated or plicated. This is most readily accomplished by the McCall culdoplasty (62) or a modification (63) (Fig. 32.2). A sacrospinous vault suspension is a procedure of choice for vault prolapse, allowing good support while maintaining an adequate vaginal canal (64). The overall success rate functionally and anatomically is close to 90%, but it is not without risk (65).

Iliococcygeus (prespinous) fascia fixation is an attractive alternative to sacrospinous vault suspension because it does not place the pudendal vessels or sciatic and pudendal neuromuscular bundles at risk, and in contrast the vaginal axis is straight (66). All existing and potential pelvic floor defects

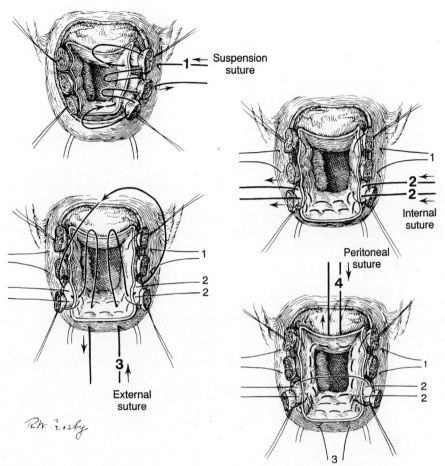

Figure 32.2.   Posterior culdoplasty to correct or prevent enterocele at the time of vaginal hysterectomy and to support the vaginal vault. (1) A continuous delayed-absorbable suture is placed through the lateral vaginal wall and adjacent peritoneum to include the distal portions of the cardinal and uterosacral ligaments before returning through the vaginal wall. (2) A posterior culdoplasty permanent suture is placed through the uterosacral ligament, cul-de-sac peritoneum, and opposite uterosacral ligament. This forms an internal suture, and a second one is placed slightly higher in position. (3) External culdoplasty absorbable sutures are placed through the posterior fornix and pass through each uterosacral ligament before returning through the peritoneum to the posterior fornix. (4) A purse-string suture closes the peritoneum. (From Mattingly RF, Thompson JB, eds. Malpositions of the uterus. In: TeLinde's operative gynecology, 6th ed. Philadelphia: Lippincott, 1985: 541–567.)

should be repaired (67). Anterior wall defects may occur in 20% of patients who have had a sacrospinous vault suspension if attention is not directed in this area (68–70). Posterior repair and rebuilding of the perineal body further supports the repair and is crucial to its long-term success (66, 71).

A pessary (72), Sims' speculum (73), or vaginal pack (74) has been used preoperatively during urodynamic testing or as a clinical test in patients with severe cystocele, vault prolapse, or procidentia to detect potential stress incontinence. The incidence of potential stress incontinence is significant at 20–60% (60, 74, 75). These patients or those with GSI even without reduction of the prolapse require correction of the urethrovesical junction defect at the time of surgery for prolapse. This can be accomplished by the modified Pereyra procedure or similar needle procedures. Reported risks factors for intrinsic sphincter deficiency include age greater than 50, previous pelvic irradiation, and a history of previous antiincontinence surgery (76–79). Preoperative testing will assist in detecting intrinsic urethral sphincter deficiency (ISD), in which case a suburethral sling may be the preferred method for repair of the urethrovesical junction defect (78, 80). Alternatively, periurethral collagen injections are the treatment of choice for elderly with ISD and a nonmobile bladder neck (81–83).

Some surgeons prefer an abdominal approach for repair of vault prolapse (abdominal sacrocolpopexy), attaching synthetic material to the top of the vagina and fixing it to the sacral promontory (84). For patients with incontinence, an abdominal repair is performed along with obliteration of the cul-de-sac to correct or prevent enterocele. Abdominal surgery preserves vaginal length, but it cannot adequately repair posterior defects or large enterovaginal defects.

Elderly patients frequently recover rapidly from vaginal surgery or procedures when organs are not removed. If bladder neck repair is performed, bladder drainage may best be achieved by the use of suprapubic catheter because some of these patients require prolonged catheterization. When bladder suspension is not performed, a Foley catheter may be used and removed early in the postoperative course. Patients must be checked for adequacy of bladder emptying to avoid bladder distension. Fecal impaction can cause urinary retention, and this is to be avoided by diligent attention to fiber diet, liquid intake, and monitoring of bowel activity.

Despite advancing age, many patients are medically fit for surgery, although medical and anesthetic consultation should be regularly obtained. Mortality in the very elderly may be as low as 1.6% (85) or 3.8% in nursing home patients (86). Major complications include a high rate of psychiatric decompensation, including profound depression, in this age group. Risk factors associated with low mortality include elective surgery, American Society of Anesthesiologist class 3 or less, and the use of spinal or local anesthesia (86). Compared with the general population, survival at 2–5 years is the same in patients aged 90 or more who undergo surgery as with those who do not (85).

Urinary Tract Infections

Urinary tract infections are the most common cause of acute bacterial sepsis in elderly patients. The incidence of bacteriuria increases with age and immobility (87), and the two major risk factors responsible are a decrease in bladder emptying and diminished natural host defenses (Table 32.8) (88). The former may result from age-related altered nerve conduction and decreased concentration of central nervous system neurotransmitters, which include bladder and urethral dysfunction. The latter may result from altered vaginal flora secondary to increased vaginal pH as a result of hypoestrogenic changes. Cellular changes include smoother cell surfaces and altered enzyme concentrations. Altered immune function is also present, resulting in increased susceptibility to infection. Incontinence of bladder or bowel and chronic catheter use are significant risk factors (87). Asymptomatic bacteriuria for many older people is intermittent with spontaneous acquisition and resolution. Only one third of patients with asymptomatic bacteriuria still have persistent bacteriuria 18 months later (27).

The best urine sample for culture is a suprapubic aspirate, but a catheterized specimen is acceptable. Midstream specimens have a false-positive rate of 17% (27). Considerable skill is required to obtain a useful midstream urine. In a survey of their unit, Claque and Horan (89) found that only 19% of nurses identified the correct technique. Significant bacteriuria for a midstream clean catch specimen has been defined as greater than 100,000 colony forming units per ml (cfu/mL). Suprapubic aspirates or catheter specimens are considered significant with a pure growth of 100 cfu/mL. Bacterial wall invasion has been noted with lower levels of bacteria. The organisms are most frequently gram-negative bacilli, with *E. coli* as the

Table 32.8. Prevalence of Bacteriuria in Females

Age (y)	Prevalence (%)
40–50	<5
65–70[a]	20
Over 80	23–50

[a]Age over 65.
Community, 18%; nursing home, 25%; hospitalized, 33%.
From Zilkoski MW, Smucker DR, Mayhew HE. Urinary tract infections in elderly patients. Postgrad Med 1988;84: 191–206.

predominant isolate. Functionally impaired nursing home patients have bacteriuria caused by the following: *E. coli* 32%, *Proteus* species 30%, other gram-negative 12%, providencia 10%, *Pseudomonas aeruginosa* 9%, and *Klebsiella* 7% (90). Hospitalization or indwelling catheters increase the risk of *Proteus, Klebsiella, Pseudomonas,* and enterococci. Screening may be performed by examining an unstained uncentrifuged urine under 40×. The presence of bacteria is abnormal; white cells, if present, are strongly suggestive of infection.

Microscopy may be a satisfactory test of cure, but culture and sensitivity of a catheterized specimen are required in the elderly for treatment. Elderly patients with asymptomatic bacteriuria do not require treatment. Eberle et al. (87) demonstrated no evidence of significant adverse outcomes resulting directly from the bacteriuric state. High mortality was the result of underlying functional impairment and severity of illness rather than the presence or persistence of asymptomatic bacteriuria. Similarly, Abrutyn et al. (91) showed that asymptomatic bacteriuria in elderly community dwelling women does not require treatment and is not an independent risk factor for mortality. Furthermore, a 12-year observational longitudinal study of 1000 noncatheterized adults with asymptomatic bacteriuria found little evidence of progressive renal disease in the absence of obstruction or preceding hypertension (92).

Concern has been raised by Reid's study (93) demonstrating that despite the presence of antibiotics, adherent viable bacteria were found on bladder cells of 94% of specimens. This obviously raises serious concerns over the emergence of highly drug-resistant strains.

Bacterial cystitis does require treatment, and patients should be rechecked for cure after treatment. Successful treatment has been documented with short-term antibiotic therapy (94–96). With all antibiotics, single-dose therapy appears to be less efficient than a 3- or 5-day treatment (96, 97). Also, single-dose therapy appears to be more successful in premenopausal patients, although with the new fluoroquinolones, good cure rates have been demonstrated in the postmenopausal age group. Pfau and Sacks (98) demonstrated a 90% cure in postmenopausal

patients treated with a single dose of two tablets of Ofloxacin (400 mg) or Ciprofloxacin (500 mg), although cure rates were once again higher in the premenopausal patients. A 3-day course of therapy is probably advisable in most patients (94). A 3-day regimen of trimethoprim-sulfamethoxazole is effective and is less expensive than similar regimens of nitrofurantoin, cefadroxil, or amoxicillin (95).

If the first line of treatment is ineffective, culture and sensitivity are required and appropriate therapy should be given for 7–14 days. Pyelonephritis may develop insidiously, and 50% of patients will not experience the classic signs of flank tenderness or fever. Some patients present with gastrointestinal and pulmonary symptoms, and 22% may present in shock. Intravenous cephalosporin or aminoglycoside is usually given, although enterococcus, which is sensitive to ampicillin, could be present. Pseudomonas is frequently found in catheterized or hospitalized patients and requires an extended spectrum penicillin, such as ticarcillin. Patients are treated until afebrile for 48–72 hours and then continued on oral therapy to complete 14 days of treatment.

Patients with recurrent infections may be placed on prophylaxis with nitrofurantoin 50 mg, trimethoprim 100 mg, or one regular trimethoprim-sulfamethoxazole tablet at night. Quinolones have also been shown to appreciably lower the number of gram-negative pathogens in the introital flora, making their use as prophylaxis attractive (98). Estrogen therapy appears to have a role in the prevention of recurrent urinary tract infections. In a randomized, double blind, placebo-controlled trial, topical intravaginal estradiol cream significantly reduced the incidence of symptomatic urinary tract infections compared with that in the group given placebo (7).

Those patients with high residuals need to be assessed for diabetes and taught double voiding techniques or intermittent self-catheterization.

Patients often ask about drinking cranberry juice to prevent urinary tract infections. A recent study by Avorn et al. (99) suggests a scientific basis to this folklore. In a randomized, double-blind, placebo-controlled trial, they demonstrated that cranberry juice decreased the frequency of bacteriuria with pyuria. The effect was not seen until 4–8 weeks and persisted thereafter. Its effects were more pronounced in converting urine samples out of the state of bacteriuria with pyuria compared with preventing the conversion of noninfected urine samples to bacteriuric ones (99). Thus, it may have a role in those patients with chronic bacteriuria who are at increased risk of recurrent urinary tract infections.

In chronically catheterized patients, the prevalence of polymicrobial bacteriuria is significantly associated with the duration of catheterization. Chronic pyelonephritis and chronic renal inflammation are also associated with long-term catheter use (100). Significant bacteremia upon catheter removal and reinsertion appears to be a rare event, and prophylactic antibiotics do not appear necessary (101). In the presence of urinary tract symptoms and fever, these patients should be treated with appropriate antibiotics.

Incontinent Disorders

Incontinent disorders in the elderly are known to incur a large financial burden and social stigma resulting from loss of urinary control. Disorders to be discussed include GSI, DI, combined GSI and DI, and overflow incontinence.

GSI

The etiology, diagnosis, and treatment of GSI have been discussed elsewhere in the text. Essential diagnostic tests in the elderly have also been discussed. A standing simple cystometrogram to rule out DI and urethral closure pressure profiles to confirm the diagnosis and rule out an impaired urethral sphincter should be performed when operative intervention is contemplated. Treatment for GSI in the elderly should first be approached with conservative measures. Nonspecific measures to treat associated medical disorders such as chronic bronchitis, asthma, diabetes, restriction of smoking, and weight loss may help. Weight loss may improve the technical ease of surgery, but there is little

evidence to suggest improvement of urinary symptoms, per se. In fact, obesity promotes estrogen production in peripheral fatty tissues, and this may prevent sequelae of estrogen deficiency in the obese patient.

Pelvic floor exercises initially introduced by Kegel (102) performed diligently over a 3-month interval will improve GSI in a high percent of cases (103). A metaanalysis of studies of pelvic floor exercises indicate cure rates between 31 and 73% (104). Compliance is a key factor, and Henderson and Taylor (105) noted better compliance in older than younger patients. Biofeedback may be superior to the "verbal only" (106) method, but this issue is not fully resolved (107). The role of resistive devices (i.e., perineometer) is unclear (108, 109). The individual needs mental competence to follow directions and reasonably good health to be able to expend the energy necessary to locate the muscles and practice the exercises.

Functional electrical stimulation, like pelvic floor exercises, requires a cooperative patient. Short-term transvaginal electrical stimulation may be an effective form of therapy, and patients can expect to see improvement in 6 weeks (110, 111). In a multicenter placebo-controlled trial (pre- and postmenopausal patients) involving 15 weeks of active pelvic floor stimulation or a sham device, patients using the active device showed significantly greater improvement in daily and weekly leakage episodes, pad testing, and vaginal muscle strength than controls. Pad testing showed cure or improvement in 62% of patients (112). Other studies report improvement rates of 71–89%. Most studies have not documented as yet the duration of improvement; however, it has been suggested that maintenance therapy may be required for most patients, although some remain cured after an initial 6-week course. Stimulation frequency is a crucial factor, and because of to the contractile properties of the fast and slow motor units, 50–100 Hz has been recommended for the treatment of stress incontinence (113).

Weighted vaginal cones are now available to stimulate the pelvic floor. Contraction of the pelvic floor is required to retain the cone, plus the feeling of "falling out" initiates a pelvic floor contraction and acts as a biofeedback response. Sixty to 70% improvement rates are reported (114). Although not specifically studied in the geriatric population, it appears cones may be as effective and less labor intensive than office electrical stimulation therapy (115).

Estrogen alone subjectively improves incontinence, but objective improvement has been difficult to demonstrate. There is no strong evidence of an effect on urodynamic parameters (58). As mentioned in the section on hypoestrogenism, oral or vaginal estrogen when combined with phenylpropanolamine (50 mg twice a day) in postmenopausal patients, particularly in those where estrogen was given before the addition of phenylpropanolamine, can result in a marked improvement or cure in many patients (55, 56, 67).

Surgery is undertaken in patients in whom the risk-benefit ratio favors an operative intervention. There is no "best surgery," and each surgery must be tailored to the patient's needs and presence or absence of medical disability. There is obvious appeal for vaginal procedures that allow concomitant pelvic floor repair for prolapse. Operative time tends to be less, and the immediate postoperative recovery is easier. With special reference to the elderly, Gillon and Stanton (116) showed a cure rate of approximately 90% with retropubic culposuspension. Holschneider et al. (117), in their 15-year follow-up of the modified Pereyra, did not find age as a significant independent risk factor for failure. Peattie and Stanton (118), however, found a 40% success rate for the Stamey in women over 65 compared with an 89% success with the retropubic urethropexy in a similarly elderly population.

In a comparative analysis of the patients older and younger than 65 undergoing the Raz bladder suspension, Nitti et al. (119) found no statistical difference in outcome with age and a subjective cure rate of 85%. Similarly, Raz et al. (120) found no correlation between age and success in their review of 206 Raz suspensions. In contrast, Korman et al. (121) reporting on their experience with the modified Pereyra noted that patients with poor outcome were significantly older. In a prospective study of patients over 65 years treated with the Raz procedure, Stanton et al. (122) found an objective cure rate of 46% over 2 years. Results were poorer in those with preoperative DI, history of previous

surgery, or nulliparity. Thus, the picture is somewhat cloudy, but based on objective cure rates, in healthy elderly patients, the retropubic urethropexy would be the procedure of choice with the needle procedures reserved for the medically less fit where operative time is of prime importance and in those patients with marked pelvic relaxation who have potential stress incontinence.

ISD

Recently, Horbach et al. (76) in a study of 263 stress incontinent patients identified age greater than 50 as the only independent variable that could predict the presence of intrinsic sphincter deficiency. Numerous authors had previously reported higher failure rates in these patients treated with the standard antiincontinence procedures (77, 78, 81, 123, 124). Sand et al. (78) showed a threefold increase failure rate, and Koonings et al. (123) showed a 33% failure rate in these patients treated with the Burch procedure. Similarly, Richardson et al. (124) and Koonings et al. (123) reported failure rates of 50–60% with standard needle suspensions.

For those patients with a mobile urethrovesical junction (cotton swab greater than 30°, opening and descent of the urethrovesical junction on urethroscopy), a suburethral sling has been recommended (80, 81, 125, 126). Success rate for this procedure is greater than 80%. The absence of urethral hypermobility has been suggested as a predictor of higher failure rates with the sling procedure (81). It is currently recommended that these patients be treated with periurethral collagen injections. Success rates as defined as cure or significant help are reported at 65–90% (82, 83). This procedure is particularly appealing in this age group because it is an office procedure with minimal morbidity.

DI

In elderly women with incontinence, the finding of DI may exceed 50% (10, 29, 30, 127, 128). A high incidence of DI is not necessarily associated with UTI, urethral syndrome, or interstitial cystitis. Conditions may coexist, and it is believed that when a sensory disorder is associated with a stable detrusor, there is increased bladder discomfort during filling and, therefore, a reduced capacity (129).

The diagnosis and therapy for DI are discussed elsewhere in the text. The following comments relate specifically to the geriatric patient.

Treatment commences with management of fluids if appropriate. Self-recorded daily fluid intake in a study of 333 incontinent community living elderly ranged from 385 to 3852 mL and averaged 1749 mL (61). These extremes suggest diverse beliefs on the effect of drinking on incontinence. The fluid requirement depends on body size and activity but averages 16–20 mL/lb. As caffeine is a diuretic, restriction of caffeine may be appropriate.

Because of the potential risk of complications and the fact that side effects are common with medication in this age group, bladder retraining (or drills) is particularly appealing (130). In a study of 131 community dwelling women with urinary incontinence, bladder retraining reduced the number of incontinent episodes by 57% (131). Prompted voiding has also been successful in the nursing home setting (132, 133).

Medications are probably still the mainstay of therapy (134). Dicyclomine hydrochloride (Bentyl) possesses a direct smooth muscle relaxant effect in addition to an anticholinergic action. It appears to be the most well-tolerated drug in the elderly, with doses commencing at 10 mg twice a day to a maximum of 20 mg three to four times a day. Oxybutynin chloride (Ditropan) possesses the above activities plus a local anesthetic activity. In postmenopausal women, it has been shown to be significantly more effective than placebo in reducing the symptoms of urgency and urge incontinence but at the expense of an increased residual and considerable side effects. In one study, only 7 of 37 patients (19%) continued to take the medication after the trial (135). Starting doses of 2.5 mg twice or three times per day are recommended.

Imipramine has potent anticholinergic effects, weak antimuscarinic effects, and a strong direct inhibitory effect on the bladder smooth muscle. A single nighttime dose of 10–25 mg is often useful. Care with dosing needs to be exercised because the half-life has been shown to be prolonged in the elderly (136). Rarely does a maximum dose of 50 mg need to be exceeded. Weakness, fatigue, and postural hypotension can be particularly severe. Ray et al. (137) reported a threefold increase in hip fractures in elderly patients taking imipramine.

The calcium channel antagonist, terodiline, has been used extensively in Europe (138, 139), and recently a multicenter, randomized, placebo-controlled trial was conducted in the United States (140). The terodiline group showed a 70% decrease in the mean number of incontinent episodes per week with only one drop-out from side effects. An unusual form of cardiac arrhythmia has been reported as possibly associated with terodiline, particularly in patients with cardiac risk factors or concomitant drug therapy (141). Thus, open trials have been suspended until this is further evaluated.

Desmopressin acetate given intranasally in the dose of 20–40 µg has been shown to decrease nocturnal urine production, and long-term safety and effectiveness has been demonstrated for adult nocturnal enuretics (142).

Functional electrical stimulation is also used for patients with DI. In Europe, maximal electrical stimulation (i.e., 5–10 Hz) with a current intensity to the threshold of "unpleasant" for 20 minutes once or twice weekly has shown clinical and urodynamic cures of 50% and a significant improvement in 33% (143). Caputo et al. (144) in a study of 76 patients with incontinence treated with maximal electrical stimulation at 20 Hz weekly for 6 weeks demonstrated a 63% subjective and 73% objective improvement in patients with DI. With home therapy, a frequency of 10–20 Hz is administered twice daily for 6 weeks or longer. In a study of 45 patients with GSI, DI, or both, Bent et al. (110) showed a subjective success of 70% for the subset of patients with pure DI treated with twice daily electrical stimulation.

In nursing homes or in general, Foley catheter drainage should be avoided if at all possible because the catheter increases bladder irritability and infection. Pad and urine absorbing diapers and pants are helpful and protective creams for the perineum are recommended.

COMBINED GSI AND DI

Because the incidence of DI increases with age, combined GSI and DI exist in a large number of elderly patients. The approach for the combined problem is to first make an accurate diagnosis and then to manage the individual conditions. Estrogen replacement therapy, Kegel exercises, a bladder relaxant, or a urethral constrictor may be commenced. Imipramine has a dual action for reducing bladder contractility in addition to its alpha-adrenergic activity on the urethral smooth muscle to improve stress incontinence. This medication has significant side effects as noted previously as well as postural hypotension, restlessness, tachycardia, and altered sensorium.

Bladder retraining may be useful. Fantl et al. (131) demonstrated a decrease in the number and severity of incontinent episodes in patients with mixed incontinence using scheduled voiding based on the patient's baseline daytime voiding intervals. Biofeedback with instruction in pelvic floor muscle rehabilitation combined with bladder retraining drills may be the most useful conservative approach.

Some patients respond well to functional electrical stimulation. A frequency of 10–20 Hz has been recommended for the DI component and 50 Hz for the GSI, but there is probably overlap. The device can be set for the dominant disability.

Some patients will still come to surgery secondary to the disabling GSI despite coexisting DI. Studies indicate postoperative resolution of DI in 30–66% (119, 120). Some will require continued medication for the DI component, and patients should be counseled regarding this preoperatively.

OVERFLOW INCONTINENCE

Overflow incontinence is diagnosed by history and by postvoid residual urine measurements. It is unusual to have incontinence with a residual urine less than 400; however, residuals of greater than 150–200 can cause recurrent urinary tract infections and aggravate the symptoms associated with GSI and DI. The prevalence of nursing home patients with postvoid residuals greater than 100 mL has been estimated at approximately 28–48% (145, 146). The relationship between large postvoid residuals and incontinence is uncertain. Diokno (147) did not find any difference in continence status with various postvoid residuals, whereas Ouslander et al.

(146) showed more frequent incontinence with increasing postvoid residuals. The most common cause of overflow incontinence in the elderly may be age-related changes that cause a decreased concentration of central nervous system neurotransmitters and altered nerve conduction resulting in sensory and motor voiding dysfunction. Many other causes exist (Table 32.9), and reversible causes must be ruled out by thorough history and examination.

Once reversible causes have been eliminated, treatment consists of surgery to relieve mechanical obstruction; an alpha-adrenergic blocker, prazosin hydrochloride (Minipress); cholinomimetic, bethanechol chloride (urecholine) (not useful orally); and indwelling or intermittent catheterization. Most female elderly patients, even those with associated diseases, can learn intermittent self-catheterization. A retrospective analysis of 65 patients aged 60–80 years found 94% successful at mastering intermittent self-catheterization with minimal complications (148). Most will develop bacteriuria, but few will develop sepsis. The technique requires some degree of mental aptitude and manual dexterity. A 10–14F self-intermittent catheter is recommended, and this can be kept in a plastic toothbrush case or resealable bag between uses. The technique is clean but not sterile. If necessary, the catheter is lubricated with 2% lidocaine gel or water and then washed clean with tap water after use and returned to the toothbrush case or plastic bag. Catheter and case can be boiled at midweek or a new catheter can be used once or twice weekly. Asymptomatic bacteriuria should not be treated nor should prophylaxis be used unless two symptomatic infections occur within a 3-month interval (149).

Care should be exercised in making the diagnosis of overflow incontinence as incontinence is still more likely because of urgency or stress incontinence or may merely reflect impaired mobility and dependence.

Chronic Indwelling Catheter Patients

In a study of patients 65 years and older in a randomized selection of Maryland nursing homes, 10% of females was using this form of

Table 32.9.   Causes of Overflow Incontinence

General Problem	Specific Cause
Hypotonic bladder	Diabetes mellitus
	Alcoholic problem
	Overdistention associated with surgery, i.e., fractured hip or radical hysterectomy
	Altered nerve supply and conduction with aging
	Sequelae of herpes virus infection
Drug related	Anticholinergic
	Alpha-adrenergic
	Tranquilizers/sedatives
	Narcotic analgesics
Detrusor sphincter dyssynergia	Multiple sclerosis
	Radical pelvic surgery
	Psychologic/psychiatric
Bladder outlet obstruction	Mechanical compression (rare)
	Malignancy, fibroid
Impairment of sensation to void	Fecal impaction
	Acute illness
	Immobility
	Confusional state
	Psychologic

Adapted from Ouslander JG. Lower urinary tract disorders in the elderly female. In: Raz S, ed. Female urology. Philadelphia: WB Saunders, 1983:308–325.

Table 32.10.   Estimated Incidence of Bacteriuria Associated with Various Urine Collection Devices

Device	New Episodes Per 100 Days Used
Urethral	8
Intermittent	3
External	
Women	3
Men	1

From Warren JW. Urine-collection devices for use in adults for urinary incontinence. J Am Geriatr Soc 1990;38: 364–367.

urinary drainage device (150). Thus, at any point in time, more than 80,000 nursing home patients are using urethral catheters.

The indication for chronic catheter drainage include (*a*) management and prevention of decubitus ulcers or other skin wounds, (*b*) pain on movement that would make frequent changes of clothing and linens difficult, (*c*) decision by patient or family that dryness overweighs the risk of catheterization, and (*d*) overflow incontinence (151). The complications of urethral catheter drainage include chronic bacteriuria with subsequent sepsis, stones, and chronic cystitis. Only two efforts have proven effective in postponing bacteriuria: maintenance of a closed system and use of systemic antibiotics that postpones, not prevents, bacteriuria, which when it occurs will be most likely due to antibiotic-resistant organisms (152). Even with aseptic catheter insertion, bacteriuria occurs at a rate of 3–10% per day, and if catheterized for more than 30 days, 95% of patients are bacteriuric (100) (Table 32.10). Autopsy specimens reveal more than one third of long-term catheterized patients have acute pyelonephritis (153) and, if catheterized for more than 90 days, a 10% incidence of chronic pyelonephritis (100). The urinary tract is also the source of two thirds of febrile episodes in elderly chronically catheterized patients (154). Bacteriuria should not be treated, because clinical symptoms and bacteremia are rare events even at the time of catheter changing (101). The best method of prevention is a catheter-free state, but if not possible, then the use of clean intermittent self-catheterization is preferable. Once catheters are removed, a continence training program is initiated to assist patients to the toilet, voiding habits are monitored, pelvic floor muscle training in cooperative patients is encouraged, fecal impaction is avoided, and there is restriction of sedatives and tranquilizers. Drug therapy includes short-acting diuretics in preference to longer acting ones, when possible; estrogen replacement therapy; and pharmacotherapy for GSI and DI, which was previously discussed.

Behavioral Therapy

As discussed previously, fluid management may be appropriate. Avoiding natural
diuretics such as caffeine and xanthines
commonly found in tea, coffee, and soda is
useful. Percolated coffee has less caffeine
per milligram than drip coffee. Attention to
bowel care is important because chronic
constipation and fecal impaction may interfere with bladder emptying (61). Behavioral
therapy refers to various techniques in behavioral modification that will result in improved urinary control in elderly patients at
home or in institutions. The high percentage of patients with incontinence but normal urodynamic (10) findings suggests that
prompted voiding may have an important
role in reducing incontinence. This system
is applied during the daytime (e.g., 7:00 a.m.
to 9:00 p.m.) as follows: (*a*) patients have
hourly checks and are prompted to void;
(*b*) assistance to the toilet is provided if
required; (*c*) patients are praised for successful toileting; (*d*) social reinforcement is
provided in the form of conversation or personal services if the patient is found dry on
a scheduled check; and (*e*) the patients are
prompted to hold their urine until the next
check (132, 155). In a study of the cognitively impaired and poorly mobile (only
11% independently ambulatory), Schnelle
(132) showed that 40% will respond to the
point in which they experience less than one
incontinent episode in a 12-hour period.
Unfortunately, those patients who are the
most incontinent respond the poorest. Many
nursing homes do not use prompted voiding
because the 1- to 2-hour schedule is too
labor intensive. Data from Burgio et al. (133)
using a 3-hour schedule indicate that 3-hour
prompted voiding can improve dryness in
patients with mild to moderate incontinence. Also noteworthy is that patients
maintained their incontinence after the initial education period.

Environmental Manipulation

An environment conducive to maintaining
continence is important. Simple things such
as adequate lighting, space, nonslip floors,
easy to open doors, and location of toilets
close to bedrooms are often overlooked.
Chair design and bed height should be appropriate (156). Bedside commodes are particularly helpful at night. The most commonly
cited activity associated with falls in the
elderly is going and returning from the bathroom (157, 158).

Incontinent Appliances

Incontinent pads and appliances, discussed elsewhere in this text, comprise a
growing economic impact in providing comfort to our elderly incontinent patients when
the above methods have not controlled the
problems (156, 159). A resource guide of
incontinence aids and services is available
from Help for Incontinent People (P.O. Box
544, Union, SC 29739). Two other organizations of note that can give patients more
information, ideas, and support are Alliance
for Aging Research (2021 K Street, N.W.,
Suite 305, Washington, DC, 20006) and Simon Foundation for Incontinence (Box 835,
Wilmett, IL 60091).

Summary

Urinary tract dysfunction increases with
aging. Patients should have simplified evaluation and testing. The office or bedside cystometrogram is well tolerated and versatile in
its application and can lead to directed
therapy. Because the elderly have a high
incidence of complications due to medications, this can identify those patients for
whom medication may help. Those patients
contemplating surgical correction for stress
incontinence should have more involved
urodynamic testing because of the higher
incidence of intrinsic sphincter dysfunction.
The recent approval by Medicare of periurethral collagen injections has been a great
advance for patients in this age group because of the low morbidity of the procedure.
Patients with pelvic organ prolapse should
have preoperative testing to rule out potential stress incontinence. For those patients
with DI or mixed incontinence, behavioral therapy (bladder retraining) offers improvement and/or cure, including patients in

nursing homes. Medications in this age group should be used cautiously in view of the increased half-life and potential for side effects. A catheter-free state should be the goal of therapy.

Finally, the patient's desires and endpoints need to be considered and should guide therapy. Most patients are not expecting total continence but are happy with a significant improvement, which is certainly achievable with the methods outlined above.

REFERENCES

1. National Institutes of Health Consensus Development Conference. Urinary incontinence in adults. J Am Geriatr Soc 1990;38:265–276.
2. Hu T-W. Impact of urinary incontinence on health-care costs. J Am Geriatr Soc 1990;38:292–295.
3. Katz S, Papsideio J, Stevens R. Cost of incontinence. East Lansing, MI: Centers for Policy Analysis in Aging and Long Term Care, Michigan State University, 1982.
4. Wyman JF, Harkins SW, Fantl JA. Psychosocial impact of urinary incontinence in the community-dwelling population. J Am Geriatr Soc 1990;38:282–287.
5. Norton PA, MacDonald LD, Sedwick PM, Stanton SL. Distress and delay associated with urinary incontinence, frequency and urgency in women. Br Med J 1988;297:1187–1189.
6. Macauley AJ, Stern RS, Holmes DM, et al. Micturition and the mind: psychological factors in the etiology and treatment of urinary symptoms in women. Br Med J 1987;294:540–543.
7. Herzog AR, Diokno AC, Brown MB, Fultz NH, Goldstein NE. Urinary incontinence as a risk factor for mortality. J Am Geriatr Soc 1994;42:264–268.
8. Branch LG, Walker LA, Wetle TT, DuBeau CE, Resnik NM. Urinary incontinence knowledge among community-dwelling people 65 years of age and older. J Am Geriatr Soc 1994;42:1257–1262.
9. Horbach NS. Problems in the clinical diagnosis of stress incontinence. J Reprod Med 1990;35:751–759.
10. Yu LC, Rohner TJ, Kaltreider L, Hu T, Igou JI, Dennis PJ. Profile of urinary incontinent elderly in long-term care institutions. J Am Geriatr Soc 1990;38:433–439.
11. Rekers H, Drodendijk AC, Valkenburg HA, Riphagen S. The menopause, urinary incontinence, and other symptoms of the genito-urinary tract. Maturitas 1992;15:101–111.
12. Burgio KL, Ives DG, Locher JL, Arena VC, Kuller LH. Treatment seeking for urinary incontinence in older adults. J Am Geriatr Soc 1994;42:208–212.
13. McDowell EJ, Silverman M, Martin D, Musa D, Keane C. Identification and intervention for urinary incontinence by community physicians

and geriatric assessment teams. J Am Geriatr Soc 1994;42:501–505.
14. Mohide EA. The prevalence and scope of urinary incontinence. Clin Geriatr Med 1986:2:639–655.
15. Ouslander JG, Zarit SH, Orr NK, Muira SA. Incontinence among elderly community-dwelling dementia patients: characteristics, management, and impact on caregivers. J Am Geriatr Soc 1990;38:440–445.
16. Teasdale TA, Taffett GE, Luchi RJ, Adam E. Urinary incontinence in a community-residing elderly population. J Am Geriatr Soc 1988;36:600–606.
17. Raz R, Stamm W. A controlled trial of intravaginal estradiol in postmenopausal women with recurrent urinary tract infections. N Engl J Med 1993;329:753–756.
18. Meisels A. The menopause: a cytohormonal survey. Acta Cytol 1966;10:49–55.
19. Levy BJ, Wight TN. Structural changes in the aging submucosa: new morphologic criteria for the evaluation of the unstable human bladder. J Urol 1990;144:1044–1055.
20. Gilpin SA, Gilpin CJ, Dixon JS, Gosling JA, Kirby RS. The effect of age on the autonomic innervation of the urinary bladder. Br J Urol 1986;58:378–381.
21. Brockelhurst JC. Bladder outlet obstruction in elderly women. Mod Geriatr 1972;2:108.
22. Staskin DR. Age-related physiological and pathological changes affecting lower urinary tract functions. Clin Geriatr Med 1986;2:701–710.
23. Lewis WH Jr, Alving AS. Changes with age in renal function in adult men. Am J Physiol 1938;123:500.
24. Brockelhurst JC. The aging bladder. Br J Hosp Med 1986;35:8–10.
25. Dennis PJ, Rohner TJ, Hu T, Igou JF, Yu LC, Kaltreider DL. Simple urodynamic evaluation of incontinent elderly female nursing home patients—a descriptive analysis. Urology 1991;37:173–179.
26. Griffiths DJ, McCracken PN, Harrison GM, McEwan A. Geriatric urge incontinence: basic dysfunction and contributory factors. Neurourol Urodyn 1990;9:406–407.
27. Ouslander JG. Lower urinary tract disorders in the elderly female. In: Raz S, ed. Female urology. Philadelphia: WB Saunders, 1983:308–325.
28. Finkbeiner AE. The aging bladder—review article. Int Urogynecol J 1993;4:168–174.
29. Bent AE, Richardson DA, Ostergard DR. Diagnosis of lower urinary tract disorders in postmenopausal patients. Am J Obstet Gynecol 1983;145:218–222.
30. Keane DP, Eckford SD, Shepherd AM, Abrams P. Referral patterns and diagnoses in women attending a urodynamic unit. Br Med J 1992;305:1437–1438.
31. Brocklehurst JC, Andrews K, Richards B, Laycock PJ. Incidence and correlates of incontinence in stroke patients. J Am Geriatr Soc 1985;33:540–542.
32. Resnick NM, Yalla SV, Laurino E. The patho-

physiology of urinary incontinence among institutionalized elderly persons. N Engl J Med 1989;320:1–7.

33. Ouslander JG, Staskin D, Raz S, Su HL, Hepps K. Clinical vs. urodynamic diagnosis in an incontinent geriatric female population. J Urol 1987;137:68–71.

34. McIntosh LJ, Richardson DA. 30-minute evaluation of incontinence in the older woman. Geriatrics 1994;49:35–44.

35. Keister KJ, Creason NS. Medications of elderly institutionalized incontinent females. J Adv Nurs 1989;14:980–985.

36. Jensen JK, Nielsen FR, Ostergard DR. The role of patient history in the diagnosis of urinary incontinence. Obstet Gynecol 1994;83:904–910.

37. Ouslander J, Leach G, Abelson S, Staskin D, Blaustein J, Raz S. Simple vs. multichannel cystometry in the evaluation of bladder function in an incontinent geriatric population. J Urol 1988;140:1482–1486.

38. Wyman JS, Elswick RK, Ory MG, Wilson MS, Fantl JA. Influence of functional, urological, and environmental characteristics on urinary incontinence in community-dwelling older women. Nurs Res 1993;42:271–275.

39. Fonda D, Brimage PJ, D'Astoli M. Simple screening for urinary incontinence in the elderly: comparison of simple and multichannel cystometry. Urology 1993;42:536–540.

40. Diokno AS, Normolle DP, Brown MB, Herzog AR. Urodynamic tests for female geriatric urinary incontinence. Urology 1990;36:431–439.

41. Catalona WJ. Urothelial tumors of the urinary tract. In: Walsh PC, Retik AB, Stamey TA, Vaughan ED, eds. Campbell's urology. 6th ed. Philadelphia: WB Saunders, 1992:1094–1115.

42. Staskin DR. Age-related physiological and pathological changes affecting lower urinary tract function. Clin Geriatr Med 1986;2:701–710.

43. Bard H. The significance of asymptomatic microhematuria in women and its economic implications. A ten-year study. Arch Intern Med 1988;148:2629–2632.

44. Mohr DN, Offord KP, Owen RA, Melton LJ III. Asymptomatic microhematuria and urologic disease: a population-based study. JAMA 1986;256:224–229.

45. Howard RS, Golin AL. Long-term follow up of asymptomatic microhematuria. J Urol 1991;145:335–336.

46. Packham DA. The epithelial lining of the female trigone and urethra. Br J Urol 1971;43:201–205.

47. Ouslander JG. Diagnostic evaluation of geriatric urinary incontinence. Clin Geriatr Med 1986;2:715–730.

48. Judd HL, Cleary RE, Creasman WT. Oral estrogen replacement therapy. Obstet Gynecol 1981;58:267–275.

49. Mandel FP, Geola FL, Meldrum DR. Biological effects of various doses of vaginally administrated conjugated equine estrogens in postmenopausal women. J Clin Endocrinol Metab 1983;57:133–139.

50. Handa VL, Bachus KE, Johnston WW, Robboy SJ, Hammond CB. Vaginal administration of low-dose conjugated estrogens: systemic absorption and effects on the endometrium. Obstet Gynecol 1994;84:215–218.

51. Rigg LA, Hermann H, Yen SSC. Absorption of estrogens from vaginal creams. N Engl J Med 1978;298:195–197.

52. Fantl JA, Wyman JF, Anderson RL. Postmenopausal urinary incontinence: comparison between nonestrogen-supplemented and estrogen-supplemented women. Obstet Gynecol 1988;71:823–828.

53. Ishigooka M, Hashimoto T, Tomaru M, Nakada T, Mitobe K. Effect of hormonal replacement therapy in postmenopausal women with chronic irritative voiding symptoms. Int Urogynecol J 1994;5:208–211.

54. Walter S, Wolf H, Barlebo H, Jensen HK. Urinary incontinence in postmenopausal women treated with estrogens: a double-blind clinical trial. Urol Int 1978;33:135–143.

55. Schreiter F, Fuchs P, Stockamp K. Estrogenic sensitivity of alpha receptors in the urethral musculature. Urol Int 1976;31:13–19.

56. Hilton P, Weddell AL, Mayne C. Oral and intravaginal estrogens alone and in combination with alpha-adrenergic stimulation in genuine stress incontinence. Int Urogynecol J 1990;1:80–86.

57. Walter S, Kjaergaard B, Lose G, et al. Stress urinary incontinence in postmenopausal women treated with oral estrogens (Estriol) and an alpha-adrenoceptor-stimulating agent (Phenylpropanolamine): a randomized double-blind placebo-controlled study. Int Urogynecol J 1990;1:74–79.

58. Fantl JA, Cardozo L, McClish DK. Estrogen therapy in the management of urinary incontinence in postmenopausal women: a meta analysis. First Report of the Hormones and Urogenital Therapy Committee. Obstet Gynecol 1994;83:12–18.

59. Gilpin SA, Gosling JA, Smith ARB, Warrell DW. The pathogenesis of genitourinary prolapse and stress incontinence of urine: a histological and histochemical study. Br J Obstet Gynaecol 1989;96:15–23.

60. Smith ARB, Hosker GL, Warrell DW. The role of partial denervation of the pelvic floor in the aetiology of genitourinary prolapse and stress incontinence of urine: a neurophysiological study. Br J Obstet Gynaecol 1989;96:24–28.

61. Wells TJ. Additional treatments for urinary incontinence. Top Geriatr Rehabil 1988;3:48–57.

62. Thompson JB. Malpositions of the uterus. In: Thompson JB, Rock JA, eds. TeLinde's operative gynecology, 7th ed. Philadelphia: Lippincott, 1992:826–853.

63. McCall ML. Posterior culdeplasty. Surgical correction of enterocele during vaginal hysterectomy: a preliminary report. Obstet Gynecol 1957;10:595.

64. Nichols DH, Randall CL, eds. Massive eversion of the vagina. In: Vaginal surgery, 3rd ed. Baltimore: Williams & Wilkins, 1989:328–357.

65. Kaminski PF, Sorosky JI, Pees RC, Podezaski ES. Correction of massive vaginal prolapse in an older population: a four-year experience at a rural tertiary care center. J Am Geriatr Soc 1993;41:42–44.

66. Meeks GR, Washburne JF, McGehee RP, Wiser WL. Repair of vaginal vault prolapse by suspension of the vagina to iliococcygeus (prespinal) fascia. Am J Obstet Gynecol 1994;171:1444–1454.

67. Randall GG, Nichols DH. Surgical treatment of vaginal eversion. Obstet Gynecol 1971;38:327–332.

68. Morley GW, Delancy JOL. Sacrospinous ligament fixation for eversion of the vagina. Am J Obstet Gynecol 1988;158:872–881.

69. Shull BJ, Cappen CV, Reggs MW, Kuehl TJ. Preoperative and postoperative analysis of site-specific pelvic defects in 81 women treated by sacrospinous ligament suspension and pelvic relaxation. Am J Obstet Gynecol 1992;166:1764–1771.

70. Shull B, Benn SJ, Kuehl TJ. Surgical correction of prolapse of the anterior vaginal segment: an analysis of support defects, operative morbidity, and anatomic outcome. Am J Obstet Gynecol 1994;171:1429–1439.

71. Inmon WB. Suspension of the vaginal cuff and posterior repair following vaginal hysterectomy. Am J Obstet Gynecol 1974;120:977–982.

72. Richardson DA, Bent AE, Ostergard DR. The effect of uterovaginal prolapse on urethrovesical pressure dynamics. Am J Obstet Gynecol 1983;146:901–905.

73. Bump RC, Fantl JA, Hurt WG. The mechanism of urinary incontinence in women with severe uretovaginal prolapse: results of barrier studies. Obstet Gynecol 1988;72:291–295.

74. Ghoniem GM, Walters F, Lewis V. The value of the vaginal pack test in large cystoceles. J Urol 1994;152:931–934.

75. Rosenzweig BA, Pushkin S, Blumenfeld D, Bhatia NN. Prevalence of abnormal urodynamic test results in continent women with severe genitourinary prolapse. Obstet Gynecol 1992;79:539–542.

76. Horbach NS, Ostergard DR. Predicting intrinsic urethral sphincter dysfunction in women with stress urinary incontinence. Obstet Gynecol 1994;84:187–192.

77. McGuire EJ. Urodynamic findings in patients after failure of stress incontinence operations. Prog Clin Biol Res 1981;78:351–360.

78. Sand PK, Bowen LW, Panganiban R, Ostergard DR. The low pressure urethra as a factor in failed retropubic urethropexy. Obstet Gynecol 1987;69:399–402.

79. Stanton SL, Cardoza L, Williams JE, Ritchie D, Allen V. Clinical and urodynamic features of failed incontinence surgery in the female. Obstet Gynecol 1978;51:515–520.

80. Blaivas JG, Jacobs BZ. Pubovaginal sling for the treatment of complicated stress incontinence. J Urol 1991;145:1214–1218.

81. Summit RL, Bent AE, Ostergard DP, Harris TA. Stress incontinence and low urethral close pressure: correlation of preoperative urethral hypermobility with successful suburethral sling procedures. J Reprod Med 1990;35:877–880.

82. Appell RA, Macaluso JN, Deutsch JS, Goodman JR, Prats LJ, Wahl P. Urogynecologic control of incontinence with GAX collagen: the LSU experience. J Endourol 1992;6:275–277.

83. Herschorn S, Radomski SB, Steele DJ. Early experience with intraurethral collagen injections for urinary incontinence. J Urol 1992;148:1797–1800.

84. Drutz HP, Cha LS. Massive genital and vaginal vault prolapse treated by abdominal-vaginal sacropexy with use of Marlex mesh: review of the literature. Am J Obstet Gynecol 1987:156:387–392.

85. Hosking MP, Warner MA, Lobdell CN, et al. Outcomes of surgery in patients 90 years of age and older. JAMA 1989;261:1909–1915.

86. Keating HJ III. Major surgery in nursing home patients: procedures, morbidity, and mortality in the frailest of the frail elderly. J Am Geriatr Soc 1992;40:8–12.

87. Eberle CM, Winsemius D, Garibaldi RA. Risk factors and consequences of bacteriuria in non-catheterized nursing home residents. J Gerontol 1993;6:M266–M271.

88. Zilkoski MW, Smucker DR, Mayhew HE. Urinary tract infections in elderly patients. Postgrad Med 1988;84:191–206.

89. Clague JE, Horan MA. Urine culture in the elderly: scientifically doubtful and practically useless? Lancet 1994;344:1035–1036.

90. Jones SR, Kimbrough R. UTIs and two new antibiotics in the elderly. Geriatrics 1988;43:49–58.

91. Abrutyn E, Mossey J, Berlin JA, et al. Does asymptomatic bacteriuria predict mortality and does antimicrobial treatment reduce mortality in elderly ambulant women. Ann Intern Med 1994;120:827–833.

92. Ascher AW. Bacteriuria and kidney damage. Adv Nephrol 1977;6:333–340.

93. Reid G. Do antibiotics clear bladder infections? J Urol 1994;152:865–867.

94. Norrby SR. Short-term treatment of uncomplicated lower urinary tract infections in women. Rev Infect Dis 1990;12:458–467.

95. Hooton TM, Winter C, Tiu F, Stamm WE. Randomized comparative trial and cost analysis of 3-day antimicrobial regimens for treatment of acute cystitis in women. JAMA 1995;273:41–45.

96. Pfau A, Sacks TG, Shapiro A, Shapiro M. A randomized comparison of 1-day vs. 10-day antibacterial treatment of documented lower urinary tract infection. J Urol 1984;132:931–933.

97. Osterberg E, Aberg H, Hallander HO. Efficacy of single-dose versus seven-day trimethoprim treatment of cystitis in women. A randomized double blind trial. J Infect Dis 1990;161:942–947.

98. Pfau A, Sacks TG. Single-dose quinolone treatment in acute uncomplicated urinary tract infection in women. J Urol 1993;149:532–534.

99. Avorn J, Monane M, Gurwitz JH, Glynn J, Chood-novskiy I, Lipsitz LA. Reduction of bacteriuria and pyuria after ingestion of cranberry juice. JAMA 1994;217:751–754.

100. Warren JW, Muncie HL, Hebel JR, Hall-Craggs M. Long-term urethral catheterization increases risk of chronic pyelonephritis and renal inflammation. J Am Geriatr Soc 1994;42:1286–1290.

101. Polastri F, Auckenthaler R, Loewe F, Michel J, Lew D. Absence of significant bacteriuria during urinary catheter manipulation in patients with chronic indwelling catheters. J Am Geriatr Soc 1990;38:1204–1208.

102. Kegel AH. Progressive resistance exercise in the functional restoration of the perineal muscles. Am J Obstet Gynecol 1948;56:238–248.

103. Henalla SM, Kirwin P, Castleden CM, Hutchins CJ, Breeson AJ. The effect of pelvic floor exercises in the treatment of genuine urinary stress incontinence in women at two hospitals. Br J Obstet Gynaecol 1988;95:602–606.

104. Wells TJ. Pelvic (floor) muscle exercise. J Am Geriatr Soc 1990;38:333–337.

105. Henderson J, Taylor K. Age as a variable in an exercise program for the treatment of simple urinary stress incontinence. J Obstet Gynecol Neonat Nurs 1987;16:266–272.

106. Burgio KL, Robinson JC, Engel BT. The role of biofeedback in Kegel exercise training for stress urinary incontinence. Am J Obstet Gynecol 1986;154:54–64.

107. Burns PA, Pranikoff K, Nochajski T, Desotelle P, Howard MK. Treatment of stress incontinence with pelvic floor exercises and biofeedback. J Am Geriatr Soc 1990;38:341–344.

108. Shepherd AM, Montgomery E, Anderson R. Treatment of genuine stress incontinence with a new perineometer. Physiotherapy 1983;69:113.

109. Castleden CM, Duffin HM, Mitchell EP. The effect of physiotherapy on stress incontinence. Age Ageing 1984;13:235–237.

110. Bent AE, Sand PK, Ostergard DR, Brubaker LT. Transvaginal electrical stimulation in the treatment of genuine stress incontinence and detrusor instability. Int Urogynecol J 1993;4:9–13.

111. Plevnick S, Janez J, Vrtacnik P. Short-term electrical stimulation: home treatment for urinary incontinence. World J Urol 1986;4:24–26.

112. Sand PK, Richardson DA, Staskin DR, et al. Pelvic floor stimulation in the treatment of genuine stress incontinence: a multicenter placebo controlled trial. Presented at the annual meeting of the American Urogynecologic Society, Toronto, Canada, September, 1994.

113. Fall M, Lindstrom S. Functional electrical stimulation: physiological basis and clinical principles. Int Urogynecol J 1994;5:296–304.

114. Peattie AB, Plevnik S, Stanton SL. Vaginal cones: a conservative method of treating genuine stress incontinence. Br J Obstet Gynaecol 1988;95:1049–1053.

115. Olah KS, Bridges N, Denning J, Farrar DJ. The conservative management of patients with symptoms of stress incontinence: a randomized prospective study comparing weighted vaginal cones and interferential therapy. Am J Obstet Gynecol 1990;162:87–92.

116. Gillan G, Stanton SL. Long-term follow-up of surgery for urinary incontinence in elderly women. Br J Urol 1984;56:478–481.

117. Holschneider CH, Solh S, Lebherz TB, Montz FJ. The modified Pereyra procedure in recurrent urinary stress incontinence: a 15-year review. Obstet Gynecol 1994;83:573–578.

118. Peattie AB, Stanton SL. The Stamey operation for correction of genuine stress incontinence in the elderly woman. Br J Obstet Gynaecol 1989;96:983–986.

119. Nitti VW, Bregg KJ, Sussman EM, Raz S. The Raz bladder neck suspension in patients 65 years old and older. J Urol 1993;149:802–807.

120. Raz S, Sussman EM, Eriksen DB, Bregg KJ, Nitti VW. The Raz bladder neck suspension: results in 206 patients. J Urol 1992;148:845–850.

121. Korman HJ, Sirls LT, Kirkemo AK. Success rate of modified Pereyra bladder neck suspension determined by outcomes analysis. J Urol 1994;152:1453–1457.

122. Stanton SL, Reynolds SF, Creighton SM. The modified Pereyra (Raz) procedure for genuine stress incontinence—a useful option in the elderly or frail patient? Int Urogynecol J 1995;6:22–25.

123. Koonings PP, Bergman A, Bellard CA. Low urethral pressure and stress urinary incontinence in women: risk factor for failed retropubic surgical procedure. Urology 1990;37:245–248.

124. Richardson DA, Ramahi AJ, Chalaf E. Surgical management of stress incontinence in patients with low urethral pressures. Gynecol Obstet Invest 1991;31:106–109.

125. Horbach NS, Blanco JS, Ostergard DR, Bent AE, Cornella JL. A suburethral sling procedure with polytetrafluoroethylene for the treatment of genuine stress incontinence in patients with low urethral closure pressures. Obstet Gynecol 1988;71:648–652.

126. Drutz HP, Buckspan M, Flax S, Mackie L. Clinical and urodynamic re-evaluation of combined abdominovaginal Marlex sling operations for recurrent stress urinary incontinence. Int Urogynecol J 1990;1:70–73.

127. Brocklehurst JC, Dillane JB. Studies of the female bladder in old age. II. Cystometrograms in 100 incontinent women. Gerontol Clin 1966;8:306–319.

128. Hilton P, Stanton SL. Algorithmic method for assessing urinary incontinence in elderly women. Br Med J 1981;282:940–942.

129. Bates CP. Continence and incontinence. Ann R Coll Surg Engl 1971;49:18–35.

130. Fantl JA. Bladder changes for women. J Am Geriatr Soc 1990;38:330–331.

131. Fantl JA, Wyman JS, McClish DK, et al. Efficiency of bladder training in older women with urinary incontinence. JAMA 1991;265:609–613.

132. Schnelle JF. Treatment of urinary incontinence in nursing home patients by prompted voiding. J Am Geriatr Soc 1990;38:356–360.

133. Burgio LB, McCormick KA, Scheve AS, Engel BT, Hawkins A, Leahy E. The effects of changing prompted voiding schedules in the treatment of incontinence in nursing home residents. J Am Geriatr Soc 1994;42:315–320.

134. Wein AJ. Pharmacological treatment of incontinence. J Am Geriatr Soc 1990;38:317–325.

135. Tapp AJS, Cardozo LD, Versi E, Cooper D. The treatment of detrusor instability in postmenopausal women with oxybutynin chloride: a double-blind placebo controlled study. Br J Obstet Gynaecol 1990;97:521–526.

136. Abernathy DR, Greenblatt DJ, Shader JP. Imipramine and desipramine disposition in the elderly. J Pharmacol Exp Ther 1985;232:183–188.

137. Ray WA, Griffin MR, Schaffner W. Psychotropic drug use and the risk of hip fracture. N Engl J Med 1987;316:363–369.

138. Tapp AJS, Fall M, Norgaard DJ, et al. Terodiline—a dose titrated, multicenter study of treatment of idiopathic detrusor instability in women. J Urol 1989;142:1027–1031.

139. Gestenberg TC, Klarskov P, Ramirez D, et al. Terodiline in the treatment of urgency and motor urge incontinence: a clinical and urodynamic double-blind cross over study. Br J Urol 1986;58:129–133.

140. Norton P, Karram M, Wall LL, Rosenzweig B, Benson JT, Fantl JA. Randomized double-blind trial of terodiline in the treatment of urge incontinence in women. Obstet Gynecol 1994;84:386–391.

141. Connolly M, Estridge P, White B, Morley C, Cowan C. Torsades de pointes ventricular tachycardia and Terodiline. Lancet 1991;338:344–346.

142. Knudsen UB, Rittig S, Tedersen JB, Norgaard JP, Djaarhus JC. Long-term treatment of nocturnal enureses with Desmopressin—influence on urinary output and hematological parameters. Neurourol Urodynam 1989;8:348–349.

143. Eriksen BC, Bergmann S, Eik-Nes SH. Maximal electrostimulation of the pelvic floor in female idiopathic detrusor instability and urge continence. Neurourol Urodynam 1989;8:219–230.

144. Caputo RM, Benson TJ, McClellan E. Intravaginal maximal electrical stimulation in the treatment of urinary incontinence. J Reprod Med 1993;38:667–672.

145. Grosshans C, Passadori Y, Peter B. Urinary retention in the elderly: a study of 100 hospitalized patients. J Am Geriatr Soc 1993;41:633–638.

146. Ouslander JG, Raz S, Hepps K, Su HL. Genitourinary dysfunction in the geriatric outpatient population. J Am Geriatr Soc 1986;34:507–514.

147. Diokno AC. Diagnostic categories of incontinence and the role in urodynamic testing. J Am Geriatr Soc 1990;38:300–305.

148. Bennett CJ, Dionko AC. Clean intermittent self-catheterization in the elderly. Urology 1984;24:43–45.

149. Whitlaw S, Hammonds JC, Tragellas R. Clean intermittent self-catheterization in the elderly. Br J Urol 1987;60:125–127.

150. Warren JW, Steinberg L, Hebel JR, et al. The prevalence of urethral catheterization in Maryland nursing homes. Arch Intern Med 1989;149:1535–1537.

151. Warren JW. Catheters and catheter care. Clin Geriatr Med 1986;2:857–871.

152. Warren JW. Urine-collection devices for use in adults for urinary incontinence. J Am Geriatr Soc 1990;38:364–367.

153. Warren JW, Muncie HL, Hall-Craggs M. Acute pyelonephritis associated with bacteriuria of long-term catheterization: a prospective clinicopathological study. J Infect Dis 1988;158:1341–1346.

154. Warren JW, Damron D, Tenney JH, et al. Fever, bacteremia, and death as complications of bacteriuria in women with long-term urethral catheters. J Infect Dis 1987;155:1151–1158.

155. Hu T, Igou JF, Kiltreider DL, et al. A clinical trial of a behavioral therapy to reduce urinary incontinence in nursing homes: outcomes and implications. JAMA 1989;261:2656–2662.

156. Brink CA. Absorbent pads, garments, and management stress strategies. J Am Geriatr Soc 1990;38:368–373.

157. Morgan VR, Mathison JH, Rice JC, Clemmer DI. Hospital falls: a persistence problem. Am J Public Health 1985;75:775–777.

158. Ashley MJ, Gryfe CI, Amies A. A longitudinal study of falls in an elderly population. II. Some circumstances of falling. Age Ageing 1976;6:211–220.

159. Cottenden AM. Incontinence pads and appliances. Int Disabl Studies 1988;10:44–47.

SECTION V

Detrusor Instability

CHAPTER 33

Detrusor Instability

Joseph M. Montella

Definition

Detrusor instability (DI) (unstable bladder) describes the occurrence of uncontrolled bladder activity resulting in lower urinary tract symptoms. Objectively, the unstable bladder is one that is shown to contract spontaneously, or on provocation, during bladder filling while the patient is attempting to inhibit micturition. DI is diagnosed during provocative cystometry when one of the following conditions occurs: a true detrusor pressure rise of 15 cm H_2O or a true detrusor pressure rise of less than 15 cm H_2O in the presence of urgency or urge incontinence (1). Subthreshold detrusor contractions less than 15 cm H_2O may have clinical significance and have been shown to cause urinary incontinence in 10% and urgency in 85% of patients (2). Additionally, a urodynamic diagnosis associated with the symptom of urge incontinence in the frail elderly is detrusor hyperactivity with impaired contractility (DHIC). These patients have involuntary detrusor contractions causing incontinence but are unable to completely empty their bladders, leaving a large postvoid residual (3). The terms DI and unstable bladder are generally used interchangeably, although for this discussion, the term DI will be applied. A pressure rise during filling may represent decreased bladder compliance or insufficient time to accommodate the increase in volume, because cystometry is time dependent (4), and this would not be considered as DI in this context.

Synonyms that have been used to describe this condition include bladder dyssynergia, vesical instability, and detrusor hyperreflexia. The latter term is now used to describe DI secondary to a known neurological abnormality (1); the other synonyms should not be used. The term neurogenic bladder is reserved for spinal cord injuries and other similar defects and their impact on bladder function.

Finally, the term urge incontinence describes involuntary loss of urine associated with a strong desire to void (urgency). The urgency may be secondary to overactive detrusor function as recorded during cystometry (motor urge incontinence) or may be secondary to hypersensitivity (sensory urge incontinence). In this latter case, cystometry does not reveal detrusor contractions, even though the patient complains of incontinence associated with urgency and a pad test may confirm urine loss. In this chapter, the term urge incontinence will not be used, although European literature uses it interchangeably with DI.

Incidence

The occurrence of involuntary detrusor contractions in infancy is a normal state for bladder emptying and is later controlled by the development of cortical inhibition of reflex bladder activity. Farrar et al. (5) described the prevalence of DI as 8–50%, depending on age distribution. In over 2000 women studied by Abrams (6), DI occurred in 38% of those 65 or older and in 27% less than 65 years of age. In institutionalized women, urinary incontinence secondary to DI is greater than 80% (7). Thus, the prevalence of

DI is greatest at the extremes of life, has a 5–10% occurrence in premenopausal patients, increases to as much as 38% in the elderly, and may be over 80% in institutionalized incontinent elderly patients.

Clinical Presentation

The symptoms of DI include urgency, frequency, urge incontinence, and nocturia, as well as a history of childhood nocturnal enuresis in some patients (8). However, the clinical history has been shown to correlate poorly with the objective diagnosis of urinary incontinence. DI may coexist with genuine stress incontinence, and stressful activity may trigger a detrusor contraction. In 100 women with the urodynamic diagnosis of DI, Wiskind et al. (9) reported that although 86% of patients had symptoms of urge incontinence, 76% also complained of stress incontinence. Sand et al. (10) reported on 188 incontinent women, and of those reporting only stress incontinence, 34.9% had DI. Only 32.6% of patients reporting both urge and stress incontinence had DI.

Differential Diagnosis

Because the symptoms of frequency, urgency, and incontinence overlap with other lower urinary tract conditions, a number of other diagnoses must be entertained. Table 33.1 lists the differential diagnosis for these symptoms. A special word must be written about urethral instability, which tends to be rather poorly defined. Wise et al. (11) investigated the prevalence and significance of

Table 33.1. Differential Diagnosis of Detrusor Instability

Severe genuine stress incontinence
Uninhibited urethral relaxation
Urethral diverticulum
Urinary tract fistula
Cystitis
Bladder foreign body (stone, suture, etc.)
Bladder tumor
Urethritis

urethral instability in a group of women with idiopathic DI. This occurred in 42% of patients with DI and was strongly associated with the sequence of relaxation of the urethra before unprovoked detrusor contraction. Women with DI and a stable urethra exhibited primary contraction of the detrusor, whereas the symptom of stress incontinence was more common in women with urethral instability. They postulated that women with DI should be divided into two groups, those with and those without urethral instability, the latter group possibly benefiting from alpha agonist therapy. In addition, Petros and Ulmsten (12) found that provocative urethrocystometry revealed a rise in detrusor pressure followed by a fall in urethral pressure, both preceded by urge symptoms. They concluded that urethral instability, DI, and urge incontinence were different manifestations of a prematurely activated micturition reflex. Urethral instability may not be a separate entity but a part of urine loss associated with urge.

Etiology

Table 33.2 lists the etiologies of DI. Neurological diseases (multiple sclerosis, cere-

Table 33.2. Etiologies of Detrusor Instability

Neurological disease
  Multiple sclerosis
  Cerebrovascular disease
  Parkinsonism
  Alzheimer's disease
Local bladder or urethral irritation
  Cystitis
  Foreign bodies (stones, suture material)
Outflow obstruction
  Tumors
  Genitourinary prolapse (cystocele, vaginal
    vault prolapse)
  Previous antiincontinence surgery
Medication (parasympathomimetics)
Idiopathic
  Disorder of bladder ganglia
  Disorder of pacemaker cells
  Generalized smooth muscle disorders
  Increased sensory nerve density
  Prostacyclin deficiency

brovascular disease, parkinsonism, Alzheimer's disease), local bladder and urethral irritants (cystitis, foreign bodies, tumors), outflow obstruction (severe cystocele or vaginal vault prolapse), and medications (parasympathomimetics) must be considered as etiologies. Most cases, however, apart from those in the very young or elderly, are idiopathic in nature. Del Carro et al. (13) compared women with idiopathic DI with age-matched controls using subtracted cystometry and anal sphincter electromyography sacral reflex analysis along with other neurological tests using evoked potentials. All patients had normal neurophysiological tests, and there was no significant difference between patients and controls. Because women with idiopathic DI do not appear to have either clinical or subclinical damage of central sensory or motor pathways, other investigators have put forth their theories regarding intrinsic bladder abnormalities. These include disorders of the bladder ganglia, disorder of pacemaker cells, generalized smooth muscle disorders, increased density of sensory nerves, and deficiency in prostacyclin production.

Disorders of the Bladder Ganglia

During the past few years, the role of neuropeptides as neurotransmitters at the various levels of the peripheral and central micturition reflex arc have been evaluated (14). The sacral parasympathomimetics that originate from S2 to S4 are the major excitatory input to the urinary bladder. The corresponding ganglia lie within the bladder itself. Vasoactive intestinal polypeptide (VIP), a neuropeptide, has been found to be present in a certain proportion of cholinergic ganglion cells and functions as an inhibitory agent in this parasympathomimetic pathway. Furthermore, VIP is noted to be in reduced concentrations in detrusor muscles of patients with DI (14).

Enkephalins may also be released from certain bladder ganglia and function as inhibitory agents in central and peripheral efferents controlling bladder capacity and stability. Exogenous enkephalins have been shown to depress the release of acetylcholine from the preganglionic nerve and thus inhibit transmission in bladder parasympathomimetic ganglia. This effect is demonstrated with the administration of opiate epidural drugs. This produces urinary retention in a significant number of patients and has been demonstrated urodynamically to reduce the magnitude of detrusor contractions and increase bladder capacity (15).

Disorder of Pacemaker Cells

The bladder is never really in a complete resting state. Rather, in vitro and in vivo studies show that it is in continuous activity, with rhythmic contractions that wax and wane (16, 17). Van Duyl (18) suggested that small regional contractions from possible pacemaker cells may be the origin of large bladder contractions. In childhood, involuntary spontaneous and rhythmic contractions occur, but these are eventually suppressed via the maturation of cortical control. The persistence or reappearance of such uncontrolled contractions is possibly related to an aberrant control mechanism of pacemaker cells. In vitro studies by Kinder and Mundy (16) showed that muscle from bladders with DI, regardless of the etiology, spontaneously contract more often and with a greater amplitude than muscle from urodynamically normal bladders. This suggests a disorder of the intrinsic neuromodulatory mechanism leading to DI.

Generalized Smooth Muscle Disorder

A significant proportion of patients with irritable bowel syndrome have urinary complaints, including urgency and nocturia. Whorwell et al. (19) studied such patients urodynamically and found that 50% of these patients have DI. They suggested that this high incidence of DI is secondary to a diffuse disorder of smooth muscle or its innervation.

Increased Sensory Nerve Activity

Moore et al. (20) found that the density of subepithelial presumptive sensory nerves in the bladder wall were significantly greater in patients with DI than in normal controls using bladder biopsies stained for acetylcholinesterase activity. They suggested that a relative abundance of these nerves may serve to increase the appreciation of bladder filling, giving rise to the frequency and urgency of micturition characteristic of patients with DI.

Deficiency of Prostacyclin Production

It is also postulated that women with idiopathic DI have a deficiency in the production of prostacyclin that was observed via in vitro studies using bladder biopsies from women with DI and normal controls (21).

Local Bladder Irritation

Bladder or urethral irritation, especially in the proximal urethra and bladder trigone, aggravates and may possibly produce vesical instability via an increased sensory input that overfacilitates the detrusor reflex and results in loss of volitional control.

Outflow Obstruction/ Antiincontinence Surgery

It has been thought that outflow obstruction in the male with prostatic hypertrophy is associated with DI because the relief of this obstruction usually leads to the resolution of DI. However, recent work by Abrams (6) has shown that DI may be related to advanced age and that a postoperative decrease in instability may be due to interruption of sensory afferents. Obstruction with high outflow pressure in women is rare. Abrams studied over 2000 female patients and found only

3.7% had outlet obstruction, defined by a maximum flow rate of less than 15 m/s. Additionally, there was no increased incidence of DI in those patients with outflow obstruction.

It may be hypothesized that elevation of the vesical neck by surgical repair for stress incontinence leads to excessive urethral compression and could cause outflow obstruction, resulting in DI. However, this is not correlated with changes in peak flow rates and maximum voiding pressures. Furthermore, patients with vaginal prolapse and preexisting DI are not usually cured of their instability by repairing the prolapse (22).

The incidence of de novo DI in patients who preoperatively have only genuine stress urinary incontinence ranges from 5–18% (23, 24). It was postulated by Cardozo et al. (23) that repeat surgeries at the vesical neck interfere with the autonomic nerve supply of the bladder and result in DI. In a review of six studies of patients who had a Burch colposuspension performed for stress incontinence, Vierhout and Mulder (25) found the prevalence between 5% and 27% with 68 of 396 patients developing de novo DI.

Psychological

Various methods of behavioral modification have been used with success in treating patients with DI. These methods include bladder drills, biofeedback, and hypnotherapy (14–16). This lends evidence to a psychosomatic etiology for DI in a certain number of patients.

Diagnosis

The classic history is that of an urgency to void that when not relieved immediately or by frequent voiding, culminates in sudden urine loss. The physical examination should include a neurological evaluation of the lower sacral segments, including bulbocavernosus and anal wink reflexes. The pelvic examination is usually normal; however, severe genitourinary prolapse must be ruled out. Subjective symptoms are documented via a 24-hour voiding diary, which can reveal

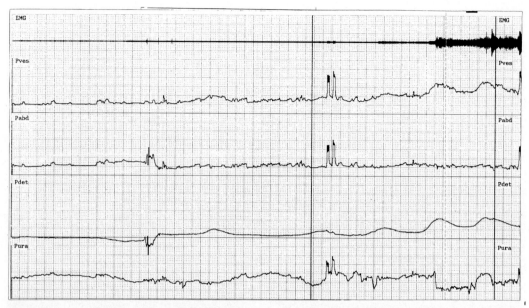

Figure 33.1. Multichannel CMG illustrating detrusor instability. The patient had a detrusor contraction after she washed her hands. Before provocation, she had no contraction.

the presence of urgency, frequency, or urge incontinence.

Objective testing includes urinalysis and culture to rule infection and hematuria, the latter of which may be indicative of a tumor or stone in the urinary tract and should be investigated by cystourethroscopy. Uroflowmetry may reveal obstructive voiding patterns secondary to severe genitourinary prolapse or tumor. Postvoid residual determination is important to document adequate detrusor function and rule out DHIC.

It is important to perform urodynamic testing on patients with complaints of DI. Wiskind et al. (9) retrospectively reviewed 100 patients with the urodynamic diagnosis of DI and found no significant correlations between the symptoms of urinary frequency and urgency and the cystometric findings. The "gold standard" of diagnosis is the standing multichannel cystometrogram, which provides information on the filling phase of bladder function and measures the pressure-volume relationships. The diagnosis of DI is made when uninhibited contractions of greater than 15 cm H_2O occur during bladder filling (motor) or when clinical symptoms coincide with rises in detrusor pressure less than 15 cm H_2O (sensory) (1).

It is also important to closely duplicate the circumstances surrounding urine loss, which would include provocative maneuvers such as coughing, positional changes, running water, hand washing, rapid filling, and temperature change of the filling medium. These can increase the sensitivity of the test (Fig. 33.1). Without provocation, DI will be undiagnosed in 30–40% of patients (9). In cases in which traditional cystometry fails to produce a diagnosis, alternative methods may be used. One such method is extramural ambulatory urodynamic monitoring. McInerney et al. (26) and Webb et al. (27) in two separate studies pronounced ambulatory monitoring as more sensitive in the diagnosis of DI than conventional cystometry. Porru and Usai (28) used this technique in 46 patients with urinary incontinence, 16 of whom had urge incontinence symptoms. Conventional cystometry identified detrusor contractions in only 50% of these patients, whereas ambulatory monitoring identified detrusor contractions in 93%. Another technique involves diuresis cystometry in which a patient is given a diuretic to fill the bladder to more closely approximate the anterograde filling phase. Van Venrooij and Boon (29) evaluated women with frequency and urge incontinence with a negative retrograde cystometrogram using diure-

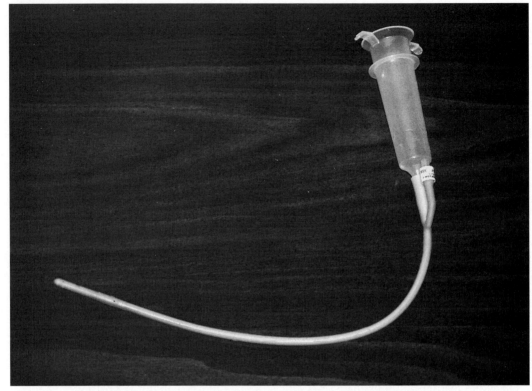

Figure 33.2. Toohey syringe attached to catheter for bedside cystometrogram.

sis cystometry and noted an increase in the detection of DI.

Finally, although multichannel standing cystometry is considered the gold standard for diagnosis, it may not always be possible to perform this test in those with poor mobility or in those who are unable to maintain a standing position. Simple cystometry at the bedside was found to have a specificity of 75% and a sensitivity of 88% compared with multichannel testing in the diagnosis of DI (30). This may be an excellent method of diagnosing DI in the frail elderly using a Toohey syringe attached to a Foley catheter (Fig. 33.2). The bladder is filled in incremental fashion and a rise in the meniscus represents a detrusor contraction.

Management

There are several methods of managing DI as listed in Table 33.3. Depending on the degree of the patient's incontinence and desires, these treatments may be used separately or in tandem.

Table 33.3. Management of Detrusor Instability

Behavioral (timed voiding)
Electrical stimulation
Medical
    Anticholinergics
    Tricyclic antidepressants
    Calcium channel blockers
Surgical
    Augmentation cystoplasty
    Bladder denervation

Bladder Training (Timed Voiding)

There are three main components to bladder training: education, scheduled voiding with systematic delay of voiding, and positive reinforcement. The education portion combines written, visual, and verbal instruction that serves to familiarize the patients with the anatomy and physiology of the lower urinary tract. Patients are then asked to resist or inhibit the sensation of urgency, to postpone voiding, and to urinate according to a timetable rather than according to the urge to void (31). In addition to this, adjustment in fluid loads and delaying voiding to increase bladder volume may be used to augment this therapy (32). The patient is also asked to complete a daily diary as illustrated in Figure 33.3.

Fantl et al. (33) conducted a controlled randomized study of 131 women with unstable detrusor function and sphincteric incompetence who either received treatment in the form of behavioral strategies to decrease urge, patient education, and a schedule of voiding. Twelve percent became dry and 75% had at least a 50% reduction in the number of incontinence episodes, with a greater effect in women with DI. Although primarily used for treatment of stress incontinence, pelvic floor muscle exercises may augment bladder training (34).

Electrical Stimulation

Nonimplantable neuromuscular electrical stimulation involves stimulating the pelvic viscera, the pelvic muscles, or the nerve supply to these structures. Electrical stimulation is used to inhibit detrusor overactivity by influencing the sacral micturition reflex arc (35). This technique is described in Chapter 41.

Medication

ANTICHOLINERGICS

Anticholinergic agents are recommended as first-line medical therapy for DI by working at the ganglionic receptor to block contraction of the normal bladder and the unstable bladder. These medications are contraindicated in patients with narrow-angle but not wide-angle glaucoma. The low dosage range is always initially used in elderly patients.

Because of the strength of the studies demonstrating its usefulness, oxybutinin is considered the anticholinergic agent of choice, combining both anticholinergic and smooth muscle relaxant properties. In five placebo-controlled studies in middle-aged outpatients, oxybutinin reduced incontinence frequency by 19–58% over placebo (36–40).

NAME _____ **DATE** _____

TIME	VOID	TIME	VOID	TIME	VOID
6 AM		2 PM		10 PM	
7 AM		3 PM		11 PM	
8 AM		4 PM		Midnight	
9 AM		5 PM		1 AM	
10 AM		6 PM		2 AM	
11 AM		7 PM		3 AM	
Noon		8 PM		4 AM	
1 PM		9 PM		5 AM	

Please place a check mark next to the time that you void.

Figure 33.3. Timed voiding record.

Side effects were noted in all studies and included dry skin, blurred vision, nausea, constipation, and marked xerostomia. The severity of side effects increased with increasing dosages, with severe xerostomia occurring in 84% of patients receiving oxybutinin in a dose of 5 mg four times a day. The recommended dosage is 2.5–5 mg taken orally three or four times a day (36).

Propantheline is the prototype of anticholinergic agents used for urological conditions because it best approximates atropine's effect on the bladder in vitro, although its central nervous system side effects are less marked. This is recommended as a second-line anticholinergic agent in doses of 7.5–30 mg three to five times per day and may need to be given in higher doses of 15–60 mg qid. Side effects include blurry vision, xerostomia, nausea, constipation, tachycardia, drowsiness, and confusion, the most common of which was xerostomia. Two studies evaluated propantheline use in nursing home patients and found a 13–17% reduction of incontinence over placebo, which was statistically significant (41, 42).

Dicyclomine hydrochloride is an anticholinergic agent with smooth muscle relaxant properties. Studies are limited, and those studies that were performed included small numbers of patients. No studies exist comparing this to other anticholinergics. However, clinical usefulness has been derived using 10–20 mg two to four times daily, and it may be a tolerable first-line approach in the elderly patient.

Flavoxate is a tertiary amine that has smooth muscle relaxant properties in vitro. Four randomized controlled studies failed to demonstrate a significant benefit over placebo (38, 43–45), and therefore this medication is not recommended for the treatment of urge incontinence.

Hyoscyamine and other oral anticholinergics are known to be used for the treatment of DI; however, there are no studies that adequately compare the effects of this medication to placebo. Dosage of this is 0.125 mg three to four times a day.

TRICYCLIC ANTIDEPRESSANTS

The effects of tricyclic antidepressants on the lower urinary tract are twofold: anticholinergic properties as described above and alpha-adrenergic properties to increase tone of the urethra and bladder neck. Two randomized controlled studies revealed the effectiveness of doxepin and imipramine in reducing nocturnal incontinence in patients with DI. Side effects noted in these studies included fatigue, xerostomia, dizziness, blurred vision, nausea, and insomnia (46, 47). The usual oral dosages are 10–25 mg one to three times per day with the daily total dose usually 25–100 mg.

NONSTEROIDAL ANTIINFLAMMATORY AGENTS

These medications are theorized to be effective for DI because of their inhibition of prostaglandin synthetase, thereby interfering with prostaglandin-mediated bladder contractions. Limited research is available, and in general the use of these medications has not been successful. Dosages that are effective in reducing bladder contractions produce extreme side effects of gastritis and ulceration.

CALCIUM CHANNEL BLOCKERS

These agents stop the influx of extracellular calcium required for the contractile process of the detrusor and also prevent the mobilization from intracellular calcium stores with resultant inhibition of excitation contraction coupling (48). They are mainly used in the treatment of angina because of their ability to prevent intracellular movement of calcium through the slow channel in a membrane; however, investigators have used these drugs in the treatment of DI because uninhibited bladder contractions have been shown to be dependent on calcium influx. No controlled studies for nifedipine, diltiazem, or verapamil have been performed, and their use for urge incontinence is not recommended at this time. Terodiline, an agent that possesses both calcium channel blocking and anticholinergic properties, has shown in vivo activity in controlling detrusor contractions, but patients had polymorphic ventricular tachycardia (torsades de pointes) when used in high doses. A randomized double-blind trial of terodiline using 25 mg twice a day showed a 70% reduction in incontinence over placebo, with no cardio-vascular side effects (49). Further investigation of other calcium channel blockers with fewer cardiovascular side effects continues.

Surgery

Surgery should be considered if behavioral or medical therapy has failed because this therapy is associated with advanced morbidity. The two procedures most commonly performed are augmentation intestinocystoplasty and bladder denervation. Augmentation cystoplasty is recommended for those with intractable severe DI or for those with low-compliance bladders. A segment of detubularized intestine is sutured to the bladder to allow low-pressure storage and bladder emptying by voluntary voiding in patients with idiopathic DI without dyssynergia. The goal of augmentation cystoplasty in patients with DI with lower motor neuron lesions or detrusor sphincter dyssynergia is to induce urinary retention and allow the patient to empty using intermittent self-catheterization. The risks of this surgery include voiding difficulties, mucus or stone formation, and metabolic problems. Contraindications include renal insufficiency, bowel disease, and inability to perform self-catheterization. Mean cure rates were 77.2%; mean cure or improvement rates were 80.9% (50–53).

Bladder denervation can be accomplished by selective sacral rhizotomy, S3 foramen injection, or paravaginal denervation. It is beyond the scope of this chapter to describe each procedure in detail. Complications include perineal hypesthesia, wound infection, and intraoperative bleeding. Long-term follow-up revealed that 50% had persistent or recurrent incontinence and an additional 20% were dry only with the addition of anticholinergic agents (54–56).

REFERENCES

1. Abrams P, Blaivas JG, Stanton SL, Anderson JT. The standardization of terminology of lower urinary tract function recommended by the International Continence Society. Int Urogynecol J 1990; 1:45–58.

2. Coolsaet BLRA, Blok C, Van Venrooij GE, et al. Subthreshold detrusor instability. Neurourol Urodyn 1985;4:309–311.

3. Resnick NM, Yalla SV, Laurino E. The pathophysiology of urinary incontinence among institutionalized elderly persons. N Engl J Med 1989; 320:1–7.

4. Coolsaet BLRA. Bladder compliance and detrusor activity during the collection phase. Neurourol Urodyn 1985;4:263–265.

5. Farrar DJ, Whiteside G, Osborne J, et al. Urodynamic analysis of micturition symptoms in the female. Surg Gynecol Obstet 1975;141: 875–877.

6. Abrams P. Detrusor instability and bladder outlet obstruction. Neurourol Urodyn 1985;4: 317–319.

7. Starer P, Libow LS. The measurement of residual urine in the evaluation of incontinent nursing home residents. Arch Gerontol Geriatr 1988;7: 75–81.

8. Fantl JA. Urinary incontinence due to detrusor instability. Clin Obstet Gynecol 1984;27: 474–489.

9. Wiskind AK, Miller KF, Wall LL. One hundred unstable bladders. Obstet Gynecol 1994;83: 108–112.

10. Sand PK, Hill RC, Ostergard DR. Incontinence history as a predictor of detrusor instability. Obstet Gynecol 1988;71:257–260.

11. Wise BG, Cardozo LD, Cutner A, Benness CJ, Burton G. Prevalence and significance of urethral instability in women with detrusor instability. Br J Urol 1993;72:26–29.

12. Petros PE, Ulmsten U. Bladder instability in women: a premature activation of the micturition reflex. Neurourol Urodyn 1993;12:235–239.

13. Del Carro U, Riva D, Comi GC, et al. Neurophysiologic evaluation in detrusor instability. Neurourol Urodyn 1993;12:455–462.

14. de Groat WC, Kawatani M. Neural control of the urinary bladder: possible relationship between peptidergic inhibitory mechanisms and detrusor instability. Neurourol Urodyn 1985;4: 285–288.

15. Rawal N, Mollefors K, Axelsson K, et al. An experimental study of urodynamic effects of epidural morphine and Naloxone reversal. Anesth Analg 1983;62:641–647.

16. Kinder RB, Mundy AR. Pathophysiology of idiopathic detrusor instability and detrusor hyperreflexia: an in vitro study of human detrusor muscle. Br J Urol 1987;60:509–515.

17. Kinder RB, Mundy AR. Inhibition of spontaneous contractile activity in isolated human detrusor muscle strips by vasoactive intestinal polypeptide. Br J Urol 1987;57:20–23.

18. van Duyl WA. Spontaneous contractions in urinary bladder smooth muscle: preliminary results. Neurourol Urodyn 1985;4:301–304.

19. Whorwell PJ, Lupton EW, Erduran D, et al. Bladder smooth muscle dysfunction in patients with irritable bowel syndrome. Gut 1986;27:1014–1017.

20. Moore KH, Gilpin SA, Dixon JS, Richmond DH, Sutherst JR. Increase in presumptive sensory

nerves of the urinary bladder in idiopathic detrusor instability. Br J Urol 1992;70:370–372.

21. Bergman A, Stanczyk FZ, Lobo RA. The role of prostaglandins in detrusor instability. Am J Obstet Gynecol 1991;165:1833–1836.

22. Stanton SL, Williams JE, Ritchie B. The colposuspension operation for urinary incontinence. Br J Obstet Gynaecol 1976;83:890–893.

23. Cardozo L, Stanton SL, Williams JE. Detrusor instability following surgery for genuine stress incontinence. Br J Urol 1979;51:204–206.

24. Langer R, Ron-el R, Newman M, et al. Detrusor instability following colposuspension for urinary stress incontinence. Br J Obstet Gynaecol 1988; 95:607–610.

25. Vierhout ME, Mulder AF. De novo detrusor instability after Burch colposuspension. Acta Obstet Gynecol Scand 1992;71:414–416.

26. McInerney PD, Vanner TF, Harris SA, Stephenson TP. Ambulatory urodynamics. Br J Urol 1991;67: 272–274.

27. Webb RJ, Ramsden PD, Neal DE. Ambulatory monitoring and electronic measurement of urinary leakage in the diagnosis of detrusor instability and incontinence. Br J Urol 1991;68: 148–152.

28. Porru D, Usai E. Standard and extramural ambulatory urodynamic investigation for the diagnosis of detrusor instability-correlated incontinence and micturition disorders. Neurourol Urodyn 1994;13:237–242.

29. van Venrooij GE, Boon TA. Extensive urodynamic investigation: interaction among diuresis, detrusor instability, urethral relaxation, incontinence and complaints in women with a history of urge incontinence. J Urol 1994;152:1535–1538.

30. Fonda D, Brimage PJ, D'Astoli M. Simple screening for urinary incontinence in the elderly: comparison of simple and multichannel cystometry. Urology 1993;42:536–540.

31. McCormick KA, Burgio K. Incontinence: an update on nursing care measures. J Gerontol Nurs 1984;10:16–23.

32. Frewen W. Role of bladder training in the treatment of the unstable bladder in the female. Urol Clin North Am 1979;6:273–277.

33. Fantl JA, Wymen JF, Harkins SW, Ellswick RK, Taylor JR. Efficacy of bladder training in older women with urinary incontinence. JAMA 1991; 265:609–613.

34. Burton J, Pearce L, Burgio KL, Engel BT, Whitehead WE. Behavioral training for urinary incontinence in elderly, ambulatory patients. J Am Geriatr Soc 1988;36:693–698.

35. Vodusek DB, Plevnik S, Vrtacmik P, Janez J. Detrusor inhibition on selective pudendal nerve stimulation in the perineum. Neurourol Urodyn 1988;6:389–393.

36. Tapp AJ, Cardozo LD, Versi E, Cooper D. The treatment of detrusor instability in postmenopausal women with oxybutinin chloride: a double-blind placebo controlled study. Br J Obstet Gynaecol 1990;97:521–526.

37. Holmes DM, Montz FJ, Stanton SL. Oxybutinin versus propantheline in the management of detrusor instability: a patient-regulated variable dose trial. Br J Obstet Gynaecol 1989;96:607–612.

38. Zeegers AGM, Kiesswetter H, Kramer AEJL, Jonas U. Conservative therapy of frequency, urgency and urge incontinence: a double-blind clinical trial of flavoxate hydrochloride, oxybutinin chloride, emepronium bromide and placebo. World J Urol 1989;5:57–61.

39. Riva D, Casolati E. Oxybutinin chloride in the treatment of female idiopathic bladder instability. Clin Exp Obstet Gynecol 1984;11:37–42.

40. Moore KH, Hay DM, Imrie AE, Watson A, Goldstein M. Oxybutinin hydrochloride (3 mg) in the treatment of women with idiopathic detrusor instability. Br J Urol 1990;66:479–485.

41. Dequeker J. Drug treatment of urinary incontinence in the elderly. Controlled trial with vasopressin and propantheline bromide. Gerontol Clin 1965;7:311–317.

42. Zorzitto ML, Jewett MAS, Fernie GR, Holliday PJ, Bartlett S. Effectiveness of propantheline bromide in the treatment of geriatric patients with detrusor instability. Neurourol Urodyn 1986;5: 133–140.

43. Meyhoff HH, Gerstenberg TC, Nordling J. Placebo—the drug of choice in female motor urge incontinence? Br J Urol 1983;55:34–37.

44. Robinson JM, Brocklehurst JC. Emepronium bromide and flavoxate hydrochloride in the treatment of urinary incontinence associated with detrusor instability in elderly women. Br J Urol 1983;55:371–376.

45. Chapple CR, Parkhouse H, Gardener C, Millroy EJ. Double-blind, placebo controlled, crossover study of flavoxate in the treatment of idiopathic detrusor instability. Br J Urol 1990;66:491–494.

46. Lose G, Jorgensen L, Thunedborg P. Doxipin in the treatment of female detrusor overactivity: a randomized double-blind crossover study. J Urol 1989;142:1024–1026.

47. Castleden CM, Duffin HM, Gulati RS. Double-blind study of imipramine and placebo for incontinence due to bladder instability. Age Ageing 1986;15:299–303.

48. Andersson KE, Sjogren C. Aspects on the physiology and pharmacology of the bladder and urethra. Prog Neurobiol 1982;19:71–89.

49. Norton P, Karram M, Wall LL, Rosenzweig B, Benson JT, Fantl JA. Randomized double-blind trial of terodiline in the treatment of urge incontinence in women. Obstet Gynecol 1994;84: 386–391.

50. Sidi AA, Becher EF, Reddy PK, Dykstra DD. Augmentation enterocystoplasty for the management of voiding dysfunction in spinal cord injury patients. J Urol 1990;143:83.

51. George NK, Russel GL. Clam ileocystoplasty. Br J Urol 1991;68:487–489.

52. Strawbridge LR, Kramer SA, Castillo OA, Barrett DM. Augmentation cystoplasty and the artificial genitourinary sphincter. J Urol 1989;142: 297–301.

53. Lockhart JL, Bejany D, Politano VA. Augmentation cystoplasty in the management of neuro-

genic bladder disease and urinary incontinence. J Urol 1986;135:9069–9072.

54. Opsomer RJ, Klarskov P, Holm-Bentzen M, Hald T. Long-term results of superselective sacral nerve resection for motor urge incontinence. Scand J Urol Nephrol 1984;18:101–105.

55. Lucas MG, Thomas DG, Clarke S, Forster DMC. Long-term follow-up of selective sacral neurectomy. Br J Urol 1988;61:218–220.

56. Hodgkinson CP, Drukker BH. Infravesical nerve resection for detrusor dyssynergia. Acta Obstet Gynecol Scand 1977;56:401–403.

CHAPTER 34

Behavioral Therapy for Detrusor Instability

Scott A. Farrell

Introduction

Despite Hodgkinson et al.'s (1) early success at identifying the role of idiopathic detrusor instability in the etiology of urgency incontinence, a definitive cure of this condition has remained elusive. Idiopathic urgency incontinence, a diagnosis made after pathological conditions are excluded, is subdivided into two categories; motor urgency (detrusor instability) and sensory urgency (2). Sensory urgency is diagnosed in the absence of cystometric evidence of detrusor instability. Many of these patients have subclinical detrusor instability (3). The clinical condition is characterized by complaints of urinary frequency, urgency, and incontinence due to an inability to inhibit spontaneous bladder emptying. Patients plagued by the most severe form of this condition are literally housebound by their fear of socially embarrassing incontinence. Traditional conservative management is based on a combination of pharmacotherapy and behavioral modification. Research has focused on the efficacy of regimens that include behavioral modification alone, drug therapy alone, scheduling regimens, biofeedback, and psychotherapy.

The challenge of managing urinary incontinence of the elderly in both the ambulatory community and nursing home settings has prompted a number of studies involving scheduling regimens. These regimens have been particularly successful at reducing incontinence in cognitively impaired nursing home patients. A strong psychological overlay of depression and neurosis often accompanies urinary incontinence problems (4). The most effective treatment regimens incorporate schedules that provide for frequent patient contact with the opportunity to provide positive reinforcement and general encouragement. Biofeedback has been used to successfully manage urgency incontinence in intelligent highly motivated patients. For many patients, supportive therapy and practical guidelines for better bladder behavior will prove to be the most effective and welcome form of treatment for this troublesome problem.

Behavioral Management of Idiopathic Detrusor Instability

Idiopathic detrusor instability (motor urgency incontinence) should be diagnosed only after a thorough evaluation has ruled out the other causes of detrusor instability. Up to 90% of detrusor instability cases may be idiopathic in etiology. A number of pathophysiological mechanisms have been proposed to explain idiopathic detrusor instability. These include local bladder irritation, uninhibited urethral relaxation, smooth muscle dysfunction, incompetent bladder neck, and a deficient cortical inhibition of sacral reflexes (2).

Jeffcoate and Francis (5) were the first to describe a form of behavioral modification that they called "bladder discipline." Their patients were admitted to the hospital for an intensive course of behavioral modification under constant nursing supervision. Adjuvant therapy included anticholinergic and anxiolytic medication. The patient was supervised through a course of strictly enforced gradually increasing voiding intervals. The goals of therapy included a voiding interval of 4 hours, relief of the symptoms of urgency, and continence. Jeffcoate and Francis reported a cure rate of 55% and an overall improvement rate of 78% in over 200 patients using this regimen.

In the wake of Jeffcoate and Francis' early success, a number of authors have reported their results using behavioral management regimens. Their work has resulted in significant modification of the original hospital regimen. A chronology of some of the more important developments in the management of idiopathic urgency incontinence follows.

1. An 86% symptomatic cure was achieved using an outpatient behavioral management regimen. This intensive program included weekly outpatient visits, the use of bladder drill cards to reinforce strict voiding intervals, and propantheline bromide as adjuvant medical therapy (6).

2. Symptomatic cure in patients with urgency incontinence usually occurs within the first few weeks of treatment and precedes the urodynamic finding of stable cystometry. Patients living in stressful circumstances are less likely to succeed with behavioral modification (7).

3. Behavioral modification alone can be used successfully to treat idiopathic urgency incontinence. Urodynamic characteristics such as peak bladder pressures, bladder capacity, and type of detrusor instability (noncompliant bladder versus unstable contractions) did not forecast response to therapy. Significant predictors of treatment failure included a history of recurrent enuresis, bladder pressure of >100 cm H_2O during voluntary interruption of voiding, and failure to improve within the first 2 weeks of treatment (8).

4. An inpatient regimen using bladder drill alone was compared with outpatient medical therapy using flavoxate sodium alone. Eighty-four percent of the bladder drill group achieved continence compared with 56% in the drug-treated group (9).

5. Patients with urgency incontinence were divided into three groups based on their urodynamic diagnosis: stable bladder, noncompliant bladder, and detrusor instability. The initial response rates to an in hospital regimen with adjuvant drug therapy were ≥90% in all three groups. Relapse rates were >40% in patients with noncompliant bladder and detrusor instability. The overall success rate at 3-year follow-up was only 50%. Careful outpatient follow-up with reinforcement by the same physician was crucial to continued success (10).

6. Treatment failures were more likely to occur in patients with urodynamically proven detrusor instability (11).

7. Patients with idiopathic sensory urgency respond well to bladder training regimens (12).

8. A retrospective review comparing the success rates of two outpatient regimens, bladder drill with adjuvant medical therapy and bladder drill alone, found no significant difference. It was concluded that anticholinergic therapy did not confer any additional benefit (13).

9. A randomized prospective clinical trial was conducted comparing 6 weeks of therapy with oxybutynin alone to 6 weeks of bladder training. Although the initial success rate with oxybutynin was high (93%), 10% of the patients dropped out because of side effects attributed to the medication, and at 6 months follow-up the cure rate had dropped to 57%. Although bladder drill had a lower initial success rate (81%), dropout rates were low and the success rate at 6 months was 70% (14).

Behavioral Modification Protocol

An effective bladder training program that has produced good results consisted of a

NAME:_____ Date: _____

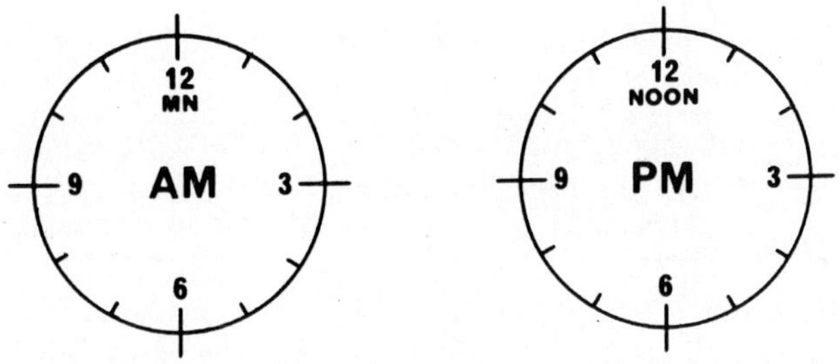

OBSERVATIONS

1) Involuntary leakage: _____

2) Bedwetting: _____

3) Nightime voiding: _____

4) Other: _____

Figure 34.1. Front and back of bladder drill card. Compliance and progress are self-reported. One card is used daily.

6-week outpatient voiding protocol (6). It is presented to the patient as a means of regaining cortical control over the detrusor and is offered as primary management for patients with idiopathic detrusor instability. Patients who are admitted to the program undergo a full urogynecological evaluation to exclude other causes of incontinence. Diagnosis of idiopathic detrusor instability is confirmed by provocative subtractive cystometry that shows an uninhibited crescendo-diminuendo curve of detrusor pressure of any amplitude associated with urinary urgency and/or incontinence or a detrusor pressure curve greater than or equal to 15 cm H_2O that may not be associated with incontinence or urgency.

The patient is given a simple explanation of the problem using tracings and figures as illustrations. Patients are assigned a voiding schedule based on their urolog voiding interval. Instructions to the patients include the following:

1. Empty your bladder at the scheduled time whether or not you feel the urge to void.
2. The amount of urine voided is irrelevant.
3. The important aspect is the voluntary initiation of voiding.
4. Avoid going to the bathroom between scheduled times.
5. Make a special effort to suppress urgency.
6. Do not feel embarrassed if you leak.

Initial voiding intervals during waking hours range from 30–60 minutes and are subsequently increased each week. The protocol requires weekly visits for 6 weeks. During each visit, monitoring of compliance and progress is made, and behavioral reinforcement is accomplished through praise and encouragement. The treatment is considered successful if the patient achieves a voiding interval of 3–4 hours, is continent, and is free from sensory symptomatology. Patients record their daily progress using preprinted cards (Fig. 34.1).

Table 34.1. Scheduling Regimens for Continence Control

Regimen	Indication	Principle
Bladder training	Ambulatory, cognitive intact patient	Reestablishment of cortical inhibition of sacral reflexes
Habit training	Ambulatory, cognitive intact patient	Toileting schedule fitted to individual's voiding pattern
Timed voiding	Neurogenic bladder, minor cognitive impairment	Fixed voiding schedule to regularly empty bladder
Prompted voiding	Severe cognitive and mobility deficits	Attention focusing on need to void with assistance to void

Behavioral Modification in the Elderly

The overall incidence of urinary incontinence increases with age. In older patients, detrusor instability, cognitive deficits, and decreased mobility are more common causes of urinary incontinence. Urinary incontinence in elderly patients may confine them to home or may be the "final straw" that precipitates admission to a nursing care facility. Urinary incontinence consumes an inordinate amount of nursing time and taxes the budgets of nursing home facilities (15).

Hadley (15) described four scheduling regimens (Table 34.1) specifically tailored to the capabilities of the patient. They ranged from behavioral modification, used in cognitively intact ambulatory patients, to prompted voiding, used in patients with severe cognitive and mobility impairments. Hu et al. (16) used a randomized prospective protocol to study the efficacy of a prompted voiding regimen in 133 institutionalized women. Using nurses aides to prompt and assist patients to void every hour for 14 hours of the day, they were able to reduce wet episodes by 0.6 per day, a reduction of 26% over baseline episodes. Ouslander et al. (17) designed a prospective study to look at the combined effects of a timed voiding schedule and oxybutynin chloride in 15 institutionalized patients with detrusor instability. In a longitudinal study design, timed voiding was implemented for the first 2 weeks alone. Oxybutynin was then added to the timed voiding regimen. Timed voiding significantly reduced the episodes of incontinence and the addition of oxybutynin chloride did not confer any additional benefit. Fantl et al. (18)

studied 123 community dwelling women aged ≥50 years using a standard bladder training protocol. They were able to reduce incontinence episodes by 57% and the quantity of fluid loss by 54% in this group of women.

Biofeedback Therapy for Urgency Incontinence

Cardozo et al. (20) used the following definition for biofeedback: "Biofeedback training is a form of learning or re-education in which the patient is placed in a closed feedback loop where one or more of her normally unconscious physiologic processes is made available to her as a visual, auditory, or tactile signal." The goal of biofeedback training is inhibition of detrusor contractions. Using a group of patients who had failed other forms of therapy for urgency incontinence, Cardozo et al. devised a system that provided both visual and auditory warning of impending detrusor contractions. They achieved an 81% improvement rate. Important observations from this study included the following: patients with severe detrusor instability did not respond well, only patients who were highly motivated and intelligent succeeded, and therapy was extremely time consuming. Kjolseth et al. (20) used biofeedback therapy in seven adults with detrusor instability who had failed other forms of treatment. They used a row of red lamps as the signal for a detrusor contraction. The number of lamps lit corresponded to the strength of the detrusor contraction. Patients were instructed to switch off the lamps by contracting the pelvic floor muscles. Over the course of one to four sessions, they were able to cure one patient and achieve moderate improvement in two others. In no cases was detrusor instability converted to a normal cystometrogram.

Burgio et al. (21) combined a timed voiding regimen with biofeedback. Using a system that gave an immediate visual feedback of bladder contractions, patients were instructed to inhibit these contractions by any means. Sessions lasted 1–2 hours and took place every 2–4 weeks. Using this regimen to treat 12 women with urgency incontinence, they achieved average improvement on a number of symptoms. Seventy-five percent of patients with detrusor instability were improved compared with 94% of patients with urgency incontinence in the absence of detrusor instability. Patients with higher mental status scores were more likely to respond to treatment.

Psychotherapy

Walters et al. (4) conducted psychological testing in patients with detrusor instability and compared the results to those from a group of continent women. They found that patients with detrusor instability scored higher than controls on the hypochondriasis, depression, and hysteria scales. These patients also reported a higher rate of sexual dysfunction.

Macaulay et al. (22) found patients with sensory urgency scored higher than normal on anxiety scales. Patients with detrusor instability had higher scores in both anxiety and hysteria. They conducted a randomized trial comparing psychotherapy, bladder drill, and propantheline bromide. The psychotherapy group were seen by a psychiatrist for 8–12 weekly sessions that lasted for approximately 50 minutes. The treatment was designed to offer nonsymptom-oriented measures of support, counseling, and anxiety reduction. Patients who underwent psychotherapy showed significant improvement in symptoms of nocturia, urgency, and incontinence. The bladder training protocol involved weekly visits with the urodynamics unit nurse for 3 months. Patients were trained to resist the urge to void other than at specific time intervals that were gradually increased in length. Patients were also taught Kegel exercises. Patients in the behavioral modification arm of the study noticed a decrease in their state of anxiety and depression. There was only modest improvement in urgency, nocturia, and urinary incontinence. Patients placed on propantheline experienced improvement in urinary frequency but did not notice improvements in any other bladder symptoms.

Conclusions

The pathophysiology of idiopathic urgency incontinence remains elusive. A pragmatic therapeutic approach includes a number of modalities that have been used successfully to treat this problem. The evidence would suggest that there is a significant element of psychological dysfunction in these patients. Therapies that address the psychological needs of the patient are more likely to be successful. The most successful behavior modification regimens have included regular contact with authority figures who provided positive reinforcement and encouragement, thereby meeting the psychological needs of the patients and enhancing therapeutic efficacy. Drugs should not be used as the first line of therapy in patients with urgency incontinence. With drug therapy alone, long-term success rates are low because of the impact of side effects on compliance rates. Adjuvant drug therapy does not significantly improve the outcomes of behavior modification therapy, and side effects from drugs may prompt patients to withdraw from all forms of therapy. Biofeedback is a labor-intensive form of treatment with the prerequisite of an intelligent and highly motivated patient. It will probably continue to play a limited role in the therapeutic armamentarium. Scheduling regimens seem to offer the best means to decrease urinary incontinence in elderly nursing home patients with both physical and cognitive impairment. Although urgency incontinence will undoubtedly persist as a thorny clinical problem, the physician treating these patients should be encouraged by the fact that supportive therapy combined with practical guidelines for better bladder behavior provide both welcome and effective therapy.

REFERENCES

1. Hodgkinson CP, Ayers MA, Drukker BH. Dyssynergic detrusor dysfunction in the apparently normal female. Am J Obstet Gynecol 1963;87: 717–728.
2. Wall LL. Diagnosis and management of urinary incontinence due to detrusor instability. Obstet Gynecol Surv 1990;45(Suppl):1S–47S.
3. Coolsaet BLRA, Elhilali MM. Detrusor overactivity. Neurourol Urodyn 1988;7:541–561.
4. Walters MD, Taylor S, Schoenfeld LS. Psychosexual study of women with detrusor instability. Obstet Gynecol 1990;75:22–26.
5. Jeffcoate TNA, Francis WJA. Urgency incontinence in the female. Am J Obstet Gynecol 1966; 94:604–618.
6. Fantl JA, Hurt WG, Dunn LJ. Dysfunctional detrusor control. Am J Obstet Gynecol 1977;129: 299–303.
7. Frewen WK. An objective assessment of the unstable bladder of psychosomatic origin. Br J Urol 1978;50:246–249.
8. Pengelly AW, Booth CM. A prospective trial of bladder training as treatment of detrusor instability. Br J Urol 1980;52:463–466.
9. Jarvis GJ. A controlled trial of bladder drill and drug therapy in the management of detrusor instability. Br J Urol 1981;53:565–566.
10. Holmes DM, Stone AR, Bary PR, Richards CJ, Stephenson TP. Bladder training—3 years on. Br J Urol 1983;55:660–664.
11. Elder DD, Stephenson TP. An assessment of the Frewen regime in the treatment of detrusor dysfunction in females. Br J Urol 1980;52: 467–471.
12. Jarvis GJ. The management of urinary incontinence due to primary vesical sensory urgency by bladder drill. Br J Urol 1982;54:374–376.
13. Fantl JA, Hurt WG, Dunn LJ. Detrusor instability syndrome: the use of bladder retraining drills with and without anticholinergics. Am J Obstet Gynecol 1981;140:885–890.
14. Colombo M, Zanetta G, Scalambrino S, Milani R. Oxybutynin and bladder training in the management of female urinary urge incontinence: a randomized study. Int Urogynecol J 1995;6: 63–67.
15. Hadley EC. Bladder training and related therapies for urinary incontinence in older people. JAMA 1986;256:372–379.
16. Hu T-W, Igou JF, Kaltreider DL, et al. A clinical trial of a behavioral therapy to reduce urinary incontinence in nursing homes. JAMA 1989;261: 2656–2662.
17. Ouslander JG, Blaustein J, Connor A, Pitt A. Habit training and oxybutynin for incontinence in nursing home patients: a placebo controlled trial. J Am Geriatr Soc 1988;36:40–46.
18. Fantl JA, Wyman JF, McClish DK, Harkins SW, Elswick RK, Taylor JR, Hadley EC. Efficacy of bladder training in older women with urinary incontinence. JAMA 1991;265:609–613.
19. Cardozo LD, Abrams PD, Stanton SL, Feneley RCL. Idiopathic bladder instability treated by biofeedback. Br J Urol 1978;50:521–523.
20. Kjolseth D, Madsen B, Knudsen LM, Norgaard JP, Djurhuus JC. Biofeedback treatment of children and adults with idiopathic detrusor instability. Scand J Urol Nephrol 1994;28:243–247.
21. Burgio KL, Whitehead WE, Engel BT. Urinary incontinence in the elderly. Bladder-sphincter biofeedback and toileting skills training. Ann Intern Med 1985;104:507–515.
22. Macaulay AJ, Stern RS, Holmes DM, Stanton SL. Micturition and the mind: psychological factors in the aetiology and treatment of urinary symptoms in women. Br Med J 1987;294:540–543.

CHAPTER 35

Surgical Therapy for Detrusor Instability

Sherif R. Aboseif and Emil A. Tanagho

Detrusor instability is a socially incapacitating disorder that can be very difficult to treat. Various terms have been used to describe it: the uninhibited, hyperreflexic, irritable, spastic, or unstable bladder. This liberal use of different terms has led to considerable confusion both in description and diagnosis. The International Continence Society defines unstable bladder as that "which is shown to contract (>15 cm H_2O) spontaneously or on provocation during the filling phase associated with the severe urge to urinate despite the patient's attempt to inhibit it" (1). This condition is sometimes difficult to diagnose with standard cystometry and may require ambulatory monitoring over a number of hours of slow filling. Detrusor instability is a normal finding in infancy and is common in old age. It may occur in association with various neurological disorders such as cerebrovascular accidents, spinal cord injury, and multiple sclerosis (detrusor hyperreflexia) or it may be a manifestation of underlying pathology in the bladder such as tumors or outflow obstruction. The latter is more commonly seen in males. In women, it may be encountered after surgery for incontinence and, in a few cases, may require urethrolysis to relieve the obstruction. In most patients, detrusor instability has no discernible underlying cause and is described as idiopathic (2), although many investigators believe this to be related to deficiency of a nonadrenergic/noncholinergic neuromodulator (3).

Although research is still ongoing to clarify the pathophysiology of this debilitating condition, we must continue to treat these patients. Nonoperative management of detrusor instability or hyperreflexia, including behavior modification alone or in combination with pharmacological therapy, can be expected to provide symptomatic relief in a significant number. However, many of these patients will either fail to improve or will be unable to tolerate medical therapy. These patients should be considered candidates for surgical treatment. Catheter drainage (suprapubic or urethral) is usually reserved for the debilitated patient with limited functional bladder capacity who is unresponsive to or cannot tolerate pharmacological therapy but who at the same time is not a surgical candidate. We herein review the surgical options available.

Bladder Hydrodistention

This was initially reported by Helmstein (4) in 1972 for the treatment of carcinoma of the bladder by compromising the blood supply and inducing tumor necrosis. Although this was subsequently replaced by more effective treatments, the technique was adopted by other investigators for detrusor instability (5, 6). In one large series from Oxford with a 7-year follow-up, patients experienced a significant increase in bladder capacity and decrease in frequency. However, although approximately one half of these patients reported symptomatic improvement initially, this relief disappeared with time and only 20% and 10% continued to report symptomatic relief after 1 and 4 years, respectively (7). A recent study by Taub and Stein (8) demonstrated that bladder hydrodistention has no role in patients with detrusor hyperreflexia (secondary to neurological disorder) and only limited success in the symptomatic relief of severe urgency, frequency, and incontinence of other origin. In addition, complications such as transient urinary retention and extraperitoneal bladder rupture have been reported. Anderson and coworkers (9) reported that bladder overdistention produced interstitial and submucosal hemorrhage initially, followed by deposition of collagen fibers; accordingly, they postulated that distention therapy would actually decrease bladder distensibility rather than increase it.

Bladder Augmentation

This is usually indicated in cases of severely spastic and contracted bladder with markedly reduced capacity under anesthesia. In these situations, all denervation procedures are associated with very poor outcome and the patients are left with the option of either augmentation cystoplasty or urinary diversion. The former should be considered only in patients who are physically and mentally capable of dealing with a reconstructed lower urinary tract. In certain situations, a patient might be best served with a simple supravesical diversion. Many patients with augmentation cystoplasty will require clean intermittent catheterization and should possess the manual dexterity and the motivation to perform it.

Selection of the appropriate bowel segment for bladder reconstruction depends on many factors, including the preference of the surgeon, the patient's renal function and anatomy, and the availability of nondiseased bowel segments. It is important to consider not only the physiological effects on the gastrointestinal tract from loss of bowel segments but also the possible metabolic consequences of adding bowel mucosa to the urinary tract.

SURGICAL TECHNIQUE

Enterocystoplasty

Through a lower midline transperitoneal incision, the desired segment of the bowel (ileum, right colon, or the sigmoid colon) is inspected, and its mobility, mesenteric length, and blood supply are assessed. A 20- to 25-cm segment of the bowel is mobilized by dividing its mesentery for a short distance, taking care not to damage its blood supply, and the continuity of the intestine is restored with staples or sutures. The bowel segment selected is partially exteriorized from the wound and irrigated until clear; it is then opened by cutting along its antimesenteric border with the electrocautery. The opened bowel is fashioned into a "U" and the adjacent margins are sutured to each other with 3-0 absorbable suture material. The reconfigured bowel either may be placed on the bladder as a flap (10) or may be further folded to form a cup (11). After the bowel segment is prepared, it is wrapped in a moist gauze and attention is turned to preparation of the bladder. The anterior surface of the bladder is gently freed from the perivesical tissues all the way down to the bladder neck. The posterior wall is dissected free from the anterior wall of the peritoneum. A transverse incision starting just superior to the trigone and the anterior-superior levels is brought up toward the superior pole of the bladder. Pediatric feeding tubes are placed in the ureters to facilitate identification and prevent injury during augmentation.

The bowel patch is brought down, taking care not to twist the vascular pedicle, and is sutured to the bladder, starting posteriorly. A two-layer closure with absorbable suture material is usually performed. A Malecot catheter is usually placed before the anterior segment is sutured in place and is brought through a separate incision away from the suture line. If possible, the drainage tube should be brought through the native bladder.

Gastrocystoplasty

The use of a gastric segment as a bladder replacement or as a means of augmentation was initially described by Sinaiko (12), Leong and Ong (13), and Rudick and associates (14). In both animals and humans, this demonstrated physiological advantages over other bowel segments: active excretion of chloride, low mucous production, favorable fibroelasticity, and low incidence of infection. These characteristics are particularly important in patients with impaired renal or hepatic function.

A gastric wedge is selected close to the cardia of the stomach with its apex close to but not including the lesser curvature. The length of the base is usually about 9–15 cm. The wedge is isolated by incising the greater omentum several centimeters below and parallel to the gastroepiploic artery. The stomach is usually repaired in two layers: an inner through-and-through running 3-0 absorbable suture (Dexon or vicryl) and an outer layer of interrupted seromuscular 3-0 silk sutures. The wedge-shaped gastric flap is brought with its blood supply retroperitoneally through the mesentery of the transverse colon and small bowel and sutured to the bladder in a fashion similar to that for ileocystoplasty.

Other Forms of Cystoplasty

The potential complications of the use of the gastrointestinal tract for augmentation cystoplasty stimulated extensive research for alternative methods.

Autoaugmentation. This approach was initially described by Cartwright and Snow (15) in 1989 as an alternative to enterocytoplasty. The detrusor muscle over the entire dome of the bladder is removed, allowing the underlying epithelium to bulge and function as a large diverticulum to enhance the storage capacity of the bladder. This technique has been adopted by many investigators with encouraging results (15–17).

Ureterocystoplasty. In the few cases with a nonfunctioning kidney on one side associated with a dilated ureter, the bladder can be augmented with the ureter. Its absorptive characteristics are probably similar to the bladder's, and thus major electrolyte imbalance is unlikely. Although ureterocystoplasty might have some advantage over other forms of cystoplasty, experience with it is very limited (18–20).

COMPLICATIONS

Complications Related to Intestinal Surgery

These are rare and include anastomotic leakage, infectious complications such as wound infection and pelvic abscess, wound dehiscence, and intestinal obstruction.

Nutritional Complications

Removal of a substantial portion of the stomach or bowel may result in significant nutritional problems, depending on the segment used. Resection of the stomach may result in the dumping syndrome. Loss of a significant segment of ileum will result in the malabsorption syndrome. Loss of the ileocecal valve may cause reflux of a large number of bacteria from the colon into the ileum, resulting in bacterial overgrowth and interference with reabsorption of fatty acid, fat-soluble vitamins such as vitamins A and D, and bile-salt interaction. Resection of the colon may result in diarrhea, as its main function is to absorb water, sodium, and chloride and to limit their loss in the stool.

Metabolic Complications

Disturbances in serum electrolytes and acid-base balance will depend on the segment used and the length of time that urine is in contact with the bowel mucosa. In general, in the presence of normal renal and hepatic function, these electrolyte abnormalities are usually corrected by normal hemostatic mechanisms. If the stomach is used, a hypochloremic metabolic alkalosis may result from hydrogen and chloride secretion. If the ileum or colon is used, hyperchloremic metabolic acidosis and hypokalemia may occur. This usually results from active reabsorption of sodium and chloride through the ileum with simultaneous loss of bicarbonate and passive loss of potassium. This is usually mild and well handled except in the presence of poor renal function. Osteomalacia has been reported in all forms of urinary intestinal diversion. The cause is probably multifactorial; it may result from chronic acidosis, vitamin D resistance, and excessive calcium loss by the kidneys. Correction of acidosis results in remineralization of the bones.

Cancer

The risk of developing cancer in patients with ureterosigmoidostomy where urine has been diverted into the intact fecal stream is well established and has been estimated between 6% and 29% (mean 11%) (21, 22). However, the risk of tumor in intestine chronically in contact with urine without fecal contamination is not known. Many reports of various tumors developing in patients with ileal conduits, colon conduits, and bladder augmentation have been described, including adenocarcinoma, undifferentiated carcinoma, squamous cell carcinoma, sarcoma, and transitional cell carcinoma (23–25).

Rupture

Spontaneous bladder rupture has been reported by many authors. The exact cause is not clear; however, overdistension of the augmented bladder either from plugging by mucus or from poor compliance with intermittent catheterization seems to be the cause in most cases (26–29). Ischemia, transmural infection, wall weakness, and trauma from external sources or during careless catheterization are other possible causes. Generally, there appears to be no direct correlation between spontaneous rupture and the age of the patient, the interval since enterocystoplasty, the site of the rupture, or the segment of bowel used (29). However, in a recent report by Scheidler and associates (30), 7 of 12 ruptures occurred in cases where the sigmoid colon was used for augmentation.

Urinary Diversion

This is usually considered the last option in patients who are not good candidates for reconstruction of the lower urinary tract. The most common method of urinary diversion is the ileal loop.

Denervation Procedures

PERIPHERAL DENERVATION

Subtrigonal Phenol Injection

Phenol is a potent neurolytic agent that in concentrations over 5% produces an irreversible denaturing of protein (31) and when administered experimentally (in rats) directly to the paravesical plexus results in denervation of the detrusor muscle (32). Subtrigonal phenol injection was introduced in 1982 by Ewing et al. (33) for the treatment of patients with detrusor instability and hyperreflexia. The rationale behind it was that the consequent damage to nerves in the paravesical pelvic plexus should result in relative hypocontractility of the detrusor and hence the abolition of unwanted contractions. Despite encouraging early reports (33, 34), a recent report and review of the literature by Chapple et al. (35) showed the benefit to be short-lived, with only a small percentage of patients (particularly those with hyperreflexic bladder) experiencing any benefit after 6 months. In addition, an overall complication rate of 11% has been reported, including urinary retention, tissue damage with fistula formation (36, 37), and local spread of phenol with severe neural damage, including sciatic nerve palsy and impotence (38). Most authors agree that subtrigonal phenol injection should be reserved only for patients with refractory hyperreflexic bladder in whom no alternative treatment is possible. It should be completely avoided in patients with extensive prior surgery or radiotherapy, as the risk of complications is higher.

Partial Bladder Denervation

This was initially described in the early 1950s in Sweden by Ingelman-Sundberg (39) for the treatment of urge incontinence in women. The same technique was later adopted by Hodgkinson and Drukker (40). Through a vaginal approach, the inferior hypogastric plexuses, which are located lateral to the rectum and usually follow the inferior vesical pedicle medially, are transected as they approach the bladder base. Patients are usually tested before the procedure by injecting 10–15 mL of bupivacaine beneath the bladder trigone transvaginally. The position of the trigone is determined by palpation of an indwelling Foley catheter balloon, which is pulled down gently at the bladder neck. If the patient reports a 6- to 24-hour period of complete freedom from any urge incontinence, the partial bladder denervation procedure will usually have about a 70% chance of symptomatic improvement for a year. If the procedure fails, early or late, a repeat operative procedure usually does not work (41).

Bladder Transection

Transection of the bladder, with division of all the inferior lateral communications including the inferior vesical vessels, was introduced for the control of detrusor instability in 1967 by Turner-Warwick and Ashken (42). The goal of this procedure is also to achieve supratrigonal sensory denervation of the bladder. The technique consisted of a circumferential bladder transection beginning 2 cm above the trigone with subsequent bladder reconstruction. Some investigators have used the same technique in patients with enuretic syndrome, frequency, urgency, and urge incontinence with a success rate ranging between 53% and 81% (43, 44).

Cystolysis

This was first described in 1973 for the alleviation of pain and control of frequency in patients with intractable interstitial cystitis (45). In their initial report, Worth and Turner-Warwick (45) recommended that the procedure should be performed only in patients with reasonable bladder capacity under anesthesia. All patients in their series achieved relief of pain and in most frequency lessened. Bladder capacity under anesthesia only improved in 50% of cases. Later, cystolysis was extended to patients with urinary incontinence secondary to uninhibited neurogenic bladder with remarkable success (46). The main goal of this procedure is to achieve a selective denervation of the detrusor muscle superior to the trigone without interfering with the sphincteric mechanism or bladder base sensation. The technique is relatively simple and consists of extensive mobilization of the bladder, leaving an intact patch of peritoneum over the dome. The plane between the posterior bladder wall and the anterior vaginal wall is developed down to the trigone. The distal 2–3 inches of the ureters are freed from all surrounding tissues, leaving the ureteral sheath intact. The superior vesical pedicle and the ascending branches of the inferior vesical, together with all the surrounding tissue, are divided as they enter the detrusor muscle. The procedure is considered complete when the bladder remains attached only to peritoneum over the dome superiorly, the ureters posteriorly, and the trigone and bladder neck inferiorly. Leach et al. (47) recommend more extensive dissection of the bladder base posteriorly with complete urethral mobilization from the anterior vaginal wall. A Burch bladder neck suspension is then performed to support the urethra. This procedure was performed on 14 patients with severe detrusor hyperreflexia secondary to severe neurological problems. Eight patients had indwelling catheters. Twelve of 14 patients experienced some relief.

CENTRAL DENERVATION

Subarachnoid Block

Since the early report by Comarr in 1959 (48), subarachnoid block with alcohol has been used in patients with severe somatic spasticity as well as severe detrusor hyperreflexia and a small functional capacity. In this technique, 5–10 mL of absolute alcohol is injected into the subarachnoid space between L4 and S1 vertebral levels. Recently, Miyata et al. (49) reported the use of 0.3–0.6 mL of 10% phenol glycerin injected into the subarachnoid space in patients with traumatic spinal cord injury. In all patients, detrusor hyperreflexia and urinary incontinence disappeared or abated significantly. However, the risk of associated erectile dysfunction is high.

Selective Posterior (Dorsal) Rhizotomy

Sacral rhizotomy has been advocated for many years as a treatment of detrusor hyperreflexia in an attempt to achieve urinary continence and protect the upper tract from high detrusor pressure. Early attempts at this form of therapy involved extensive rhizotomies and spinal cordotomies with the resultant abolition of all sacral innervation to the bladder and surrounding structures (50, 51). Although it is possible to perform total sacral neurectomy in patients with complete supraconal spinal lesion without major adverse effects, in ambulatory patients these nonselective procedures may result in flaccid bladder; erectile dysfunction; and rectal, anal, and urethral dysfunction. For this reason, selective neurectomy of the roots innervating the bladder alone has been suggested (52–54). The neural control to the bladder arises mainly from the S3 and S4 nerve roots, with S2 innervating the striated urethral sphincter (55, 56). Ideally, to increase bladder capacity, S3–S4 dorsal rhizotomy should be performed. However, due to both the intrinsic variability in bladder innervation and the patchy neural integrity in patients with spinal cord injury, one must tailor the rhizotomy on the basis of intraoperative neurostimulation and urodynamic monitoring (57–59). Selective rhizotomy results in less erectile and sphincteric dysfunction (60). To predict the success of central denervation procedures, some authors recommend temporary nerve blockade before rhizotomy to determine those patients in whom bladder capacity is increased or the onset of detrusor contraction is delayed (59, 61).

Long-term results of sacral rhizotomy have varied among different series. Rockswold et al. (62) reported a success rate of only 31% in patients with multiple sclerosis and severe urge incontinence and recommended more extensive rhizotomy if long-term success is to be achieved. Many investigators have reported recurrence of reflux detrusor activity and suggest that this is most likely due to development of reflex pathways along surviving roots (62–64) or to the sprouting of alpha-adrenergic nerve terminals at the bladder base (65). In another series, Torring et al. (66) reported excellent long-term results of selective sacral neurectomy in 12 patients with intractable urge incontinence. Excellent results were also reported recently by Gasparini et al. (60) in patients with spinal cord injury and severe reflex neuropathic bladder. It seems that this wide variation is related to selection criteria and to the technique and extent of the rhizotomy. Patients with severe spasticity and severely contracted bladders are usually not good candidates for this procedure.

Electrical Stimulation and Neuromodulation

Electrical stimulation to control bladder and urethral function has been attempted in the past with varying success. Transvaginal or transanal electrical stimulation of the pelvic floor has been used for the treatment of detrusor instability and voiding dysfunction. Although these techniques were initially promising, their long-term use has not proved very successful. In recent years, neural stimulation of the sacral roots for the control of all aspects of bladder function has attracted attention in both Europe and the United States. It has been advocated as a treatment option for various lower urinary tract dysfunctions, such as incontinence (including postprostatectomy), urge-frequency syndromes, and chronic pelvic pain syndromes (67, 68). This approach is therapeutically attractive because it uses existing physiological mechanisms to correct detrusor hyperreflexia or to modulate pelvic floor function. Electrodes can be implanted either around the whole nerve root (foramen electrode) in patients with detrusor instability and voiding dysfunction or around the ventral roots in association with selective dorsal rhizotomy in patients with spinal cord injury and severely spastic bladder. In the latter, the electrodes can be placed either intradurally (69) or extradurally (70). A neurophysiological explanation for the effectiveness of this treatment mode in detrusor instability is based on animal experiments and neurophysiological studies in humans. A natural reflex between the activity of the external sphincter and detrusor exists. Neural stimulation will use the same principle to inhibit detrusor hyperreflexia. It will initiate muscular activity, either smooth or striated muscle (71–73), thus enhancing the tone within the urethral sphincter, which will have a suppressive effect on the irritable detrusor muscle (74–77). In addition, it will improve detrusor contraction and bladder emptying.

Detrusor dysfunction in many of these patients appears to originate with unstable urethral activity by activation of the voiding reflexes. Reflex-triggered detrusor activity leads to precipitate urgency, frequency, and incontinence. Active contraction of the pelvic muscles induced by stimulation has an inhibitory effect on this muscular spasticity, with consequent reduction of symptoms. As prerequisites to neurostimulation, the sacral motoneuron pathway must be intact with no damage to the pelvic nerve and the detrusor must contract (as determined by cystometrography). Sacral nerve root anatomy and responses to stimulation vary significantly; thus, preoperative percutaneous testing and intraoperative urodynamic monitoring are very important.

PREOPERATIVE TEST (TEMPORARY) STIMULATION

This is an effective method for determining the therapeutic potential of chronic neural stimulation. Using the bony landmarks of the sacrum, one can easily identify the sacral foramina. Each foramen can be entered with an insulated needle and the response to stimulation can be tested. Visceral and sphincteric responses are monitored urodynamically. S2 stimulation results in inward rotation of the leg and flexion of the foot and the toes with little perineal activity and some urethral sphincteric response but no bladder response. S4 stimulation usually results in contraction of the levator ani with visible perineal movement, no leg or foot activity, and, not infrequently, a bladder response. S3 stimulation generally produces detrusor and sphincteric action. External signs of S3 stimulation include plantar flexion of the great toe, occasional flexion of the foot or small toes, and anal sphincteric contraction. There is a variable contribution of the S3 nerve to the pudendal nerve, leading to referred sensation in the external genitalia and groin. Some patients will report a pulling sensation in the pelvis.

After proper identification of S3, a fine insulated wire electrode is placed into the foramen through the testing needle and is connected to an external stimulator. The response to stimulation is carefully assessed after a trial period of 5 days. If a subjective improvement of more than 50% is observed, the patient is considered for permanent electrode implantation.

PLACEMENT OF PERMANENT ELECTRODES

The patient is placed, well padded, in a prone position on a Wilson frame with both hips and knees flexed to 65°. An S-shaped or a midline sacral incision is carried through the skin and subcutaneous tissue down to the sacral spine. With a Shaw knife blade to control bleeding without diathermy, an incision is made on the side of the spinal processes to separate all fascial muscular structures attached to the spine. Less bleeding is encountered if one stays very close to the bone. Once this plane is developed, blunt dissection is quite helpful in retracting most of the musculotendinous structures, exposing the entire back of the sacrum and sacral foramen.

Placement of Foramen Electrodes

A 22-gauge 3.5-inch spinal needle, insulated except for the tip, is passed into the desired foramen. Its direction should be slightly downward and outward to follow the course of the foramen. Intraoperative stimulation is performed. If a good response consistent with S3 is obtained, the needle is removed and a permanent foramen electrode (Medtronic, Inc., Minneapolis MN) is inserted into the foramen. The electrode is fixed over the outside of the sacrum and its lead is tunneled under the skin to the anterior abdomen. It is then connected to a stimulator that is embedded under the skin.

Sacral Electrodes with Dorsal Rhizotomy

Sacral laminectomy adequate to expose the distal end of the dura and sacral roots is performed. Upon entrance to the sacral canal in the extradural space, the fatty vascular tissue surrounding the sacral roots is dissected free, exposing them bilaterally. Under continuous urodynamic monitoring, the appropriate nerve roots are selected with the aid of in situ electrical stimulation. The sacral nerve root that provoked an adequate detrusor contraction is mobilized freely, and, under magnification, its ganglion and dorsal components are separated from the ventral components. Dorsal rhizotomy is then performed. (Some authors suggest that rhizotomy is better accomplished intradurally [78]. Sauerwein et al. [79] recommend intradural dorsal rhizotomy and extradural electrode implantation.) Electrodes are then placed around the ventral component either intra- or extradurally and fixed in place. Usually three to four electrodes are implanted. The leads are then tunneled under the skin to the anterior abdomen to be attached to the receiver.

RESULTS

Tanagho and Schmidt (80) reported an 81% success rate in 43 patients, all of whom had urge incontinence that was intractable to conventional management. It appears that patients with severe spasticity caused by neurological disease and mild forms of reflex instability are amenable to neural stimulation. Recently, Bosch and Groen (81) studied the effect of sacral (S3) nerve stimulation in patients with severe urge incontinence due to detrusor instability or hyperreflexia refractory to drug treatment. They reported a success rate of 83% (61% with greater than 90% and 22% with a 50–90% decrease in pad use and/or incontinent episodes). This effect appears to be durable, lasting for longer than 2 years.

RISKS AND COMPLICATIONS

The intradural approach carries the risk of cerebrospinal fluid leakage and arachnoiditis. Few studies have investigated the potential harmful effects of long-term stimulation, but some have suggested that very high levels of current density produce nerve damage (82, 83). These studies were performed largely on the brain unprotected by its meningeal wrapping. Peripheral nerves are presumed to be more resistant because of the protection of a thick epidural cover. It has been demonstrated that stimulation amplitudes less than 4 mA applied at a frequency of 20 Hz are safe (84). Erectile and rectal dysfunction are potential risks after dorsal rhizotomy (60, 85). Neuromodulation is a valuable new technology for patients with detrusor instability and

urge incontinence. The low complication rate and absence of reports of irreversible changes to bladder or nerves are major advantages over other alternatives, such as augmentation or denervation.

REFERENCES

1. Abrams P, Blaivas JG, Stanton SL, Andersen JT. The standardization of terminology of lower urinary tract function. Scand J Urol Nephrol 1988; 114:5–19.
2. Fantl JA, Hurt WG, Dunn LJ. Dysfunctional detrusor control. Am J Obstet Gynecol 1977;129: 299–303.
3. de Groat WC, Kawatani M. Neural control of the urinary bladder: possible relationship between peptidergic inhibitory mechanisms and detrusor instability. Neurourol Urodyn 1985;4:285–300.
4. Helmstein K. Treatment of bladder carcinoma by a hydrostatic pressure technique. Br J Urol 1972; 44:434–450.
5. Dunn M, Smith JC, Ardran GM. Prolonged bladder distension as a treatment of urgency and urge incontinence. Br J Urol 1974;46:645–652.
6. Ramsden PD, Smith JC, Dunn M, Ardran GM. Distension therapy for the unstable bladder: later results including as assessment of repeat distensions. Br J Urol 1976;48:623–629.
7. Smith JC. The place of prolonged bladder distension in the treatment of bladder instability and other disorders. A review after 7 years. Br J Urol 1981;53:283.
8. Taub HC, Stein M. Bladder distention therapy for symptomatic relief of frequency and urgency: a ten-year review. Urology 1994;43:36–39.
9. Anderson JD, England HR, Mollard EA, Blandy JP. The effects of overstretching on the structure and function of the bladder in relation to Helmstein's distension therapy. Br J Urol 1975;47:835–840.
10. Tasker JH. Ileo-cytoplasty: a new technique. Br J Urol 1953;25:349–357.
11. Goodwin WE, Winter CC, Barker WF. Cup patch technique of ileocystoplasty for bladder enlargement or partial substitution. Surg Gynecol Obstet 1959;108:370–372.
12. Sinaiko E. Artificial bladder from segment of stomach and study of effect of urine on gastric secretion. Surg Gynecol Obstet 1956;102: 433–438.
13. Leong CH, Ong GB. Gastrocystoplasty in dogs. Aust NZ J Surg 1972;41:272–279.
14. Rudick J, Schonholz S, Weber HN. The gastric bladder: a continent reservoir for urinary diversion. Surgery 1977;82:1–8.
15. Cartwright PC, Snow BW. Bladder autoaugmentation: partial detrusor excision to augment the bladder without use of bowel. J Urol 1989;142: 505–508.
16. Kennelly MJ, Gormley EA, McGuire EJ. Early clinical experience with adult bladder autoaugmentation. J Urol 1994;152:303–306.
17. Stothers L, Johnson H, Arnold W, Coleman G, Tearle H. Bladder autoaugmentation by vesi-

comyotomy in the pediatric neurogenic bladder. Urology 1994;44:110–113.

18. Wolf JS, Turzan CW. Augmentation ureterocystoplasty. J Urol 1993;149:1095–1098.

19. Landau EH, Jayanthi VR, Khoury AE, et al. Bladder augmentation: ureterocystoplasty versus ileocystoplasty. J Urol 1994;152:716–719.

20. Hitchcock RJ, Duffy PG, Malone PS. Ureterocystoplasty: the "bladder" augmentation of choice. Br J Urol 1994;73:575–579.

21. Schipper H, Decter A. Carcinoma of the colon arising at ureteral implant sites despite early external diversion: pathogenetic and clinical implications. Cancer 1981;47:2062–2065.

22. Stewart M, Macrae FA, Williams CB. Neoplasia and ureterosigmoidostomy: a colonoscopic survey. Br J Surg 1982;69:414–416.

23. Filmer RB, Spencer JR. Malignancies in bladder augmentations and intestinal conduits. J Urol 1990;143:671–678.

24. Egbert BM, Kraft JK, Perkash I. Undifferentiated sarcoma arising in an augmented ileocystoplasty patch. J Urol 1980;123:272–274.

25. Nurse DE, Mundy AR. Assessment of the malignant potential of cystoplasty. Br J Urol 1989;64:489–492.

26. Sheiner J, Kaplan G. Spontaneous bladder rupture following enterocystoplasty. J Urol 1988;140:1157–1158.

27. Elder JS, Snyder HM, Hulbert WC, Duckett JW. Perforation of the augmented bladder in patients undergoing clean intermittent catheterization. J Urol 1988;140:1159–1162.

28. Rushton HG, Woodard JR, Parrott TS, Jeffs RD, Gearhart JP. Delayed bladder rupture after augmentation enterocystoplasty. J Urol 1988;140:344–346.

29. Dixon MC, Filmer RB, Chang CH, et al. Spontaneous perforation of bladder augmentation in pediatric patients [abstract]. J Urol 1989;141:195A.

30. Scheidler DM, Brito CG, Rink RC. Insight into bladder rupture following lower urinary tract reconstruction [abstract]. J Urol 1989;141:195A.

31. Nathan PW, Sears TA, Smith MC. Effects of phenol on the nerve roots of the cat: an electrophysiologic and histologic study. J Neurosci 1965;2:7–29.

32. Parkhouse HF, Gilpin SA, Gosling JA, Turner-Warwick RT. Quantitative study of phenol as a neurolytic agent in the urinary bladder. Br J Urol 1987;60:410–412.

33. Ewing R, Bultitude MI, Shuttleworth KE. Subtrigonal phenol injection for urge incontinence secondary to detrusor instability in females. Br J Urol 1982;54:689–692.

34. Blackford HN, Murray K, Stephenson TP, Mundy AR. Results of transvesical infiltration of the pelvic plexuses with phenol in 116 patients. Br J Urol 1984;56:647–649.

35. Chapple CR, Hampson SJ, Turner-Warwick RT, Worth PH. Subtrigonal phenol injection. How safe and effective is it? Br J Urol 1991;68:483–486.

36. Nordling J, Steven K, Meyhoff HH. Subtrigonal phenol injection: lack of effect in the treatment of detrusor instability. Neurourol Urodyn 1986;5:449–451.

37. Wall LL, Stanton SL. Transvesical phenol injection of pelvic nerve plexus in females with refractory urge incontinence. Br J Urol 1989;63:465–468.

38. McInerney PD, Vanner TF, Matenhelia S, Stephenson TP. Assessment of the long term results of subtrigonal phenolisation. Br J Urol 1991;67:586–587.

39. Ingelman-Sundberg A. Partial denervation of the bladder. A new operation for the treatment of urge incontinence and similar conditions in women. Acta Obstet Gynecol Scand 1959;38:487–502.

40. Hodgkinson CP, Drukker BH. Intravesical nerve resection for detrusor dyssynergia. Acta Obstet Gynecol Scand 1977;56:401–408.

41. Wan J, McGuire EJ, Wang JC, Cerny JC, Hodgkinson CP. Ingelman-Sundberg denervation for detrusor instability. J Urol 1991;145:358A.

42. Turner-Warwick RT, Ashken MH. The functional results of partial, subtotal and total cystoplasty with special reference to ureterocystoplasty, selective sphincterotomy, and cystocystoplasty. Br J Urol 1967;39:3–12.

43. Parsons KF, O'Boyle PJ, Gibbon NO. A further assessment of bladder transection in the management of adult enuresis and allied conditions. Br J Urol 1977;49:509–514.

44. Hindmarsh JR, Essenhigh DM, Yeates WK. Bladder transection for adult enuresis. Br J Urol 1977;49:515–521.

45. Worth PHL, Turner-Warwick RT. The treatment of interstitial cystitis by cytolysis with observations on cystoplasty. Br J Urol 1973;45:65–71.

46. Freiha FS, Stamey TA. Cystolysis: a procedure for the selective denervation of the bladder. J Urol 1980;123:360–362.

47. Leach GE, Goldman D, Raz S. Surgical treatment of detrusor hyperreflexia. In: Raz S, ed. Female urology. Philadelphia: WB Saunders, 1983:326–333.

48. Comarr AE. The practical urological management of the patient with spinal cord injury. Br J Urol 1959;31:29–31.

49. Miyata M, Mizunaga M, Kaneko S, Morikawa M, Yachiku S, Watabe Y. Urologic management of spinal cord injury by subarachnoid phenol block. Jpn J Urol 1990;81:841–846.

50. Meirowsky AJ, Scheibert CD, Hinchey TR. Studies on the sacral reflexic arch in paraplegia. J Neurosurg 1950;7:33–38.

51. Brendler H, Krueger G, Lerman J, et al. Spinal root section in treatment of advanced paraplegic bladder. J Urol 1953;70:223–229.

52. Mosak SJ, Bunts RC, Ulmer JL, Eagles WM. Nerve interruption procedures in the urologic management of paraplegic patients. J Urol 1962;88:392–401.

53. Rockswold GL, Bradley WE, Chou SN. Differential sacral rhizotomy in the treatment of neurogenic bladder dysfunction. J Neurosurg 1973;38:748–754.

54. Gargour GW, Toczek SK, McCullough DC. Selective sacral rootlet section for experimental detrusor inhibition. J Neurosurg 1973;38:494–498.

55. Juenemann KP, Lue TF, Schmidt RA, Tanagho EA.

Clinical significance of sacral and pudendal nerve anatomy. J Urol 1988;139:74–80.

56. Schmidt RA, Senn E, Tanagho EA. Functional evaluation of sacral nerve root integrity. Urology 1990;35:388–392.

57. Torrens MJ, Griffith HB. The control of the uninhibited bladder by selective sacral neurectomy. Br J Urol 1974;46:639–644.

58. Toczek SK, McCullough DC, Gargour GW, Kachman R, Baker R, Luessenhop AJ. Selective sacral rootlet rhizotomy for hypertonic neurogenic bladder. J Neurosurg 1975;42:567–574.

59. Diokno AC, Vinson RK, McGillicuddy J. Treatment of the severe uninhibited neurogenic bladder by selective sacral rhizotomy. J Urol 1977;118:299–301.

60. Gasparini ME, Schmidt RA, Tanagho EA. Selective sacral rhizotomy in the management of the reflex neuropathic bladder: a report on 17 patients with long-term followup. J Urol 1992;148:1207–1210.

61. Muller SC, Frohneberg D, Schwab R, Thuroff JW. Selective sacral nerve blockade for the treatment of unstable bladders. Eur Urol 1986;12:408–412.

62. Rockswold GL, Chou SN, Bradley WE. Revaluation of differential sacral rhizotomy for neurological bladder disease. J Neurosurg 1978;48:773–778.

63. Torrens MJ, Griffith J. Management of the uninhibited bladder by selective sacral neurectomy. J Neurosurg 1976;44:176–185.

64. Lucas MG, Thomas DG, Clarke SJ, Forster DM. Long term follow-up of selective sacral rhizotomy. Br J Urol 1988;61:218–220.

65. Sundin T, Dahlstrom A, Norlen L, Svedmyr N. The sympathetic innervation and adrenoreceptor function of the human lower urinary tract in the normal state and after parasympathetic denervation. Invest Urol 1977;14:322–328.

66. Torring J, Petersen T, Klemar B, Sogaard I. Selective sacral rootlet neurectomy in the treatment of detrusor hyperreflexia. Technique and long-term results. J Neurosurg 1988;68:241–245.

67. Tanagho EA. Induced micturition via intraspinal sacral root stimulation: clinical implications. In: Hambrecht FT, Reswick JB, eds. Functional electrical stimulation. New York: Marcel Dekker, 1977.

68. Schmidt RA. Applications of neurostimulation in urology. Neurourol Urodyn 1988;7:585–588.

69. Brindley GS, Polkey CE, Rushton DN, Cardozo L. Sacral anterior root stimulators for bladder control in paraplegia: the first 50 cases. J Neurol Neurosurg Psychiatry 1986;49:1104–1114.

70. Tanagho EA, Schmidt RA, Orvis BR. Neural stimulation for control of voiding dysfunction. J Urol 1989;142:340–345.

71. Schmidt RA, Bruschini H, Tanagho EA. Urinary

bladder and sphincter responses to stimulation of dorsal and ventral sacral roots. Invest Urol 1979;16:300–304.

72. Tang PC, Walter JS. Voiding in conscious spinal dogs induced by stimulating sacral and coccygeal roots with the "volume conduction" method. Neurourol Urodyn 1984;3:43.

73. Walter J, Robinson CJ, Wheeler JS, Bolam JM, Wurster RD. Monopolar stimulation of sacral nerve roots effectively evacuates the bladder of the chronic spinal male dog [abstract]. Federation Proc 1986;45:172.

74. Godec C, Cass AS, Ayala GF. Electrical stimulation for incontinence: technique, selection and results. Urology 1976;7:388–392.

75. Mahony DT, Laferte RO, Blais DJ. Incontinence of urine due to instability of micturition reflexes. I. Detrusor reflex instability. Urology 1980;15:229–239.

76. Mahony DT, Laferte RO, Blais DJ. Incontinence of urine due to instability of micturition reflexes. II. Pudendal nucleus instability. Urology 1980;15:379–388.

77. Riddle PR, Hill DW, Wallace DM. Electronic techniques for the control of adult urinary incontinence. Br J Urol 1969;14:205–210.

78. Light JK. Electrical stimulation to modify detrusor function. Adv Neurol 1993;63:303–309.

79. Sauerwein D, Ingunza W, Fischer J. Extradural implantation of sacral anterior root stimulators. J Neurol Neurosurg Psychiatry 1990;53:681–684.

80. Tanagho EA, Schmidt RA. Surgery for voiding dysfunction by neurostimulation. In: Droller M, ed. Surgical management of urologic disease. An anatomic approach. Chicago: Mosby/Year Book, 1992:1095–1111.

81. Bosch JLHR, Groen J. Sacral (S3) segmental nerve stimulation as a treatment for urge incontinence in patients with detrusor instability: results of chronic electrical stimulation using an implantable neural prosthesis. J Urol 1995;154:504–507.

82. Angew WF, Yuen TGH, McGreery DB. Morphologic changes after prolonged stimulation of the cat's cortex at defined charge densities. Exp Neurol 1983;79:397.

83. Pudenz RH, Bullara LA, Tallaa A. Electrical stimulation of the brain. Surg Neurol 1975;4:389–400.

84. Angew WF, Yuen TGH, McGreery DB, Bullara LA. Histologic evaluations of peripheral nerves implanted with stimulating electrodes. Presented at the 30th Congress of the International Union of Physiological Scientists, Vancouver, July 1986.

85. Schmidt RA, Aboseif SA, Gleason C. Role of dorsal rhizotomy in management of patients with spastic neurogenic bladder [abstract]. J Urol 1992;148:58.

CHAPTER 36

Genuine Stress Incontinence: An Overview

Robert L. Summitt, Jr., and Alfred E. Bent

The International Continence Society defines stress incontinence as a symptom, a sign, and a condition (1). The symptom is the patient's complaint of involuntary urine loss with physical exercise. The sign is the observation of urine loss from the urethra immediately upon increasing intraabdominal pressure, (e.g., coughing). The condition genuine stress incontinence is the involuntary loss of urine that occurs when intravesical pressure exceeds maximal urethral pressure in the absence of detrusor activity.

The state of urinary continence involves the interplay of several complex mechanisms. Not only are normal central nervous system function and a normal bladder wall required, but anatomic and functional integrity of the urethra and vesical neck are necessary. At the level of the urethra, urinary continence exists when pressure in any part of the urethra is the same or exceeds the pressure in the bladder (2). Factors that contribute to the maintenance of this pressure differential, in both the resting and stressed states, include an intact urethral sphincteric mechanism and proper anatomic support of the urethra and urethrovesical junction (3). For urine to pass, the maximum urethral pressure must be lower than the bladder pressure. This fact provides a pathophysiological basis for the development of genuine stress incontinence.

Historical Background

Lapides et al. (4) proposed one of the first theories for the pathophysiology of stress incontinence. It stated that the abnormality common to all women with stress incontinence was a urethra that was extremely short in the standing position. This concept resulted from comparative measurement studies using a Foley catheter and was based on the principle that the resistance of a tubular structure varied directly with the length of the tube. Surgery thus succeeded by lengthening the urethra. However, subsequent reports have shown no statistically significant difference in urethral length between continent controls and patients with stress incontinence (5–10). Furthermore, the functional length of the urethra is not consistently changed by corrective surgery (10–13).

Jeffcoate and Roberts (14) stated that stress incontinence was the result of a loss of the normal posterior urethrovesical angle as observed by lateral chain urethrocystography. This theory was strengthened by Green (11), who showed that the anatomic factors contributing to the development of stress incontinence were the loss of the posterior urethrovesical angle and the loss of the angle of inclination of the urethral axis. According to this theory, any operation that restored these angles would cure stress incontinence. More recently, however, several reports have shown overlap in radiological findings between continent women and those with stress incontinence. Kitzmiller et al. (15) demonstrated that 28% of continent women had abnormal posterior urethrovesical angles and 26% of women with stress incontinence had normal angles. Fantl et al. (16) reviewed cystourethrograms and determined that 98% of women with genuine stress incontinence had lost the posterior urethrovesical angle but also that 94% of patients with only detrusor instability had lost the angle.

Hodgkinson (17, 18) proposed that stress incontinence was the result of displacement of the urethrovesical junction to a position in which it was the most dependent portion of the bladder. Thus, it was in a position of highest hydrostatic pressure. Subsequently, however, 30–70% of continent patients have also been shown to demonstrate this sign radiographically (15, 16).

Finally, Hutch (19) presented the theory that continence was the result of a structure called the base plate, representing an internal urethral sphincter. When this base plate was flat, continence was maintained. When the base plate descended into a space between the symphysis and the anterior vaginal wall, stress incontinence occurred because of funneling of the sphincter. Again, later radiographic studies showed that although 98% of patients with stress incontinence lack the flat base plate, 100% of patients with detrusor instability also show funneling (16).

Mechanism of Continence

The primary etiological factor producing genuine stress incontinence is the incomplete transmission of abdominal pressure to the proximal urethra due to displacement from its intraabdominal position (5–7, 17, 20, 21). Other less well-understood functional and anatomic deficiencies in the urethra and its supporting structures may also be involved (22–24). To fully understand the factors involved in the development of genuine stress incontinence, one must be aware of the mechanisms that maintain continence. A review of these mechanisms follows.

Urinary continence exists, in both the resting and stressed states, when intraurethral pressure equals or exceeds intravesical pressure. Specifically, the components that prevent stress incontinence by maintaining intraurethral pressure and pressure transmission are an internal urethral sphincteric mechanism, an extrinsic urethral sphincter, proper anatomic support of the urethrovesical junction, and intact innervation to these components, providing modulation of their function (2, 3).

The internal urethral sphincteric mechanism maintains adequate resting urethral closure pressure over a specific length (3). It also provides a mucosal seal through coaptation of mucosal surfaces. Components of the internal mechanism that provide these functions include urethral mucosa, elastic and connective tissue of the urethral wall, smooth muscle fibers in the urethral wall, and the vascular content of the submucosal cavernous plexus (2, 3, 6, 20, 25). These structures are estrogen dependent. Coaptation of the mucosa, providing a watertight seal, is a result of the rich folds of the urethral lining accompanied by tension from the submucosal cavernous plexus (3). Contributing to maintenance of resting closure pressure are the smooth muscle component, submucosal cavernous plexus, and connective tissue. The smooth muscle of the female urethra consists of small bundles running longitudinally and obliquely in the urethral wall (26). The contribution of smooth muscle to closure pressure depends on this anatomic arrangement of fibers along with the physiological ability to exert constant tonus and the neurological modulation of its response (3). The urethra has rich autonomic innervation, especially with sympathetic receptors (20). The submucosal vascular plexus is considered as a cylindrical cushion and contributes to compression of the urethral lumen (2). This contribution can be limited by urethral scarring and menopausal status.

The extrinsic urethral sphincteric mechanism is anatomically composed of periurethral striated muscle fibers (sphincter urethrae) and muscles of the urogenital diaphragm or perineal membrane (2, 23). The sphincter urethrae extends from the trigonal plate posteriorly and passes distally, fanning out into connective tissue of the urogenital diaphragm (2). It is composed primarily of slow-twitch striated fibers innervated by the pelvic (splanchnic) efferent nerves. They are arranged in a circular disposition external to the smooth muscle component and are thickest in the middle third. These slow-twitch fibers are capable of maintaining contraction over long periods of time and actively contribute to tone that closes the urethra and maintains both passive continence and a margin to prevent incontinence during stress (26). The muscular contribution from the perineal membrane consists of two bands of striated muscle, the compressor urethrae and the urethrovaginal sphincter. Originating near the lower third of the urethra, these muscles arch over the ventral aspect of the urethra, forming a single band and blending with the circular fibers of the sphincter urethrae. This striated muscle contribution consists primarily of fast-twitch fibers innervated by the perineal branch of the pudendal nerve (24, 26). Lying in the region from 60% to 80% of the urethral length in the perineal membrane, the compressor urethrae and urethrovaginal sphincter may be responsible for reflex contraction with cough, increasing urethral resistance (24–26). Based on the timing of this rise in pressure, these muscles may contract in preparation for a cough rather than as a reflex (23, 27). The compressor urethrae, urethrovaginal sphincter, and sphincter urethrae combined have been termed the striated urogenital sphincter (23).

Support of the proximal urethra and urethrovesical junction, maintaining an intraabdominal position, is provided by the contributions of a number of anatomic structures. Most important is a sling formed beneath the middle and upper portions of the urethra by a segment of anterior vaginal wall fused with pubocervical fascia (23, 28). This segment of anterior vaginal wall is attached laterally to the muscles of the pelvic diaphragm, its overlying endopelvic fascia, and the arcus tendineus fascia pelvis. When the pelvic diaphragm contracts, the vaginal wall moves anteriorly, drawing the proximal urethra toward the pubic bone. Medial divisions of the pelvic diaphragm (levator ani muscle group) and fascial attachments of the vagina to the arcus tendineus fascia pelvis prevent posterior displacement of the urethra, maintaining it above the levator plate. Additional support to the proximal urethra, preventing posterior rotational descent, has been ascribed to the pubourethral ligaments. However, others question whether true ligamentous attachment of the urethra to the pubic bone exists (23). Instead, urethral support is provided in a common fashion by those attachments of the anterior vaginal wall to the pelvic

diaphragm, its superior fascia, and the arcus tendineus fascia pelvis. They consist of collagen, elastin, and smooth muscle. The sum of the contributions to the support of the proximal urethra elevate it above the pelvic floor and subject it to increases in intraabdominal pressure, thus allowing compression and maintenance of continence (6).

The neurological integrity of the anatomic components maintaining continence is extremely important. Intact innervation of the periurethral striated muscles and pelvic floor musculature by the pelvic efferent nerves and pudendal nerve, respectively, serve to modulate resting tone and reflex increases in urethral pressure with stress (26). Voluntary increases in urethral pressure by the muscles of the perineal membrane are elicited via upper motor neuron pathways (pyramidal tracts), initiated from the cerebral cortex (29). Interruption of or damage to the innervation of these various structures can cause dysfunction at any level.

Urodynamic Assessment of Stress Incontinence

Various means to measure the functional integrity of the components that prevent stress incontinence have long been studied and modified. As noted above, the primary factor in the development of stress incontinence is the displacement of the urethra from the intraabdominal position, which leads to impaired pressure transmission during stress. One of the most accurate means of measuring urethral function, sphincteric capacity, and the support that provides pressure transmission is the urethral pressure profile obtained by using multichannel urodynamic testing (9). Urodynamics, initially developed by Enhorning in 1961 (6), allows simultaneous measurement of intravesical, intraurethral, and intraabdominal pressures. The introduction of microtip pressure transducers by Asmussen and Ulmsten (30) has allowed precise and reproducible recording of these measurements.

The parameters measured with urodynamic testing allow both quantitative and qualitative assessments of the contribution to continence made by the internal and external sphincteric components and the supporting pelvic structures. The urethral closure pressure profile reflects the urethral closure pressure over the entire functional urethral length (length of the urethra over which intraurethral pressure exceeds intravesical pressure). The resting urethral pressure profile primarily reflects intrinsic urethral pressure (e.g., the urethral closure pressure), which maintains continence at rest. The anatomic components that contribute to resting urethral closure pressure include smooth muscle fibers in the urethra, periurethral striated muscle fibers, the submucosal cavernous plexus, and, to some extent, urethral mucosa and elastic and connective tissue of the urethral wall (2, 6, 20, 25). Using curarization followed by clamping of the common iliac arteries at the time of radical hysterectomy, Rud et al. (31) showed that resting urethral closure pressure resulted primarily from the first three of these anatomic structures. Their contributions to closure pressure were smooth muscle with connective tissue, one third; striated muscle fibers, one third; and submucosal cavernous plexus, one third. These relative contributions can vary considerably depending on patient age, parity, previous surgery, integrity of innervation, and medications (20). Statistically significant differences in the maximum resting urethral closure pressure have been noted between continent controls and patients with genuine stress incontinence (5, 6, 9, 32). The patients with stress incontinence have lower closure pressures. However, after surgery in these patients, there is frequently no significant change in resting closure pressure despite restored continence (9, 12, 13). Therefore, resting urethral closure pressure is not as significant a determinant for stress incontinence as intraabdominal pressure transmission. Instead, resting urethral closure pressure may be more closely related to the severity of symptoms (5).

The urethral pressure profile performed during stress maneuvers (e.g., coughing, Valsalva maneuver) reflects the positional, mechanical, and dynamic factors contributing to continence. A cough pressure profile is performed by withdrawing the dual microtransducer through the urethra as the patient coughs continuously. The resulting profile can demonstrate the adequacy of pelvic support, represented by pressure transmission, and the possible reflex contraction of the pelvic floor musculature, reflected by augmentation of transmitted pressure. In continent patients, the cough profile shows that the pressure increment rises significantly higher in the urethral compartment than in the bladder, thus maintaining a positive urethral closure pressure (Fig. 36.1) (6, 9). This occurs by virtue of the fact that the urethrovesical junction and proximal urethra are above the pelvic floor, positioned properly in the abdominal sphere (6). This positioning allows equal transmission of sudden intraabdominal pressure to the bladder and to the proximal urethra (2, 6, 17). The maintenance of the positive urethral closure pressure due to equal pressure transmission is reflected in measurement of the transmission ratio (the ratio of change in intraurethral pressure to change in intravesical pressure during coughing). In studying transmission ratios in continent and incontinent patients, Hilton and Stanton (5) showed that continent patients maintained transmission ratios exceeding 95% in some parts of the urethra. There was greater maintenance of the transmission ratio in the proximal urethra, with accentuation in the midurethra to values greater than 100%. Bump et al. (33) showed similar findings, stating that a pressure transmission ratio less than 90% was associated with stress urinary incontinence. However, both Rosenzweig et al. (34) and Summitt et al. (35) showed no threshold transmission ratio associated with genuine stress incontinence.

Although the transmission ratio is not a diagnostic tool for evaluating stress incontinence, it does reflect the integrity of pelvic-supporting structures and may represent reflex muscle activity of the pelvic floor. Simultaneous pressure recordings in continent patients show that a cough-induced rise in intraurethral pressure precedes and exceeds the rise in abdominal pressure as it is transmitted to the bladder and urethra (1, 25, 27). Specifically, an augmentation of transmitted pressure occurs in the urethra, generating urethral pressures during stress that are greater than those expected from direct transmission of intraabdominal pressure. This is

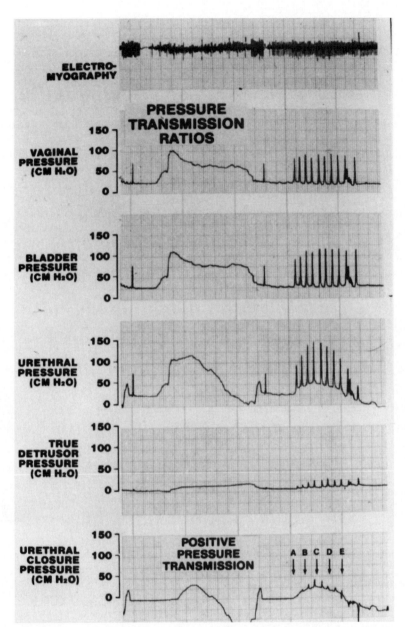

Figure 36.1. Urethral pressure profiles from a continent patient. The cough profile illustrates maintenance of a positive urethral closure pressure, a function of the positive pressure transmission ratio.

possibly the result of a cough-induced reflex contraction of fast-twitch fibers of the levator ani and periurethral striated muscles. Therefore, continence is maintained not only by passive transmission of pressure to the urethra, but an active, reflex muscle contraction also takes place that increases pressure transmission to greater than 100% (9, 27).

Mechanism of Stress Incontinence

With an understanding of how urodynamic testing measures the contribution to continence by the internal and external urethral sphincteric mechanisms and the pelvic-supporting structures, multichannel urody-namics can also demonstrate how various etiological factors produce stress inconti-nence. The resting urethral pressure profile reflects the constant tonus and margin to incontinence provided by the components of the internal urethral sphincteric mechanism and the external urethral sphincter. The cough pressure profile reflects the function of sphincteric and supporting components un-der dynamic conditions. In addition to the cough profile, the measurement of leak point pressures has been used to assess urethral resistance under stressful maneuvers (36). In most cases, the abdominal pressure neces-sary to produce leakage is measured. How-ever, methodology for making this test con-sistent among researchers awaits further refinement.

Urethral hypermobility, or downward dis-placement of the urethra, is the most com-mon cause of genuine stress incontinence. The transmission ratio, obtained during the cough profile, not only demonstrates how intraabdominal pressure transmission to the proximal urethra plays a major role in maintaining continence with stress, but it also demonstrates how anatomic displace-ment of the urethra results in reduced pres-sure transmission and is the major etiol-ogical factor in producing stress inconti-nence (Fig. 36.2). When showing that all continent patients had transmission ratios greater than 95%, Hilton and Stanton (5) revealed that only 3 of 120 women with stress incontinence demonstrated ratios greater than 95%. In fact, it was shown that transmission ratios of incontinent patients

URETHRAL PRESSURE PROFILES

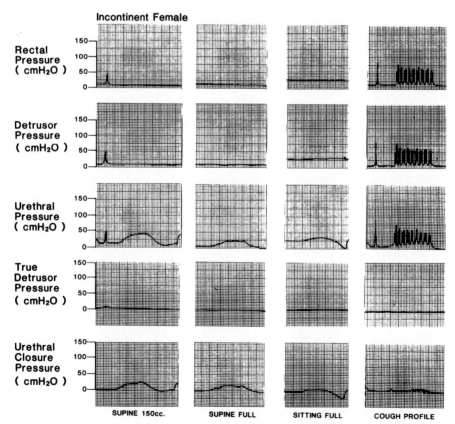

Figure 36.2. Urethral pressure profiles from an in-continent patient. Resting profiles demonstrate de-terioration of urethral closure pressure. The cough profile illustrates pressure equalization.

demonstrated a linear decrease from the urethrovesical junction to the external meatus.

Anatomic descent of the urethra and urethrovesical junction can result from a number of causes. The trauma of childbirth is one of the primary etiological factors that can result in pelvic floor weakness. Descent of the fetal head distends the genital hiatus and levator muscles and stretches the pubocervical fascia, the pubourethral ligaments, and the urogenital diaphragm. This weakening then leads to descent and posterior rotation of the proximal urethra and bladder base. Other causes for pelvic floor weakness include aging and neurological deficits. Using single-fiber electromyogram studies of the anal sphincter in women with stress incontinence, Anderson (21) demonstrated evidence of chronic denervation, reflecting damage to peripheral branches of the pudendal nerve. In another study in which terminal motor latencies of pelvic efferent nerves and the perineal branch of the pudendal nerve were measured in patients with stress incontinence, slowing in each was consistent with damage to the nerves and thus denervation of their respective muscles (24). Most likely, damage to these nerves is the result of traction injury from childbirth or chronic straining. A denervated muscle is an abnormal muscle and thus may function less efficiently. This lack of efficiency may account for reduced pressure transmission and impaired reflex contraction of the pelvic floor (21, 24).

The muscular dysfunction resulting from childbirth and aging may also impair the reflex augmentation of transmitted intraabdominal pressure to the urethra. Various studies showed that this reflex contraction and the ability to augment closure pressure are lost with stress incontinence (9, 25, 37). Therefore, the anatomic defect predisposing to poor pressure transmission may also place the urethra and its surrounding musculature in a suboptimal position to effect adequate pressure augmentation.

In patients with stress incontinence, the resting urethral closure pressure has been found to be significantly lower than in continent controls (Fig. 36.2). This lower intraurethral pressure at rest is presumed not to result from lower transmission of pressure from surrounding tissues but is due to decreased contribution from components of the urethral wall and sphincter (6, 35). A group of patients with genuine stress incontinence and low urethral closure pressures (<20 cm H_2O in the sitting position with a full bladder) has been identified (7, 22, 38). Researchers have shown that these patients, with low urethral closure pressure, are at significantly higher risk for surgical failure with the standard Burch colposuspension (54% objective failure rate) (22, 38). They represent a group of patients in which the urethra no longer maintains sphincteric function. An anatomic defect with downward urethral displacement may not exist.

A broader term, intrinsic sphincter deficiency (ISD), is now being used to include patients with impaired sphincteric function, with or without adequate anatomic support of the urethra. No consensus agreement has been developed to precisely define ISD. Currently, this definition is subject to individual clinical interpretation, usually based on a combination of historical, physical, and objective findings, often including tests such as maximum urethral closure pressure measurements, leak point pressures, and video or static radiographic studies.

Various etiological factors can predispose to impairment of the internal urethral sphincteric mechanism and external sphincter as they contribute to resting tonus and continence during stress. These same factors also produce ISD. In studying 120 women with urodynamically proven stress incontinence, Hilton and Stanton (5) found that repeated unsuccessful incontinence operations were associated with the finding of low urethral pressure. Previous surgery may result in scar formation around and within the delicate urethral structures. Menopause may also contribute to lower urethral pressure. Hypoestrogenism can result in atrophy of urethral epithelium, urethral smooth muscle and the submucosal cavernous plexus (2, 3, 39, 40). Although not the major contributing factor to stress incontinence, resultant low urethral pressure may in some instances reduce the margin to incontinence such that only minor anatomic changes can result in urine loss with stress.

Stress Incontinence: The Scope of the Problem

Urinary incontinence, whether present in the elderly or young woman, can have devastating effects on self-esteem, psychological well being, and overall physical health. Awareness of the prevalence and scope of incontinence, specifically stress incontinence, is of great value to both the physician and patient.

Among women between the ages of 15 and 64 years, the prevalence of urinary incontinence ranges from 10% to 25% (41). The prevalence of urinary incontinence among elderly patients in long-term care facilities has been noted to range from 40% to 60% (42). However, most of these cases are related to urge incontinence, often associated with stroke or senile dementia. Among noninstitutionalized elderly patients, the statistics are somewhat different. Diokno et al. (43) surveyed a population-based group of men and women, 60 years of age and older, as to urinary incontinence and other urological disorders. Of the women surveyed, 37.7% experienced some form of urinary incontinence. Stress incontinence was reported as the primary cause for leakage by 26.7%, and 55.5% reported mixed incontinence as their cause for urine loss. Only 9% reported pure urge incontinence. Of the women with urinary incontinence, 63.7% graded it as moderate to severe in quality.

Younger healthy patients may also manifest stress incontinence. In a survey of Danish women 45 years of age, the prevalence of stress incontinence was found to be 22% (44). However, only 3% of these women sought medical help. When 356 nulliparous student nurses were questioned, 40% admitted to some degree of stress incontinence (45).

Urinary incontinence is associated with a high incidence of health problems and poor health status (42). It is associated with exorbitant health costs, with estimates for direct costs of caring for all ages in the community of $7 billion and in nursing homes of $3.3 billion (46). Incontinence becomes more severe with advancing age. Patients often avoid seeking medical treatment either because of embarrassment or the misconception that their condition is a normal consequence of aging and gender. Physician awareness of the magnitude of the problem will lead to improved diagnosis and care. Not only should patients with complaints of stress incontinence be dealt with in an appropriate and organized fashion, but asymptomatic patients should be screened for a history of urine loss. Although treatment is not recommended for stress incontinence unless it is socially unacceptable, educating the patient as to its consequences and possible therapeutic options is of great value.

Diagnosis of Stress Incontinence

The diagnosis of stress incontinence is based on demonstrating objective loss of urine with physical exertion and ruling out other causes of urine loss. The differential diagnosis (Table 36.1) not only includes functional disorders such as detrusor instability and overflow incontinence but anatomic abnormalities such as urogenital fistulae and ectopic ureters.

A thorough evaluation consisting of a history, neurological and physical examinations, and selected clinical testing will allow an expeditious diagnosis of stress incontinence and avoid an incomplete workup. The history centers on the patient's complaints of urine loss. Particular attention is directed toward menopausal status, history of previous surgery, and medication intake. A urinalysis is obtained to rule out

Table 36.1. Differential Diagnosis of Stress Incontinence

Genuine stress incontinence
   Anatomic
   Intrinsic sphincter deficiency (ISD)
Detrusor instability
Reflex incontinence
   Detrusor hyperreflexia
   Involuntary urethral relaxation
Overflow incontinence
Extraurethral incontinence
   Fistulae
   Ectopic ureter

the presence of bacteriuria, pyuria, or hematuria. Neurological examination centers
on the functional aspects of anatomic areas
innervated by the sacral nerve roots S2–S4.
Abnormalities should be noted and proper
referrals made. The physical examination
notes the presence of pelvic relaxation: uterine prolapse, cystocele, rectocele, enterocele. Cotton swab testing evaluates for the
presence of urethral hypermobility. Postvoid
residual urine volume should be determined
by either catheterization or ultrasound. Cystometry is of paramount importance to rule
out the presence of detrusor instability.
Bladder capacity and compliance may also
be noted during this test.

Objective tests for the demonstration of
urine loss with physical exertion include the
cough stress test and various pad tests. The
cough stress test is performed when the patient has a full bladder, most easily after
screening cystometry (47). While standing,
one leg is elevated on a stool and the patient
coughs vigorously several times. The patient
with stress incontinence will leak in spurts
simultaneously with coughing. Care must be
taken in this evaluation because patients
with cough-induced detrusor instability may
leak several seconds after a cough. A multitude of various pad tests have been described
to demonstrate urine loss. The 1-hour pad
test, introduced by the International Continence Society, is the most commonly used
(1). After a 1-hour battery of physical activities, a preweighed pad is reweighed for evidence of urine loss.

In the patient demonstrating objective
urine loss with stress a normal cystometrogram and normal neurological findings, a
diagnosis of stress incontinence can easily be
made. However, a large number of patients
may exhibit mixed symptoms and clinical
findings. These patients require specialized
testing to confirm a diagnosis of stress incontinence and exclude other causes of urine
loss. Other patients who may require specialized tests, such as multichannel urodynamics, include postmenopausal patients and
patients with previous incontinence surgery.

Management Based on Mechanism of Incontinence

The mechanisms that lead to the development of stress incontinence can serve as a
basis to guide therapeutic management. The
success obtained with various management
techniques serves to emphasize these etiological mechanisms as they contribute to
stress incontinence. Historically, the treatment of stress incontinence has been divided
into nonsurgical and surgical therapy (Table
36.2). A nonsurgical approach has been reserved for mild to moderate forms of stress
incontinence, whereas surgery has been applied to all degrees.

Impaired sphincter activity, resulting in
reduced urethral pressure and a reduced
margin to incontinence, may be improved
enough to restore continence even when an
anatomic defect is present. In postmenopausal women, estrogen use has been found
to increase urethral closure pressure as much
as 50–90%, resulting in symptomatic improvement (7, 48). Although noting no improvement in resting closure pressure, Hilton
and Stanton (40) found an increase in pressure transmission and stress closure pressure
after 4 weeks of vaginal estrogen use. This
was believed to result from improved function of paraurethral supporting structures
and pelvic floor muscles. These results occurred primarily in women with mild to
moderate stress incontinence, possibly reflecting the less significant role of urethral

Table 36.2. Treatment of Stress Incontinence

Nonsurgical therapy
  Avoidance techniques
  Vaginal pessary
  Medical therapy
    Estrogen
    Alpha-adrenergic drugs
  Pelvic floor exercise (Kegel exercises)
  Functional electrical stimulation
Surgical therapy
  Retropubic urethropexy
    Burch procedure
    Marshal-Marchetti-Krantz procedure
  Anterior colporrhaphy
  Needle procedures
    Modified pereyra procedure
    Stamey procedure
  Pubovaginal sling procedures
  Periurethral bulking agents

sphincteric activity in producing stress incontinence.

Conservative therapy to correct pelvic floor weakness and reduced reflex contractile ability has shown success in mild to moderate stress incontinence, emphasizing the role of a pure anatomic defect in the pelvic floor. Kegel exercises show symptomatic improvement through hypertrophy of fast-twitch pubococcygeal muscle fibers (49). This results in improved reflex augmentation of transmitted abdominal pressure. Functional electrical stimulation produces a similar effect.

The results of incontinence surgery emphasize the concept of incomplete pressure transmission to the proximal urethra, due to anatomic descent, as the major etiological factor in stress incontinence. The goal of surgery is to restore the proximal urethra and urethrovesical junction to their normal intraabdominal location (6). Surgical correction has been shown to restore transmission ratios to normal despite the fact that no significant increase occurred in closure pressure or functional length (6, 7, 20). For women with ISD, standard incontinence operations have been shown to have higher failure rates (22). When ISD is accompanied by urethral hypermobility, suburethral sling procedures have success rates greater than 90% (50). However, when hypermobility is lacking, even sling procedures may have a high failure rate. For the woman with ISD and a lack of urethral mobility, periurethral bulking agents provide a successful alternative to abdominal or vaginal surgery. Gluteraldehyde cross-linked collagen was approved by the Food and Drug Administration within the last 2 years, showing promising results for correcting incontinence when used as a periurethral injection.

Summary

The primary components that prevent urinary stress incontinence in the female include an internal urethral sphincteric mechanism, an external urethral sphincter, and proper anatomic support of the urethra and urethrovesical junction. Genuine stress incontinence is a consequence primarily from a defect in pelvic support of the urethrovesical junction, resulting in impaired transmission of intraabdominal pressure to the proximal urethra and urethrovesical junction. Secondary defects that may contribute to stress incontinence include impaired function of the urethral sphincteric mechanism that produces ISD and dysfunction of reflex contraction of the pelvic floor, resulting in reduced augmentation of transmitted pressure. Individualized therapies directed toward these defects correct or improve urodynamically measured parameters that correlate with stress incontinence.

REFERENCES

1. Bates P, Bradley WE, Glen E, et al. The standardization of terminology of lower urinary tract function. J Urol 1979;121:551–554.
2. Asmussen M, Miller ER. Clinical gynaecology and urology. London: Blackwell Scientific Publications, 1983.
3. Staskin DR, Zimmern PE, Hadley HR, et al. The pathophysiology of stress incontinence. Urol Clin North Am 1985;12:271–278.
4. Lapides J, Ajemian EP, Stewart BH, et al. Physiopathology of stress incontinence. Surg Gynecol Obstet 1960;3:224–231.
5. Hilton P, Stanton SL. Urethral pressure measurement by microtransducer: the results in symptom-free women and in those with genuine stress incontinence. Br J Obstet Gynaecol 1983;90: 919–933.
6. Enhorning G. Simultaneous recording of intravesical and intra-urethral pressure. Acta Chir Scand 1961;76(suppl):1–68.
7. McGuire EJ, Lytton B, Pepe V, et al. Stress urinary incontinence. Am J Obstet Gynecol 1976;47: 255–264.
8. Toews HA. Intraurethral and intravesical pressures in normal and stress-incontinent women. Am J Obstet Gynecol 1967;29:613–624.
9. Faysal MH, Constantinou CE, Rother LF, et al. The impact of bladder neck suspension on the resting and stress urethral pressure profile: a prospective study comparing controls with incontinent patients preoperatively and postoperatively. J Urol 1981;125:55–60.
10. Gleason DM, Reilly RJ, Bottaccini MR, et al. The urethral continence zone and its relation to stress incontinence. J Urol 1974;112:81–88.
11. Green TH. Development of a plan for the diagnosis and treatment of urinary stress incontinence. Am J Obstet Gynecol 1962;83:632.
12. Obrink A, Bunne G, Ulmsten U, et al. Urethral pressure profile before, during and after pubococcygeal repair for stress incontinence. Acta Obstet Gynecol Scand 1978;57:49–61.
13. Henricksson L, Ulmsten U. A urodynamic evaluation of the effects of abdominal urethrocystopexy and vaginal sling urethroplasty in women

with stress incontinence. Am J Obstet Gynecol 1978;131:77–82.

14. Jeffcoate TNA, Roberts H. Observations on stress incontinence of urine. Am J Obstet Gynecol 1952; 64:721–738.

15. Kitzmiller JL, Manzer GA, Nebel WA, et al. Chain cystourethrogram and stress incontinence. Obstet Gynecol 1972;39:333–340.

16. Fantl JA, Hurt WG, Beachley MC, et al. Bead-chain cystourethrogram: an evaluation. Obstet Gynecol 1981;58:237–240.

17. Hodgkinson CP. Stress urinary incontinence-1970. Am J Obstet Gynecol 1970;108:1141–1168.

18. Hodgkinson CP. Recurrent stress urinary incontinence. Am J Obstet Gynecol 1978;132:844–860.

19. Hutch JA. A new theory of the anatomy of the internal urinary sphincter and the physiology of micturition. V. The base plate and stress incontinence. Am J Obstet Gynecol 1967;30:309–317.

20. Asmussen M. Static and dynamic pressures of the lower urinary tract as measured by simultaneous urethral cystometry. In: Ostergard DR, ed. Gynecologic urology and urodynamics: theory and practice. Baltimore: Williams & Wilkins, 1985:133–165.

21. Anderson RS. A neurogenic element to urinary genuine stress incontinence. Br J Obstet Gynaecol 1984;91:41–45.

22. Sand PK, Bowen LW, Panganiban R, et al. The low pressure urethra as a factor in failed retropubic urethropexy. Obstet Gynecol 1987;69:399–402.

23. DeLancey JOL. Structural aspects of the extrinsic continence mechanism. Obstet Gynecol 1988;72:296–301.

24. Snooks SJ, Badenoch DF, Tiptaft RC, et al. Perineal nerve damage in genuine stress urinary incontinence: an electrophysiological study. Br J Urol 1985;57:422–426.

25. Constantinou CE. Resting and stress urethral pressures as a clinical guide to the mechanism of continence in the female patient. Urol Clin North Am 1985;12:247.

26. Gosling J. The structure of the bladder and urethra in relation to function. Urol Clin North Am 1979;6:31–38.

27. Constantinou CE, Govan DE. Spatial distribution and timing of transmitted and reflexly generated urethral pressures in healthy women. J Urol 1982;127:964–969.

28. Richardson AC, Edmonds PB, Williams NL. Treatment of stress urinary incontinence due to paravaginal fascial defect. Obstet Gynecol 1981; 57:357–362.

29. Ostergard DR. Neurological control of micturition and integral voiding reflexes. In: Ostergard DR, ed. Gynecologic urology and urodynamics: theory and practice. Baltimore: Williams & Wilkins, 1985:29–42.

30. Asmussen M, Ulmsten U. Simultaneous urethrocystometry and urethral pressure profile measurement with a new technique. Acta Obstet Gynecol Scand 1975;54:385–386.

31. Rud T, Andersson KE, Asmussen M, et al. Factors maintaining the intraurethral pressure in women. Invest Urol 1980;17:343–347.

32. Awad SA, Bryniak SR, Lowe PJ, et al. Urethral pressure profile in female stress incontinence. J Urol 1978;120:475–479.

33. Bump RC, Fantl JA, Hurt WG. Dynamic urethral pressure profilometry pressure transmission ratio determinations after continence surgery: understanding the mechanism of success, failure, and complications. Obstet Gynecol 1988; 72:870–874.

34. Rosenzweig BA, Bhatia NN, Nelson AL. Dynamic urethral pressure profilometry pressure transmission ratio: what do the numbers really mean? Obstet Gynecol 1991;77:586–590.

35. Summitt RL, Sipes DR, Bent AE, Ostergard DR. Evaluation of pressure transmission ratios in women with genuine stress incontinence and low urethral pressure: a comparative study. Obstet Gynecol 1994;83:984–988.

36. McGuire EJ, Fitzpatrick CC, Wan J, et al. Clinical assessment of urethral sphincter function. J Urol 1993;150:1452–1454.

37. Bhatia NN, Ostergard DR. Urodynamics in women with stress urinary incontinence. Obstet Gynecol 1982;60:552–559.

38. Bowen LW, Sand PK, Ostergard DR, et al. Unsuccessful Burch retropubic urethropexy: a case controlled urodynamic study. Obstet Gynecol 1989;160:452–458.

39. Slate WG. Disorders of the female urethra and urinary incontinence. Baltimore: Williams & Wilkins, 1982.

40. Hilton P, Stanton SL. The use of intravaginal oestrogen cream in genuine stress incontinence. Br J Obstet Gynaecol 1983;90:940.

41. Thomas TM, Plymat KR, Blannin J, Meade TW. Prevalence of urinary incontinence. Br Med J 1980;281:1243–1245.

42. Palmer MH. Incontinence. The magnitude of the problem. Nurs Clin North Am 1988;23:139–157.

43. Diokno AC, Brock BM, Brown MB, et al. Prevalence of urinary incontinence and other urological symptoms in the noninstitutionalized elderly. J Urol 1986;136:1022–1025.

44. Hording U, Pedersen K, Sidenius K, et al. Urinary incontinence in 45-year old women. Scand J Urol Nephrol 1986;20:183.

45. Scott JC. Stress incontinence in nulliparous women. J Reprod Med 1969;2:96.

46. Urinary Incontinence Guideline Panel. Urinary incontinence in adults: clinical practice guideline. Rockville, MD: U.S. Department of Health and Human Services. AHCPR Publication No. 92-0038. March 1992.

47. Scotti JR, Ostergard DR. Practical guide for triage of patients with lower urinary tract symptoms. In: Ostergard DR, ed. Gynecologic urology and urodynamics: theory and practice. Baltimore: Williams & Wilkins, 1985:45–58.

48. Faber P, Heidenreich J. Treatment of stress incontinence with estrogen in postmenopausal women. Urol Int 1977;32:221–223.

49. Bergman A. Nonsurgical treatment of stress urinary incontinence. In: Ostergard DR, ed. Gynecologic urology and urodynamics: theory and practice. Baltimore: Williams & Wilkins, 1985: 419–435.

50. Summitt RL, Bent AE, Ostergard DR, Harris TA. Stress incontinence and low urethral closure pressure: correlation of preoperative urethral hypermobility with successful suburethral sling procedures. J Reprod Med 1990;35:877–880.

CHAPTER 37

Nonsurgical Management of Stress Urinary Incontinence

John J. Klutke and Arieh Bergman

Introduction

The first cures for incontinence were achieved surgically. Howard Kelly and other superb aggressive pelvic surgeons set a strong precedent, and for nearly a century the treatment for stress urinary incontinence was primarily surgical.

Medical costs have altered this course abruptly. The magnitude of the problem of incontinence and its cost, about $10 billion per year in the United States, has opened our eyes to effective and relatively inexpensive nonsurgical alternatives for treating stress urinary incontinence. The current recommendation of the Agency for Health Care Policy and Research is to attempt a nonsurgical therapy in nearly all patients with stress incontinence before surgery (1). We predict that changes in reimbursement will reflect this policy.

Surgery has the greatest success in curing stress urinary incontinence but limits future options. When an antiincontinence procedure fails, subsequent surgery has poor outcome. Conservative estimates predict that nonsurgical therapy will cure 10% of patients with stress incontinence and substantially improve another 40% (2). When 50 women with stress incontinence were randomly treated with either surgery or exercises, almost half of the conservatively treated group were improved or cured (3). Those patients that failed the conservative treatment still had the option of surgery.

Many women are suited to nonsurgical therapy. They include frail elderly patients who face a prohibitive surgical risk and young patients who want to have children in the future. Many younger women do not want to deal with prolonged convalescence after surgery. Surgery for stress incontinence remains an elective procedure in all cases.

Estrogen

Treating incontinence often falls within the much broader context of treating the menopausal woman. Estrogen-replacement therapy in postmenopausal women has a well-established substantial role in reducing cardiovascular disease and osteoporosis (4–7).

Menopause is associated with a general weakening of connective tissue due to impaired synthesis and metabolism of collagen (8). The density of bone and dermal thickness, for example, decline in parallel after the menopause (9). Collagen is the main constituent of these tissues and is also the key structural component in the support of the pelvic organs. Fibroblasts in the pelvic ligaments produce and secrete collagen and have estrogen receptors (10, 11). Lack of estrogen, therefore, may explain an accelerated rate of pelvic organ prolapse in the menopause. Defective anatomic support of the bladder neck is largely responsible for stress incontinence (12).

Table 37.1. Effect of Estrogen Supplementation on Incontinence: Randomized Placebo-Controlled Studies

Author	Number of Patients	Duration (mo)	Estrogen	Route	Response
Judge[48]	20	1	Quinestradiol	Oral	Improved incontinence
Walter et al.[49]	29	4	Estradiol and estriol	Oral	Improved urge incontinence
Samsioe et al.[50]	34	3	Estriol	Oral	Improved urge and mixed incontinence
Wilson et al.[51]	36	3	Piperazine estrone sulfate	Oral	No change
Foidart et al.[52]	109	6	Estriol	Vaginal	Improved frequency

As a short-term remedy for the stress incontinent woman, estrogen's role remains unproven. Only a few randomized trials have prospectively studied the effect of estrogen on genuine stress incontinence (Table 37.1). Most of these trials assess this effect in an insufficient number of patients to give the results sufficient statistical power. Furthermore, the type and route of estrogen varies substantially between studies, making comparisons difficult.

PHYSIOLOGICAL EFFECTS OF ESTROGEN AND ALPHA-ADRENERGIC MEDICATIONS ON THE BLADDER AND URETHRA

If estrogen has a theoretical basis in anatomic support, its effect on the urethra's intrinsic function is clear. Intrinsic urethral function describes the component of urinary continence not dependent on anatomic support of the urethra (13). The physiological factors responsible for this function include the periurethral striated muscle, neurological tone of the bladder neck, urethral vascularity, and mucosal surface tension. All of these factors depend on estrogen stimulation.

The lower urinary tract and vagina develop from a common primordial structure. The histochemical similarities between mature vaginal and urethral tissue include a high concentration of estrogen receptors (14, 15). Estrogen stimulation causes maturation of the mucosa of the urethra, with a concomitant improvement in lower urinary tract symptoms, such as incontinence (16, 17). Estrogen replacement therapy in the patient with atrophic vaginitis improves blood flow to the pelvis, manifested as decreased dyspareunia and increased vaginal lubrication (18).

Estrogen seems to potentiate alpha-adrenergic transmission in the urethra. This has been clearly demonstrated in animal tissue preparations. Levin et al. (19) reported a decreased sensitivity to alpha-adrenergic stimulation of the rabbit urethra after castration removed the source of estrogen. This effect disappeared after estrogen was administered exogenously. Other studies described an increase in the density of adrenergic receptors in rabbit lower urinary tract tissue after estrogen administration (20, 21).

The combination of alpha-adrenergic agonists with estrogen in women with stress incontinence improves estrogen's effectiveness both subjectively and in terms of specific urodynamic parameters. Beisland et al. (22) treated 18 postmenopausal women with stress incontinence in a prospective randomized crossover trial. Oral phenylpropanolamine and vaginal estriol were given separately and in combination. With combined treatment, eight patients became completely continent and nine were considerably improved. Similar cure rates were reported in another prospective clinical trial using norepinephrine in combination with oral estradiol (23). Kinn and Lindskog (24) carried out a randomized crossover trial with 36 postmenopausal women with stress incontinence. Additive effects of combination treatment with oral estriol and phenylpropanolamine reduced the number and amount of leakage episodes by 40%. Finally, Ahlstrom et al. (25) studied 29 postmenopausal women with stress incontinence in a randomized double-blind trial. They showed that a combination treatment of phenylpropanolamine and oral estriol was more effective than estriol alone in treating the incontinence.

Medications with alpha-adrenergic properties are common constituents of over-the-counter diet suppressants (Table 37.2). We prescribe ornade spansules, one tablet orally twice a day. Imipramine and other tricyclic antidepressants have anticholinergic effects in addition to alpha-adrenergic effects. We prefer imipramine in patients with mixed incontinence. Patients may be given up to 150 mg daily. A trial of 8 weeks is allowed for these medications.

Until evidence disproves estrogen's role in stress urinary incontinence, we recommend its use in all estrogen-deficient women without contraindication to estrogen-replacement therapy. Urodynamic effects of pharmacological treatment are illustrated in Figures 37.1 and 37.2. We prefer conjugated equine estrogen cream, 2 g intravaginally every other day, with the dose reduced by half once a response is demonstrated. Ideally, patients are simultaneously prescribed alpha-sympathomimetic drugs. These latter medications, however, affect the vascular tone, which can frequently contraindicate their use in postmenopausal patients. They should be used with caution, particularly in patients with hypertension or cardiac disease.

Pelvic Floor Musculature

The anatomy of the pelvic floor has been dealt with elsewhere. In terms of the continence mechanism, the striated pelvic floor muscles perform both a supportive and a sphincteric function (26). Striated muscle is composed of two distinct muscle fiber types: slow-twitch or type I fibers, which use aerobic oxidative metabolism in their function to maintain tone and support, and fast-twitch or type II fibers, which use anaerobic glycolytic metabolism for rapid forceful contractions in response to sudden increases in intro abdominal pressure.

Muscle fibers with greater aerobic oxidative capacity have less resistance to fatigue, and vice versa. The periurethral levator ani muscle is composed of 70% type I fibers and 30% type II fibers. The levator ani supports the pelvic organs and forms the scaffolding to which the pelvic ligaments attach (27). The striated urethral sphincter muscle contains almost exclusively type I or slow-twitch fibers and is important in intrinsic urethral function and passive continence (28).

The strength of muscular contraction depends on the muscle's cross-sectional area. Partial denervation of the pelvic floor muscles occurs with aging and childbirth (29). Delayed conduction of impulses to the pelvic floor muscles is present in women with stress urinary incontinence (30). Denervated muscle tissue atrophies, resulting in weaker muscular contractions and more rapid onset of fatigue. Both types of fibers, but especially the slow-twitch fibers, are capable of hypertrophy with appropriate training. Exercises that cause hypertrophy of the pelvic floor muscles will improve the efficiency of their supportive and sphincteric actions.

Arnold Kegel (31) posited that denervation injury occurs with childbearing and was the first to develop a method to "reconstruct" the pelvic floor muscles by exercising them. In Kegel's original publication, he recognized the importance of segregation, guidance, and

Table 37.2. Currently Available Dietary Suppressants Containing Phenylpropanolamine

Drug	How Supplied[a]	Phenylpro-panolamine (mg)	Caffeine (mg)
		Dosages	
Anorexin	C	25	100
Anorexin One-Span	C, SR	50	200
Appedrine	T	25	100[b]
Contac	C, SR	75	—[c]
Control	C, SR	75	—
Dexatrim	C, SR	50	200
Dexatrim Extra Strength	C, SR	75	200
Dexatrim	C, SR	75	—
Diet Gard	C, T	25	—
Dietac	C, SR	50	200
Dietac	T	25	—
Dietac	D	25	—
E-Z Trim	C, SR	75	—
Ornade	C, SR	75	—
Prolamine	C	37.5	140[c]
Super Odrinex	T	25	100

[a]C, capsule; SR, sustained release; T, tablet; D, drops.
[b]Also contains vitamins.
[c]Also contains chlorpheniramine.

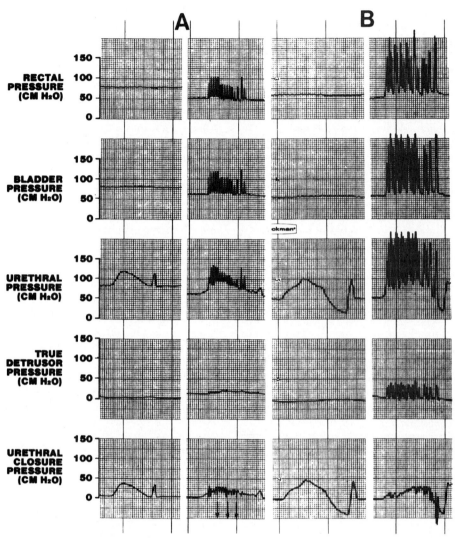

Figure 37.1. Urethral pressure profile and urethral pressure cough profile before treatment (**A**) and at 12 weeks during estrogen treatment (**B**). Note positive urethral closure pressure, with pressure equalization between bladder and urethra at times of stress (*arrows*) and negative urethral cough pressure profile after estrogen treatment.

progression in pelvic floor muscle training. These principles are often forgotten when pelvic floor exercises are prescribed. Indeed, because the appropriate muscles are anatomically hidden and not normally noted in daily activity, inadequate instruction in their identification may be counterproductive to controlling incontinence. Patients frequently contract muscles like the rectus abdominis that promote loss of urine. Bump et al. (32) showed that more than half of a series of patients with stress incontinence contracted inappropriate muscles after brief verbal instruction in Kegel exercises (32).

Digital vaginal examination with the other hand on the patient's abdomen should confirm contraction of the pubococcygeus and not the abdominal muscles. We instruct our patients to sit on the toilet seat at home and try to stop the flow of urine without moving their legs, thereby isolating the pubococcygeus muscle. This is only used to identify the correct muscles, and patients should never practice the exercise by stopping urine flow. Patients are instructed to hold the contraction for 10 seconds in groups of 10 contractions, three times daily. To train both fast-and slow-twitch fibers, sustained maximal contractions should be combined with "quick flicks," that is, brief forceful contractions. Patients should perform the contractions in different positions to limit Valsalva-type efforts. Patients will need close follow-up and frequent positive reinforcement for the exercises to be optimally effective. The exercises are supervised by a dedicated physiotherapist, and ideally, follow-up will be twice weekly in the initial sessions. Patients who improve should note a change within 2–3 months.

A study recently assessed the effect of Kegel exercises in an objective manner. Fifty-six percent of stress incontinent women considered their problem substantially improved or cured when Kegel exercises were performed under optimal conditions (N = 36) (33). Other researchers reported similar success rates of 47–67% in patients treated with Kegel exercises for stress incontinence (34–36).

Peattie and Plevnik (37) used a novel and ingenious technique to strengthen the pelvic floor muscles. Patients insert a weighted

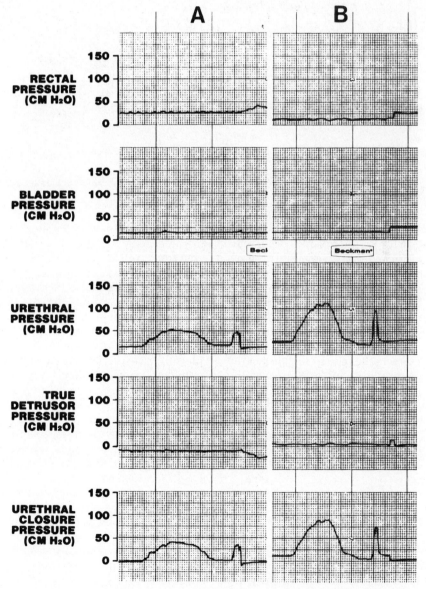

Figure 37.2. Urethral pressure profiles before treatment (**A**) and at 3 months after imipramine treatment (**B**).

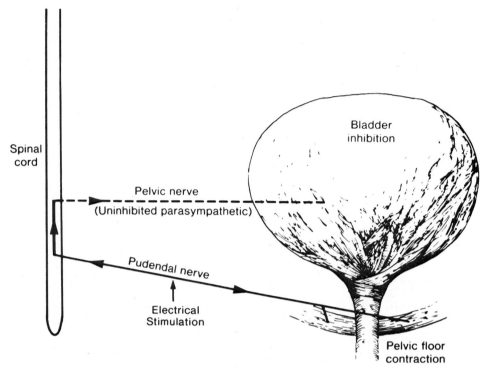

Figure 37.3. Electrical stimulation. Pudendal nerve stimulation can cause a direct pelvic floor contraction, an increase in urethral pressure, and, through the spinal cord, a reflex pelvic nerve stimulation, which results in inhibition of bladder activity.

vaginal cone in the vagina, tip down, and retained it for 15 minutes. Cones of increasing weights from 20–100 g were used progressively. Because the cone orients vertically with the apex pointing downward, lateral pressure from contraction of the pubococcygeus causes retention while force directed at the base (Valsalva) causes it to slip out. The tactile feedback of the cone slipping out of the vagina directs the patient to contract the pelvic floor muscles while she relaxes the muscles that cause a Valsalva. Seventy percent of women participating reported significant improvement after using these cones for 1 month. Similar results were reported by other groups (38–40).

Biofeedback

Filling and storage of urine requires accommodation of increasing volumes of urine without bladder contraction in the presence of a competent bladder outlet. Detrusor control and contraction of the striated muscle sphincter are learned processes, making incontinence a kind of behavioral deficit. Biofeedback, a behavioral therapy, effectively facilitates the learning of skills necessary to overcome this deficit.

As a therapeutic process, biofeedback furnishes the information on the state of a physiological variable to enable the individual to gain voluntary control over the variable being monitored. The goal in applying biofeedback specifically to stress incontinence is to increase the voluntary control of the pelvic floor muscles. The application of biofeedback to pelvic floor muscle exercises is not new and dates back to Kegel's original work (31). Kegel's technique involved monitoring the intravaginal pressure with a device called a perineometer. Patients were able to progressively increase the efficiency of their pelvic floor muscle exercises using the visual feedback of intravaginal pressure. Kegel reported a 90% improvement in 455 patients treated.

Another variable monitored and "fed back" to the patient is vaginal electrical activity. The electromyogram activity of the pelvic floor contraction can be detected with a surface electrode and furnished to the patient as an auditory or visual signal. This technique has the advantage of reflecting pelvic floor muscular activity only, independent of abdominal muscle contraction. A recent publication investigated this technique in patients with stress urinary incontinence and reported a 76% reduction in incontinence (41). Like pelvic floor muscular exercises, all forms of biofeedback require a highly motivated patient and the supervision of a trained therapist.

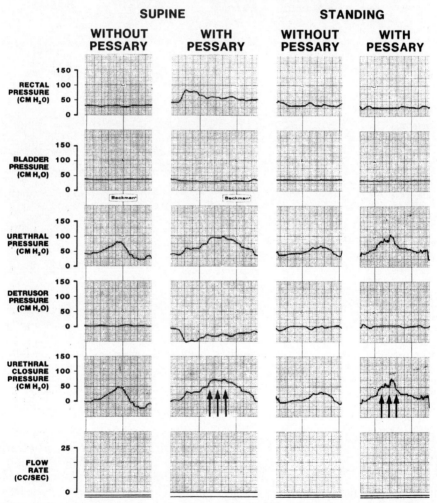

Figure 37.4.   Effect of the vaginal pessary on urethral closure pressure profiles in a patient with stress urinary incontinence in the supine and standing positions. The arrows point to the increased area of positive closure pressure under the profile curve. The upper three tracings are direct pressure measurements by microtip transducers placed in the rectum, bladder, and urethra. The next lower two channels are electronically subtracted, that is, true detrusor pressure (2 - 1) and urethral closure pressure (3 - 2). The bottom channel is for uroflow recording. (From Bhatia N, Bergman A, Gunning J. Urodynamic effects of a vaginal pessary in women with stress urinary incontinence. Am J Obstet Gynecol 1983;147:876.)

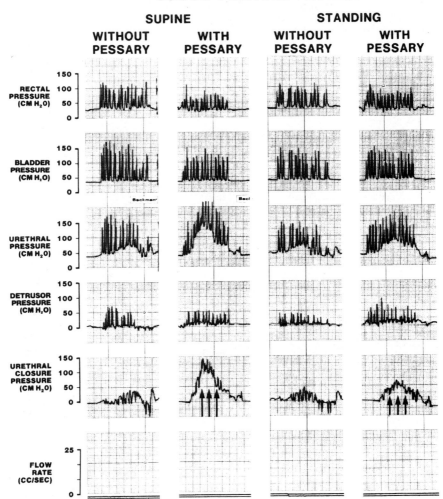

Figure 37.5. Cough pressure profiles in a patient with stress urinary incontinence in the supine and standing positions with various degrees of bladder filling, before and after placement of the vaginal pessary. The arrows point to the large area of positive closure pressure created under the curve of the cough profile by the vaginal pessary. (From Bhatia N, Bergman A, Gunning J. Urodynamic effects of a vaginal pessary in women with stress urinary incontinence. Am J Obstet Gynecol 1983;147:876.)

Functional Electrical Stimulation

Functional electrical stimulation is based on the premise that electrical stimulation of the pelvic floor results in a reflex contraction of the periurethral and paraurethral striated muscles with inhibition of detrusor activity (Fig. 37.3). The technique is therefore a passive one in that it does not require the active participation of the patient. Functional electrical stimulation may be particularly suited to mixed incontinence because of the simultaneous detrusor inhibition. Like pelvic floor muscular exercise, however, at least partial innervation of the pelvic floor musculature must exist for the technique to be effective.

Bors (42) first described the effect of electrical stimulation on the bladder neck, and Caldwell and associates (43) demonstrated its effectiveness in the treatment of incontinence. Early attempts, although effective, were cumbersome technically. In the technique described by Caldwell et al., electrodes were surgically implanted in the pelvic floor. Since then, sophisticated and reliable apparatuses have evolved. Electrodes are removable, in the form of vaginal pessaries or vaginal and anal plugs. Treatment can be given in the office or with portable battery-operated devices that the patient takes home. To date, the effectiveness and the optimal parameters for treatment have not been established, but encouraging results have been reported (see Chapter 41).

Stationary office devices apply maximal electrical stimulation as determined by the patient's level of pain tolerance. Treatment is given on a weekly basis. One clinical trial, although uncontrolled, showed an 89% improvement in patients with stress urinary incontinence after six sessions of maximal stimulation (44). Portable devices for home treatment (such as the Microgyn II device; InCare Medical Products, Libertyville, IL) provide long-term or chronic stimulation. This stimulation is of such low voltage that the sensory threshold is not crossed. An improvement in 50% of patients appears to be feasible (45).

Mechanical Devices

Vaginal pessaries have been used to prevent stress incontinence. Several pessaries, such as the Smith, Hodge, and Gellhorn types, provide support to the proximal urethra. These pessaries restore continence in some women by stabilizing the bladder base and increasing functional urethral length (Figs. 37.4 and 37.5) (46). It is difficult to predict which women will benefit from this effect. Because pessaries are effective in some women with stress urinary incontinence, they merit consideration as a conservative modality of treatment. Several pessaries are now marketed specifically for stress incontinence, including the Cook continence ring and the bladder neck support prosthesis marketed by Johnson and Johnson. A urethral plug has been developed and appears to be effective in a preliminary report (47).

Summary

A trial of nonsurgical therapy is recommended in virtually all patients with stress incontinence. Up to 50% of patients treated in this conservative fashion may improve enough to forego surgery.

The various conservative modalities for treating stress incontinence each aim at a different aspect of the continence mechanism. These modalities can thus be combined for optimal benefit.

Estrogen forms a cornerstone in the treatment of the postmenopausal woman. Estrogen has recognized physiological effects on the lower urinary tract. Estrogen in conjunction with alpha-adrenergic medications appears to be effective in treating mild genuine stress incontinence by improving intrinsic urethral function.

The muscles of the pelvis promote continence through a supportive and sphincteric function. Loss of this function occurs with the denervation injury of childbirth and aging. Pelvic muscle training in the form of Kegel exercises or with weighted vaginal cones is effective in improving this function. Pelvic floor exercises can be optimized with biofeedback or with functional electrical stimulation, which creates a "passive Kegel" contraction of the pelvic floor muscles.

REFERENCES

1. Urinary Incontinence Guideline Panel. Urinary incontinence in adults: clinical practice guidelines. Rockville, MD: U.S. Department of Health and Human Services. AHCPR Publication no. 92-0038. March 1992.
2. Richardson DA. Conservative management of urinary incontinence: a symposium. J Reprod Med 1993;38:659–661.
3. Klarskov P, Belving D, Bischoff N, et al. Pelvic floor exercise versus surgery for female urinary incontinence. Urol Int 1986;41:129–132.
4. Genant HK, Baylink DJ, Gallagher JC. Estrogens in the prevention of osteoporosis in postmenopausal women. Am J Obstet Gynecol 1989;17: 201–223.
5. Ernster VL, Bush TL, Huggins GR, Hulka BS, Kelsey JL, Schottenfeld D. Benefits and risks of menopausal estrogen and/or progestin hormone use. Prev Med 1988;20:47–63.
6. Stampfer MJ, Colditz GA. Estrogen replacement therapy and coronary artery disease: a quantita-

tive assessment of the epidemiologic evidence. Prev Med 1991;20:47–63.

7. Barrett-Conner E, Bush TL. Estrogen and coronary heart disease in women. JAMA 1991;265:1861–1867.

8. Albright F, Smith PH, Richardson AM. Postmenopausal osteoporosis—its clinical features. JAMA 1941;116:2465–2474.

9. Brincat M, Moniz CF, Kabalan S, et al. Decline in skin collagen content and metacarpal index after the menopause and its prevention with sex hormone replacement. Br J Obstet Gynaecol 1987;94:126–129.

10. Dube JY, Lesage RL, Tremblay RR. Androgen and estrogen binding in rat skeletal and perineal muscles. Can J Biochem 1976;54:50–55.

11. Dionne FT, Lesage RL, Dube JY. Estrogen binding proteins in rat skeletal and perineal muscles: in vitro and in vivo studies. J Steroid Biochem 1979;11:1073–1080.

12. Enhorning G. Simultaneous recording of intra urethral and intra vesical pressure: a study on urethral closure in stress incontinent women. Scand J Urol Nephrol 1978;12:105–119.

13. Blaivas JG, Klutke CG, Raz S, Webster GD. When sphincter failure is the cause of female stress incontinence. Contemp Urol 1993;1–11.

14. Batra S, Iosif S. Functional estrogen receptors in the female urethra. Proceedings of the 2nd Joint Meeting of ICS and Urodynamic Society, Aachen, 1983:548.

15. Iosif S, Batra S, Ek A, Astedt B. Estrogen receptors in the human female lower urinary tract. Am J Obstet Gynecol 1981;141:817–820.

16. Salmon UJ, Walter RI, Geist SA. The use of estrogens in the treatment of dysuria and incontinence in postmenopausal women. Am J Obstet Gynecol 1941;42:845–851.

17. Bergman A, Karram MM, Bhatia NN. Changes in urethral cytology following estrogen administration. Gynecol Obstet Invest 1990;29:211–213.

18. Sarrel PM. Sexuality and menopause. Obstet Gynecol 1990;75:26S–32S.

19. Levin RM, Jacobowitz D, Wein AJ. Autonomic innervation of rabbit urinary bladder following estrogen administration. Urology 1981;17:449–453.

20. Hodgson BT, Dumas S, Bolling DR, et al. Effect of estrogen on sensitivity of rabbit bladder and urethra to phenylephrine. Invest Urol 1978;16:67–69.

21. Levin RM, Shofer FS, Wein AJ. Cholinergic, adrenergic and purinergic response of sequential strips of rabbit urinary bladder. J Pharmacol Exp Ther 1980;212:536–540.

22. Beisland HO, Fossberg E, Moer A, et al. Urethral sphincteric insufficiency in postmenopausal females: treatment with phenylpropanolamine and estriol separately and in combination. A urodynamic and clinical evaluation. Urol Int 1984;39:211–216.

23. Ek A, Andersson KE, Gullberg B, et al. Effects of oestradiol and combined norephedrin and oestradiol treatment on female stress incontinence. Zentralbl Gynaekol 1980;102:839–844.

24. Kinn A, Lindskog M. Estrogens and phenylpro-

panolamine in combination for stress urinary incontinence in postmenopausal women. Urology 1988;32:273–280.

25. Ahlstrom K, Sandahl B, Sjoberg B, et al. Effect of combined treatment with phenylpropanolamine and estriol, compared with estriol treatment alone, in postmenopausal women with stress urinary incontinence. Gynecol Obstet Invest 1990;30:37–43.

26. Delancy JO, Richardson AC. Anatomy of genital support. In: Benson JT, ed. Female pelvic floor disorders, investigation and management. New York: WW Norton, 1992:19–26.

27. Zacharin R. The suspensory mechanism of the female urethra. J Anat 1963;97:423–427.

28. Eriksen BC. Electrical stimulation. In: Benson JT, ed. Female pelvic floor disorders, investigation and management. New York: WW Norton, 1992:222.

29. Peterson I, Franksson C, Danielson GO. Electromyography of the pelvic floor and urethra in normal females. Acta Obstet Gynecol Scand 1955;34:273–285.

30. Snooks SJ, Badenoch DF, Tiptaft RC, et al. Perineal nerve damage in genuine stress urinary incontinence: an electrophysiologic study. Br J Urol 1985;57:422–426.

31. Kegel AH. Progressive resistance exercise in the functional restoration of the perineal muscles. Am J Obstet Gynecol 1948;56:238–248.

32. Bump RC, Hurt WG, Fantl JA, Wyman JF. Assessment of Kegel pelvic muscle exercises after brief verbal instruction. Am J Obstet Gynecol 1991;165:322–327.

33. Elia G, Bergmann A. Pelvic muscle exercises: when do they work? Obstet Gynecol 1993;81:283–286.

34. Henalla SM, Kirwan P, Castleden CM, et al. The effect of pelvic floor exercises in the treatment of genuine urinary stress incontinence in women at two hospitals. Br J Obstet Gynaecol 1988;95:602–606.

35. Mouritsen L, Frimodt-Moller C, Moller M. Long-term effect of pelvic floor exercises on female urinary incontinence. Br J Urol 1991;68:32–37.

36. Hahn I, Milsom I, Fall M, Ekelund P. Long-term results of pelvic floor training in female stress urinary incontinence. Br J Urol 1993;72:421–427.

37. Peattie AB, Plevnik S, Stanton SL. Vaginal cones: a conservative method of treating genuine stress incontinence. Br J Obstet Gynecol 1988;95:1049–1053.

38. Olah KS, Bridges N, Denning J, Farrar DJ. The conservative management of patients with symptoms of stress incontinence: a randomized, prospective study comparing weighted vaginal cones and interferential therapy. Am J Obstet Gynecol 1990;162:87–92.

39. Wilson PD, Borland M. Vaginal cones for the treatment of genuine stress incontinence. Aust NZ J Obstet Gynaecol 1990;30:157–160.

40. Kato K, Kondo A, Hasegawa S, et al. Pelvic floor muscle training as treatment of stress incontinence. The effectiveness of vaginal cones. Nippon Hinyokika Gakkai Zasshi 1992;88:498–504.

41. McIntosh LJ, Frahm JD, Mallett VT, Richardson

DA. Pelvic floor rehabilitation in the treatment of incontinence. J Reprod Med 1993;38:663–666.

42. Bors E. Effect of electric stimulation of the pudendal nerves on the vesical neck: its significance for the function of cord bladders: a preliminary report. J Urol 1952;67:925–935.

43. Caldwell KPS, Flack FC, Broad AF. Urinary incontinence following spinal injury treated by electronic implants. Lancet 1965;1:846–847.

44. Caputo RM, Benson JT, McClellan E. Intravaginal maximal electrical stimulation in the treatment of urinary incontinence. J Reprod Med 1993;38:9: 667–671.

45. Doyle PT, Edwards LE, Harrison NW, et al. Treatment of urinary incontinence by external stimulating devices. Urol Int 1974;29:456–457.

46. Bhatia N, Bergman A, Gunning J. Urodynamic effects of a vaginal pessary in women with stress urinary incontinence. Am J Obstet Gynecol 1983; 147:876.

47. Nielsen KK, Walter S, Maegaard E, Kromann-Andersen B. The urethral plug II: an alternative treatment in women with genuine urinary stress incontinence. Br J Urol 1993;72:428–432.

48. Judge TG. The use of quinestradiol in elderly incontinent women. Gerontol Clin 1969;11: 159–164.

49. Walter S, Wolf H, Barlebo H, et al. Urinary incontinence in postmenopausal women treated with oestrogens: a double blind clinical trial. Urol Int 1978;33:135–143.

50. Samsioe G, Jansson I, Mellstrom D, Svanborg A. Occurrence, nature and treatment of urinary incontinence in a 70 year old female population. Maturitas 1985;7:335–342.

51. Wilson PD, Faragher B, Butler B, Bu-Lock D, Robinson EL, Brown AD. Treatment with oral piperazine oestrone sulphate for genuine stress incontinence in postmenopausal women. Br J Obstet Gynaecol 1987;94:568–574.

52. Foidart JM, Vervliet J, Buytaert PH. Efficacy of sustained-release vaginal estriol in alleviating urogenital and systemic climacteric complaints. Maturitas 1991;13:99–107.

CHAPTER 38

Evaluation of Different Surgical Procedures

Mary T. McLennan, Alfred E. Bent, and David A. Richardson

In an attempt to determine the best approach to managing incontinent patients, one must wade through voluminous urogynecological literature inundated with contradictions, unsubstantiated opinions, and speculative assertions. Adequate comparison of results, even with the same procedure, are generally not available.

The primary difficulty in literature analysis lies in four areas:

1. Lack of uniform diagnostic criteria;
2. Lack of uniform outcome criteria (i.e., "cure");
3. Failure to identify preoperative bladder instability;
4. Failure to control for relevant independent variables.

Diagnostic Criteria

It is obviously difficult to compare outcomes if one is unsure of what is actually being treated. The terms stress incontinence and genuine stress incontinence (GSI) are not interchangeable. The former can be a symptom, a sign, or a diagnosis. The latter is a diagnosis reached after testing has excluded other causes for incontinence. Jensen et al. (1), in a recent literature analysis, showed that reliance on history alone to demonstrate GSI resulted in a misdiagnosis in 25% of cases.

Intrinsic sphincter deficiency (ISD) has also been defined in variable ways: low maximal urethral closure pressure (MUCP)

less than 20 cm H_2O, leak point pressure less than 65 cm H_2O, or by some clinical criteria such as history of severe or total incontinence without urethrovesical junction mobility and with endoscopic evidence of an open bladder neck and fixed urethra. It is difficult to compare outcomes between groups of patients where preoperative criteria are so different.

The literature suggests that patients with decreased mobility have higher failure rates, but few articles report on preoperative mobility (2). A description of the extent of the dissection, the areas of fixation, and the type and number of sutures or sling material used is needed, and there should be consistency in operative technique. One recent study on laparoscopic bladder neck suspensions described three different suture attachment sites, making any comparison of outcomes impossible.

To allow an objective outcomes comparison, preoperative assessment must include a thorough history, including previous surgeries; physical examination, including directed neurological residual urine determination, urinalysis, or culture; assessment of urethrovesical junction mobility; stress test at a defined volume; and cystometrogram.

Outcome Criteria

Comparison of surgical outcomes is difficult because of a disparity in the definition of cure, lack of objective evaluation, and variable length of follow-up. Most articles report subjective evaluation. Many report on "good symptomatic relief" without defining whether this is dry or improved. Cure rates based on retrospective chart reviews have inherent inaccuracies because they rely on the question and depend on the accuracy and completeness of charting. In a retrospective review of the Stamey procedure, Stamey (3) reported a 91% cure. In contrast, Walker and Texter (4), using a questionnaire-based study, found 40% reported cure and 81% improved. Both the physician and the patient are potential sources of bias. The physician may not listen to the patient or ask questions and patients may be afraid to be honest for fear of letting their doctor down or because they are afraid of further surgery. Patients may also fail to follow-up for review. The dropout rate must be critically appraised in any study. A 30% dropout rate will vastly lower success rates (5).

Objective cure rates typically are lower than subjective cures. Karram et al. (6) reported that 82% of postoperative patients denied any urinary leakage but only 63% were continent at urodynamic testing. The method of objective assessment needs to be defined. Repeat urodynamic testing certainly allows for assessment of risk factors for those having failed surgery but is probably not necessary on all patients. Stress testing at a known bladder volume and pad testing are reproducible defined outcome measures. If one is to have a category of improved, then there must be some objective criteria (e.g., reduction in incontinent episodes).

A defined minimum length of follow-up may allow better standardization. Because of the decline in cure rates with time, Stanton and Cardozo (7) believed a minimum of 5 years was necessary. Bergman and Elia (8) noted 1-year success rates of 63%, 65%, and 89% for the anterior repair, Pereyra procedure, and Burch procedure, respectively. At 5 years, the success rates had declined to 37%, 43%, and 82%, respectively. Alcalay et al. (9) noted a declining success rate for Burch colposuspension over 10–12 years. Analyzing articles in the English literature, Jarvis (10) found objective results available on 4801 (23.5%) of 20,481 patients reported (Table 38.1).

Articles may not report complications, and the patient who develops urinary retention, detrusor instability (DI), graft rejection, or chronic incisional pain may not consider the surgery to be successful.

Detrusor Instability

The incidence of DI in the community is variable, with a reported incidence of 10–50%, which increases with age. Although the complaint of stress loss of urine is sensitive in predicting GSI, Jensen et al. (1) in their review noted a 9–52% incidence of stress-induced detrusor activity. Reliance on history alone would have resulted in the misdiagnosis of GSI in 25% of patients (1). Obviously, these patients would have been included in the surgical failure group when surgery had not failed but was inappropriate.

Hodgkinson (11), Jorgensen et al. (12), Karram and Bhatia (13) reported cure rates of 37%, 31%, and 59%, respectively, in unselected patients with DI. Raz et al. (14) noted worsening of urgency and urge incontinence in 7.5% of patients. Beck et al. (15) noted an 84% resolution of DI in those patients with mixed incontinence whose DI was previously unresponsive to medical therapy. Generally, studies indicate a 30–60% resolution of DI in patients with mixed incontinence (14, 16).

Patients need to be extensively counseled regarding the persistence of their irritative voiding symptoms and/or urge incontinence postoperatively.

Table 38.1. Objective Cure Rates for Various Procedures

Procedure	Objective[a]
MMK	443 (89.2)
Colposuspension	2300 (84.3)
Needle	729 (70.7)
Sling	720 (85.3)
Kelly type[b]	490 (72.0)
Injectables	133 (60.2)
Total	4815

From Jarvis GJ. Surgery for genuine stress incontinence. Br J Obstet Gynaecol 1994; 101:371.
[a]Values are n, with percents in parentheses.
[b]Mixed group.

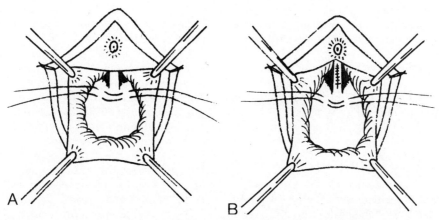

Figure 38.1. **A.** Kelly plication. **B.** Kelly–Kennedy modification.

Independent Variables

In the evaluation of any surgical procedure, there are a number of independent variables that have an impact on success. One of the most important of these is operator skill. Age has been found to be a significant factor in certain types of surgery. Peattie and Stanton (17) found a 40% success for the Stamey procedure in women greater than 65 years of age compared with an 89% success in those having retropubic procedures. Korman et al. (18) and Kursh (19) noted similar findings, whereas Nitti et al. (20) and Raz et al. (14) found similar success rates in this age group than in younger patients.

The effect of obesity is questionable. Alcalay et al. (9) found a preoperative weight greater than 80 kg a bad prognostic feature, whereas Stanton et al. (21) found no relationship. The number of patients greater than 80 kg in both reports was small. Available evidence supports the use of permanent suture (22).

Many studies reported lower success rates in patients with failed previous surgeries (10, 23, 24), urethral hypomobility (2), and low pressure urethra/type III incontinence/ISD (25–28). Sand et al. (25) showed a threefold increase and Koonings et al. (27) a 33% failure rate with the Burch colposuspension in patients with ISD. Horbach and Ostergard (29) identified age greater than 50 as a risk factor for ISD. Performing urethral closure pressure profiles and/or leak point pressures, particularly in patients over the age of 50, will identify this at-risk subgroup.

Anterior Colporrhaphy

At one time, the anterior colporrhaphy (Kelly plication or Kelly–Kennedy modification) was the mainstay of treatment for stress incontinence (Fig. 38.1) (30, 31). The purpose of these operations was to repair the injured or torn sphincter that we now know to be an anatomically incorrect assumption.

In both randomized and nonrandomized studies, Bergman and Elia (8), Zirkovic et al. (32), and Van Geelen et al. (33) compared the anterior repair with other surgical techniques, reporting cure rates of 63%, 59%, and 43%, respectively. In contrast, Bergman and Elia (8) and Van Geelen et al. (33) reported success rates of 89% and 85% for the Burch procedure. Bergman and Elia (8) also reported a marked fall-off in success at 5 years to 37% for anterior repair versus 82% for the Burch procedure. At 5 years, Zivkovic et al. (32) also published success rates of 96% for the Burch compared with 59% for the anterior repair. Both Van Geelen et al. (33) and Zivkovic et al. (32) demonstrated higher failure rates in association with higher degrees of incontinence.

Beck et al. (15) are among the few authors reporting continued good success with anterior colporrhaphy. In their review of 519 patients, they reported a cure rate of 94%. They did admit the reason for increased success compared with their original series (75%) was a directional and depth change in suture placement under and around the urethra. In their series, the needle was placed so that the long axis was inserted deeper and at right angles into the fascia below, lateral, and above the urethra. This probably provides better fixation and high elevation of the bladder neck.

Complication rates for anterior colphorraphy are low (1–3%) (15, 34). DI appears to occur infrequently (2–6%) (15, 33), but the true incidence may be understated.

Retropubic Urethropexy

The first described retropubic procedure was in 1949 by Marshall, Marchetti, and Krantz (MMK) in which the periurethral tissue was sutured to the back of the symphysis. Burch in 1962 modified the procedure by fixing the periurethral tissue to Cooper's ligament (Fig. 38.2) (35). It is generally accepted that the cure rate is similar for both procedures (10, 35, 36). The complication rate appears higher with the MMK, which is more obstructive (voiding difficulties in up to 28%), and it has the unique complication of osteitis pubis in up to 5% (36–39).

The Burch urethropexy is the best studied procedure with good objective and long-term follow-up. Short-term objective success rates of 75–90% are reported (8, 33, 34). Because of the decline in cure rates with time, Stanton and Cardozo (7) believed a minimum of 5 years (33) follow-up was necessary. Van Geelen et al. (33) reported a subjective cure of 78% at 5 years (1) and Kjolhede and Ryden (24) reported 63% at a median of 6 years (range 2–10 years). Bergman and Elia (8), Zivkovic et al. (32), and Eriksen et al. (40) found objective success rates of 82%, 86%, and 71%, respectively, at 5 years. Four 10-year follow-up reports (3 with objective data) have been recently published. Alcalay et al. (9) noted a decline for 10–12 years, at which time a plateau of 69% was reached. Feyereisl et al. (41) demonstrated an 82.6% cure based on postoperative urodynamic criteria, and Herbertsson and Isof (42) reported an objective success rate of 90%. Laursen et al. (43) reported a subjective success (questionnaire based) of 54% at 18 years.

The most frequent complications reported are DI (5–18%) (9, 35, 40) and voiding difficulties (8–22%) (9, 24, 35, 44). Colposuspension with its high anterior elevation seems to aggravate posterior wall weakness. The incidence of enterocele ranges from 5 to 17% (40, 45). Kjolhede and Ryden (24) reported a 15% reoperation rate for posterior wall prolapse.

Poor outcomes have been reported in the elderly (over 65 years) (21, 45). In contrast, Gillion and Stanton (46) reported a 90% cure rate in selected patients over 65. Alcalay et al. (9) and Eriksen et al. (40) showed no significance difference in long-term success with patients greater than 65 years of age.

An increased risk of failure has been reported with patients with a low MUCP (25, 27, 47). Feyereisl et al. (41) showed a high failure rate with patients with an MUCP lower than that corresponding to the patient's age, regardless of whether it was higher or lower than 20 cm H_2O.

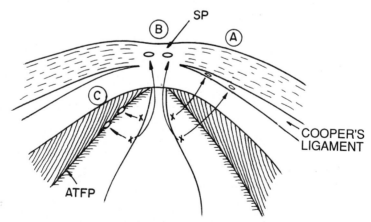

Figure 38.2. A. Burch colposuspension with sutures attached to Cooper's ligament. **B.** MMK procedure with sutures attached to the symphysis pubis. **C.** Richardson paravaginal approach with sutures attached to the arcus tendineus fascia pelvis.

MODIFIED PEREYRA   GITTES   STAMEY

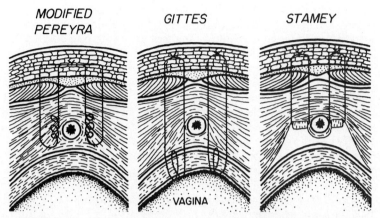

Figure 38.3. Three variations of the needle urethropexy procedure.

The paravaginal or Richardson repair largely used for the treatment of cystocele secondary to lateral defects has been advocated for the treatment of GSI. Here the endopelvic fascia is reattached to the arcus tendinous fascia pelvis (white line) or obturator internus fascia. Richardson et al. (48) reported an 81% and Shull and Baden (49) a 97% subjective success rate with this procedure. In Shull and Baden's series, the middle two sutures were placed through Cooper's ligament, so this was not strictly a paravaginal repair. To date there are no objective outcomes studies on this procedure.

Needle Urethropexy

Pereyra (50) introduced the first needle suspension in 1959. Since that time, the general procedure has undergone many modifications. In general terms, the needle procedures avoid a large abdominal incision. Through a small suprapubic incision, a needle is passed through the space of Retzius to the vagina. Sutures are placed in the periurethral endopelvic fascia and attached to the rectus fascia (Fig. 38.3). In 1973, Stamey (51) added endoscopy to the procedure and supported the vaginal sutures with the use of a buttress. In 1980, he reviewed 203 patients and reported a 91% cure rate (52). Raz (53) attached the supporting suture in a helical manner to the fascia adjacent to the bladder neck rather than using a bolster. In 1987, Gittes and Loughlin (54) eliminated the vaginal incision based on their laboratory observation that sutures tied under tension cut through the skin and became internalized without inflammation. With this particular procedure, a helical suture is placed directly into the vaginal wall in an attempt to prevent the suture cutting through the endopelvic fascia.

Needle procedures have been extensively reported in the urological literature. Their advantages are the shorter operative times, decreased hospital stays, and less postoperative pain while allowing correction of other vaginal defects. However, there appears to be a lower success rate, particularly over the long term.

Reported success rates have shown a great variation. Subjective cure rates have varied from 47 to 93% (Stamey [52], 1980, 91%; Jones et al. [55], 1989, 68%; Kursh et al. [56], 1991, 94%; Hilton and Mayne [57], 1991, 53%; Karram et al. [6], 1992, 82%; Korman et al. [18], 1994, 47%). Objective assessment once again is less commonly reported and with generally lower success rates (Karram et al. [6], 1992, 63%; Loughlin et al. [58], 1990, 83%; Hilton and Mayne [57], 1991, 83%). Caution needs to be exercised in interpretation because most objective assessments were reported at 3 months or 1 year.

Conflicting results have also been noted in the elderly. Peattie and Stanton (17) reported a 68% subjective and 40% objective success at 3 months in patients older than 65 years. Korman et al. (18) reported significantly worse outcomes in older patients, and Kursh (19) noted all his failures were in postmenopausal patients. In contrast, Nitti et al. (20)

and Raz et al. (14) noted success rates similar to younger patients, whereas Hilton and Mayne (57) and Griffith-Jones and Abrams (59) reported high success in the elderly. The concern is that the vaginal sutures may more easily pull through poor supporting tissues in the elderly postmenopausal patient.

In the only long-term study with a mean follow-up of 9.8 years, Trockman et al. (60) reported a subjective cure of only 49% for needle urethropexy. Notably, 22% of patients underwent one or more subsequent antiincontinence procedures. The first repeat procedure was performed an average of 4 years postoperatively, once again underscoring the importance of long-term follow-up.

Risk factors for high failure rates include previous failed surgery (23, 55, 58), severe grades of incontinence (14, 20, 60), and low MUCP (6, 23, 56).

The incidence of immediate postoperative complications is high, the most common being infectious (1–18%) (6, 14, 16, 23), obstructive voiding (2–15%) (6, 17, 23, 40, 58), de novo DI (7–25%) (6, 14, 20, 56), and persistent pain (0.7–13%) (14, 56, 57, 59).

In an attempt to reduce suture pull through, a vaginal wall sling procedure was developed. A distal island of vaginal wall over the urethrovesical junction is left attached, and four helical sutures incorporating periurethral endopelvic fascia are anchored to the four corners for better support. Initial subjective short-term success rates are reported at 94–100% (61, 62).

Laparoscopic Retropubic Urethropexy

Patient demand for less invasive procedures and the push for shorter hospital stays by insurance companies have been driving forces for the development of laparoscopic bladder neck suspension.

The problem with the current operative procedure is the basic lack of uniformity of technique in its performance. Although most authors attach the periurethral endopelvic fascia to Cooper's ligament in a manner similar to the standard Burch (63–66), some have attached it centrally (similar to MMK) (67,

68) or to the arcus tendinous fascia pelvis (67). One cannot place three different attachment sites into one surgical group. It is also difficult to compare the procedure with the standard Burch when it is unknown whether the sutures are placed in exactly the same manner as with the open technique (i.e., number of bites) suture only versus the addition of stapling devices, mesh, and so on. Liu and Paek (64) performed 107 laparoscopic Burch procedures with an objective success (stress test) at 6 months of 100% and a 97.2% subjective success rate overall, with follow-up ranging from 3 to 27 months. In a small comparative but nonrandomized study, Polascik et al. (63) showed a short-term subjective success of 83% with a mean follow-up of 20.8 months for the laparoscopic route versus 70% success for the open technique. Follow-up, however, was significantly longer in the latter group with a mean of 35.6 months. Karram et al. (65) in a pilot study of 24 patients showed an objective success rate of 87.5% at 3 months. Radomski et al. (66) also demonstrated good success (85%) at a mean of 17.3 months but found that in 26% (12 of 46 cases), the laparoscopy could not be completed and the technique was converted to open. This was due to access failure and scarring (11 patients) and bladder perforation (1 case). Patients with a history of either previous pelvic or bladder surgery must be consented for a possible open procedure. Midline scars make an extraperitoneal approach particularly difficult. In the only randomized comparative study, Burton (69) demonstrated a significantly worse outcome for the laparoscopic group both on subjective and objective testing (73 versus 97% cure).

Laparoscopic surgery, particularly the intraperitoneal approach with its extensive need for dissection, has a learning curve. Operative times for the laparoscopic Burch are longer (63, 67) but decrease with experience (65, 66). This must be balanced against shorter hospital stays (63–65, 67), less analgesia (64, 67), and early resumption of normal activity (63, 64).

Inadvertent bladder injury has been the most common complication reported (3.7–8.3%) (64–67). Of the few studies that comment on the incidence of DI, it appears comparable with the open technique (10–12%) (63, 66).

It is difficult to unconditionally recommend this procedure to a patient until larger studies, preferably randomized and with long-term follow-up, are available. It is reasonable to counsel the patient as to what is known and allow them to make an informed decision.

Sling Procedures

Suburethral slings have been typically reserved for patients with ISD, recurrent incontinence (failed previous surgery), stress incontinence associated with a neurogenic bladder, and stress incontinence associated with poor mobility. These differing indications make a heterogeneous study population that may influence complication and success rates. For example, McGuire et al.'s (70) large study of 82 patients included 9 with myelodysplasia (8 of whom had associated bladder augmentation procedures), 6 with fistulas, and 19 with bladder and urethral dysfunction (trauma, radical surgery, radiation, spinal cord injury). This group is obviously not comparable with that of Chin and Stanton (71), who treated women with GSI or GSI/DI only.

Originally reported by Goebel in 1910 (72), the sling has undergone many modifications both with types of materials used and technique. Both organic material (rectus fascia, fascia lata) and synthetic material (Mersilene, Marlex, Silastic, Gore-Tex) are currently used. Obviously, the use of different materials makes direct comparison of success and complications also difficult.

Organic materials have been criticized because of the increased operative time required for harvest, increased patient discomfort, and inadequate length and inconsistent strength and quality. Synthetic materials have uniformly caused increased problems with infection, graft rejection, and an increased incidence of obstructive voiding and urinary retention.

Delayed voiding is the most common complication. Reports suggest the incidence of retention may be higher with synthetic materials (2.2–16%) (71, 73, 74). Long-term need for self-catheterization occurs in 1.5–7.8% (75, 76). Urodynamic studies confirm increased outflow resistance as the mechanism (76). Patients must be counseled preoperatively regarding this complication, but for the patient constantly wet or with multiple surgeries, this may be a small price to pay.

Graft infection, rejection, erosion, and removal are serious concerns with the use of synthetic materials. Summit et al. (77) reported a 12.5% and Bent et al. (78) a 23% removal rate with a polytetrafluoroethylene (Gore-Tex) sling. Chin and Stanton (71) reported an 11% erosion rate with Silastic, Morgan et al. (79) a much lower rate of 0.7% with Marlex, and Young et al. (73) 1.8% with Mersilene. Obviously, this problem does not occur with organic materials.

The incidence of DI appears to be no higher than with the standard retropubic urethropexy (6–25%) (70, 71, 75).

The most impressive characteristic of the sling is its success rate for patients with recurrent incontinence (i.e., failed previous surgery). Success rates of 72–99% are reported. A metaanalysis of studies reporting on objective cures showed that the sling had a mean success of 86.1% for the treatment of recurrent incontinence (10). Morgan et al. (79) reported a subjective success rate of 72%, and Chin and Stanton (71) an objective success of 68% at 5 years for patients who had two or more failed surgeries. However, Chin and Stanton did note that women with three or more failed operations had a decreased success rate with an objective cure of 33%. Long-term follow-up studies indicate the durability of the sling with most failures occurring within 3 years (71).

Comparative Studies

To our knowledge, there are six groups who have conducted truly randomized trials: Henriksson and Ulmsten, 1978 (80); Milani et al., 1985 (81) and 1991 (82); Stanton and Cardozo, 1979 (83); Hilton, 1989 (84); Bergman et al., 1989 (85) and 1995 (8); and Columbo et al., 1994 (36) (Table 38.2). Both anterior repair and needle urethropexy showed lower success rates than other procedures. The advantage of these studies is that the patients were prospectively randomized and had objective testing at defined

Table 38.2. Randomized Comparative Trials: Objective Cure

	Anterior Colporrhaphy (%)	Retropubic (%)		Needle (%)	Sling (%)
		Burch	MMK		
Henriksson and Ulmsten (80)			100		100
Stanton and Cardozo (83)	36				84
Hilton (84)				80	90
Bergman and Elia (8)	37			43	82
Colombo et al. (36)		80	65		

intervals. In the longest follow-up to date, Bergman and Elia (8) found a significant drop-off in success between 1 and 5 years with the Burch having the least fall-off, 7% versus 26% and 22%, respectively, for the anterior repair and needle procedures.

Summary

The number of procedures and studies is endless. At a minimum, each report needs to document patient characteristics, such as age, parity, weight; number and type of previous procedures; a normal physical examination, including postvoid residual; the nature and type of the incontinence through preoperative studies, including assessment of the urethral sphincter with leak point pressure or MUCP and the degree of mobility; and the procedure, including suture type and any concomitant repairs. Follow-up needs to be objective and subjective. The latter is important because demonstrating leakage at 700 mL may be objective evidence of failure, but if the patient is dry with all activities, then it is a surgical success for the patient. Objective criteria need to be defined (i.e., stress test at a set volume, pad test, urodynamics). Length of follow-up needs to be stated with a minimum follow-up reported (i.e., 1 year and ideally 5 years). Complications, including postoperative DI and voiding disorders, need to be documented. Only through rigid, preoperative, intraoperative, and postoperative documentation will informed recommendations to patients be made.

REFERENCES

1. Jensen JK, Nielsen FR, Ostergard DR. The role of patient history in the diagnosis of urinary incontinence. Obstet Gynecol 1994;83:904–910.

2. Summit RL, Bent AE, Ostergard DR, Harris TA. Stress incontinence and low urethral closure pressure: correlation of preoperative urethral hypermobility with successful suburethral sling procedures. J Reprod Med 1990;35:877–880.

3. Stamey TA. Endoscopic suspension of the vesical neck for urinary incontinence in females. Report on 203 consecutive patients. Ann Surg 1980;192:465–471.

4. Walker GT, Texter JH Jr. Success and patient satisfaction following the Stamey procedure for stress urinary incontinence. J Urol 1992;147:1521–1523.

5. Herbertsson G, Iosif CS. Surgical results and urodynamic studies 10 years after retropubic colpourethrocystopexy. Acta Obstet Gynecol Scand 1993;72:298–301.

6. Karram MM, Angel O, Koonings P, Tabor B, Bergman A, Bhatia N. The modified Pereyra procedure: a clinical and urodynamic review. Br J Obstet Gynaecol 1992;99:655–658.

7. Stanton SL, Cardozo L. Results of colposuspension operation for incontinence and prolapse. Br J Obstet Gynaecol 1979;86:693–697.

8. Bergman A, Elia G. Three surgical procedures for genuine stress incontinence: five-year follow-up of a prospective randomized study. Am J Obstet Gynecol 1995;173:66–71.

9. Alcalay M, Monga A, Stanton SL. Burch colposuspension: a 10–20 year follow-up. Br J Obstet Gynaecol 1995;102:740–745.

10. Jarvis GJ. Surgery for genuine stress incontinence. Br J Obstet Gynaecol 1994;101:371–374.

11. Hodgkinson CP. Recurrent stress incontinence. Am J Obstet Gynecol 1978;131:844–860.

12. Jorgensen L, Lose G, Mousted-Pedersen L. Vaginal repair female motor urge incontinence. Eur Urol 1987;13:382–385.

13. Karram MM, Bhatia NN. Management of coexistent stress and urge urinary incontinence. Obstet Gynecol 1989;74:4–7.

14. Raz S, Sussman EM, Erickson DB, Bregg KJ, Nitti VW. The Raz bladder neck suspension: results in 206 patients. J Urol 1992;148:845–850.

15. Beck RP, McCormick S, Nordstrom L. A 25-year experience with 519 anterior colporrhaphy procedures. Obstet Gynecol 1991;78:1011–1018.

16. Nitti VW, Bregg KJ, Sussman EM, Raz S. The Raz bladder neck suspension in patients 65 years and older. J Urol 1993;149:802–807.

17. Peattie AB, Stanton SL. The Stamey operation for correction of genuine stress incontinence in the elderly women. Br J Obstet Gynaecol 1989;96:983–986.

18. Korman HJ, Sirls LT, Kirkemo AK. Success rate of modified Pereyra bladder neck suspension determined by outcomes analysis. J Urol 1994;152:1453–1457.
19. Kursh ED. What factors influence the outcome of a no-incision urethropexy [abstract]? J Urol 1991;145:322A.
20. Nitti VW, Bregg KJ, Sussman EM, Raz S. The Raz bladder neck suspension in patients sixty-five years and older. J Urol 1993;149:802–807.
21. Stanton SL, Cardozo L, Williams JE, Ritchie D, Allen V. Clinical and urodynamic features of failed incontinence surgery in the female. Obstet Gynecol 1979;51:515–520.
22. Korn AP. Does use of permanent suture material affect outcome of the modified Pereyra procedure? Obstet Gynecol 1994;83:104–107.
23. Holschneider CH, Solh S, Lebherz TB, Montz FJ. The modified Pereyra in recurrent stress urinary incontinence: a 15-year review. Obstet Gynecol 1994;83:573–578.
24. Kjolhede P, Ryden G. Prognostic factors and long-term results of the Burch colposuspension. A retrospective study. Acta Obstet Gynecol Scand 1994;73:642–647.
25. Sand PK, Bowen LW, Panganiban R, Ostergard DR. Low pressure urethra as a factor in failed retropubic urethropexy. Obstet Gynecol 1987;69:399–402.
26. McGuire EJ, Lytton B, Pepe V, Kohorn EI. Stress urinary incontinence. Obstet Gynecol 1976;47:255–264.
27. Koonings PP, Bergman A, Ballard CA. Low urethral pressure and stress urinary incontinence in women: risk factor for failed retropubic surgical procedure. Urology 1990;36:245–248.
28. McGuire EJ. Urodynamic findings in patients after failure of stress incontinence operations. Prog Clin Biol Res 1981;78:351–360.
29. Horbach NS, Ostergard DR. Predicting intrinsic urethral sphincter dysfunction in women with stress urinary incontinence. Obstet Gynecol 1994;84:187–192.
30. Kelly HA, Dunn VM. Urinary incontinence in women, without manifest injury to the bladder. Surg Gynecol Obstet 1914;18:444–450.
31. Kennedy WT. Incontinence of urine in the female, the urethral sphincter mechanism, damage of function, and restoration of control. Am J Obstet Gynecol 1937;34:576–587.
32. Zivkovik F, Pieber D, Tamussino K, Ralph G. 5-year results of three incontinence operations according to their preoperative degree of stress incontinence [abstract]. Int Urogynecol J 1995;6:302.
33. Van Geelen JM, Theevwes AGM, Eskeo LAB, Martin C. The clinical and urdynamic effects of anterior vaginal repair and Burch colposuspension. Am J Obstet Gynecol 1988;159:137–144.
34. Peters VA, Thornton WN. Selection of the primary operative procedure for stress urinary incontinence. Am J Obstet Gynecol 1980;137:923–930.
35. Burch JC. Cooper's ligament urethrovesical suspension for stress incontinence. Am J Obstet Gynecol 1968;100:764–774.
36. Colombo M, Scalambrino S, Magginoni A, Milani R. Burch colposuspension versus modified Marshall-Marchetti-Krantz urethropexy for primary genuine stress urinary incontinence: a prospective, randomized clinical trial. Am J Obstet Gynecol 1994;171:1573–1579.
37. Mainprize TC, Drutz HP. The Marshall-Marchetti-Krantz procedure: a critical review. Obstet Gynecol Surg 1988;43:729–742.
38. Lee RA, Symmonds RE, Goldstein RA. Surgical complications and results of modified Marshall-Marchetti-Krantz procedure for urinary incontinence. Obstet Gynecol 1979;53:447–450.
39. Persky L, Guerriere K. Complications of Marshall-Marchetti-Krantz urethropexy. Urology 1976;8:467–471.
40. Eriksen BC, Hagen B, Eik-Nes SH, Molne K, Mjolnerod D, Romslo I. Long-term effectiveness of the Burch colposuspension in female urinary stress incontinence. Acta Obstet Gynecol Scand 1990;69:45–50.
41. Feyereisl J, Dreher E, Haenggi W, Zikmund J, Schneider H. Long-term results after Burch colposuspension. Am J Obstet Gynecol 1994;171:647–652.
42. Herbertsson G, Iosif CS. Surgical results of urodynamic studies 10 years after retropubic colpourethropexy. Acta Obstet Gynecol Scand 1993;72:298–301.
43. Laursen H, Farlie R, Rasmussen KL, Aagard J. Colposuspension Burch—an 18 year follow-up study [abstract]. Neurourol Urodyn 1994;13:445.
44. Lose G, Jorgensen L, Mortensen SO, Monsted-Pedersen L, Kristensen JK. Voiding difficulties after colposuspension. Obstet Gynecol 1987;1:33–38.
45. Stanton SL, Williams JE, Ritchie D. The colposuspension operation for urinary incontinence. Br J Obstet Gynaecol 1976;83:890–895.
46. Gillon G, Stanton SL. Long-term follow-up of surgery for urinary incontinence in elderly women. Br J Urol 1984;56:478–481.
47. Bowen LW, Sand PK, Ostergard DR, Franti CE. Unsuccessful Burch retropubic urethropexy: a case-controlled urodynamic study. Am J Obstet Gynecol 1989;160:452–458.
48. Richardson AC, Edmonds PB, Williams NL. Treatment of stress urinary incontinence due to paravaginal fascial defect. Obstet Gynecol 1981;57:357–362.
49. Shull BL, Baden WF. A 6-year experience with paravaginal defect repair for stress urinary incontinence. Am J Obstet Gynecol 1989;160:1432–1440.
50. Pereyra AJ. A simplified surgical procedure for the correction of stress incontinence in women. West J Surg Obstet Gynecol 1959;67:223–227.
51. Stamey TA. Endoscopic suspension of the vesical neck for urinary incontinence. Surg Gynecol Obstet 1973;136:547–554.
52. Stamey TA. Endoscopic suspension of the vesical neck for urinary incontinence in females. Report of 203 consecutive patients. Ann Surg 1980;192:265–271.
53. Raz S. Modified bladder neck suspension for female stress incontinence. Urology 1981;17:82–85.

54. Gittes RF, Loughlin KR. No-incision pubovaginal suspension for stress incontinence. J Urol 1987; 138:568–570.

55. Jones DJ, Shah PJR, Worth PHL. Modified Stamey procedure for bladder neck suspension. Br J Urol 1989;63:157–161.

56. Kursh ED, Angell AH, Resnick MI. Evolution of endoscopic urethropexy: seven-year experience with various techniques. Urology 1991;37: 428–431.

57. Hilton P, Mayne CJ. The Stamey endoscopic bladder neck suspension: a clinical and urodynamic investigation, including actuarial follow-up over four years. Br J Obstet Gynaecol 1991;98: 1141–1149.

58. Loughlin KR, Whitmore WF, Gittes RF, Richie JP. Review of an 8-year experience with modifications of endoscopic suspension of the bladder neck for female stress urinary incontinence. J Urol 1990;143:44–55.

59. Griffith-Jones MD, Abrams PH. The Stamey endoscopic bladder neck suspension in the elderly. Br J Urol 1990;65:170–172.

60. Trockman BA, Leach GE, Hamilton J, Sakamoto M, Santiago L, Zimmern PE. Modified Pereyra bladder neck suspension: 10-year mean follow-up using outcomes analysis in 125 patients. J Urol 1995;154:1841–1847.

61. Couillard DR, Deckard-Janatpour KA, Stone A. The vaginal wall sling: a compressive suspension procedure for recurrent incontinence in elderly patients. Urology 1994;43:203–208.

62. Juma S, Little NA, Raz S. Vaginal wall sling: four years later. Urology 1992;37:424–428.

63. Polascik TJ, Moore RG, Rosenberg MT, Kavoussi LR. Comparison of laparoscopic and open retropubic urethropexy for treatment of stress urinary incontinence. Urology 1995;45:647–652.

64. Liu CY, Paek W. Laparoscopic retropubic colposuspension (Burch procedure). Gynecol Laparoscopic 1993;1:31–34.

65. Karram MM, Miklos JR, Schull BL, Summit R. Laparoscopic Burch colposuspension for stress incontinence—a pilot study [abstract]. Int Urogynecol J 1994;5:379.

66. Radomski SB, Herschorn S. Laparoscopic Burch bladder neck suspension: early results. J Urol 1996;155:515–518.

67. McDougall EM, Klutke CG, Cornell T. Comparison of transvaginal versus laparoscopic bladder neck suspension for stress urinary incontinence. Urology 1995;45:641–646.

68. Vancaillie TG, Schuessler W. Laparoscopic bladder neck suspension. J Laparoendosc Surg 1991; 1:169–173.

69. Burton G. A randomized comparison of laparoscopic and open colposuspension [abstract]. Neurourol Urodyn 1996;13:497–498.

70. McGuire EJ, Bennett CJ, Konnak JA, Sonda LP, Savastano JA. Experience with pubovaginal slings for urinary incontinence at the University of Michigan. J Urol 1987;138:525–526.

71. Chin YK, Stanton SL. A follow-up of silastic sling for genuine stress incontinence. Br J Obstet Gynaecol 1995;102:143–147.

72. Goebel R. Zur operativen Beseitigung der Angelborenen Incontinenz Vesicae. Zsch F Gynakol U Urol 1910;2:187.

73. Young SB, Rosenblatt PL, Pingeton DM, Howard AE, Baker SP. The Mersilene mesh suburethral sling: a clinical and urodynamic evaluation. Am J Obstet Gynecol 1995;173:1719–1726.

74. Ghoniem GM, Shaaban A. Sub-urethral slings for treatment of stress urinary incontinence. Int Urogynecol J 1994;5:228–239.

75. Blaivas JG, Jacobs BZ. Pubovaginal fascial sling for the treatment of complicated stress incontinence. J Urol 1991;145:1214–1218.

76. Spence-Jones C, DeMarco E, Lemieux M-C, Drutz HP. Modified urethral sling for the treatment of genuine stress incontinence and latent incontinence. Int Urogynecol J 1994;5:69–75.

77. Summitt RL, Bent AE, Ostergard DR, Harris TA. Suburethral sling procedure for genuine stress incontinence and low urethral closure pressure: a continued experience. Int Urogynecol J 1992;3: 18–21.

78. Bent AE, Ostergard DR, Zwick-Zuffutom M. Tissue reaction to expanded polytetrafluro ethylene suburethral sling for urinary incontinence: clinical and histological study. Am J Obstet Gynecol 1993;169:1198–1204.

79. Morgan JE, Farrow GA, Stewart FE. The Marlex sling operation for the treatment of stress urinary incontinence: a 16-year review. Am J Obstet Gynecol 1985;151:224–226.

80. Henriksson L, Ulmsten U. A urodynamic evaluation of the effects of abdominal urethrocystopexy and vaginal sling urethroplasty in women with stress incontinence. Am J Obstet Gynecol 1978;131:77–82.

81. Milani R, Scalambrino S, Quadri G, Algeri M, Marchesin R. Marshall-Marchetti-Krantz procedure and Burch colposuspension in the surgical treatment of female urinary incontinence. Br J Obstet Gynaecol 1985;92:1050–1053.

82. Milani R, Maggioni A, Colombo M, Pisani G, Quinto M. Burch colposuspension versus modified Marshall-Marchetti-Krantz for stress incontinence. Neurourol Urodyn 1991;9:454–455.

83. Stanton SL, Cardozo LD. A comparison of vaginal and suprapubic surgery in the correction of incontinence due to urethral sphincter incompetence. Br J Urol 1979;51:497–499.

84. Hilton P. A clinical and urodynamic study comparing the Stamey bladder neck suspension and suburethral sling procedures in the treatment of genuine stress incontinence. Br J Obstet Gynaecol 1989;96:213–220.

85. Bergman A, Ballard CA, Koonings PP. Comparison of three different surgical procedures for genuine stress incontinence: prospective randomized study. Am J Obstet Gynecol 1989;160: 1102–1106.

CHAPTER 39

Retropubic Surgical Approach for Correction of Genuine Stress Incontinence

Michelle M. Germain and Donald R. Ostergard

There is still considerable debate about the best surgical approach for the treatment of genuine stress incontinence (GSI). However, retropubic urethropexy is considered by most to be the gold standard for surgical correction of GSI. As our understanding of the pathophysiology of GSI has grown, our appraisal of the optimal treatment for GSI has changed. Proper urethral function and maintenance of continence requires that the proximal urethra is positioned, and well supported, within the abdominal cavity. The displacement of the urethra from its normal intraabdominal position and the loss of anatomic support are the primary disturbances that cause the changes in the urethral axis during stress and result in urinary incontinence. In GSI, the urethral muscular sphincter function is normal, but because of urethral hypermobility, an unequal transmission of pressure occurs during stress between the bladder and the proximal urethra. Thus, bladder pressure exceeds the maximal urethral pressure, and leakage results.

The goal of antiincontinence procedures is to reestablish the proper intraabdominal location of the proximal urethra. However, crucial to the success of these procedures is the avoidance of excessive elevation of the urethrovesical junction (UVJ). Urinary retention and detrusor instability can occur as a result of urethral obstruction because of overcorrection of the anatomic defect.

With all retropubic procedures, there is risk of formation of postoperative enterocele. This occurs because the retropubic procedure changes the axis of the vagina, so that the posterior wall is exposed to the pressure of the intraabdominal organs. In fact, Burch (1) reported a 7.6% incidence of enterocele formation and therefore strongly advocated concurrent obliteration of the cul-de-sac. This can be accomplished via a Moschowitz or a McCall's type culdoplasty, depending on the other procedures performed. If the retropubic urethropexy is the only procedure performed, the patient should be thoroughly counseled for the risk of enterocele formation. In these cases, the physician must weigh the risks and benefits of laparotomy to prevent the small incidence of postoperative enterocele.

Preoperative Evaluation

Before initiating surgical intervention, a complete urogynecological evaluation is essential. This should include thorough history and physical examination, including a cotton swab test; determination of the postvoid residual urine volume; and demonstration of urine loss with stress. Although stress loss after simple bladder filling is highly predictive of GSI (2), a single-channel cystometrogram is recommended to provide diagnostic certainty (3). In a recent study, a positive cough stress test alone was 77% sensitive and 100% specific for the diagnosis of GSI, whereas observed urine loss with cough during a multichannel cystometrogram had a sensitivity of 91% and a specificity of 100% for GSI (4). For patients with mixed urinary incontinence symptoms and patients with prior incontinence procedures, a multichannel urodynamic evaluation is recommended.

The major goal of this evaluation is to exclude all other causes of incontinence and to identify those women at risk for intrinsic sphincter deficiency of the urethra. In a recently published study, women over age 50 and women with a history of prior antiincontinence surgery were at the highest risk for the presence of intrinsic sphincter deficiency (5). Therefore, women with these characteristics should have an evaluation of urethral function by urethral closure pressure profiles, augmented by leak point pressures, as part of their preoperative urodynamics. For patients without demonstrable urethral hypermobility and those with low urethral pressures, retropubic urethropexies are contraindicated. In one study, patients with low urethral pressures had a 54% failure rate after retropubic urethropexy (6).

Access to the Retropubic Space

The patient is positioned either in modified dorsal lithotomy or frog-legged position to allow easier access to the vagina. A Pfannenstiel skin incision is used unless concurrent surgical procedures, such as exploratory laparotomy and/or abdominal hysterectomy, require another type of incision. The rectus muscles are carefully separated from the underlying transversalis fascia, taking care to avoid injury to the inferior epigastric vessels. A self-retaining retractor is placed, with the bladder blade superior, to retract the intraabdominal organs, and the lateral blades under the rectus abdominus muscles.

The retropubic space is developed, under direct visualization, using blunt dissection;

sharp dissection may be necessary if the patient has had prior incontinence surgery. The surgeon places the nondominant hand in the vagina to elevate the perivaginal fascia and to identify the UVJ. The UVJ is located by placing gentle traction on the catheter and palpating the lower edge of the Foley balloon. Perivaginal fascial fat is removed with forceps, and then the bladder is mobilized superiorly using a sponge with strokes parallel to the urethra. Fat is removed from this fascia to facilitate identification of landmarks and to promote fibrosis. The midline area, including the 2 cm on each side of the urethra, are not dissected. Special care must be taken to avoid injuring the aberrant obturator vessels that are found approximately 5 cm lateral to the pubic tubercles. In addition, attention must be paid to the vessels that run parallel to the bladder at the level of the UVJ so as not to damage them. However, if damaged, the bleeding from these vessels is usually controlled when the figure of eight urethropexy sutures are tied (see Fig. 39.1).

Marshall-Marchetti-Krantz Urethropexy

This procedure was first reported in 1949 (7) and was the mainstay of therapy for stress urinary incontinence. The original authors, as well as other researchers, reported a number of modifications of this procedure, most of which were directed at reducing urethral injury. The authors of the original procedure described placement of double bites through the vaginal and the lateral urethral walls with chromic sutures that were secured to the symphysis pubis. Additionally, the bladder muscle was sutured to the posterior rectus fascia (7). Modifications included changes in suture to delayed absorbable and nonabsorbable material and changes to help visualize the UVJ (8).

The original authors reported a greater than 90% subjective success rate in a retrospective report, with an average follow-up of 45.7 months (9). In a metaanalysis that reviewed 56 retrospective articles about the Marshall-Marchetti-Krantz (MMK) proce-

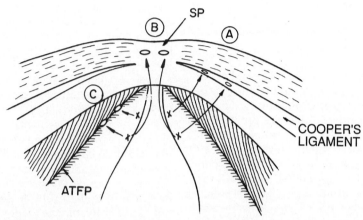

Figure 39.1. **A.** Burch colposuspension with sutures attached to Cooper's ligament. **B.** Marshall-Marchetti-Krantz procedure with sutures attached to the sym- physis pubis (*SP*). **C.** Richardson paravaginal approach with sutures attached to the arcus tendineous fascia pelvis.

dure, most of which did not have objective postoperative data, the overall success rate was 86.1% in 2712 cases, with 92.1% success in primary repairs and 84.5% in secondary procedures (8).

As described below, the periosteum of the symphysis pubis is used to elevate and stabilize the bladder neck. Osteitis pubis, a noninfectious inflammatory condition, results from trauma and impaired circulation to the periosteum of the symphysis (10). It is a rare, but serious, complication that occurs in patients undergoing this procedure (8).

SURGICAL TECHNIQUE

Entry into the space of Retzius is accomplished as described above. A Foley catheter bulb is used to identify the bladder neck. Although the initial report described placement of sutures through the lateral urethral wall, the authors subsequently recommended that this be avoided (11). Permanent sutures are placed lateral to the urethra and then placed through the periosteum and tied down (Fig. 39.1). No specific details were originally given about the degree of tension when tying the sutures; however, one of the authors described bringing "the urethra and bladder in close apposition to the posterior surface of the symphysis" (12). We recommend that to prevent overcorrection, there is sufficient space for the operator to place a

finger easily between the symphysis pubis and the perivaginal fascia.

Burch Retropubic Urethropexy

In 1961, Burch (13) described a new technique for urethropexy that he developed while attempting to perform an MMK. He reported that Cooper's ligament was ideal for "passing and holding a suture" and that tying to Cooper's ligament "produced a most satisfactory restoration of the normal anatomy of the bladder neck." Indeed, the objective cure rate for this operation, by urodynamic evaluation, is reportedly as high as 98% at 1 year (14). Additionally, the problem of osteitis pubis is avoided in this surgical technique.

In 1976, Tanagho (15) described a modification of this technique in which he recommended that dissection be avoided in the midline over the urethra. He also recommended placement of sutures far lateral to the urethra and tying of sutures so that two fingers could easily be inserted between the fascia and the symphysis. We advocate using this modification of the Burch retropubic urethropexy. As seen in Figure 39.2, this technique restores normal anatomy, avoids urethral compression, and limits urethral mobility.

SURGICAL PROCEDURE

After the retropubic space has been entered and dissected as described above, Cooper's ligament is identified and cleared of all fat. The UVJ is then identified with the aid of the vaginal hand and the bulb of the Foley catheter. Using flexible permanent suture, a figure of eight stitch is placed through the vaginal wall, excluding the vaginal mucosa, 2 cm lateral to the UVJ. A second suture is placed at the level of the midurethra. This is performed bilaterally. As seen in Figure 39.1, the free ends of the sutures are placed through Cooper's ligament in a staggered fashion so that the ligament is not easily torn. The distal stitches are placed first, approximately 3 cm lateral to the symphysis. The proximal urethral stitches are then placed, approximately 1 cm more laterally. Gelfoam is placed laterally in the retropubic space. With the assistant's hand in the vagina, the sutures are tied down. Appropriate tension is determined by estimating a cotton swab resting angle of 0 to +10 degrees from the horizontal. With tying, a banjo-string effect occurs because the fascia is not brought up to Cooper's ligament but is placed in apposition to the pelvic side wall where it will permanently fibrose.

Paravaginal Repair

In an attempt to more clearly define relaxation of the anterior vaginal wall, Richardson et al. (16) described four defects of the anterior pelvis, lateral, transverse, midline, and pubourethral. The lateral defect is the most common. Paravaginal repair of this defect produced good results in 95% of cases at 2–8 years of follow-up; however, the authors did not clearly define surgical success (17). The paravaginal repair was originally designed to correct the defect of a cystourethrocele; Richardson (18) does not consider the paravaginal repair a procedure to correct GSI. In a series of 149 incontinent women, Shull and Baden (19) reported a 97% subjective success rate for cure of stress urinary incontinence using the paravaginal repair. However, they placed Burch stitches bilaterally, in addition to the paravaginal stitches.

Patients can be evaluated for paravaginal defects during their routine pelvic examination. Originally, tongue blades were used for the evaluation. Ring forceps, or a paravaginal defect analyzer, can be placed parallel to the vaginal axis on either sides of the vagina and used to elevate the lateral portion of the anterior vaginal wall. If the anterior vaginal wall defect disappears using this maneuver, when the patient strains, the defect is considered to be lateral. If there is still a bulge present, a midline defect exists.

SURGICAL PROCEDURE

The paravaginal repair is begun as all other retropubic procedures described previously. The operator's hand is placed within the vagina and is used to identify the lateral sulci of the vagina. The fat is removed from the perivaginal fascia and the pelvic side wall down to the level of the pelvic floor. The arcus tendineous fascia pelvis (ATFP), also known as the "white line," runs from the symphysis pubis to the ischial spine. It is located 1.5–2 cm below the obturator canal. It may be attenuated and difficult to identify in elderly women.

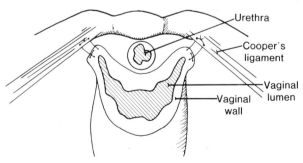

Figure 39.2. The retropubic space is free, without urethral compression, after sutures are tied. (Redrawn from Tanagho EA. Colpocystourethropexy: the way we do it. J Urol 1976;116:751–753.)

The object of the procedure is to reattach the lateral sulcus of the vagina to the pelvic sidewall at the level of the ATFP (18). The bladder is held medially and superiorly with a sponge stick. Permanent suture is used, and the first stitch is placed through the perivaginal fascia at the level of the lateral sulcus. Subsequent sutures are placed at 1-cm intervals, dorsally and ventrally. As can be seen in Figure 39.1, after placement of all perivaginal fascial sutures bilaterally, the sutures are then placed through the ATFP on the lateral pelvic wall. If the ATFP is not identifiable, sutures are placed through the obturator internus fascia. Sutures are tied sequentially and at the corresponding levels bilaterally. There is risk that the repair will be uneven if the sutures are first tied on one side and then on the other.

Laparoscopic Urethropexy

The goal of all laparoscopic surgery is to provide equally effective surgical treatment that is associated with decreased morbidity and cost when compared with the open technique. Review of the literature reveals several series using multiple different laparoscopic techniques for the treatment of GSI (20–24). Some studies do not truly replicate the open retropubic procedures and therefore should not be used for comparison. These laparoscopic studies have variable intervals for follow-up and different criteria for determination of surgical success (also see Chapter 49).

Access to the space of Retzius has been achieved using the preperitoneal and the transperitoneal approaches (20). The laparoscopic MMK technique has been described by a number of authors; however, only a few performed a true MMK. The clinical success rate for a true laparoscopic MMK reported by Vancaillie and Shuessler (21) was 100%, but there was limited follow-up. Liu (22) reported that the laparoscopic Burch urethropexy, mimicking the open technique, resulted in a 94.8% subjective success rate at 6–22 months. A similar technique using a stapling device to attach mesh to the paravaginal tissue and Cooper's ligament also has

reportedly good short-term results (23). However, in a prospective randomized study, Burton (24) reported that laparoscopic urethropexy had a significantly higher failure rate on both subjective and objective testing than the open Burch technique at 1 year of follow-up.

Endoscopy

After all retropubic procedures, it is appropriate to perform cystoscopy to exclude the presence of suture material in the bladder and to ensure the functioning of both ureters. For the urethropexies in which a suprapubic catheter is placed, suprapubic cystoscopy (teloscopy) is performed. This is done with the patient in the Trendelenberg position by placing a purse-string suture and a stab incision in the dome of the full bladder and inserting a 30-degree telescope from any endoscopic setup. Indigo carmine, given intravenously, is used to confirm ureteral function. The suprapubic catheter is inserted through a separate skin incision and then either passed through the cystotomy made for the endoscope or guided by transurethral cystoscopy into the bladder.

Summary

There are many procedures for the treatment of urinary incontinence, but the long-term results of some are unfavorable, because the displacement of the UVJ recurs. The retropubic urethropexies provide permanent correction of the anatomic defect, without damage to the urethra, which is the key to the success of antiincontinence surgery. The paravaginal repair compliments the urethropexy by treating coexistent anterior vaginal wall defects. Surgery near the urethra and UVJ can result in fibrosis, denervation, and devascularization, all of which profoundly affect urethral sphincteric function. In addition, the permanent success of these procedures depends on the postoperative period of modified activity for as long as 3 months. Scarification and fibrosis are as important as suture choice and placement for the long-term success of these procedures.

Gynecological laparoscopic surgery has made great advances during the past decade. Laparoscopic surgery for incontinence may hold great promise for the future, because of reduced morbidity and cost of extended hospital stays. The postoperative recovery time is shorter because of decreased pain. However, the postoperative period for modified activity should not be altered.

REFERENCES

1. Burch JC. Cooper's ligament urethrovesical suspension for stress incontinence: nine years' experience—results, complications, technique. Am J Obstet Gynecol 1968;100:764–774.
2. Wall LL, Wiskind AK, Taylor PA. Simple bladder filling with a cough stress test compared with subtracted cystometry for the diagnosis of urinary incontinence. Am J Obstet Gynecol 1994;171:1472–1479.
3. Summitt RL, Stovall TG, Bent AE, Ostergard DR. Urinary incontinence: correlation of history and brief office evaluation with multichannel urodynamic testing. Am J Obstet Gynecol 1992;166:1835–1844.
4. Swift SE, Ostergard DR. Evaluation of current urodynamic testing methods in the diagnosis of genuine stress incontinence. Obstet Gynecol 1995;86:85–91.
5. Horbach NS, Ostergard DR. Predicting intrinsic urethral sphincter dysfunction in women with stress urinary incontinence. Obstet Gynecol 1994;84:188–192.
6. Sand PK, Bowen LW, Panganiban R, Ostergard DR. The low pressure urethra as a factor in failed retropubic urethropexy. Obstet Gynecol 1987;69:399–402.
7. Marshall VF, Marchetti AA, Krantz KE. Correction of stress incontinence by simple vesicourethral suspension. Surg Gynecol Obstet 1949;88:509–518.
8. Mainprize TC, Drutz HP. The Marshall-Marchetti-Krantz procedure: a critical review. Obstet Gynecol Surv 1988;43:724–729.
9. Parnell JP, Marshall VF, Vaughan ED Jr. Primary management of urinary stress incontinence by the Marshall-Marchetti-Krantz vesicourethropexy. J Urol 1982;127:679–682.
10. Lentz SS. Osteitis pubis: a review. Obstet Gynecol Surv 1995;50:310–315.
11. Marchetti AA, Marshall VF, Shultis LD. Simple vesicourethral suspension: a survey. Am J Obstet Gynecol 1957;74:57–63.
12. Marchetti AA. Urinary incontinence. JAMA 1956;162:1366–1368.
13. Burch JC. Urethrovaginal fixation to Cooper's ligament for correction of stress incontinence, cystocele, and prolapse. Am J Obstet Gynecol 1961;81:281–290.
14. Bhatia NN, Bergman A. Modified Burch versus Pereyra retropubic urethropexy for stress urinary incontinence. Obstet Gynecol 1985;66:255–261.
15. Tanagho EA. Colpocystourethropexy: the way we do it. J Urol 1976;116:751–753.
16. Richardson AC, Lyon JB, Williams NL. A new look at pelvic relaxation. Am J Obstet Gynecol 1976;126:568–573.
17. Richardson AC, Edmonds PB, Williams NL. Treatment of stress urinary incontinence due to paravaginal fascial defect. Obstet Gynecol 1981;57:357–362.
18. Richardson AC. How to correct prolapse paravaginally. Contemp OB/GYN 1990;35:100–114.
19. Shull BL, Baden WF. A six-year experience with paravaginal defect repair for stress urinary incontinence. Am J Obstet Gynecol 1989;160:1432–1440.
20. Lyons TL. Minimally invasive treatment of urinary stress incontinence and laparoscopically directed repair of pelvic floor defects. Clin Obstet Gynecol 1995;38:380–391.
21. Vancaillie TG, Shuessler W. Laparoscopic bladder neck suspension. J Laparoendosc Surg 1991;3:169–171.
22. Liu CY. Laparoscopic retropubic colposuspension (Burch procedure): a review of 58 cases. J Reprod Med 1993;38:526–530.
23. Ou CS, Presthus J, Beadles E. Laparoscopic bladder neck suspension using hernia mesh and surgical staples. J Laparoendosc Surg 1993;3:553–556.
24. Burton G. A randomised comparison of laparoscopic and open colposuspension. Neurourol Urodyn 1994;13:497–498.

CHAPTER 40

Needle Procedures for Stress Incontinence

Jeffrey L. Cornella

Introduction

The year 1989 marked the 30th anniversary of the introduction of a new approach in the treatment of female urinary stress incontinence, the needle suspension procedure by Pereyra (1). Pereyra spent two decades experimenting with operative materials and various surgical techniques, revising his needle suspension procedure into the form we recognize today, the modified Pereyra procedure (2). Indications for the operation include the primary treatment of urinary stress incontinence, the secondary treatment of stress incontinence in patients who have failed prior operation but continue to demonstrate mobility of the urethrovesical junction, and as a component of vault repair in patients with prolapse or procidentia who demonstrate the onset of stress incontinence during manual reduction of the prolapsed tissues. The needle suspension is not the procedure of choice for patients who have intrinsic sphincteric deficiency.

In recent years, variations to the techniques described by Pereyra have been added (3–6). The foundation for these procedures is the original and modified Pereyra procedure. A historical understanding of the development of the modified Pereyra procedure indicates that most significant modifications in the needle suspension procedure were performed by Pereyra initially. A knowledge of the modified Pereyra procedure technique is intrinsic to performing the variety of needle suspension procedures that exist today.

Historical Perspective: Development and Modification of the Pereyra Procedure

Armand J. Pereyra's life was one of service. In 1956, he retired from a 26-year career in the United States Navy, which included a residency in Obstetrics and Gynecology. He became chief medical officer at the California Institution for Women. The women's prison was the unlikely site for the development of a new operation for female incontinence. Many women suffering from urinary incontinence had been previously treated with a Marshall-Marchetti-Krantz (MMK) approach. Thoughtful consideration by Pereyra allowed realization that the correction of urinary stress incontinence need not involve retropubic dissection. Pereyra performed several transitional operations that culminated in a new approach, the needle suspension procedure (1). Thirty-one patients were followed for 14 months; 28 operations were judged successful and 2 were complete failures.

The original technique described passage of a special needle carrier through an abdominal stab incision without prior dissection. The needle carrier would pass retropubically and penetrate the undissected vaginal wall. Extension of a stylet would result in a "Y" shape and double unilateral vaginal penetration (Fig. 40.1). Subsequent placement of

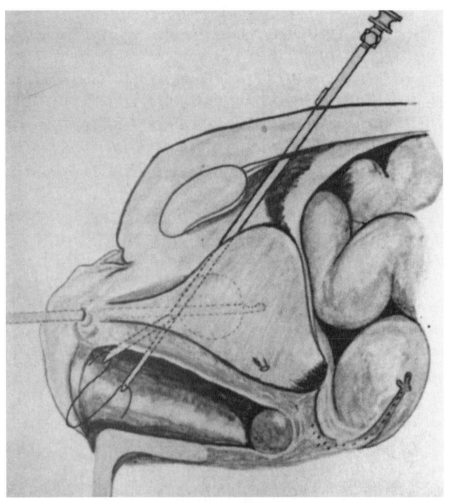

Figure 40.1. Lateral view of the pelvis with cannula and trochar points protruding paraurethrally through the anterior vaginal wall and threaded with suture (Pereyra's own drawing for historical interest).

suture and needle carrier withdrawal would result in vaginal wall elevation. The suture material (no. 30 steel wire) would later penetrate the epithelium into the fibrous tissue of the vaginal wall.

Pereyra began to collaborate with another gynecologist, Thomas B. Lebherz. They worked jointly on several reports of surgical results and techniques (7–9). The first collaboration included vaginal dissection and contiguous placement of the needle carrier against the vaginal index finger for direct periurethral delivery into the vagina, thus decreasing the risk of bladder injury. The article reported 210 patients and indicated an initial success rate of 94.3% (7). The failure rate increased to 16% as Pereyra followed patients for months to years. Pereyra and Lebherz concluded that this was secondary to suture failure. Nonabsorbable sutures would pull through or penetrate the tissues, and absorbable sutures would often subsequently break and give way (10). A method that used nonabsorbable sutures in a manner that prevented tissue penetration was required.

Pereyra and Lebherz spent an additional decade experimenting with various suture materials, baffles, instrumentation, and techniques (Table 40.1). From 1974 to 1976, the procedure evolved to the form recognized today as the modified Pereyra procedure. The surgical description and results of this procedure were published in two separate texts in the years 1978 and 1979 (2, 8). The 1978 report described a revision that included detachment of the endopelvic fascia from the pubic rami and "helix" binding of periurethral tissues. A helix suture was placed to bind "pubourethral ligaments" and musculofascial tissues (Fig. 40.2). This suture was delivered to the abdominal site by a new needle carrier developed in 1975 (Fig. 40.3).

At a symposium on disorders of the urethra and urinary incontinence in Wilmington, Delaware in November of 1976, Pereyra reported results of 29 patients operated on with this technique. The symposium's attendant monograph was published in 1979 and included a chapter by Pereyra (2) illustrating a midline epithelial vaginal incision and dissection, followed by penetration of the urogenital diaphragm and suture incorporation of the pubourethral ligaments and musculofascial tissues. An abdominal incision was made, and the revised ligature carrier was introduced through the rectus fascia, contacting the surgeon's finger. "Retropubic transfer of helical suture ends" (2) was then accomplished, and traction resulted in elevation of the tissues. The sutures were secured to the abdominal fascia. Pereyra wrote (2)

These colligated P-U supports, with the anterior musculofascial surfaces previously denuded of epithelium, when elevated retropubically by the suspensory sutures anchored to the suprapubic abdominal fascia, are held firmly against the posterior pubis. As a result, the musculofascial tissues produce fibrous union over a broad area of posterior pubic periosteum without tension between opposing forces.

A similar description was reported (8); however, the pubourethral ligaments were not emphasized as a component of the bound tissues.

The needle suspension, as it is performed today, was developed by 1976, reported in a symposium the same year, and subsequently published with case results in the years 1978 and 1979. Included in the modified procedure was a contribution made by Dr. Thomas Stamey in 1973 (3). This was the use of endoscopy during the needle suspension procedure.

THE MODIFIED PEREYRA PROCEDURE

The method of Pereyra and Lebherz summarized from the second edition of Buchsbaum and Schmidt (11) is as follows.

Technique

The patient is positioned in the dorsal recumbent position, and a no. 18 Foley catheter is placed within the bladder. Gentle traction and palpation of the catheter allows delineation of the urethrovesical junction. Sterile normal saline solution is injected subepithelially from the level of the junction to 2 cm proximal to the urinary meatus. The injection is continued laterally on each side of the urethra to the pubic rami. This detaches the epithelium from the underlying endopelvic fascia.

A half-circle incision is made through the epithelium 2 cm superior to the lower urethral meatus. A vertical incision is made through the freed epithelium over the urethra, beginning at the middle of the half-circle incision and extending down to the urethrovesical junction. Using Metzenbaum scissors, the epithelium is mobilized laterally on each side to the sites of insertion of the endopelvic fascia into the pubis. A fingertip directed against the inferior posterolateral pubic ramus is inserted through the endopelvic fascia at its site of attachment to the ramus 3–4 cm lateral to the urethrovesical junction on each side of the patient (Fig. 40.4).

Once a proper opening into the space of Retzius is made, the retropubic space is

Table 40.1. Modifications of the Original Pereyra Procedure

Date	Description	Reference
1967	Vaginal and periurethral dissection into the space of Retzius. Contiguous guidance of the needle carrier by surgeon's (vaginal) finger.	7
1974[a]	Detachment of endopelvic fascia from pubic rami and "helix" binding of pubourethral ligaments and musculofascial tissues. (Incise vaginal epithelium maintaining endopelvic fascia on the bladder.)	2 and 8

[a]1974 revision published 1978 and 1979.

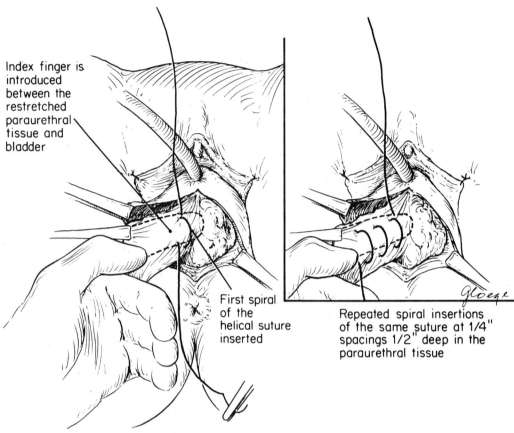

Index finger is introduced between the restretched paraurethral tissue and bladder

First spiral of the helical suture inserted

Repeated spiral insertions of the same suture at 1/4" spacings 1/2" deep in the paraurethral tissue

Figure 40.2. Repeated spiral insertions of the same suture at one quarter-inch spacings in periurethral tissue. (From Pereyra AJ, Lebherz TB. Revised Pereyra procedure. In: Buchsbaum HJ, Schmidt JD, eds. Gynecologic and obstetric urology. Philadelphia: WB Saunders, 1978:212.)

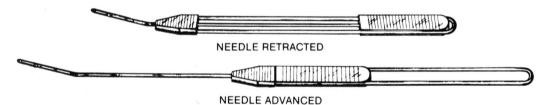

NEEDLE RETRACTED

NEEDLE ADVANCED

Figure 40.3. The Pereyra ligature carrier, 1975. (From Pereyra AJ, Lebherz TB. The modified Pereyra procedure. In: Buchsbaum HJ, Schmidt JD, eds. Gynecologic and obstetric urology. 2nd ed. Philadelphia: WB Saunders, 1982:260.)

explored with an index finger, rotating medially as far as the urethra and laterally down to the level of the urethrovesical junction. With the retropubic spaces exposed bilaterally, the operator frees any adhesions that exist.

The right index finger is extended along the left side of the urethra until it abuts against the catheter bulb, which has been drawn toward the urethrovesical junction by trac-

tion and deflected to the patient's right side. The fingertip is flexed medially to hook around the posterior pillar of the ligament. The pillars are grasped with Allis forceps and held aside. The process is repeated on the opposite side of the patient.

A no. 0 Prolene suture, 30 inches long, is introduced through one pillar near its attachment to the urethra. The suture is inserted three to four times in a helical fashion transversely through the endopelvic fascia, with each bite taken increasingly lateral to the previous one (Fig. 40.5). Tension on the suture ends indicate whether the bound tissues will hold. The tissues are reinforced as required. The process is repeated on the opposite side of the patient with an additional Prolene suture.

A transverse 4-cm skin incision is made 2 cm above the symphysis pubis. The special needle carrier is introduced through the lateral aspect of the abdominal incision, and the point of the angulated needle is advanced through the abdominal fascia at its attachment to the crest of the pubis, 3 cm lateral to the symphysis pubis.

The operator inserts the index finger vaginally, contacting rectus muscle under the advancing needle and guiding the needle along the posterior pubis, avoiding the bladder (Fig. 40.6A). The long needle shaft is advanced retropubically into the vagina, where the elongated eye near the point is threaded with the two unilateral Prolene suture ends (Fig. 40.6B). The needle is withdrawn suprapubically, and the process is repeated on the opposite side of the patient.

The pubourethral supports are elevated retropubically by pulling on both pairs of suprapubic Prolene suture ends. The vaginal wall is closed, and an attendant cystocele repair may be accomplished, if indicated.

The Foley catheter is removed, and a urethroscope is inserted. The four suture ends are tied together over the abdominal fascia when the suture tension results in partial closure of the lower edge of the urethral internal meatus. Alternately, the function of the elevation can be tested by increasing intravesical pressure using suprapubic pressure with 350 mL within the bladder and observing for urine loss.

Results

In 1982, Pereyra and Lebherz published results of 82 patients treated for stress urinary incontinence using the modified Pereyra procedure (9). Of 54 women treated with this procedure as a primary operation for anatomic stress urinary incontinence, 47 (87%) showed complete cure and 4 (7.4%) showed marked improvement 4–6 years postoperatively. In 28 patients with a history of previous incontinence surgery, 23 (82%) were cured and 2 (7.1%) were markedly improved. Three of six failures noted were in patients who underwent polyglactin absorbable su-

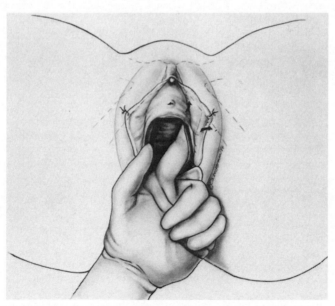

Figure 40.4. An index finger develops the periurethral avascular space. The fingertip is directed against the inferior, posterolateral pubic ramus, penetrating the urogenital diaphragm at its attachment. (From Cutner LP, Ostergard DR. The modified Pereyra procedure. In: Ostergard DR, ed. Gynecologic urology & urodynamics, 2nd ed. Baltimore: Williams & Wilkins, 1985:530.)

ture suspensions early in the study (Table 40.2). Each had repeat modified procedures using no. 0 polypropylene nonabsorbable suspensory sutures with successful 4-year results.

This was followed by a larger study of 162 patients. Of these, 108 had primary operations, 34 had secondary procedures, and 20 had two or more previous procedures for incontinence. The patient follow-up was a minimum of 1 year. Of the total population, 143 patients had no evidence of stress incontinence in the supine or squatting position when straining or coughing. There were eight patients markedly improved with subjective cure, but drops of urine were noted with coughing on objective testing. In 11 patients, the procedure was considered a failure (Table

40.3). Pereyra and Lebherz stated, "It would appear the modified Pereyra procedure is effective in 94% of patients operated on for stress urinary incontinence" (11).

Most of the literature shows attrition of the cure rate with time. Lebherz would later publish a retrospective article with a mean follow-up of 36 months showing a cure rate of 81.6% in low-risk patients and 43.8% in high-risk patients. High risk was defined as patients with low urethral pressure (< 20 cm H_2O), detrusor instability on preoperative testing, neurogenic incontinence, or a negative cotton swab test.

Riggs (12) reported his personal experience with long-term follow-up in patients treated with retropubic urethropexy and needle suspension. Two hundred fifty-two patients re-

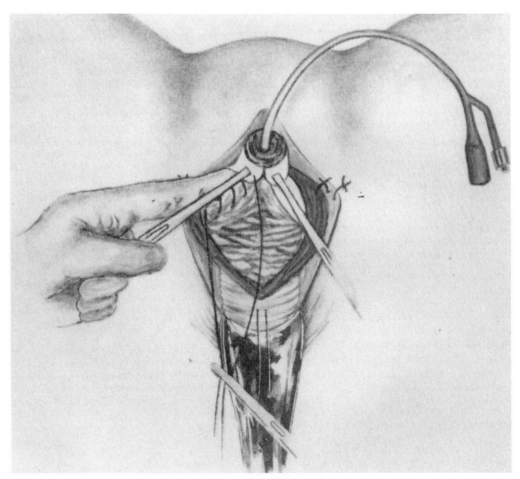

Figure 40.5. Allis forceps grasp the posterior pillars of the ligaments with helical sutures, binding pillars, and endopelvic fascia. (From Pereyra AJ, Lebherz TB. The modified Pereyra procedure. In: Buchsbaum HJ, Schmidt JD, eds. Gynecologic and obstetrical urology. Philadelphia: WB Saunders, 1978:269.)

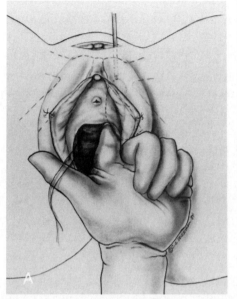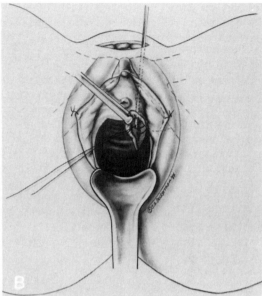

Figure 40.6.   A. The vaginal finger positioned retro-pubically makes contact with the tip of the carrier needle. This contact is maintained as the needle is advanced and the finger withdrawn. The direct needle contact of finger and needle aids in the pre-vention of bladder injury. **B.** The ends of the helical sutures are threaded through the aperture in the emerging needle carrier. (From Cutner LP, Ostergard DR. The modified Pereyra procedure. In: Ostergard DR, ed. Gynecologic urology and urodynamics. 2nd ed. Baltimore: Williams & Wilkins, 1985:532–533.)

Table 40.2.   Results: Modified Pereyra Procedure (1976–1982)[a]

No. of Previous Operations	No. of Patients	Cured[b]	Improved[c]	Failed
None	54	47 (87%)	4 (7.4%)	3 (5.5%)
1 or more	28	23 (82%)	2 (7.1%)	3 (10.7%)
Total	82	70	6	6

[a]Pereyra AJ, Lebherz TB, Growdon WA, Powers JA. The pubourethral supports in perspective: a modified procedure for stress urinary incontinence. Obstet Gynecol 1982;59:643.
[b]No recurrence of stress urinary incontinence reported; no loss of urine with stress test on coughing.
[c]Occasional escape of few drops of urine reported. Loss of less than 5 mL of urine noted on stress test.

Table 40.3.   Cure Rates for Modified Pereyra Procedure[a]

Type of Procedure	No. of Patients	Markedly Improved	Improved	Failed
Primary	108	94 (87%)	6 (5.6%)	8 (7.4%)
Secondary	34	32 (94%)	1 (2.9%)	1 (2.9%)
Tertiary	20	17 (85%)	1 (5%)	2 (10%)
Total	162	143	8	11

[a]Modified from Pereyra AJ, Lebherz TB. The modified Pereyra procedure. In: Buchsbaum HJ, Schmidt JD, eds. Gynecologic and obstetric urology. 2nd ed. Philadelphia: WB Saunders, 1982:274.

ceived a modification of the Pereyra proce-dure and 490 patients underwent a MMK procedure. Riggs placed sutures vertically with small bites from the urethral meatus to the urethrovesical junction, incorporating the stretched pubourethral ligaments and endopelvic fascia. At a 10- to 15-year follow-up, 65.9% of the Pereyra patients were clini-cally cured compared with 81.6% of the MMK patients.

Reviews of the Pereyra procedure must consider the technique used. Procedures ac-complished before 1976 did not use the tech-nique of the modified Pereyra procedure described by Pereyra and Lebherz (Table 40.1). An example is that of Park and Miller (13), who reported a comparison of the Kelly plication, MMK, and Pereyra procedures in 1988. It is difficult to extrapolate these data to results reported with the modified Pereyra procedure. The patients were not randomized, a mixture of absorbable and nonabsorbable suture materials was used, and it appears the original Pereyra technique was used in most patients.

The optimum evaluation of an operative procedure for the treatment of urinary stress incontinence includes the use of preoperative and postoperative urodynamic studies (Table 40.4). Several reviews report results without indicating whether this type of urodynamic testing was performed (3–6).

Bhatia and Bergman (14) reported a study using preoperative and postoperative urodynamic assessment in 1989. This was a non-randomized comparison of the modified Pereyra procedure and the Tanagho modification of the Burch procedure. All clinical and urodynamic studies were repeated during the 1-year follow-up. Only those patients who demonstrated negative cough profiles were considered cured. The cure rate was 98% (43 of 44) in patients undergoing the Burch procedure and 85% (17 of 20) for women undergoing the modified Pereyra procedure. All failures experienced previous unsuccessful incontinence surgery.

Bergman et al. (15) and Bergman and Elia (16) subsequently published long-term prospective randomized studies of the modified Pereyra procedure objectively documenting an increased failure rate with time. The modified Pereyra procedure was compared with the Burch urethropexy and the anterior colporrhaphy. Patients with a history of failed incontinence surgery or a requirement for concomitant gynecological surgery were excluded. All procedures were accomplished with absorbable suture material in the form of no. 0 Vicryl. After 1 year, of the 127 women randomized, 107 were available, and at 5 years, 93 were available for evaluation for the report of Bergman and Elia (16). The respective objective cure rates for the anterior colporrhaphy, modified Pereyra procedure, and Burch urethropexy were 37%, 43%, and 82%, respectively. The respective decreases in success rates for the procedures over 4 years were 26%, 22%, and 7%.

Korn (17) reviewed 14 case-series reports to determine whether suture material affected outcome in the modified Pereyra procedure. The relative risk of objective failure with absorbable suture was 1.6 times higher than with permanent suture.

In 1991, Kelly et al. (18) reported a physician-directed follow-up of 145 women undergoing the modified Pereyra bladder neck suspension from 1980 to 1986 with permanent suture material. Two helical no. 1 polypropylene sutures were used for each procedure. Median follow-up was 3.5 years, and 70% of patients had follow-up between 3 and 4 years. Fifty-one percent of patients reported no subjective stress incontinence, and 76% reported their sense of control was better. The onset of incontinence was experienced more than 2 years postoperatively in 23% of the incontinent group.

Karram et al. (19) reported a 12-month follow-up of 93 patients with preoperative and postoperative urodynamic testing. Overall, 82% of patients were subjectively cured, whereas only 63% were objectively cured. A high-risk group for failure could not be defined. There were no significant differences in age, parity, menopausal status, urethral functional length, or pressure transmission ratio between success and failure groups. There was no difference in cure

Table 40.4. Objective Results of Modified Pereyra Procedure Using Preoperative and Postoperative Urodynamic Testing

Author(s)	No. of Patients	Failure Rate (%)	Year
Bhatia and Bergman (14)	20	15	1985
Leach et al.	20	10	1987
Penttinen et al.	19	21	1989
Bergman et al. (15)	98	30	1989
Karram et al.[a] (19)	93	36.6	1992

[a] Indicates absorbable suture.

between premenopausal and postmenopausal women. This is consistent with another needle suspension study by Nitti et al. (20) that showed no difference in cure between patients under and over the age of 65 years.

Korman et al. (21) conducted a questionnaire-based outcome analysis of the modified Pereyra procedure at his institution. The mean follow-up of 151 patients with an objective diagnosis of type II incontinence (urethrovesical junction mobility in the absence of intrinsic sphincteric deficiency) was 25 months. Cure was strictly defined as no urine leakage under any circumstance. Fifty patients (47%) reported cure of the stress urinary incontinence, 68 (64%) reported subjective improvement, and 27 (26%) remained the same. Eleven (10%) were subjectively worse after the bladder neck suspension.

Complications

The technique of the original Pereyra procedure places the bladder at increased risk of injury relative to the technique used in the modified Pereyra procedure. The latter allows vaginal and space of Retzius dissection, direct atraumatic needle placement, and cystourethroscopic visualization.

In their study of 54 patients, Leach and Raz (22) reported that no patient experienced bladder or urethral injuries.

Bergman and Elia (16) noted that three subjects demonstrated detrusor instability during their prospective 5-year study and were considered failures. No voiding difficulties were documented 5 years postoperatively. Two patients developed cystoceles presenting at the introitus after the needle suspension. Cotton swab tests performed after 5 years were negative in >90% of Burch patients. Most women who underwent the needle suspension or Kelly procedure demonstrated positive swab tests or bladder neck hypermobility. Korn (17) noted that complications of fistula, intravesical suture, wound infection, granulation reactions, and abscess were reported in 25 of 509 operations using permanent suture and 20 of 478 operations using absorbable suture.

Karram et al. (19) noted retention of urine as the most frequent complication in their series of 93 patients; however, this was defined as a requirement for suprapubic drainage for more than 7 days after surgery. At 1-year follow-up, all patients were voiding spontaneously with low residual volumes. Six patients required blood transfusions, and two patients had incidental cystotomies.

In Nitti et al.'s study (20) of 92 patients, de novo urgency and urgency incontinence occurred in 24% and 13% of the patients, respectively.

Miyazaki and Shook (23) reported seven cases of ilioinguinal nerve entrapment after 402 needle suspension procedures. These cases were taken from a 27-month time period at a large medical group practice. Diagnoses were made secondary to symptoms of pain localized to the medial groin, mons, labia majora, and inner thigh. Three of seven patients were treated with suture removal, of which two experienced pain relief. Four patients were observed and noted eventual resolution of pain. The authors note that the ilioinguinal nerve is most vulnerable to entrapment near its exit from the superficial inguinal ring, which lies directly superior to the pubic tubercle. Needle suspension suture placement lateral to the tubercle may entrap the nerve.

Series by Nitti and Raz (24) and Foster and McGuire (25) reported management of postoperative urethral obstruction with transvaginal urethrolysis. These series described a combined total of 89 patients, of which 30 were obstructed secondary to performance of a previous needle suspension.

THE RAZ TECHNIQUE

In 1981, Raz (6) reported a modification of the Pereyra procedure. This modification is the modified Pereyra procedure reported in the Slate monograph with one or possibly two exceptions: an inverted U-shaped incision is made in the vagina to initiate the procedure and the helix suture passes through full thickness vagina (excluding mucosa).

In 1992, Raz et al. (26) reported a retrospective study of 206 patients with a mean follow-up of 15 months. Two helical no. 1 polypropylene sutures were used for each procedure. Successful outcome was reported in 90.3% of patients. However, the definition of successful outcome was cure (no stress incontinence) or the presence of stress incontinence not requiring pads. Patients with persistent irritative voiding symptoms were included in the successful outcome group. Thirty-eight percent of 90 patients had persistent significant urgency postoperatively. Twenty of 58 patients had continued urgency incontinence postoperatively with worsening noted in 7.5% of these patients. Overall, surgery decreased the numbers of patients experiencing urgency, urgency incontinence, and frequency of urination. In patients with moderate incontinence, the success rate was 93%, and in patients with severe incontinence (loss with gravity or slight exertional stresses), the subjective success rate was 65%.

Complications occurred in 30 patients, for a complication rate of 15% (26). Secondary prolapse was the most common complication. Enterocele occurred in seven patients (3%), six of whom underwent operative repair. Other forms of prolapse included four moderate cystoceles and two patients with uterine descensus, with five of these patients undergoing subsequent prolapse surgery. Suprapubic pain occurred in seven (3.5%) patients. Persistent pain in another patient was relieved by suture removal. Dyspareunia occurred in three patients (1.5%), wound infection in two (1%), and clitoral anesthesia in one (0.5%).

GITTES TECHNIQUE

In September of 1987, Gittes and Loughlin (4) published an article on no-incision pubovaginal suspension for stress incontinence (4). This procedure is identical to the original needle suspension procedure described by Armand Pereyra in 1959, with four minor variations: *(a)* nonabsorbable monofilament no. 2 hydroxypropylene suture is used in the place of no. 30 steel wire; *(b)* a Stamey needle carrier replaces the original Pereyra ligature carrier, making two penetrations through the rectus fascia on each side of the patient; *(c)* a full-thickness bite is taken through a portion of the vaginal wall that stretches between the first and second perforations; and *(d)* each suture is tied unilaterally in the abdominal stab incisions rather than tying the two sutures in the midline stab incision as originally described by Pereyra.

There is no vaginal dissection described in either operation. Pereyra and early workers performing the original Pereyra procedure noted that the suture material would pull through the vaginal epithelium and become embedded in the vaginal fibrous tissue (10). This has also been demonstrated experimentally (4).

Technique

The patient is placed in the lithotomy position; routine preparation includes placement of a Foley catheter and scrubbing of the abdomen and vagina. After appropriate draping, a small puncture is made with a no. 15 scalpel blade in the suprapubic subcutaneous tissue 2 cm superior to the pubic bone and 5 cm lateral to the midline.

A Stamey needle punctures the rectus fascia and musculature and is directed along the posterior aspect of the pubic bone. At the same time, the operator's other hand elevates the anterior vaginal wall lateral to the Foley balloon and bladder neck. This directs needle penetration through the vagina. A long no. 2 hydroxypropylene monofilament suture is threaded into the eye of the passed needle and withdrawn into the abdominal incision. The suture is removed from the needle and tagged. The free needle then makes a second pass, entering the rectus fascia 1 cm lateral to the original penetration. The needle is directed through the vaginal wall 2 cm cephalad to the original vaginal penetration. The alternate end of the original suture is threaded into a no. 6 Mayo needle, and a full-thickness anchoring bite is taken through the portion of the vaginal wall that stretches between the first and second vaginal perforations (Fig. 40.7). The Mayo needle is unthreaded, and the free end of the suture is now placed through the stylet of the Stamey needle, which is again withdrawn. The suture is secured for subsequent tying, and the process is repeated on the opposite side of the patient.

Cystourethroscopy is done to detect any bladder damage or penetration by suture material. A 70-degree cystoscope allows inspection of the lateral wall just inside the bladder neck and allows for direct visualization during suprapubic catheter placement. The monofilament sutures are now tied

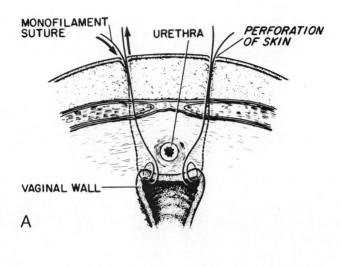

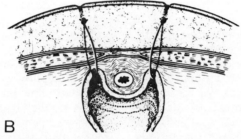

Figure 40.7. Position of transvaginal suspensory monofilament sutures in cross-section at level of female bladder neck is shown before (**A**) and after (**B**) tying into suprapubic fat to bury the knot. (From Gittes RF, Loughlin KR. No-incision pubovaginal suspension for stress incontinence. J Urol 1987;138: 568.)

tightly into the stab incision, resulting in elevation of the anterior vaginal wall. The tied sutures are pulled upward and trimmed just above the knot, which then retracts below the skin. The tension on the tissues has been noted to relax slightly after 1–2 days.

Results

Gittes and Loughlin (4) reviewed 38 patients with a total of 40 operations. The ages of the patients ranged from 36 to 80 years. All patients were initially cured of their stress incontinence, although six patients noted recurrence within 1 year. The authors indicated that the six failures occurred early in the series, before the introduction of an extra pass of the suspending suture through the vaginal wall. In the group of six failures, one patient was reported continent after a repeat procedure. The overall cure rate was reported as 87%. There is no indication that objective preoperative and postoperative urodynamic evaluations were performed on these patients.

Morales and VanCott (27) operated on 57 patients, using the technique described by Gittes and Loughlin, although three full-thickness passes were made through the vaginal wall by the suture before suspension. Complete elimination of urinary incontinence was obtained in 52 patients.

Benson et al. (28) reported 34 patients followed for 13 months postoperatively. The objective cure rate was 91% with a mean follow-up of 9.5 months. This degree of success has not been reported in studies with longer follow-up.

Narushima and Kondo (29) compared the Gittes and Stamey procedures in 394 patients. The subjective continence rate for the Stamey procedure was 78% at 51 months and for the Gittes procedure was 69% at 19 months. The 7-year continence rate was 77% for the Stamey procedure and the 3-year continence rate was 38% for the Gittes. The authors stated that the Stamey procedure was significantly more useful than the Gittes procedure.

Foster and O'Reilly (30) reviewed a series of 20 patients. Follow-up was between 9 weeks and 8 months. Twelve patients (60%) were cured, and 2 (10%) were significantly improved. Failure occurred in 6 of 20 patients (30%).

Kil et al. (31) reported transvaginal ultrasound and objective urodynamic assessment after suspension operations. They compared the methods of Gittes (18 patients), Stamey (13 patients), and Burch (29 patients). The initial cure rate comparison between the Stamey and Gittes techniques was equal at 3 months but demonstrated an increased difference with longer follow-up. The largest decrease in continence was noted in the Gittes procedure, with 44% continent at 14.7 months. The continence rate for the Burch group was 86% at 30.5 months. Elevation did not appear to be preserved in the Gittes group. The authors postulated the sutures may cut through the paraurethral tissues and that the suspension is partially lost. This was also the assertion made by Pereyra in his initial experience with the 1959 no-incision procedure, and it resulted in the subsequent modifications. Evidence indicates that the Gittes procedure may be inferior to other needle suspension procedures for long-term stress incontinence cure.

Complications

Complications include bladder spasm, urinary retention, and prolonged urgency symptomatology (4, 17).

THE LEACH TECHNIQUE

In May of 1988, Leach (5) reported a bone fixation technique for transvaginal needle suspension. The technique was a modified Pereyra procedure with essentially one variation: the pubic tubercle was used instead of the anterior rectus fascia as the fixation point for the suspension sutures. The advantage of bone fixation cited by

Leach was the avoidance of postoperative anterior abdominal wall discomfort. He indicated that patients treated with transvaginal needle suspensions for urinary incontinence often experienced prolonged postoperative discomfort and a "pulling" sensation radiating to the groin and leg. The bone fixation method was developed to avoid this discomfort and secure sutures without the use of synthetic pledget material.

Technique

An inverted U-shaped anterior vaginal wall incision is made, and sharp dissection is directed laterally to the pubic rami beneath the vaginal epithelium. The urogenital diaphragm is penetrated. A helical suture is placed, using no. 1 polypropylene and incorporating three bites of full-thickness anterior vaginal wall, excluding epithelium. A 4- to 5-cm suprapubic incision is made just cephalad to the pubic bone and carried down to the anterior rectus fascia. The suspension sutures are then transferred bilaterally to the suprapubic position, using a ligature carrier (Fig. 40.8). Gloves are changed, and the suprapubic wound is irrigated with antibiotic solution. Each pubic tubercle is then exposed, and the suture driven into it with a no. 6 Mayo needle. The vaginal wall is closed, and the suspension sutures are tied without excessive tension.

Results

Leach (5) reported 115 cases using the bone fixation technique over 2 years. He found no evidence of osteitis pubis. The early operative success rate was reported as 95% with few complications. Complications or the specific duration of postoperative follow-up relative to failures was not reported. There is no indication that preoperative urodynamic evaluations were performed in these patients.

THE STAMEY ENDOSCOPIC SUSPENSION OF THE VESICAL NECK

In 1973, Stamey (3) reported endoscopic suspension of the vesical neck for urinary incontinence. The emphasis of the report was an endoscopic visualization during the needle suspension to aid in correct suture placement and avoidance of bladder injury. Although more emphasis is noted in subsequent papers (32–34), the use of a Dacron buttress is an optional adjunct in the original description. Stamey wrote

If the pubocervical tissue is poor and unlikely to hold, the nylon suture can be passed through a 1 centimeter length of 5 millimeter knitted Dacron arterial graft, to buttress the vaginal loop.

Subsequent papers authored or coauthored by Stamey include the buttress as a component of the procedure and deviate only slightly from the original description (32–34) (Fig. 40.9). The collation of these descriptions follows.

Technique

Under general or regional anesthesia, the patient is placed in the modified lithotomy position. The patient is prepared and draped, excluding the rectum from the operative field. A weighted posterior vaginal speculum and urinary Foley catheter are placed. Two symmetrical 2- to 3-cm incisions are made 2–4 cm from the midline and three finger breadths above the pubis. The anterior rectus fascia is exposed by blunt dissection.

The anterior vaginal mucosa is incised transversely midway between the urethral meatus and bladder neck. It is separated from the urethra by gently spreading curved Metzenbaum scissors, with the instrument parallel to the floor, tips directed downward.

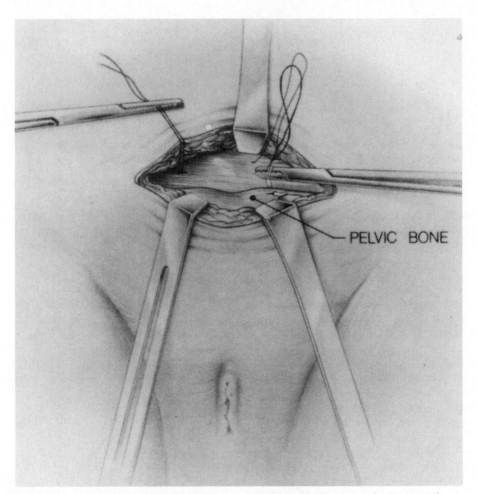

Figure 40.8. After exposure of pubic tubercle, one end of ipsilateral suspension suture is driven deeply into bone using a no. 6 Mayo trochar needle on a box needle hold. (From Leach GE. Bone fixation technique for transvaginal needle suspension. Urology 1988;31:388.)

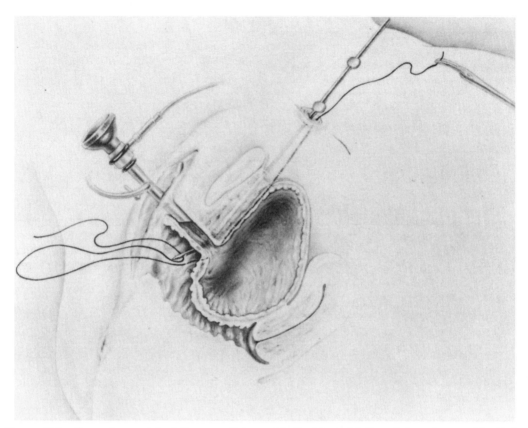

Figure 40.9. Figure from original Stamey article showing passage of the Stamey needle approximately 1–2 cm from the original suture. (From the Franklin H. Martin Memorial Foundation. Stamey TA. Endoscopic suspension of the vesical neck for urinary incontinence. Surg Gynecol Obstet 1973;136:547.)

A vertical incision is made, resulting in a T-shaped incision (26) (Fig. 40.10). The vaginal dissection is complete when it allows the tip of the surgeon's index finger to rest against the bladder neck on each side of the catheter.

A long special needle is introduced through the rectus fascia and directed along the posterior aspect of the symphysis pubis and downward along the vesical neck. Both straight needles and needles angled at either 15 or 30 degrees are useful (3). The Foley catheter is grasped in the palm of one hand, and the index finger is placed into the vaginal incision adjacent to the internal vesical neck. Excess tension on the catheter and resultant deviation of the bladder neck should be avoided. The needle point is directed by the surgeon's left index finger along the vesical neck, through the endopelvic and pubocervical fascia, and into the periurethral tissues next to the balloon of the Foley catheter, presenting in the vaginal incision (Fig. 40.11).

Accurate placement of the needle at the vesical neck is the primary reason for using the cystoscope (3). After removal of the catheter, a cystoscope with a right-angle or 70-degree lens is positioned at the vesical neck. If the needle is in the correct position at the urethrovesical junction, it will indent the ipsilateral vesical neck when the suprapubic end is moved slowly from left to right. If the needle has been incorrectly placed in a proximal position, the indentation will be seen between the bladder neck and the ureteral orifices (19). It is critical to ascertain whether the needle lies within the bladder wall or if any injury has occurred. Ideally, the bladder wall should be smooth without indentation by the needle at moderate degrees of filling (250 mL or less) (34). If the bladder is overfilled, an indentation will also be noted in a properly positioned needle. The weighted speculum should be removed during needle placement to avoid distortion of the tissues and resultant improper needle placement. A needle in an undesirable location can be repositioned before threading.

The cystoscope is withdrawn, and the needle is threaded with a no. 2 monofilament nylon suture. The needle is withdrawn suprapubically, and the suture ends are clamped with hemostats. The Foley catheter is replaced, and the free needle introduced a second time through the rectus fascia, 1–2 cm lateral to the initial placement. This second needle placement is also as close to the vesical neck area as possible, 1 cm lateral to the previous needle exit site in the periurethral tissues (33). Each needle passage must be at the level of the urethrovesical junction to avoid either pulling the urethral meatus cephalad, which may occur when a suspension suture is placed distal to the appropriate site, or inadequate urethrovesical junction elevation, which may occur when a suspension suture is placed proximal to the appropriate site.

The speculum is replaced, and the vaginal end of the nylon suture is threaded through a 1-cm tube of a 5-mm knitted Dacron arterial graft to buttress the vaginal tissue. If the Dacron tube is grasped lengthwise with an Allis clamp while the needle is pulled suprapubically, the two ends of the nylon suture can be balanced in the suprapubic incision, and the Dacron tube can be visually guided into the area of the urethrovesical junction (34). The procedure is repeated on the opposite side of the patient. A band of periurethral tissue is now within the nylon loop on each side of the vesical neck (Fig. 40.12).

Schaeffer and Stamey state "One of the major advantages of this procedure is that adequate suspension of the internal vesical neck can now be determined both anatomically and physiologically before tying the suspending nylon sutures" (34). The foroblique lens is put into the distal third of the urethra to evaluate symmetrical closure of the vesical neck. Functional closure can be tested by filling the bladder with 300 mL of irrigating fluid and removing the cystoscope while gently pushing in a posterior direction to remove the tension of the nylon loop. A stream of fluid may flow from the meatus, but it stops abruptly with minimal elevation of either or both of the suspending sutures (33). If functional or anatomic closure cannot be demonstrated, the suture placement should be reassessed.

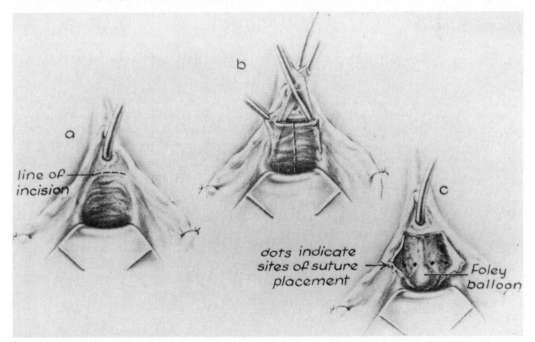

Figure 40.10. Illustration of the vaginal "T" incision made beneath the urethra during endoscopic suspension. (From Shortliffe LM, Stamey TA. Newer approaches to the correction of urinary stress incontinence in female patients. Surg Clin North Am 1982;62:1035.)

The vaginal incision is irrigated with an antibiotic solution and closed, burying the Dacron buttresses well below the suture line. The bladder is examined with a cystoscope, and a suprapubic catheter is placed under direct visualization. The weighted retractor is removed from the vagina, and the suspending sutures are lifted until the loops are taut. The sutures are then tied without tension, placing the knot against the rectus fascia. The abdominal incision is closed.

Ganabathi et al. (35) reported use of a Martius flap concomitantly with the Stamey procedure. The Martius flap was postulated to provide a buttress of well-vascularized adipose tissue that supports the proximal urethra and bladder base. The authors state that it may allow some free movement of the vaginal wall relative to the bladder during stress episodes.

Results

Stamey (32) reported 203 patients operated on between 1973 and 1979. In this referral population, 188 patients had a previous operation for urinary incontinence, 119 patients lost urine with simple physical activity, and 41 patients were classified as totally incontinent. The minimum follow-up was 6 months, although 47 patients were followed for over 4 years. The cure rate was noted to be 91%; 19 failures were reported. Of these 19 failures, 47% were totally incontinent before operation. The presence or absence of a uterus did not affect the results. Although preoperative urodynamic testing was accomplished, there is no indication that postoperative urodynamic studies were performed in these patients.

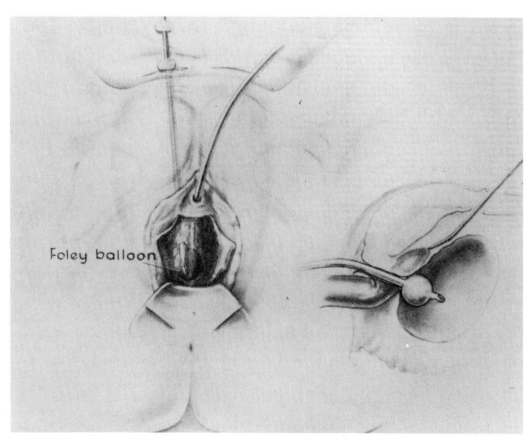

Figure 40.11. The needle is shown at the urethrovesical junction after the first medial pass. The needle is guided alongside the vesical neck by a finger elevating the periurethral tissues. (From Shortliffe LM, Stamey TA. Newer approaches to the correction of urinary stress incontinence in female patients. Surg Clin North Am 1982;62:1035.)

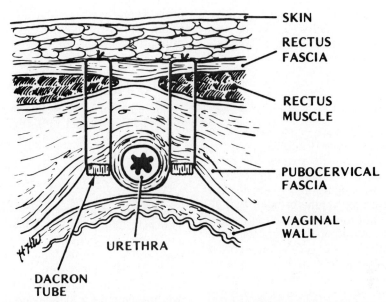

SKIN

RECTUS FASCIA

RECTUS MUSCLE

PUBOCERVICAL FASCIA

VAGINAL WALL

URETHRA

DACRON TUBE

Figure 40.12.   Schematic illustration of the suspending nylon loops on either side of the urethra at the internal vesical neck. (From Stamey TA. Endoscopic suspension of the vesical neck for urinary incontinence in females: report on 203 consecutive patients. Ann Surg 1980;192:465.)

Gaum et al. (36) used preoperative and postoperative evaluation in 60 patients who underwent endoscopic bladder neck suspension. In this series, 82% of the patients were cured of urinary stress incontinence, with a minimum follow-up of 6 months. Of the 11 patients treated unsuccessfully, 82% demonstrated recurrent urinary stress incontinence, whereas 18% experienced detrusor instability.

Mundy (37) prospectively compared the Stamey procedure and the Burch urethropexy followed by postoperative objective assessment at 1 year. One year after operation, objective evaluation with video urodynamics revealed that 85% of the Burch patients were dry (7.5% rate of persistent genuine stress incontinence and 7.5% rate of detrusor instability in 26 patients). In the Stamey group, 64% of patients were dry (16% had persistent genuine stress incontinence and 20% had detrusor instability in 25 patients). Twice as many patients in the Stamey group (24%) had low flow rates and high residual urine than the Burch patient group (12%).

Additional studies were performed on postoperative objective evaluation after the Stamey procedure (Table 40.5) (31, 38–40). Walker and Texter (41) performed a long-term

Table 40.5.   Objective Postoperative Results of Stamey Procedure

Authors	No. of Patients	Cure (%)	Follow-up (mo)
English and Fowler (38)	45	58	9
Hilton and Mayne (39)	100	83	3
Athanassopoulos et al. (40)	32	78	11
Ki et al. (31)	13	64	34

follow-up survey to determine patient satisfaction after Stamey suspension. The response rate for the survey was 72% (192 of 284). Overall improvement was reported in 82% of patients with approximately 41% of patients claiming to be dry. There was a gradual increase in failure with time. Only 70% of patients reported improvement after 5 years of follow-up. Sixty-five percent of the respondents said they would go through the experience again.

O'Sullivan et al. (42) sent questionnaires to 67 patients after the Stamey procedure. Immediately after surgery, 70% of patients were dry and 15% were much improved. At 6 months, 56% of patients were dry and 21% were much improved. This decreased to 31%

and 28%, respectively, after postoperative year 1. The authors concluded that the procedure should not be used as a first-line procedure for incontinence.

Complications

The synthetic bolsters or sleeves caused an increased incidence of foreign body reaction than other needle suspension techniques. Patients have required removal of sutures due to migration or erosion of the buttress into the vagina or bladder (20). Bihrle and Tarantino (43) reported seven women with suture/bolster migration seen at the Lahey Clinic. Evans et al. (44) reported bladder calculus formation due to migration of the Stamey suture/Dacron bolster in three patients. Richardson et al. (45) reported a delayed reaction to the Dacron bolster in 5% of 163 patients after receiving the Stamey procedure. Patients complained of pain, dyspareunia, vaginal discharge, and induration of the abdominal incision.

Huland and Bucher (46) noted a 15.2% rate of fistulas around the Stamey sutures in 86 consecutive patients. Spencer et al. (47) noted an 8.2% rate of postoperative suture removal in 41 patients.

Mundy (37) noted a high incidence of voiding difficulties both in the early postoperative period and after longer follow-up. Twenty percent of patients became unstable after the procedure. This is assessed further by a study by Pope et al. (48), who performed serial cystometrograms on alternate days after spontaneous postoperative micturition was established in 20 patients. Eighteen of 20 patients became dry immediately. Their mean preoperative voiding pressure was 26 ± 8 cm H_2O, rising to 42 ± 6 cm H_2O ($P < 0.001$) after 3 days of spontaneous voiding. Their voiding pressure at 21 days was 50 ± 8 cm H_2O. Twelve months later, no further significant changes occurred. Three women developed bladder instability; their voiding pressures exceeded 70 cm H_2O. Pope et al. (48) suggested that the risk of detrusor instability may be secondary to iatrogenic outflow obstruction. Pope et al.'s study of patients did demonstrate increased voiding pressures and reduced flow rates, suggesting some degree of obstruction from the Stamey proce-

dure. There has been at least one report of pubic osteomyelitis after the Stamey procedure (49).

THE HADLEY/KARRAM TECHNIQUE

The concept of using a patch was introduced by Hadley et al. (50), who used a rectus fascia patch. However, the rectus fascia is often attenuated in patients with incontinence and/or prolapse.

In March of 1990, Karram and Bhatia (51) reported a fascia lata patch modification for the transvaginal needle suspension. This technique was a modified Pereyra procedure with essentially one variation: the helix suture was attached to a patch of fascia lata placed suburethrally. The fascia lata patch offers the material strength of a suburethral hammock to the needle suspension. Patients with a thin vaginal vault or those with previous anterior vaginal wall dissections may benefit from the added strength of the patch.

Technique

A 5×7 cm piece of fascia lata is removed via a 3-cm incision placed four finger breadths above the midpatella lateral to the knee and the lower thigh. The modified Pereyra dissection is then performed with penetration into the space of Retzius via the vaginal route. The patch is sewn under the urethra and bladder base with multiple 4-0 Dexon sutures. The patch should cover an area from just distal to the midurethra to approximately 1 cm beyond the bladder neck. In a helical fashion, a no. 1 prolene suture is passed through the long axis of the patch, taking at least four bites. Each of these bites also incorporates endopelvic fascia. The helical stitch is continued down to the level of the bladder neck. A similar suture is placed on the opposite side. The sutures are then elevated into the abdominal incision in the usual fashion and cystoscopy is performed to ensure no bladder injury or stitch penetration has occurred. The vaginal incision is then closed with a running absorbable suture before tying the prolene sutures via the transverse abdominal incision (Fig. 40.13).

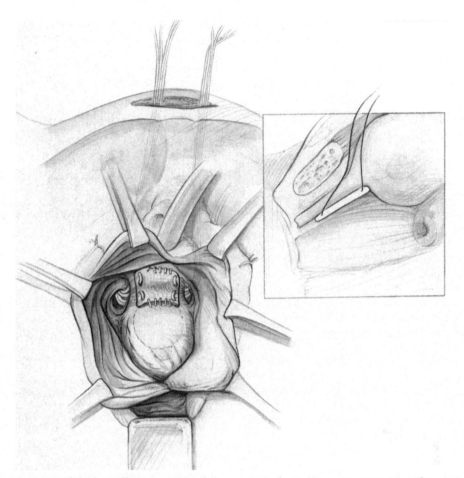

Figure 40.13. Combined needle suspension sling procedure in which suburethral patch of fascia is suspended with permanent sutures to the anterior rectus fascia. (From Karram MM, Walters MD. Clinical urogynecology. St. Louis, MO: Mosby, 1993.)

Results

Karram and Bhatia (51) originally reported on 10 patients, using a fascia lata patch to support the bladder base and the urethra. Nine of 10 patients were objectively continent at 1–2 years postoperatively. Preoperative and postoperative urodynamics were compared, and a significant increase in urethral closure pressure, functional urethral length, and abdominal pressure transmission in the proximal urethra were demonstrated. The authors noted that intraoperative and postoperative morbidity were minimal.

Summary

Armand J. Pereyra introduced a new approach, which did not require abdominal retropubic dissection, in the treatment of female urinary stress incontinence. This operation and subsequent modifications by Pereyra serve as the foundation for various needle suspension procedures. The reported cure rates for the modified Pereyra procedure and its variations have exceeded 85% in several short-term studies. Objective studies have shown a significantly higher failure rate at 1 year. There is strong evidence of increasingly high failure rates with long-term objective follow-up.

This evidence is present in both the gynecological and urological literature. Objective studies looking at failure in more detail show a high recurrence of urethrovesical junction rotation in patients with a history of needle suspensions relative to retropubic urethropexy, such as the Burch procedure. Although procedures performed with permanent suture appear to have a greater success rate, the failure rates remain high compared with the Burch urethropexy.

The reasons for the increased failure rate appear to be the same that Pereyra noted in the late 1960s and early 1970s. The sutures either pull through the tissue or, less commonly, break with stress. The primary method of dealing with this difficulty has been to incorporate larger and stronger amounts of endopelvic/musculofascial tissue in the helix suture. Many studies have not addressed adding one or two additional sutures to add strength on each side of the urethra. Muzsnai et al. (52) reported a technique of using three permanent sutures on each side of the urethra with apparent success in decreasing incontinence failure rates. This should be strongly considered by surgeons performing the needle suspension procedure. Bone-anchoring techniques are less helpful because suture failure most commonly occurs at the connection to the vaginal wall. Intuitively it seems difficult to understand why the procedures should offer less strength than a urethropexy. Benson and McClellan (53) showed increased evidence of pudendal neuropathy secondary to vaginal surgery when compared with the abdominal route. One postulate would be increased neurological and pelvic support damage during vaginal dissection in comparison with abdominal retropubic dissection. Although some authors have suggested retropubic scarification is important in incontinence cure and increases with the retropubic approach, one could argue that all previous incontinent patients show maintenance of anterior tissue attachment to the posterior aspect of the pelvic brim despite recurrent incontinence and often despite the route of previous incontinence surgery.

The Pereyra procedure has a role in the treatment of incontinence during vaginal correction of procidentia if multiple permanent sutures are used. It is accomplished with concomitant anterior colporrhaphy in patients who have demonstrated immediate and nonsustained stress leakage during prolapse reduction.

The modified Pereyra procedure is one of four basic surgical approaches to stress incontinence in the female. Additional long-term objective studies are needed to assess this and other operative approaches for incontinence. This will allow improved and precise treatment of this difficult condition in the female patient.

REFERENCES

1. Pereyra AJ. A simplified surgical procedure for the correction of stress urinary incontinence in women. West J Surg Obstet Gynecol 1959;67:223–226.
2. Pereyra AJ. The revised Pereyra procedure using colligated pubourethral supports. In: Slate WG, ed. Disorders of the female urethra and urinary incontinence. Baltimore: Williams and Wilkins, 1979:143–159.
3. Stamey TA. Endoscopic suspension of the vesical neck for urinary incontinence. Surg Gynecol Obstet 1973;136:547–554.
4. Gittes RF, Loughlin KR. No-incision pubovaginal suspension for stress incontinence. J Urol 1987;138:568–570.
5. Leach GE. Bone fixation technique for transvaginal needle suspension. Urology 1988;31:388–390.
6. Raz S. Modified bladder neck suspension for female stress incontinence. Urology 1981;17:82–85.
7. Pereyra AJ, Lebherz TB. Combined urethrovesical suspension and vaginourethroplasty for correction of urinary stress incontinence. Obstet Gynecol 1967;30:537–546.
8. Pereyra AJ, Lebherz TB. The revised Pereyra procedure. In: Buchsbaum HJ, Schmidt JD, ed. Gynecologic and obstetric urology. Philadelphia: WB Saunders, 1978:208–222.
9. Pereyra AJ, Lebherz TB, Growdon WA, Powers JA. The pubourethral supports in perspective: a modified procedure for urinary incontinence. Obstet Gynecol 1982;59:643–648.
10. Cornella JL, Pereyra AJ. Historical vignette of Armand J. Pereyra and the modified Pereyra procedure: the needle suspension for stress incontinence in the female. Int J Urogynecol 1990;1:25–30.
11. Pereyra AJ, Lebherz TB. The modified Pereyra procedure. In: Buchsbaum HJ, Schmidt JD, eds. Gynecologic and obstetric urology, 2nd ed. Philadelphia: WB Saunders, 1982:259–277.
12. Riggs JA. Retropubic cystourethropexy: a review of two operative procedures with long-term follow-up. Obstet Gynecol 1986;68:98.
13. Park GS, Miller EJ. Surgical treatment of stress urinary incontinence: a comparison of the Kelly plication, Marshall-Marchetti-Krantz, and Pereyra procedures. Obstet Gynecol 1988;71:575–579.
14. Bhatia NN, Bergman A. Modified Burch versus Pereyra retropubic urethropexy for stress urinary incontinence. Obstet Gynecol 1985;66:255–261.
15. Bergman A, Ballard CA, Koonings PP. Comparison of three different surgical procedures for genuine stress incontinence: prospective randomized study. Am J Obstet Gynecol 1989;160:1102–1106.

16. Bergman A, Elia G. Three surgical procedures for genuine stress incontinence: five-year follow-up of a prospective randomized study. Am J Obstet Gynecol 1995;173:66–71.

17. Korn AP. Does use of permanent suture material affect outcome of the modified Pereyra procedure? Obstet Gynecol 1994;83:104–107.

18. Kelly MJ, Roskamp D, Knielsen K, Leach GE, Bruskewitz R. Symptom analysis of patients undergoing modified Pereyra bladder neck suspension for stress urinary incontinence. Pre- and postoperative findings. Urology 1991;37:213–219.

19. Karram MM, Angel O, Koonings P, et al. The modified Pereyra procedure: a clinical and urodynamic review. Br J Obstet Gynaecol 1992;99:655–658.

20. Nitti VW, Bregg KJ, Sussman EM, Raz S. The Raz bladder neck suspension in patients 65 years old and older. J Urol 1993;149:802–807.

21. Korman HJ, Sirls LT, Kirkemo AK. Success rate of modified Pereyra bladder neck suspension determined by outcomes analysis. J Urol 1994;152:1453–1457.

22. Leach GE, Raz S. Modified Pereyra bladder neck suspension after previously failed anti-incontinence surgery. Urology 1984;23:359–362.

23. Miyazaki F, Shook G. Ilioinguinal nerve entrapment during needle suspension for stress incontinence. Obstet Gynecol 1992;80:246–248.

24. Nitti VW, Raz S. Obstruction following anti-incontinence procedures: diagnosis and treatment with transvaginal urethrolysis. J Urol 1994;152:93–98.

25. Foster HE, McGuire EJ. Management of urethral obstruction with transvaginal urethrolysis. J Urol 1993;150:1448–1451.

26. Raz S, Sussman EM, Erickson DB, Bregg KJ, Nitti VW. The Raz bladder neck suspension: results in 206 patients. J Urol 1992;148:845–850.

27. Morales A, VanCott GF. The Gittes procedures as an improved simplification of current techniques for vesical neck suspensions. Surg Gynecol Obstet 1988;167:243–245.

28. Benson JT, Agosta A, McClellan E. Evaluation of a minimal-incision pubovaginal suspension as an adjunct to other pelvic-floor surgery. Obstet Gynecol 1990;75:844–847.

29. Narushima M, Kondo A. Needle suspension of the bladder neck for stress urinary incontinence: surgical results of 394 patients operated on with quantitative procedures. Jpn J Urol 1995;86:1051–1059.

30. Foster MC, O'Reilly PH. Early experience of the Gittes "no-incision" pubovaginal suspension for stress urinary incontinence. Br J Urol 1989;64:590–593.

31. Kil PJ, Hoekstra JW, van der Meijden AP, et al. Transvaginal ultrasonography and urodynamic evaluation after suspension operations: comparison among the Gittes, Stamey and Burch suspensions. J Urol 1991;146:132–136.

32. Stamey TA. Endoscopic suspension of the vesical neck for urinary incontinence in females: report on 203 consecutive patients. Ann Surg 1980;192:465–471.

33. Shortliffe LM, Stamey TA. Newer approaches to the correction of urinary stress incontinence in female patients. Surg Clin North Am 1982;62:1035–1045.

34. Schaeffer AJ, Stamey TA. Endoscopic suspension of vesical neck for urinary incontinence. Urology 1984;23:484–494.

35. Ganabathi K, Abrams P, Mundy AR, et al. Stamey-Martius procedure for severe genuine stress incontinence. Br J Urol 1992;69:34–37.

36. Gaum L, Riccioti NA, Fair WR. Endoscopic bladder neck suspension for stress urinary incontinence. J Urol 1984;132:1119–1121.

37. Mundy AR. A trial comparing the Stamey bladder neck suspension procedure with colposuspension for the treatment of stress incontinence. Br J Urol 1983;55:687–690.

38. English PJ, Fowler JW. Video urodynamic assessment of the Stamey procedure for stress incontinence. Br J Urol 1988;62:550–552.

39. Hilton P, Mayne CJ. The Stamey endoscopic bladder neck suspension: a clinical and urodynamic investigation, including actuarial follow-up over four years. Br J Obstet Gynaecol 1991;98:1141–1149.

40. Athanassopoulos A, Melekos MD, Speakman M, et al. Stamey endoscopic vesical neck suspension in female urinary stress incontinence: results and changes in various urodynamic parameters. Int Urol Nephrol 1994;26:293–299.

41. Walker GT, Texter JH Jr. Success and patient satisfaction following the Stamey procedure for stress urinary incontinence. J Urol 1992;147:1521–1523.

42. O-Sullivan DC, Chilton CP, Munson KW. Should Stamey colposuspension be our primary surgery for stress incontinence? Br J Urol 1995;75:457–460.

43. Bihrle W, Tarantino AF. Complications of retropubic bladder neck suspension. Urology 1990;35:213–214.

44. Evans JW, Chapple CR, Ralph DJ, Milroy EJ. Bladder calculus formation as complication of the Stamey procedure. Br J Urol 1990;65:580–582.

45. Richardson DA, Bent AE, Ostergard DR, Cannon D. Delayed reaction to the Dacron buttress used in urethropexy. J Reprod Med 1984;29:689–692.

46. Huland H, Bucher H. Endoscopic bladder neck suspension (Stamey-Pereyra) in female urinary stress incontinence. Long-term follow-up of 66 patients. Eur Urol 1984;10:238–241.

47. Spencer JR, O'Conor VJ Jr, Schaeffer AJ. A comparison of endoscopic suspension of the vesical neck with suprapubic vesicourethropexy for treatment of stress urinary incontinence. J Urol 1987;137:411–415.

48. Pope AJ, Shaw PJR, Coptcoat MJ, Worth PHL. Changes in bladder function following a surgical alteration in outflow resistance. Neurourol Urodyn 1990;9:503–508.

49. Wheeler JS Jr. Osteomyelitis of the pubis: complication of a Stamey urethropexy. J Urol 1994;151:1638–1640.

50. Hadley RH, Zimmern PE, Staskin DR, Raz S. Transvaginal needle bladder neck suspension. Urol Clin North Am 1985;12:299–303.
51. Karram MM, Bhatia NN. Patch procedure: modified transvaginal fascia lata sling for recurrent or severe stress urinary incontinence. Obstet Gynecol 1990;75:461–463.
52. Muzsnai D, Carrillo E, Dubin C, Silverman I. Retropubic vaginopexy for correction of urinary stress incontinence. Obstet Gynecol 1982;59:113–117.
53. Benson JT, McClellan E. The effect of vaginal dissection on the pudendal nerve. Obstet Gynecol 1993;82:387–389.

CHAPTER 41

The Treatment of Female Urinary Incontinence by Functional Electrical Stimulation

Božo Kralj

Introduction and Historical Data

Although numerous conservative methods for treatment of female urinary incontinence are available, functional electrical stimulation (FES) is of increasing importance in the conservative treatment of urinary incontinence. FES applied vaginally or rectally to the pelvic floor muscles is especially successful in those kinds of urinary incontinence that are most frequently found in urogynecological practice (i.e., stress and urge incontinence).

Electrical stimulation for the correction of urinary incontinence in humans was first introduced by Caldwell in 1963 (1). He used an implantable radio-linked electrical stimulator with the electrodes fixed to the periurethral musculature. However, implantable systems were too complicated technically, and the results were successful in only 50% of cases. In 1968, Alexander and Rowan (2) presented some examples of electrical non-implantable stimulators with a vaginal or anal plug and an external housing for the circuitry and battery. In 1974, Suhel (3) developed the automatic vaginal electrical stimulator. The results of maximal perineal electrical stimulation were presented by Glen and colleagues in 1976 (4).

In 1977, Kralj et al. (5) published the first results in the treatment of urge incontinence and urgency with acute maximal functional electrical stimulation (AMFES).

To understand the actual status of FES in the management of female urinary incontinence, it is necessary to review the development of FES, especially over the last 20 years. This development resulted from the combination of research undertaken in two fields, technical and medical.

Numerous technical problems had to be solved to provide the actual indication areas, efficiency, and safety for the treatment of female urinary incontinence. New parameters for FES were established. After prolonged use of stimulators, corrosion of electrodes did not only initiate the search for new materials but also resulted in transition from monophasic to biphasic stimulation. We designed vaginal and rectal plugs, which are by far more physiological, and new electrodes. The automatic vaginal stimulator, Vagicon-X, also resulted from our research. New stimulators for AMFES have been made to maintain unchanged intensity of current throughout the 20 minutes of stimulation, regardless of the tissue impedance. Currently, we only use stimulators for external application, either vaginal or rectal.

Medical knowledge in this field has been

improved by numerous clinical, neuro-physiological, and urodynamic findings. Neurophysiology has contributed the important finding that FES applied on the pelvic floor muscles has a predominantly reflexogenic effect. The important clinical and uro-dynamic finding was that the micturition center in S2 to S4 responds to the stimulus physiologically, that is, by the contraction of the pelvic floor muscles and relaxation of the bladder detrusor (6). These findings helped to indicate the role of FES in the management of female urinary incontinence. Clinical practice has confirmed the efficiency of FES treatment in the management of individual types of female urinary incontinence and thus supports the proper direction of research (7).

Mode of Action of FES

FES applied to the pelvic floor muscles (vaginally or rectally) has a twofold action: contraction of pelvic floor muscles and relaxation or inhibition of bladder activity. At lower currents (<35 mA), only the pelvic floor muscles are affected; both effects (contraction of pelvic floor muscles and inhibition of the bladder activity) are achieved by application of a stronger current (>65 mA vaginally or >40 mA rectally).

A twofold effect on the lower urinary tract is achieved by changing the current setting at the same frequency of electrical stimulation (20 Hz). Erlandson et al. (8) determined, on the basis of experimental data, that optimal frequencies were between 20 and 50 Hz for sphincter closure and 5 and 10 Hz for bladder inhibition. Practically, it seems that the use of 5, 10, or 20 Hz produced no difference for bladder inhibition in patients (9).

At the same frequency of electrical stimulation, the same effect is achieved by only changing the current setting; therefore, our stimulators have the same parameters of stimulation irrespective of the kind of incontinence. Consequently, only the power of the applied current changes. Trontelj et al. (10) investigated the action of FES applied to the pelvic floor muscles (needle electrodes, vaginal or rectal probes) from the

neurophysiological point of view. Single-fiber electromyography was used to analyze responses of the pelvic floor muscles to electrical stimulation applied for the treatment of urinary incontinence. It has been shown that the largest proportion of the resulting motor effect is due to the polysynaptic reflex responses. This implies several important advantages as compared with direct stimulation of motor axons, for example, the physiological recruitment order of the motor units and the coordination and plasticity of the response. Direct stimulation tends to activate a limited number of motor units within the physical reach of the stimulus. Reflex stimulation, on the other hand, can activate a number of muscles from a single stimulation site. A further advantage is that the position of the electrodes is less critical than is the case with direct stimulation.

FES applied to the pelvic floor muscles primarily elicits a reflexogenic response. The electrical impulse runs along the afferent limb of the pudendal nerve to the sacral nerve roots and by the efferent pathway back to the pelvic floor muscles. Not only single motor units but almost all muscle fibers connected with the same reflex arc are activated by the electrical impulse (10). This fact is of vital importance because the reflex pathway must be essentially intact if successful FES treatment is to be achieved. At most, only a minor denervation of pelvic floor muscles is allowed. For this reason, a neurophysiological examination (electromyography) before FES treatment is recommended. Stimulation of pudendal afferents has been shown to induce bladder inhibition due to pudendal-to-hypogastric (11) and pudendal-to-pelvic spinal reflexes (12). The latter is assumed to be important for detrusor inhibition in humans. The same reflex mechanisms were activated by intravaginal electrical stimulation in cats (13), which was shown to activate the sympathetic (hypogastric) vesicoinhibitory neurons and inhibit the parasympathetic vesical motor neurons (14).

The effect of FES applied either vaginally or rectally to the pelvic floor muscles can be monitored by the changes in urodynamic parameters. Urethral pressure profile (UPP) and the cystometric curve are changed by FES application.

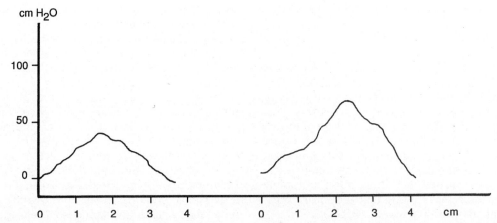

Figure 41.1. Urethral pressure profile (UPP) in female stress incontinence. *Left:* UPP before the application of functional electrical stimulation (FES).

Right: UPP during application of FES with the Vagicon-X 35 mA.

CHANGES IN UPP

When FES is applied to the pelvic floor muscles, there is an increase in the maximum urethral pressure. At the same time, the pressure along the entire urethra is increased. These changes are notable in patients with low UPP and stress incontinence. With a current of up to 35 mA, all or nearly all motor units of the pelvic floor muscles are stimulated. The success of the treatment of stress incontinence with FES does not depend solely on an increase in the UPP. More important is the reflex stimulation of the pelvic floor muscles, which improves pressure transmission to the urethra during stressful activity such as coughing (Fig. 41.1).

CHANGES IN THE CYSTOMETRIC CURVE

The cystometric curve is not significantly changed during application of chronic FES (i.e., stimulation of pelvic floor muscles using up to 35 mA current). The changes show only after the vaginal application of a current greater than 65 mA. In the treatment of incontinence secondary to detrusor overactivity, we use AMFES, which is generally applied only once. Spasms of detrusor muscle, as demonstrated by sudden increases in bladder pressure, disappear during the application of AMFES in most cases. The cystometric curve becomes smooth during application of AMFES and remains normal afterward. The bladder capacity increases two to five times in patients who respond to the treatment. Very large increases in bladder ca-

pacity are observed mostly in patients with a neurogenic bladder. In treatment with AMFES, the bladder capacity between the point of first sensation to the point of imperative need for urination is increased by 80–120 mL. Simultaneously, the bladder pressure of the full and empty bladder decreases to <20 cm H_2O in successfully treated patients.

Characteristically, the changes in the cystometric curve appear during the application of AMFES. If there are no urodynamic changes during application of AMFES, we can predict that therapy with AMFES will not be successful. Cystometric changes attained during and after AMFES treatment are no guarantee that the detrusor will keep its normal action. Twenty-six percent of patients receiving AMFES treatment for detrusor overactivity require two or more treatments (Fig. 41.2).

It is not known why the stability of the detrusor is preserved for so long after AMFES treatment for idiopathic motor urge incontinence and why for neurogenic motor urge incontinence it lasts only for a short while.

Parameters of FES for the Stimulation of Pelvic Floor Muscles

The impulse is biphasic and rectangular, frequency is 20 Hz, duration of impulse is 1 ms, and the current is 35–100 mA.

Description of Pelvic Floor Muscle Stimulator

The nonautomatic stimulator (Vagicon, Recticon) consists of two parts. The container carried in the underwear by the patient contains the impulse generator and battery. This is connected by a cable to the vaginal or rectal plug. A special button on the container allows the patient to adjust the desired power of the current in the stimulator. The current needed for stimulation of pelvic floor muscles is individualized for each patient.

In an automatic vaginal stimulator, the impulse generator and the battery are contained in the vaginal plug. Thus, the patient has the entire unit in the vagina, and there is no need for the container to be carried in the underwear. This stimulator is very practical, but it is also heavier, and it can fall out in patients with descensus of the vagina. In these cases, it is advisable to use it in the supine position.

The choice of vaginal or rectal stimulator for the treatment of urinary incontinence depends on local changes. Relative contraindications for the application of the vaginal plug are a short vagina (after radical surgery or radiation), severe vaginal descensus, or prolapse of the uterus. In women who can use

both plugs, we choose the one that better stimulates the levator ani muscles. This can be distinguished by simple palpation of the levator ani or in the urodynamic laboratory, when we assess the change of UPP after the application of the stimulator.

Serially produced stimulators with current limited to 35 mA are used twice daily for 1.5–2 hours. These stimulators require a special testing device to ensure that the current is alternating. If the light of the tester does not blink, the stimulator is broken. Provided that the stimulator is regularly tested and properly used, the vaginal or rectal tissue cannot be damaged. The results of stimulation are not affected by the choice of stimulator. We select the vaginal stimulator for those women with normal vaginal anatomy or for those women with abnormal anatomy who can use it in a supine position (Figs. 41.3–41.5).

Stimulators of pelvic floor muscles in which the current is limited to 35 mA are intended for the treatment of genuine stress incontinence. The treatment of detrusor overactivity (urge incontinence, detrusor instability, detrusor hyperreflexia) requires a stimulator with the current setting over 65 mA but limited to 100 mA. Such stimulation, which we refer to as AMFES, can only be applied for 20 minutes to prevent tissue damage.

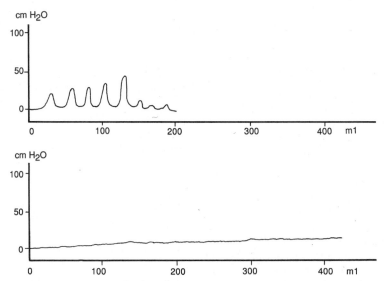

Figure 41.2. Cystometric curve typical of neurogenic motor urge incontinence (*top*). Change of cystometric curve during the application of AMFES (*bottom*).

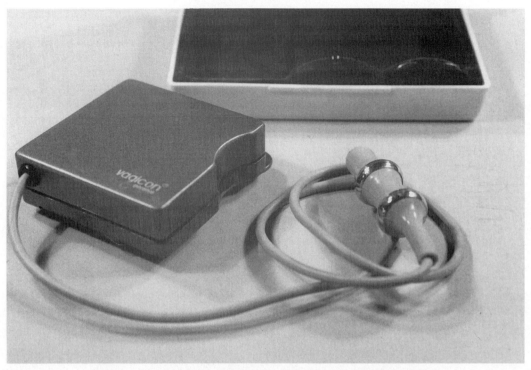

Figure 41.3. Vagicon, nonautomatic. Under the container for the battery and impulse generator, there is the device for testing.

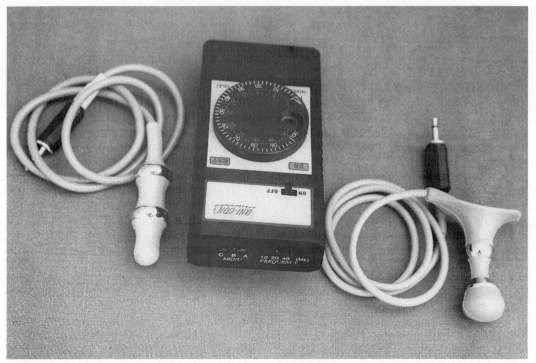

Figure 41.4. Personal stimulator for home use, the Uni-Con, is one-channel; impulse is symmetrical biphasic; duration of impulse is 0.8–1 ms; frequency of 10, 20, and 40 Hz; constant current from 0 to 100 mA, regardless of tissue impedance. It has a timer and automatic detector for the slipped out electrode. With all these capacities it provides three possibilities of application (AMFES, chronic, and intermittent).

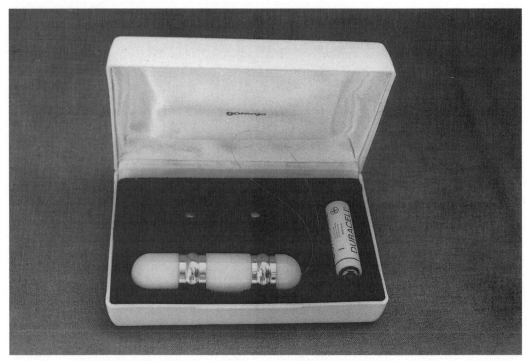

Figure 41.5. Vagicon X. The stimulator contains a battery and an impulse generator in the vaginal plug. In the stimulator case, two buttons for testing regular function of the stimulator are seen.

The maximal electrical current used is individualized according to the pain threshold. In the first years of stimulation to obtain such power, we applied three pairs of electrodes (vaginal plug, rectal plug, and needle electrodes) to pelvic floor muscles (15). Needle electrodes were soon dropped because they did not add considerably to the current. As current of such magnitude (over 65 mA) applied suddenly can be painful, we changed the method of application so that the current was gradually increased, and AMFES was no longer painful. Afterward, we changed from two-channel stimulation (vaginal and rectal) to one-channel stimulation with vaginal or rectal stimulator only. The results were the same as in two-channel stimulation. Our new stimulators for AMFES maintain unchanged intensity of current throughout the 20 minutes of stimulation regardless of the tissue impedance.

As the recurrences after treatment of urge incontinence are frequent (26%) and the results of the treatment of incontinence in neurogenic bladder are short-lived, an idea was conceived to make a new AMFES stimulator that could be used by patients very frequently at home. Until then, AMFES stimulators were only used for clinical application in the urodynamic laboratory. As neurogenic bladder is often found in patients whose walking is also handicapped, we wanted to have an AMFES stimulator that could be used by the patient at home. Thus, stimulators for AMFES stimulation were created with a vaginal or rectal plug. Patients can apply the stimulator for AMFES treatment 20 minutes daily, for 5 days consecutively. After a few days, the stimulation can be repeated. With good control and careful use for no more than 20 minutes at a time, no local damage or other adverse reactions were observed.

DEVICES

We made a new stimulator, Uni-Con, for home use. For hospital and/or outpatient use, we constructed a two-channel stimulator (Fig. 41.4). These new stimulators permit the use of vaginal or rectal electrodes. In France and the Scandinavian countries, they also use stimulators of their own production.

In the United States, the stimulators Microgyn II™ (6) and Innova are used. The parameters of Microgyn II™ are as follows: impulse is rectangular and biphasic, duration of impulse is 1 ms with maximum current of 30 mA, and frequency of stimulation is 20 or 50 Hz. The parameters of Innova are as follows: impulse is rectangular and biphasic, pulse width is 0.3 ms, frequency of stimulation is 12.5 and 50 Hz, and current ranges from 0 to 100 mA (Fig. 41.6).

Indications for Treatment of Urinary Incontinence with FES

Indications for treatment are as follows:

1. Stress incontinence
   a. Without severe vaginal descensus
   b. Recurrence after surgery

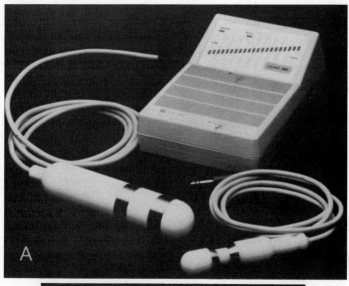

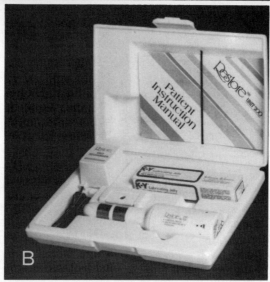

Figure 41.6. Two functional electrical stimulation units available in the United States and Canada. **A.** Microgyn II. (Distributed by In-Care Medical Products, a division of Hollister Incorporated). **B.** Restore Unit 200 (Interactive Medical Technologies, Inc., Ventura, CA). [Not shown: Liberty-Utah Medical Products Inc., Midvale, UT; Innova-Empi Inc., St. Paul, MN.]

   c. After radical pelvic surgery
   d. After pelvic radiation treatment
2. Urge incontinence
   a. Motor urge incontinence
   b. Sensory urge incontinence
3. Mixed (stress and urge) incontinence
4. Some types of neurogenic bladder incontinence
5. Vesicourethral dyssynergia
6. Frequency
7. Micturition disturbances caused by urethral instability

Contraindications for the Treatment of Urinary Incontinence with FES

There are no absolute contraindications. We consider severe urinary retention and vesicoureteral reflux as relative contraindications. The device should not be used in patients with a pacemaker or during heavy menstruation and during pregnancy.

Guidelines for Treatment by External Electrostimulation

Before deciding on the treatment of the pelvic floor (vaginal or rectal), it is necessary to make clinical and laboratory investigations to classify the type and degree of urinary incontinence. Therefore, we take a patient's precise history and perform pelvic and urological examinations. Pelvic examination provides the evaluation of vaginal and uterine malpositions, whereas in patients after gynecological surgery, especially after a radical one, it provides the evidence of the short vagina with scar tissue. In the latter case and in patients with severe vaginal prolapse or with subtotal uterine and vaginal prolapse, we use rectal stimulators, because it is impossible to use vaginal stimulators.

Before FES treatment, it is mandatory to have urine culture results because a urinary tract infection should be treated first. Hypoestrogenic changes of the vaginal mucosa should be treated before electrostimulation (16). A pad test constitutes a compulsory part

of investigations preceding the FES treatment because it enables the objective evaluation of both the degree of urinary incontinence and the outcome of treatments. Urodynamic investigations, which should always precede the introduction of FES treatment, provide the exact diagnosis of the type of urinary incontinence and/or micturition disturbances.

Electromyography (EMG) of the pelvic floor muscles is mandatory only in the patients with suspected disturbed innervation of the pelvic floor muscles and in those with central nervous system diseases. Because of the principally reflexogenic activity of FES, EMG is in these cases obligatory.

When chronic stimulation is required, it is important to motivate a patient for this mode of treatment. Therefore, these patients are often invited to follow-up visits, mainly to encourage them in continuation of treatment until favorable results are achieved.

Results of Treatment of Stress Incontinence by FES

Patients with pure stress incontinence of a mild degree without considerable vaginal prolapse are treated by chronic FES, in most cases with a vaginal stimulator (and the rectal one only rarely) with current limited to 35 mA, applied daily for 1.5–2 hours. The outcome can only be evaluated after 3 months of treatment. Of 111 patients treated, 56 patients (50.5%) were cured, 26 patients (23.4%) were improved, and 29 patients (26.1%) were unchanged.

Nearly the same outcome of treatment was found in a smaller group of patients treated by AMFES 20 minutes daily for 5 consecutive days, repeated after a 2-day pause for several weeks (B. Kralj, unpublished data).

Treatment of Urge Incontinence by FES

Because a current over 65 mA causes inhibition of detrusor activity, urge incontinence is treated by application of electric current

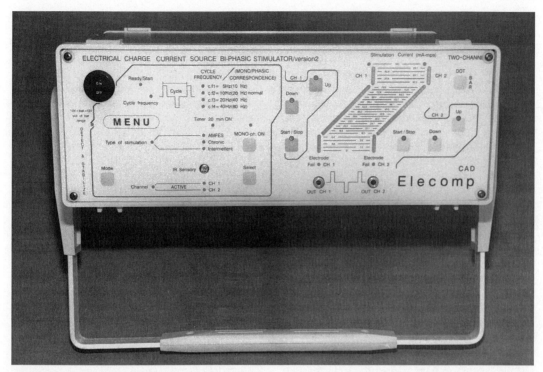

Figure 41.7. The latest AMFES treatment stimulator: two-channel, impulse is symmetrical mono- or biphasic, duration of impulse is 0.8–1 ms, frequency of 5–100 Hz, constant current from 0 to 100 mA, regardless of tissue impedance. It has a timer, automatic detector for the slipped out electrode, and meter and display of real current of stimulation. With all these capacities it provides three possibilities of application (AMFES, chronic, and intermittent).

from 65 to 100 mA. The same change on the UPP is achieved by application of a strong current as by application of a low current (35 mA); nevertheless, an essential difference in the bladder detrusor is observed. In this way, a relaxation or inhibition of the detrusor occurs. Electric current is applied using AMFES by means of a vaginal or rectal plug.

Parameters of Stimulation

The impulse is rectangular, the duration of impulse is 1 ms, and the frequency of stimulation is 20 Hz. The impulse is biphasic (to exclude corrosion of the electrodes and to ensure absolute safety from tissue damage). The new stimulator is a current generator, which retains the same current by changeable tissue impedance for the duration of stimulation. We use a simple plug electrode (vaginal or rectal). The applied current is gradually increased as long as the stimula-

tion is painless (i.e., to the threshold of pain). We stimulate daily for 20 minutes for 5 successive days (Fig. 41.7).

In patients with urge incontinence, the UPP is not changed by application of AMFES (UPP is normal in patients with pure urge incontinence). However, the cystometric curve is dramatically changed. In patients with motor and sensory urge incontinence, the capacity of the bladder increases four- to sixfold in some patients. During stimulation, the capacity of the bladder between the first sensation to void and imperative sensation to void (unable to hold any longer) is increased. During AMFES stimulation for motor urge incontinence, the uninhibited detrusor contractions disappear. The cystometric changes persist after successful AMFES treatment unless there is recurrence of the clinical disorder (Figs. 41.8 and 41.9).

Similar changes are observed in patients with neurogenic motor urge incontinence during AMFES treatment. However, recurrence is usual after only a short time interval.

Result of Treatment of Urge Incontinence by AMFES

Table 41.1 presents the overall results and does not differentiate between the two types of idiopathic urge incontinence, motor and sensory. Tables 41.2 and 41.3 present the results of motor and sensory urge incontinence, respectively. The results of treatment show no significant difference between the two types of idiopathic urge incontinence (chi square = 2.29, $P < 0.13$). Had the cured patients alone been taken into account, the difference would have almost been significant (chi square = 4.22, $P < 0.04$) (7).

Recurrence of urge incontinence after AMFES treatment is found in 26% of patients. Recurrences seldom occur earlier than 3 months, and most are observed between 3 and 6 months after AMFES treatment.

Mild (stress and urge) incontinence is an extremely frequent indication for application of FES (6, 16). The most favorable results are achieved in the treatment of moderate stress and urge incontinence. In these cases, AMFES is the method of choice. It is essential that AMFES can be applied at home, and therefore hospitalization or visits to the urodynamic laboratory are not necessary. AMFES should be applied 20 minutes daily for 5 consecutive days. The treatment is to be

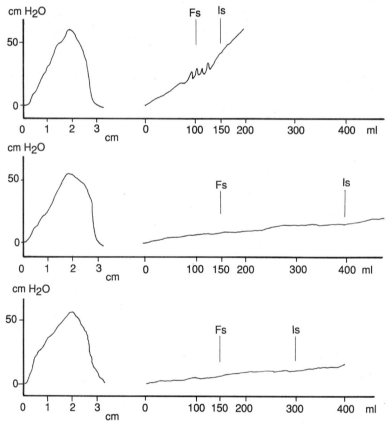

Figure 41.8. A female patient with idiopathic motor urge incontinence. *Top left:* Normal urethral pressure profile (UPP). *Top right:* Cystometric curve characteristic for idiopathic motor urge incontinence. First sensation for micturition (*Fs*) and imperative sensation to void (*Is*) are very close. The curve is spastic. Pressure = 55 cm H_2O. *Middle:* Urodynamic changes during the application of AMFES. UPP remains unchanged, but the cystometric curve changes. Bladder capacity increases from 200 to almost 500 mL. The curve is flat. Fs and Is are separated. Pressure is normal (<10 cm H_2O). *Bottom:* The same patient 3 months after AMFES treatment. Urodynamic parameters remain the same as during the application of AMFES; only the capacity of the bladder is lessened.

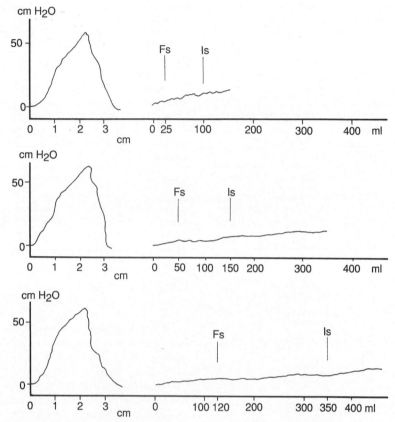

Figure 41.9. Female patient with idiopathic sensory urge incontinence. *Top left:* UPP is normal; cystometric curve is characteristic for sensory urge incontinence. Bladder capacity is only 180 mL. Bladder capacity at first sensation for micturition is only 25 mL; imperative sensation for micturition is at 100 mL. Cystometric curve is flat, and pressure is normal. *Middle:* Urodynamic changes during the application of AMFES, UPP remains unchanged. The bladder capacity is augmented to 360 mL. First sensation for micturition is at 50 mL, and imperative sensation occurs at 150 mL. *Bottom:* Urodynamic changes in the same patient 3 months after AMFES treatment. Characteristics of UPP and cystometry are the same as during the application of AMFES. The separation of Fs and Is are even greater.

Table 41.1.   Result of Treatment of Urge Incontinence by AMFES

Outcome	No. of Patients	Percent
Cured	64	72.7
Improved	8	9.1
Unchanged	16	18.2
Total	88	100.0

Table 41.2.   Results of Treatment of Motor Urge Incontinence by AMFES

Outcome	No. of Patients	Percent
Cured	22	55.0
Improved	8	20.0
Unchanged	10	25.0
Total	40	100.0

repeated after a 2-day pause for several weeks.

The application of FES is also advisable in the treatment of mixed incontinence in which stress incontinence is the prevailing component. These patients are treated with AMFES before surgery, and after surgery AMFES is applied in all patients in whom urge incontinence occurs either before or after surgery (Table 41.4) (17).

FES treatment has shown favorable results in elderly women (over 65 years) in whom urge incontinence has a high incidence. Drug treatment in these women is frequently contraindicated, whereas FES treatment has no contraindications. The results of FES treat-

Table 41.3.   Results of Treatment of Sensory Urge Incontinence by AMFES

Outcome	No. of Patients	Percent
Cured	42	87.5
Improved	0	0.0
Unchanged	6	12.5
Total	48	100.0

Table 41.5.   Results of Treatment for Patients Experiencing Frequency by AMFES

Outcome	No. of Patients	Percent
Cured	30	71.4
Improved	7	16.7
Unchanged	5	11.9
Total	42	100.0

Table 41.4.   Results of Treatment of Mixed Incontinence by AMFES

Outcome	No. of Patients	Percent
Cured	24	57.2
Improved	8	19.0
Unchanged	10	23.8
Total	42	100.0

Table 41.6.   Results of Treatment of Unstable Urethra by AMFES

Outcome	No. of Patients	Percent
Cured	22	56.4
Improved	9	23.1
Unchanged	8	20.5
Total	39	100.0

ment in elderly women are the same as in younger women. We found that a high percentage of women (79%) can use a stimulator by themselves. We consider FES a new and efficient mode of treatment in elderly incontinent women (18).

Treatment of Frequency

Patients experiencing frequency are treated by AMFES (Table 41.5) (19).

Treatment of Micturition Disturbances Caused by Unstable Urethra

After clinical and urodynamic investigations of 919 patients suffering from micturition disturbances, unstable urethra was found in 39 (4.2%) patients.

Micturition disturbances caused by unstable urethra were manifested as mixed (stress and urge) incontinence in 24 (61.5%) patients, as urge incontinence in 6 (15.4%), as stress incontinence in 5 (12.8%), and as frequency in 4 (10.3%) patients. All patients were treated by AMFES (Table 41.6).

Micturition disturbances caused by unstable urethra represent a new and efficient indication for treatment by FES (20, 21).

Conclusions

FES is a new and efficient method in the management of female micturition disturbances, with practically no contraindications. The mode of treatment has proved extremely efficient with urge incontinence (recurrence of the disease in one fourth of patients), frequency, and with micturition disturbances caused by unstable urethra. Without any serious contraindications, FES is more frequently used in the treatment of micturition disturbances in elderly women.

REFERENCES

1. Caldwell KP. The electrical control of sphincter incompetence. Lancet 1963;2:174–175.
2. Alexander S, Rowan D. Electrical control of urinary incontinence by radioimplant: a report of 14 patients. Br J Surg 1968;55;358–364.
3. Suhel P. Adjustable nonimplantable electrical stimulators for correction of urinary incontinence. Urol Int 1976;31:115–123.
4. Glen ES, Samuels BS, MacKenzie IM, Rowan D. Maximum perineal stimulation for urinary incontinence. Urol Int 1976;31:134–136.
5. Kralj B, Plevnik S, Janko M, Vrtačnik P. Urge incontinence and maximal electrical stimulation. Presented at the 7th annual meeting of the International Continence Society, Portorož, 1977.
6. Bent AE, Sand PK, Ostergard DR, Brubaker LT. Transvaginal electrical stimulation in the treatment of genuine stress incontinence and detrusor instability. Int Urogynecol J 1993;4:9–13.
7. Kralj B. Actual possibilities and perspectives for external application of functional electrical stimulation in treatment of female urinary incon-

tinence. Presented at the Ljubljana FES Conference, Ljubljana, 1993.

8. Erlandson BE, Fall M, Carlsson CA. The effect of intravaginal electrical stimulation on the feline urethra and urinary bladder: electrical parameters. Scand J Urol Nephrol 1977;44(Suppl 1):5–18.

9. Vereecken R, Das J, Grisar P. Electrical sphincter stimulation in the treatment of detrusor hyperreflexia of paraplegics. Neurourol Urodynam 1984;3:145–154.

10. Trontelj JV, Janko M, Godec C, Rakovec S, Trontelj M. Electrical stimulation for urinary incontinence: a neurological study. Urol Int 1974;29: 213–220.

11. Sundin T, Carlsson CA. Reconstruction of several dorsal roots innervating the urinary bladder. An experimental study in cats. I. Studies on the normal afferent pathways in the pelvic and pudendal nerves. Scand J Urol Nephrol 1972;6: 176–184.

12. Sundin T, Carlsson CA, Kock NG. Detrusor inhibition induced from mechanical stimulation of the anal region and from electrical stimulation of pudendal nerve afferents. Invest Urol 1974;11: 374–378.

13. Fall M, Erlandson BE, Carlsson CA, Lindstrom S. The effect of intravaginal electrical stimulation on the feline urethra and urinary bladder: neurological mechanisms. Scand J Urol Nephrol 1977; 44(Suppl 2):19–30.

14. Lindstrom S, Fall M, Carlsson CA, Erlandson BE. The neurophysiological basis of bladder inhibition in response to intravaginal electrical stimulation. J Urol 1983;129:405.

15. Kralj B. Neurogenic urge incontinence. In: Salamoto S, Tojo S, Nakayourus T, eds. Gynecology and obstetrics. Amsterdam: Excerpta Medica, 1980:652–654.

16. Fall M, Madersbacher H. Peripheral electrical stimulation. In: Mundy AR, Stephenson TP, Wein AJ, eds. Urodynamics. Principles, practice and application, 2nd ed. London: Churchill Livingstone, 1994:495–520.

17. Kralj B, Šuhel P. The results of treatment of female urinary incontinence by functional electrical stimulation. Presented at the Third Mediterranean Conference on Biomedical and Biological Engineering, Portorož, 1983.

18. Kralj B, Lukanovič A. Urinary incontinence in elderly women—treatment with functional electrical stimulation. In: Proceedings of the Seventh Congress of the International Society of Electrophysiological Kinesiology, Held and Enschede. Amsterdam: Excerpta Medica, 1988:161–164.

19. Kralj B. Zdravljenje urgentne inkontinence s funkcionalno električno stimulacijo. In: Vodušek DB, ed. Motnje kontinence in potence pri nevroloških bolnikih, urodinamska diagnostika, konzervativno zdravljenje urinske inkontinence, operativno zdravljenje urinske inkontinence. Drugi jugoslovanski simpozij o nevrourologiji in urodinamiki. Zbornik. Ljubljana: Univerzitetni klinični center, 1987:121–122.

20. Kralj B. Terapia della sindrome dell'uretra instabile con la stimolazione elettrica funzionale. In: Secondo Congresso Nazionale dell'Associazione Italiana di Urologia Ginecologica. L'Uretra Femminile, Roma 1992:145–148.

21. Kralj B. Treatment of urethral and detrusor instability with functional electrical stimulation. Presented at the Fourth Vienna Workshop on Functional Electrostimulation, Baden/Vienna, Austria, 1992.

CHAPTER 42

Suburethral Sling Procedures

Nicolette S. Horbach

Introduction

Suburethral sling procedures have traditionally been reserved for the treatment of recurrent stress urinary incontinence. This is because of the technical difficulties of the operation and the increased reported complications after a sling procedure. More recently, sling procedures have gained popularity as a treatment option for women with intrinsic urethral sphincter deficiency, especially in the presence of concomitant urethrovesical junction hypermobility. The physician who undertakes the evaluation and management of urinary incontinence must be cognizant of the indications for a suburethral sling procedure and must consider this surgical option when designing a management plan.

Historical Background

Suburethral sling procedures for the treatment of stress urinary incontinence were first introduced by von Giordano in 1907 using a gracilis muscle flap (1). Since that time, numerous modifications of both the surgical approach and the materials used for the sling have been published. Early pyramidalis muscle slings were ultimately abandoned because of the difficulty in maintaining the muscle's blood supply and the mechanical problems associated with incorporating a bulky tissue beneath the urethra. To alleviate these problems, Aldridge (2) chose to use two transverse strips of rectus fascia, which were detached at their lateral margins and then sutured below the urethra via a separate vaginal incision. Studdiford (3) modified the

Aldridge approach by passing a single continuous strip of rectus fascia attached at one lateral margin under the urethra. He then reattached the free end to the rectus fascia on the contralateral side. Given the difficulty of harvesting rectus fascia in women with prior abdominal surgery, several investigators attempted to use other autologous materials. In 1949 Shaw used fascia lata as the sling material, which can be harvested using a Masson or Wilson fascial stripper (1). The most recent advance is the use of a vaginal wall patch as a sling to support the urethra as advocated by Raz et al. (4).

Although organic tissues offer the advantages of being readily accessible and rarely rejected, mobilization of autologous fascia is at times difficult because of poor tissue quality or inadequate fascial length. Thus, some investigators attempted to use synthetic materials to serve as the sling. Nylon or Mersilene (polyethylene) strips, 0.5 cm in diameter, were initially chosen because they were thought to provide improved tensile strength compared with fascia (5, 6). However, under tension, these grafts formed a taut narrow cord, which resulted in urethral obstruction and a number of urethral transections (7).

Moir (7) substituted Mersilene gauze, 2.5 cm in diameter, for the narrow Mersilene ribbon and showed a decreased incidence of postoperative complications. Marlex mesh (polypropylene) was preferred by Morgan (8) because of its inert properties and its ability to be incorporated into the surrounding tissue without the extensive scarring associated with Mersilene gauze. The results of several studies using an inert Silastic band (9) or a Gore-tex (polytetrafluoroethylene) (10, 11) sling have been published. Theoretically, their porous nature makes these materials less prone to infection or rejection than the traditional synthetic meshes. The silastic band prevents adhesion formation; this allows the sling tension to be adjusted on follow-up visits if necessary. Obviously, the ideal material—one that is easily accessible; provides adequate tensile strength; and carries no risk of infection, rejection, or excessive scarring—has yet to be discovered.

Mechanism

In most patients, genuine stress incontinence is due to loss of the normal anatomic support of the urethra and urethrovesical junction that prevents stabilization of this area during increases in intraabdominal pressure associated with coughing, lifting, exercise, or straining (12). Standard retropubic incontinence procedures are designed to restore the normal function of the urethral continence mechanism by stabilization of the adjacent vaginal supportive tissues. Sudden increases in intraabdominal pressure are then transmitted equally to the proximal urethra and to the bladder. The urethral pressure continues to exceed intravesical pressure, and urinary continence is maintained. Unfortunately, at least 5–15% of patients experience persistent or recurrent stress incontinence after retropubic procedures, often despite successful anatomic positioning of the urethra (13).

The purpose of a suburethral sling procedure is to restore normal urethrovesical junction support (similar to the retropubic operations) and to mechanically compress or kink the proximal urethra during increases in intraabdominal pressure. This compression results in an increase in urethral outflow resistance that is believed to contribute to a successful surgical outcome but also accounts for many of the complications associated with a sling procedure (14–19).

Indications

In the past, sling procedures were advocated solely for the treatment of recurrent stress incontinence, especially in those women with decreased mobility of the ure-

Table 42.1. Indications for Suburethral Sling Procedures

Recurrent genuine stress incontinence
Intrinsic urethral sphincteric deficiency
Urethrovesical junction hypermobility
Fixed urethra and urethrovesical junction[a]
Medical conditions that may predispose to surgical failure
Chronic bronchitis
Asthma
Chronic steroid use
Congenital tissue weakness
Severe obesity
Recreational or occupational heavy lifting or high impact

[a]Patients with this condition may not be good candidates for a sling; see text for explanation.

thra secondary to postoperative scarring (19, 20). Many believed that patients with a fixed nonfunctioning urethra were not good candidates for a repeat retropubic procedure, preferring instead a suburethral sling procedure due to the partially obstructive nature of the operation (21). It now appears that the sling procedure is indicated in women with intrinsic urethral sphincteric dysfunction, especially those with urethrovesical junction hypermobility, and may be indicated as a primary procedure in a select group of high-risk patients (10, 22, 23). Table 42.1 lists the current indications for a sling procedure.

Numerous investigators attempted to delineate risk factors associated with failure of standard antiincontinence procedures for stress incontinence and to determine preoperatively which patients should be considered for an alternative surgical approach such as a suburethral sling procedure. In 1981, McGuire (13) reported that 75% of his patients who failed multiple surgical procedures for stress incontinence had evidence of poor intrinsic urethral function with or without loss of anatomic support as indicated by low (<20 cm H_2O) urethral closure pressures. He achieved surgical success in these patients with low urethral pressures after a fascial sling operation (22). Similarly, in a retrospective study of 86 patients, Sand et al. (24) reported a threefold increased risk of failure of a Burch retropubic urethropexy in patients with low preoperative urethral closure pressure (≤20 cm H_2O) compared with patients with normal pressure urethra.

As a result of McGuire's initial reports, other investigators examined the surgical outcome of women with low urethral pressures after a variety of surgical procedures as shown in Table 42.2. Clearly, women with low preoperative urethral closure pressure implying poor intrinsic sphincteric function comprise a high-risk group for failing standard surgery. However, another question remains: what is the impact of performing incontinence surgery in women with a well-supported urethra as indicated by a negative cotton swab test regardless of intrinsic urethral sphincter function? Bergman et al. (25) reported a fivefold increased risk of failing a Burch urethropexy or a Pereyra needle suspension in women with a negative cotton swab test that was unrelated to their preoperative urethral closure pressure. Summitt et al. (26) reported a 20% cure rate in women with low urethral pressures and a well-supported urethra compared with a 93% cure rate in the same group of women with a urethrovesical junction hypermobility after a suburethral sling procedure. Thus, it appears that intrinsic urethral function is not the only determinant of surgical outcome. Women with intrinsic urethral deficiency in the presence of a well-supported urethra may not be good candidates for a number of the standard operations, including a sling procedure, unless intraoperative urethrolysis is performed to remobilize this tissue at the time of the sling. Rather, these patients with fixed support and intrinsic urethral dysfunction may be better treated with periurethral injections of bulking agents.

Women with conditions that make them high risk for failing standard incontinence procedures may also be considered for a suburethral sling procedure. Severe chronic pulmonary disease such as bronchitis or asthma may lead to repetitive coughing or the use of steroids. High-impact recreational or occupational activities or congenital tissue weakness may also compromise a standard surgical repair. A sling procedure may be an alternative for these women with predisposing medical or lifestyle factors, although the data in this area are sparse.

Contraindications

A number of clinical conditions exist that are relative contraindications to a sling procedure as shown in Table 42.3 (21, 27). It is, therefore, essential that an adequate preoperative evaluation be completed to detect these potential problems before proceeding with surgery. Given the risk of postoperative voiding difficulties after a sling procedure, a patient must be both mentally and physically willing and able to perform intermittent self-catheterization. This should be addressed with the patient preoperatively, and she should be able to demonstrate her ability to perform self-catheterization before undergoing surgery.

Women with large atonic or areflexic bladders and high postvoid residuals may develop complete urinary retention after surgery. These patients must consider themselves candidates for lifelong intermittent

Table 42.2. Surgical Outcome in Women With Low Urethral Pressure After Various Incontinence Procedures

Author	Burch	Burch-Ball	Pereyra	Stamey	Sling
Bergman (1989)	65%				
Bergman (1991)		90%			
Koonings (1990)	67%		77%		
Richardson (1991)	85%			40%	
Summitt (1992)					82%

Table 42.3. Contraindication for a Suburethral Sling Procedure

Unwillingness or inability to perform self-catheterization
Atonic or areflexic bladder with elevated postvoid residual
Neurogenic bladder
Severe detrusor instability
Vesicoureteral reflux
History of pelvic radiation[a]
Vesico- or urethrovaginal fistula[a]

[a]Sling may be considered if concomitant Martius graft is performed to ensure adequate tissue between the sling and the urethra.

self-catheterization postoperatively. A history of pelvic irradiation or the presence of a urinary fistula may predispose the operative site to tissue breakdown. To prevent this, a Martius muscle flap may be mobilized and inserted between the urethra and vaginal mucosa at the time of the sling procedure.

Considerable debate exists in the literature regarding whether the sling operation should be recommended in women with mixed stress and urge incontinence. McGuire (21) found that 40% of patients with preoperative detrusor instability had resolution of their urge incontinence after abdominal retropubic surgery. He was unable to predict preoperatively on the basis of the degree of detrusor instability which patients would have a favorable surgical outcome. He also found that in 10–15% of cases, the detrusor instability worsened postoperatively. Given the obstructive nature of the sling procedure, it should not be unexpected to encounter worsening of detrusor instability after this operation.

The concern in patients with de novo or persistent detrusor instability postoperatively is the development of a hypertrophic detrusor muscle, because it contracts against a partially obstructed urethra, leading to more voiding dysfunction. High amplitude (over 40 cm H_2O) uninhibited detrusor contractions that occur in the presence of an obstructed or partially obstructed urethra may also predispose the patient to vesicoureteral reflux. The ureter becomes the low-pressure outlet in this situation. Ureteral reflux places the patient at risk for recurrent infections and/or upper tract injury. Because of the concern of worsening detrusor instability and vesicoureteral reflux, some experts recommend that a suburethral sling procedure should only be performed in patients with mixed incontinence after aggressive medical management of detrusor instability. Women who experience persistent uninhibited detrusor contractions despite medical intervention should undergo a sling procedure only if the contractions occur at >200 mL bladder volume and/or are less than 40 cm H_2O in amplitude. If a patient experiences large amplitude contractions at <200 mL volume, the surgeon should reconsider proceeding with a sling operation. If a sling is used, consideration should be made to per-

forming it concomitantly with hypogastric nerve resection or bladder augmentation to eliminate the detrusor instability. The patient should be instructed that she will probably require chronic self-catheterization postoperatively. The use of a sling procedure is also discouraged in patients with a neurogenic bladder because of the same risks of obstructive voiding and vesicoureteral reflux.

Preoperative Evaluation

It is essential that patients complete a thorough preoperative evaluation before surgery is contemplated to ensure that the diagnosis of genuine stress incontinence is correct. Other causes for urinary leakage that may not be amenable to surgery must be excluded, including significant detrusor instability, overflow incontinence secondary to an atonic bladder, a urethral or bladder fistula, or urethral dysfunction such as uninhibited urethral relaxation. Contraindications for a sling operation should also be sought. A history, physical examination, postvoid residual, urine culture, assessment of urethrovesical junction mobility (cotton swab test), cystourethroscopy, and multichannel urethrocystometry with urethral pressure profilometry and/or leak point pressure should be performed in all patients before undergoing a sling procedure. Preoperative voiding patterns must be determined to detect patients at risk for significant postoperative retention. Patients must be warned of the need for prolonged postoperative bladder drainage, and the possibility of intermittent self-catheterization on a temporary or permanent basis should be discussed. Patients unwilling to learn self-catheterization are not candidates for a sling operation.

Technique

The descriptions of most sling procedures are similar and differ in only three essential factors. First, organic or inorganic materials may be chosen as the sling. In contrast to organic slings, synthetic materials are far more accessible but are associated with the increased risk of graft infection or rejection. Second, the surgery may be performed entirely through an abdominal incision with tunneling under the urethra and bladder base, or a combination vaginal and abdominal approach may be preferred. The use of a separate vaginal incision reduces the likelihood of urethral trauma, and in the antibiotic era, it does not appear to increase the risk of significant postoperative infection. Finally, although most investigators recommend securing the sling to the rectus fascia, some have advocated an alternative attachment site, the ileopectinal ligament, because of the success of the Burch retropubic urethropexy (8).

Rectus Fascia Sling

A suburethral sling procedure using rectus fascia as advocated by McGuire and Wan (28) can be performed in the following manner. After routine intraoperative abdominal-perineal-vaginal preparation, the anterior vaginal submucosal layer is infiltrated with normal saline or dilute vasopressin in saline solution (1:10 dilution). The anterior vaginal mucosa is incised from near the vaginal apex to 1.5 cm proximal to the urethral meatus. The vaginal mucosa is dissected from the underlying tissue laterally to the descending pubic ramus. A 16–18F Foley catheter is then inserted to drain the bladder and delineate the urethra and urethrovesical junction.

Transvaginal perforation of the endopelvic fascia is accomplished by blunt dissection with the surgeon's finger along the posterior surface of the inferior pubic ramus (Fig. 42.1). If scarring is present from a prior retropubic operation, access to the retropubic space may be gained by sharp dissection with a tonsil clamp or Metzembaum scissors. To avoid bladder injury during entry, it is essential that no tissue is present between the surgeon's finger or clamp and the posterior pubic ramus. The position of the urethra should be confirmed by palpation of the catheter within the urethra. Excess medial dissection will result in injury to the urethra. However, dissection that proceeds lateral to the pubic tubercle increases the risk of injury to the

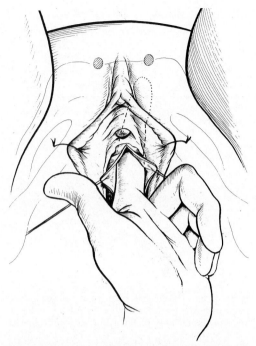

Figure 42.1. The anterior vaginal wall has been opened and the vaginal mucosa reflected laterally. With the surgeon's finger at approximately a 45-degree angle against the posterior pubic symphysis, the endopelvic fascia is perforated to enter the retropubic space. (From Stanton SL, Tanagho EA (eds). Surgery of female incontinence. 2nd ed. Berlin: Springer-Verlag, 1986.)

ilioinguinal nerve. Using delayed absorbable suture, the suburethral tissue is plicated, preferably in two layers, over the future graft site and correction of any cystocele is accomplished in the usual manner. The vaginal field is then packed while the abdominal aspect of the surgery proceeds.

A suprapubic incision is made and carried down to the rectus fascia. The fascia is opened and a 10- to 15-cm-long tapered fascial strip is mobilized from the lower aspect of the rectus incision as shown in Figure 42.2. Use of the upper aspect of the fascial incision to create the sling may make subsequent closure of the rectus fascia more difficult. The fascial strip should be approximately 0.5 cm wide at the ends and 1–1.5 cm wide in the middle. This wider portion is placed under the urethrovesical junction and proximal urethra to distribute the upward force of the sling over a wider area, decreasing the risk of urethral transection that may

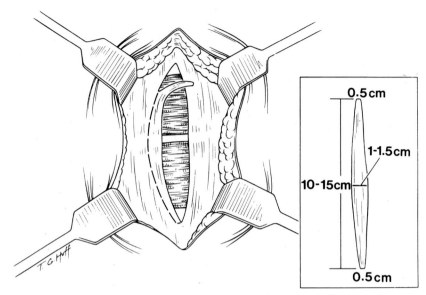

Figure 42.2. The fascial strip for the sling is harvested from the lower aspect of the fascial incision. Note the dimensions of the sling with the tapered ends and wider central portion. (From Hurt WG [ed]. Urogynecologic surgery. Gaithersburg, MD; Aspen, 1992.)

occur if a narrower sling is used. Once harvested, nonabsorbable sutures are sewn into each end of the sling perpendicular to the long axis of the graft or at such an angle that the sutures will not tear out of the longitudinally oriented fascial fibers.

The abdominal side of the sling tunnel is located by retracting the lateral aspect of the rectus muscle medially near its insertion into the pubic bone. Dissection of the overlying tissues in this area allows access to the lateral retropubic space. With the vaginal surgeon's finger pushing upward into the retropubic space, a uterine packing forceps is advanced from the abdominal field. The vaginal finger then guides the packing forceps from the abdominal incision through the retropubic space into the vaginal field as shown in Figure 42.3. Because of the lateral nature of the sling passage, the surgeon must be cognizant of the location of the obturator foreamen to avoid trauma to its contents. The sutures at the ends of the fascial graft are grasped and elevated through the retropubic space into the abdominal field (Fig. 42.4). The suture ends are brought out through small stab incisions in the lower aspect of the rectus fascia and then passed through a small pledget of fascia or synthetic material (Fig. 42.5). Before tying down the sling and closing

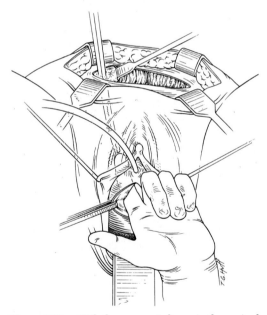

Figure 42.3. With the surgeon's finger in the vaginal tunnel, the packing forceps is guided through the retropubic space into the vaginal field. (From Hurt WG [ed]. Urogynecologic surgery. Gaithersburg, MD: Aspen, 1992.)

the incisions, cystoscopy must be performed to rule out bladder or urethral injury and to aid in the determination of correct sling tension. Partial closure of the urethrovesical junction with elevation of the sling should be documented during urethroscopy. Complete closure of the junction will result in an increased risk of postoperative voiding dysfunction. The four corners of the suburethral portion of the sling are sutured in place beneath the proximal urethra using absorbable suture and the vaginal incision closed. The rectus fascia is closed. The sutures at the end of the sling are then tied down to the predetermined tension. Excess tension should be avoided. A suprapubic catheter is inserted, and a vaginal pack placed for 24 hours. Prophylactic intravenous antibiotics (cephalosporin) may be administered as indicated. Voiding trials can begin on postoperative day 2–3. Removal of the suprapubic catheter occurs once postvoid residuals remain below 100 ml and do not exceed one fourth of the volume spontaneously voided for 12–24 hours.

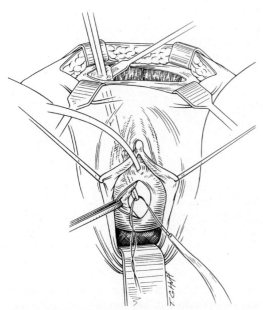

Figure 42.4. The sutures at the end of the sling are grasped and the packing forceps elevated to pass the sling ends into the abdominal field. (From Hurt WG [ed]. Urogynecologic surgery. Gaithersburg, MD: Aspen, 1992.)

Other Sling Procedures

Other organic or synthetic materials may be substituted as the sling. This may be necessary in women who have undergone numerous lower abdominal procedures where the rectus fascia is expected to be severely scarred and immobile. Fascia lata may be harvested using a Masson or Wilson fascial stripper. Alternatively, 2.0- to 3.0-cm-wide strips of Marlex, Silastic, or polytetrafluoroethylene may be used. The vaginal mucosa is opened, reflected laterally, and the endopelvic fascia perforated from below similarly to the rectus fascia sling. A smaller abdominal incision is made because the ends of the sling are brought into the abdominal field more medially through the rectus muscles as illustrated in Figure 42.6. Cystoscopy is performed to ensure that no injury has occurred and to determine correct tension of the sling before suturing the sling into place below the urethra and to the rectus fascia with nonabsorbable sutures.

Another variant on the sling procedure is that described by Karram and Bhatia (29) in which a patch of fascia lata is used suburethrally. Sutures are placed through the lateral margin of the patch, brought out through the

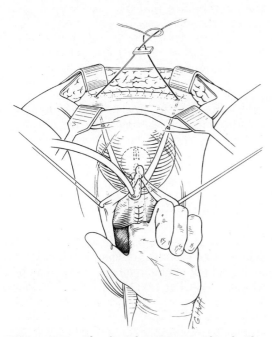

Figure 42.5. The fascial incision is closed. The sutures have been placed through the lower aspect of the rectus incision and will be tried down over a pledget. (From Hurt WG [ed]. Urogynecologic surgery. Gaithersburg, MD: Aspen, 1992.)

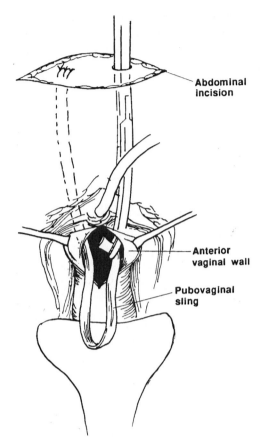

Abdominal
incision

Anterior
vaginal wall

Pubovaginal
sling

Figure 42.6. The strip of fascia lata has been passed through the retropubic tunnels and will be secured to the rectus fascia. Note that the incisions on the rectus fascia are more medial than in the procedure described by McGuire. (From Benson JT [ed]. Female pelvic floor disorders: investigation and management. New York: Norton, 1992.)

retropubic tunnel, and subsequently secured to the rectus fascia. This approach can also be done with a synthetic patch to minimize the amount of foreign material used. In 1989, Raz et al. (4) published their technique of a four-corner vaginal patch sling procedure.

Cure Rates

The surgical success rate of sling procedures reported in the current literature ranges from 70 to 100% (19, 22, 30–33). For organic slings, subjective cure rates vary from 75 to 100%. Only Low (31) and Parker et al. (32) have evaluated surgical outcome on the basis of objective criteria with 95% and 84% rates, respectively. The cure rates using inorganic sling materials are similar to those seen with autologous grafts. Subjective cure rates range from 59 to 95%, whereas objective rates are 70–85% (7–11, 33). Some authors note an improvement rate of 4–25% over and above those patients who were surgically cured (33). Most authors stress that an improvement in the surgical outcome is often obtained as the surgeon gains experience with the procedure.

The variation in reported surgical cure rates is influenced by a number of factors. Multiple modifications of the sling procedure have been described in the literature, and this makes it difficult to compare the results of one author's experience with another's. Reports may include patients with both primary and recurrent stress incontinence. Because of the poorer surgical outcome in women with a prior history of unsuccessful antiincontinence surgery (13, 22), studies including mainly patients with recurrent incontinence often report a higher failure rate. Few studies control for other preoperative variables that may predispose the patient to surgical failure. This is especially true of coexistent detrusor instability. The length of follow-up varies widely in the published series, from 3 months to over 15 years in one report. Finally, the definition and method of assessing cure is inconsistent in the literature. Ideally, specific guidelines defining surgical cure should be established to facilitate comparison of the many sling materials and procedures.

Urodynamic Changes

Numerous studies examined the effect of surgery on objective urodynamic parameters in an attempt to elucidate the mechanism of surgical cure (10, 14–18, 22, 34). Surgical success could not be consistently predicted on the basis of changes in the static measurements of functional urethral length or maximum urethral closure pressure. The two postoperative changes that do appear to be consistent throughout the literature are an improvement in pressure transmission ratios and a reduction in peak flow rate during voiding. Three reports that have measured the differential changes in pressure transmission to the urethra and the bladder found a postoperative ratio of 100% or more compared with preoperative values of 70–90% (16–18). The improvement is seen primarily in the proximal one half to three quarters of the urethra and appears to be correlated with surgical success. These results are in keeping with the proposed mechanism of cure for the sling procedure. The postoperative reduction in peak flow rate during voiding implies an increase in urethral outflow resistance after the sling operation (17, 18).

Complications

Sling procedures are usually associated with a greater incidence of intraoperative and postoperative complications than other incontinence operations. Sling procedures with inorganic materials tend to have more complications than those with organic materials as illustrated in Table 42.4. Because of its effect on urethral outflow resistance, the most common problems associated with the sling operation are voiding difficulties and urinary retention (6, 20). This is especially true in patients who are unable to generate a detrusor contraction during voiding preoperatively. Patients may complain of urgency and frequency symptoms in the absence of true voiding dysfunction (8, 10). Recurrent

urinary tract infections are also a problem that can be exacerbated by elevated postvoid residuals (8, 10, 27). Urethral injuries may be prevented by careful dissection in the vaginal field with a urethral catheter in place. An intraoperative cystotomy, especially in the patient with a history of retropubic surgery, can often be avoided by entering the retropubic space abdominally by sharp dissection under direct visualization. It is crucial that any suspected bladder injury or the presence of the sling in the bladder be evaluated intraoperatively by cystoscopy. If necessary, removal and repositioning of the sling can be accomplished. Adequate postoperative bladder drainage ensures satisfactory healing of the injury without the need to close to cystotomy.

A number of complications appear to be associated with the use of a synthetic material for the sling. The need for sling removal due to erosion (6, 9, 18) through the urethra or due to abdominal sinus tract formation (10) has been encountered in a small group of patients. Poor healing of the vaginal mucosa over the inert sling material has also been reported (33, 35, 36). To prevent this, overzealous thinning of the vaginal mucosa during dissection should be avoided. If the mucosa is thin, a layer of submucosal vaginal tissue can be brought over the sling to interpose tissue between the sling and the vaginal mucosa. Because of the difficulties with inorganic slings, some authors have recommended only using autologous materials for the graft until a better synthetic substitute is found.

Table 42.4.   Summary of Complication Rates After Suburethral Sling Procedures

Complication	Organic Sling (%) (n = 656)	Inorganic Sling (%) (n = 956)
Urinary retention	7.8 ± 0.2	8.1 ± 3.2
Detrusor instability		
De novo	3.4 ± 0.1	14.5 ± 6.6
Persistent	8.6 ± 2.9	8.8 ± 1.3
Frequency	6.6 ± 5.3	20.7 ± 8.9
Wound infection	2.6 ± 1.8	7.8 ± 1.9
Urinary tract infection	8.6 ± 0.3	11.9 ± 0.1
Urethral/bladder injury	4.2 ± 1.8	6.5 ± 2.5
Sling erosion	0.5 ± 0.5	9.4 ± 3.1
Sling revision	3.3 ± 0.1	24.2
Sling removal	0	6.6 ± 1.3
Fistula tract	1.5 ± 1.6	3.7 ± 0.6

Summary

The suburethral sling procedure is indicated in patients with recurrent genuine stress incontinence, intrinsic sphincter deficiency, or in high-risk patients with primary incontinence. An adequate preoperative evaluation is essential. The choice of sling material and operative approach should be at the surgeon's discretion, realizing the advantages and disadvantages of each decision. Surgical outcome, especially in cases of recurrent leakage, is often better than that obtained by standard retropubic procedures. Postoperative complications can be minimized by meticulous preoperative evaluation and attention to the details of surgical technique.

REFERENCES

1. Hofenfellner R, Petrie E. Sling procedures in surgery. In: Stanton SL, Tanagho E, eds. Surgery of female incontinence. 2nd ed. Berlin: Springer-Verlag, 1986:105–113.
2. Aldridge AH. Transplantation of fascia for relief of urinary stress incontinence. Am J Obstet Gynecol 1942;44:398–411.
3. Studdiford WE. Transplantation of abdominal fascia for relief of urinary stress incontinence. Am J Obstet Gynecol 1944;47:764–775.
4. Raz S, Siegel AL, Short JL, Synder JA. Vaginal wall sling. J Urol 1989;141:43–46.
5. Williams TJ, TeLinde RW. The sling operation for urinary incontinence using mersilene ribbon. Obstet Gynecol 1962;19:241–245.
6. Ridley JG. Appraisal of the Goebell-Frankenheim-Stoekel sling procedure. Am J Obstet Gynecol 1966;95:714–721.
7. Moir JC. The gauze-hammock operation: a modified Aldridge sling procedure. J Obstet Gynaecol Br Commonw 1968;75:1–13.
8. Morgan JE. A sling operation using Marlex polypropylene mesh for treatment of recurrent stress incontinence. Am J Obstet Gynecol 1970;106:369–377.
9. Stanton SL, Brindley GS, Holmes DM. Silastic sling for urethral sphincter incompetence in women. Br J Obstet Gynaecol 1985;92:747–750.
10. Horbach NS, Blanco JS, Ostergard DR, et al. A suburethral sling procedure with polytetrafluoroethylene for the treatment of genuine stress incontinence in patients with low urethral closure pressure. Obstet Gynecol 1988;71:648–652.
11. Summitt RL, Bent AE, Ostergard DR, Harris TA. Suburethral sling procedure for genuine stress incontinence and low urethral closure pressure. A continued experience. Int Urogynecol J 1992;3:18–21.
12. Enhorning G. Simultaneous recording of intraurethral and intravesical pressure: a study of urethral closure pressure and stress incontinence in women. Acta Chir Scand 1961;276(Suppl):1–68.
13. McGuire EJ. Urodynamic findings in patients after failure of stress incontinence operations. Prog Clin Biol Res 1981;78:351–360.
14. Henriksson L, Ulmsen U. A urodynamic evaluation of the effects of abdominal urethrocystopexy in women with stress incontinence. Am J Obstet Gynecol 1978;113:78–82.
15. Obrink A, Bunne G. The margin of incontinence after three types of operation for stress incontinence. Scand J Urol Nephrol 1978;12:209–214.
16. Hilton P, Stanton SL. Clinical and urodynamic evaluation of the polypropylene (Marlex) sling for genuine stress incontinence. Neurourol Urodyn 1983;2:145–153.
17. Rottenberg RD, Weil A, Brioschi PA, Bischof P, Frauer F. Urodynamic and clinical assessment of the lyodura sling operation for urinary stress incontinence. Br J Obstet Gynaecol 1985;92:829–834.
18. Hilton P. A clinical and urodynamic study comparing the Stamey bladder neck suspension and suburethral sling procedures in the treatment of genuine stress incontinence. Br J Obstet Gynaecol 1989;96:213–220.
19. Beck RP, McCormick RN, Nordstrom L. The fascia lata sling procedure for treating recurrent genuine stress incontinence of urine. Obstet Gynecol 1988;72:699–703.
20. Morgan JE, Farrow GA, Stewart FE. The Marlex sling operation for the treatment of recurrent stress urinary incontinence. A 16-year review. Am J Obstet Gynecol 1985;151:224–226.
21. McGuire EJ. Abdominal procedures for stress incontinence. Urol Clin North Am 1985;12:285–296.
22. McGuire EJ, Lytton B. Pubovaginal sling procedure for stress incontinence. J Urol 1978;119:82–85.
23. McGuire EJ, Lytton B, Pepe V, Kohorn El. Stress urinary incontinence. Obstet Gynecol 1976;47:255–264.
24. Sand PK, Bowen LW, Panganiban R, Ostergard DR. The low pressure urethra as a factor in failed retropubic urethropexy. Obstet Gynecol 1987;69:399–402.
25. Bergman A, Koonings PP, Ballard CA. Negative Q-tip test as a risk factor for failed incontinence surgery in women. J Reprod Med 1989;34:193–197.
26. Summitt RL, Bent AE, Ostergard DR, Harris TA. Stress incontinence and low urethral closure pressure. Correlation of preoperative urethral hypermobility with successful suburethral sling procedures. J Reprod Med 1990;35:877–880.
27. Beck RP. The sling operation. In: Buchsbaum HJ,

Schmidt JD, eds. Gynecologic and obstetric urology, 2nd ed. Philadelphia: WB Saunders, 1982: 285–306.

28. McGuire EJ, Wan J. Pubovaginal slings. In: Hurt WG, ed. Urogynecologic surgery. Gaithersburg: Aspen, 1992:97–105.

29. Karram MM, Bhatia NN. Patch Procedure: modified transvaginal fascia lata sling for recurrent or severe stress incontinence. Obstet Gynecol 1990; 75:461–463.

30. Ghoniem GM, Shaaban A. Sub-urethral slings for treatment of stress urinary incontinence. Int Urogynecol J 1994;5:228–239.

31. Low JA. Management of severe anatomic deficiencies of urethral sphincter function by a combined procedure with a fascia lata sling. Am J Obstet Gynecol 1969;105:149–155.

32. Parker RT, Addison WA, Wilson CJ. Fascia lata urethrovesical suspension for recurrent stress urinary incontinence. Am J Obstet Gynecol 1979; 135:843–852.

33. Kersey J. The gauze hammock sling operation in the treatment of stress incontinence. Br J Obstet Gynaecol 1983;90:945–949.

34. Poliak A, Daniller Al, Liebling RW. Sling operation for recurrent stress incontinence using the tendon of the palmaris longus. Obstet Gynecol 1984;63:850–854.

35. Nichols DH. The mersilene mesh gauze hammock for severe urinary stress incontinence. Obstet Gynecol 1973;41:88–93.

36. Bent AE, Ostergard DR, Zwick-Zaffuto M. Tissue reaction to expanded polytetrafluoroethylene suburethral sling for urinary incontinence: clinical and histological study. Am J Obstet Gynecol 1993;169:1198–1204.

CHAPTER 43

Artificial Urinary Sphincter in the Treatment of Stress Incontinence in Females

Rodney A. Appell

One of the treatment goals for urinary incontinence is to establish a normal voiding pattern while allowing the patient to become dry between voids. Procedures designed to combat bladder outlet incompetence (sphincteric incontinence) are designed to close the outflow channel or restrict it. Although this may result in the prevention of urinary leakage, these procedures may lead to an obstructive voiding pattern. Only implantation of an artificial urinary sphincter allows the obstruction to be relieved at the time of voiding such that the actual voiding pattern is normalized and the desired state of dryness is accomplished.

This concept that urinary continence can be achieved by mechanical compression of the tissues without pressure necrosis and with compensation for variability in intraabdominal pressure was described by Timm in 1971 (1) and led to the development of a mechanical device to restore continence, the artificial urinary sphincter (AUS). The first implantation of an artificial sphincter in a woman was performed by Scott et al. in 1972 (2). Since then, numerous improvements in both the design of the device and surgical technique have been produced by American Medical Systems (AMS), a subsidiary of Pfizer Pharmaceuticals. All models have a reservoir placed intraabdominally to equalize the pressure of abdominal stress (Valsalva maneuver). Each model has been designed to open partially when bladder pressures ex-

ceed physiological limits; to open fully when activated; to accept the passage of a catheter without the necessity of operating the device; and, if failure would occur, to fail in the open position.

The current device (AMS Sphincter 800) is the result of a steady evolution of design improvements and the AUS is a well-accepted and successful method for restoring urinary continence in selected patients (3–6). The ideal female patient who will benefit from the AUS is one who has genuine stress incontinence associated with normal position of the bladder base but with a poorly or nonfunctioning urethral sphincteric mechanism.

Device Description

The current device in use (AMS 800) is shown in Figure 43.1 and has replaced all earlier models.

CONTROL PUMP ASSEMBLY

The control pump assembly is placed subcutaneously in one of the labia majora. It contains the one-way valves, resistors, and poppet valve. The poppet valve controls the flow of fluid from the balloon to the cuff, and if closed, it prevents the cuff from filling. This is termed the deactivation phase and can be used to avoid tissue compression beneath the

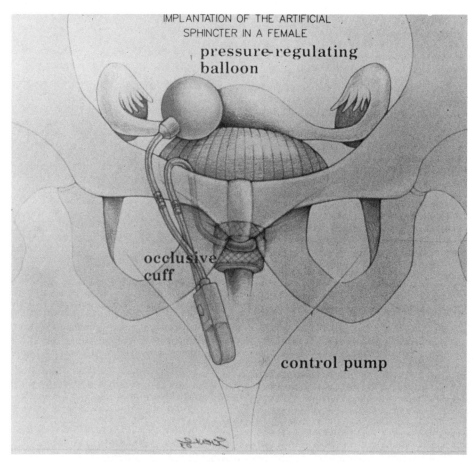

IMPLANTATION OF THE ARTIFICIAL
SPHINCTER IN A FEMALE

pressure-regulating
balloon

occlusive
cuff

control pump

Figure 43.1. The artificial urinary sphincter (AMS 800).

cuff until adequate healing has occurred. The position of the poppet valve is easily palpated through the skin because of a nipple that has been incorporated in the plastic mold of the pump-control assembly (Fig. 43.2). Pressure over this plastic nipple will close the valve, thus preventing the cuff from filling and becoming pressurized. To open the valve and activate the device requires a firm squeeze over the pump. Instrumentation of the lower urinary tract is also facilitated because the device can be deactivated by the physician or patient before cystoscopy or catheterization.

CUFF

The cuff is placed around the bladder neck and consists of an inner pliable leaflet attached to a firm Dacron backing. The smallest diameter is 4.0 cm, with increments of 0.5 cm

up to 8 cm, and then 1-cm increments up to 11 cm. The diameter of the female bladder neck in a virgin implant may vary, but the usual length required is the 7.0- or 7.5-cm cuff. Most of the mechanical failures that occurred with earlier models were secondary to a cuff leak. To address this problem, the surface-treated cuff was introduced 1983. The inner portion of the cuff is now coated with a fluorosilicone to minimize friction between the pliable leaflet and the firm Dacron backing. After introduction of this modification, cuff leaks have been nearly eliminated.

A second modification addressed the problem of pressure atrophy of the tissue beneath the cuff that, when it occurs, requires reoperation to insert a smaller cuff. To improve pressure transmission from the cuff to the lumen of the urinary tract, the Dacron backing was decreased from 2 to 1.5 cm in width. This narrow-backed cuff became available in

1987 and has further decreased the incidence of clinically significant pressure atrophy resulting in recurrence of postoperative incontinence. The currently available cuffs incorporate both the surface treatment and the narrow-back design.

BALLOON

The balloon is placed in the extraperitoneal retropubic position where it can be subjected to the effects of changes in intraabdominal pressure. This position permits the transmission of intraabdominal pressures simultaneously to the reservoir and the bladder. This feature decreases the leakage of urine in situations such as sudden straining, coughing, and sneezing. The balloon is constructed of a silicone polymer by a dipcoating process so that it provides the appropriate pressure. The thickness of the balloon wall determines the pressure. Choices of balloon pressures range from 51–60 to 71–80 cm H_2O in 10-cm H_2O increments. The choice of balloon pressure is made by the implanting surgeon. The pressure just surpassing the ac-

tive leak point pressure or voiding pressure is useful in determining which pressure-regulating balloon to use. The least amount of pressure that is capable of preventing leakage in the individual patient is desired, because erosion will occur if the cuff pressure exceeds the diastolic blood pressure.

The actual pressure of urethral closure is dependent on several factors: balloon pressure, urethral compliance, tissue perfusion, the geometric shape of the cuff, and the cuff size in relationship to the diameter of the bladder neck. The average balloon pressure used for occlusion of the bladder neck in females ranges from 51 to 70 cm H_2O and only on rare occasions does one need to use the high pressure 71- to 80-cm H_2O balloon when bladder neck tissue is extremely thickened. Once the balloon is selected, it is filled with the recommended isotonic fluid and positioned. A radiopaque contrast medium is frequently added for convenience to visualize the components in the postoperative period or for later troubleshooting, if necessary. (Information regarding the makeup of this contrast fluid is provided by American Medi-

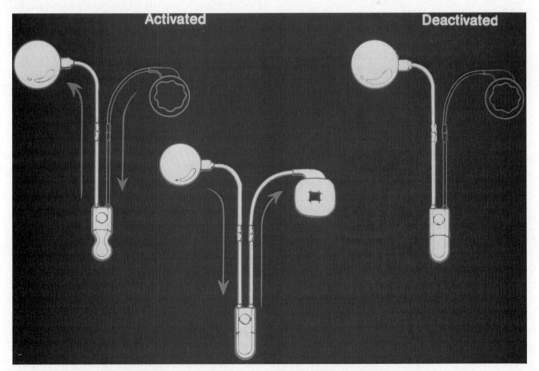

Figure 43.2. Activation and deactivation of the hydraulic system.

cal Systems, Inc., 11001 Bren Road East, Minnetonka, MN 55343.)

TUBING

Kink-resistant color-coded tubing has been added to enhance surgical implantation and decrease mechanical failure. The balloon-to-pump tubing is black, and the cuff-to-pump tubing is clear.

The device functions as follows: Squeezing the pump transfers fluid to the balloon. On releasing the pump, fluid is sucked from the cuff into the pump, and the process is repeated until the cuff is deflated as the pump flattens. The balloon begins automatic repressurization immediately, but a resistor delays the refill of the cuff sufficiently (approximately 2.5 minutes) to allow for urination. The cycle is then repeated with the next urination. The actual pressure of urethral closure, however, is dependent on multiple factors: balloon pressure, urethral compliance, tissue perfusion, the geometric shape of the cuff, and the cuff size relative to the diameter of the bladder neck.

SAFETY FEATURES

A number of safety features are inherent in the design of the device: device failure results in a decrease in pressure so that voiding can still occur, the pressure exerted by the cuff is automatically regulated by the choice of balloon, and no mechanical failure that would cause the pressure against the bladder neck to exceed the pressure generated by the balloon can occur. Because any increase in intraabdominal pressure is transmitted to the bladder, cuff, and balloon, there will be no net transfer of fluid inside the system. However, an increase in intravesical pressure alone, such as occurs during a bladder contraction, that exceeds the pressure of the balloon will overcome the resistor mechanism and fluid will flow from the cuff into the balloon, thus decreasing the occlusive pressure. The system will, therefore, release unphysiological bladder pressure caused by uninhibited bladder contractions yet will not allow stress incontinence, even though the pressures of stress usually exceed the pressure of the balloon.

Patient Selection

The AUS is most suitable for patients with pure sphincter incompetency and normal detrusor function. Patients with decreased detrusor contractility, however, may be candidates if intermittent self-catheterization or Credé voiding can be considered. The diagnosis of urethral incompetence and the status of the detrusor are determined with the use of urodynamic studies. The success of the AUS in attaining continence is definitely influenced by the presence of any bladder disease. The use of the device in the patient with a normal bladder or poor detrusor contractility with unaltered compliance is consistently associated with a high degree of success. Detrusor hyperreflexia, if found urodynamically, must be controlled before implantation of the device. Adequate bladder capacity (<125 mL) is essential, but residual urine is not a factor. Endoscopic evaluation to determine that viable tissue is present at the prospective cuff site is mandatory and also helpful in determining the proximity of the ureteral orifices to the bladder neck and the posterior segment of the urethra. The only pure contraindications to implanting the AUS are uncontrolled detrusor hyperreflexia and high-grade vesicoureteral reflux.

It is not sufficient to state that patients who have an incompetent urethra are therefore natural candidates for the AUS. They must also have adequate manual dexterity, mental capacity, and motivation to manipulate the pump mechanism each time they need to void.

Preoperative Preparation

Preoperative preparation is directed at preventing infection of the device, an obvious foreign body. Because the device is inserted into a closed space, the procedure can introduce organisms into that particular location. If there is infection after surgery, the entire device may have to be removed. Because of tissue viability, the operative site may not be as accessible to natural defense mechanisms and circulating antimicrobials. Therefore, the device and the instru-

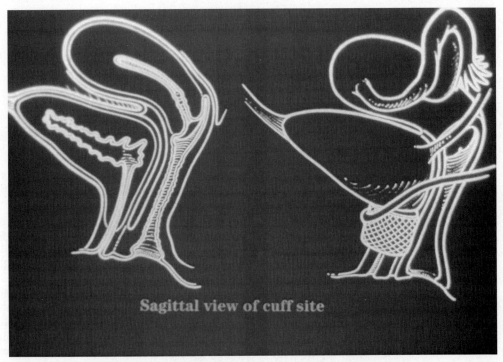

Sagittal view of cuff site

Figure 43.3. Sagittal view of cuff site and urethrovaginal septum.

ments are soaked in antimicrobials, the wound is sprayed with them, and the proper antimicrobial level is achieved in all tissues before surgery. Also, because a foreign body is being implanted, the urine must be sterile at the time of surgery. The drug, route of administration, and the length of coverage to accomplish this are a matter of individual choice, although both aerobic and anaerobic coverage is important.

Finally, it is advantageous to know whether the patient is right- or left-handed because it is much easier for the patient to operate the pump if it is placed accordingly.

Surgical Techniques

Only a small number of women have been implanted with the device because of the fear of many surgeons to approach the surgical difficulty of placing the cuff around the bladder neck. The so-called urethrovaginal septum is not a true surgical plane, and this is especially challenging in women with type III stress urinary incontinence because their urethral incompetence may occur after multiple surgical repairs for genuine stress incontinence. Even partial injury to these tissues can lead to failure related to infection or erosion of the cuff into the urethra or the vagina (Fig. 43.3). Cuff placement may be approached by means of an abdominal or a transvaginal fashion. Before describing the two approaches, it is important to recognize a few general precautions that are important regardless of the chosen approach. First, excessive handling of the device should be avoided. Silicone-coated hemostats are used for cross-clamping the tubing. This will prevent damage to the tubing and a potential leak. Second, blood must not enter the tubing because it will block the one-way valves in the pump assembly and result in device malfunction. Liberal irrigation is performed during all connections to prevent this problem. Third, avoid the use of surgical drains as these may provide access for organisms to enter and contaminate the prosthesis. Finally, antibiotic spray is used liberally throughout the procedure to prevent infection.

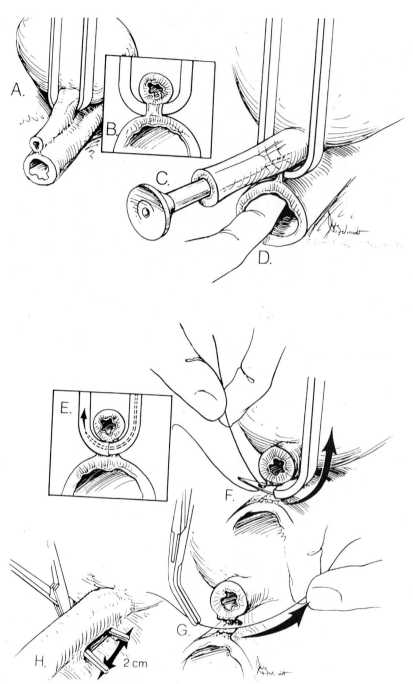

Figure 43.4.   Cutter Clamp pinches tissues for identification before cutting (**A** and **B**). Cystoscopy shows urethra clear (**C** and **D**). Cutting blade advanced into opposite limb of device (**E**). Instrument dismantled to expose blade; note "eye" for receiving suture (**F**). Instrument withdrawn with suture remaining in place to guide right-angled clamp to dilate passage for cuff placement (**G** and **H**).

After general or regional anesthesia, the patient is placed in a modified dorsal lithotomy position regardless of approach due to the fact that intraoperative cystourethroscopy is required.

ABDOMINAL APPROACH

A low Pfannenstiel incision is made down to and including the rectus fascia (5). The recti muscles are transected as described by Cherney to gain access to the retropubic space. The prevesical space is entered and dissection continued down to the level of the bladder neck. This part of the dissection may be tedious if the patient has undergone previous suprapubic suspension procedures. An indwelling 16F catheter is inserted to drain the bladder, and the balloon is inflated to aid in palpation of the bladder neck. A small incision is made in the endopelvic fascia on each side of the bladder neck to allow palpation anteriorly of both the catheter and the trigone. The vagina will lie posteriorly to this plane and can be identified with the aid of a finger in the vagina. The

trigone and catheter are then grasped between the thumb and the forefinger to separate it from the anterior vaginal wall.

Dissection proceeds in the plane between the urethra and the vagina and should be performed with care because there is no anatomic plane between these two structures. The use of right-angle scissors and a large clamp greatly facilitates this part of the operation. The use of the Cutter clamp (Lone Star Manufacturing, Houston, TX) may be extremely helpful because it is used to pinch the tissues that are to be cut and provides a means of checking placement, cutting the tissue, and providing the passage of a suture to guide instruments for dilation and creation of the passage around the bladder neck (Fig. 43.4). If, however, this subtrigonal plane cannot readily be identified, it is strongly recommended that the bladder be opened at this point well above the proposed cuff site.

Once created, the subtrigonal tunnel is gently dilated to accept a 2-cm-width cuff. The cuff size is then pulled into position with the right-angle clamp, and measurement is taken to assess the cuff length (Fig. 43.5). The cuff should be snug but not obstructive.

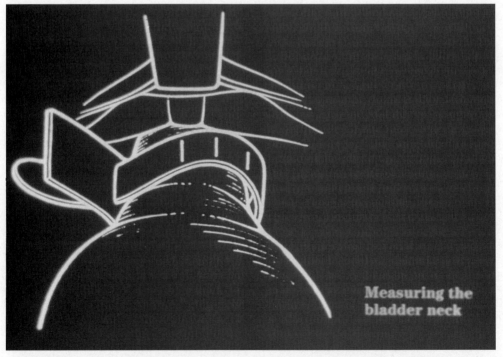

Measuring the bladder neck

Figure 43.5. Cuff sizer placed around bladder neck. (Courtesy of American Medical Systems.)

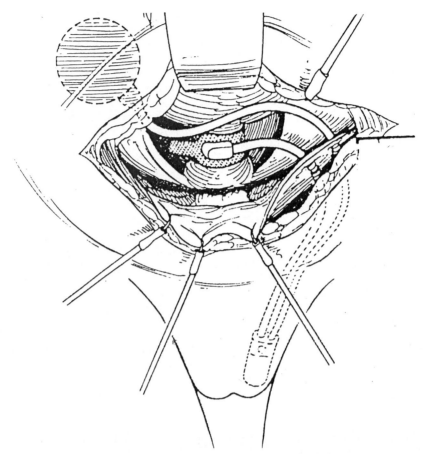

Figure 43.6. Completion of sphincter implantation.

Suture ligation readily controls the venous bleeding that almost always ensues from this dissection. The appropriately sized cuff is then slid into position, again with the use of the right-angle clamp, and snapped closed. The tubing is routed through the layers of the anterior abdominal wall to emerge in the subcutaneous position at the left-hand side of the incision with the aid of a tubing passer.

Currently, 22 mL of the appropriate solution is placed directly into the balloon, leaving the cuff empty. The balloon is then placed in the prevesical extraperitoneal space, and the tubing is routed in a similar manner to that described for the cuff.

Blunt dissection into one labium majorum is performed to create a space for the pump. The pump is then placed in this dissected space so that it rests immediately beneath the skin to allow for easy palpation and manipu-

lation by the patient. The appropriate connections between the various components are made after excising redundant tubing. A temporary connection is made between the pressure-regulating balloon and the cuff, allowing the cuff to "charge" meaning to be pressurized to its equilibrium state. This connection is then taken down, and the balloon is aspirated and refilled with exactly 22 mL of the recommended fluid. Permanent connections are then completed between the pump and the cuff and between the pump and the pressure-regulating balloon (Fig. 43.6). A functional check of the prosthesis is performed by cycling the device with cystoscopic control, and at the conclusion, the prosthesis is deactivated by squeezing the control pump to deflate the cuff completely and allowing the pump to refill partially for 10 seconds before pressing the deactivation poppet (Fig. 43.2).

Hemostasis is exceedingly important because drains are not used routinely. The abdominal incision is then closed in layers, taking care not to inadvertently puncture the prosthesis. After closure of the skin incision, the device is manipulated to ensure that no kinks have been caused by the sutures. A 14F catheter is left indwelling after completion of the procedure.

TRANSVAGINAL APPROACH

The premise underlying this approach is that deliberate opening of the anterior vaginal wall aids in placement of the cuff, thus facilitating this part of the dissection. Studies using this technique do not note any increase in device infection or cuff erosion (6, 7).

The intraoperative patient position and skin preparation is identical to that described under the abdominal approach. A posterior weighted vaginal speculum is placed in position, and an inverted "U" incision in the anterior vaginal wall is made (Fig. 43.7A).

The retropubic space is then entered between the pubic bone and the endopelvic fascia, allowing mobilization of the urethra and bladder neck. Mobilization of the urethra and bladder base is extended down to the level of the ischial tuberosity using sharp and blunt dissection. The insertion of a 14F catheter and inflation of the balloon allows easy intraoperative identification of the bladder neck. The bladder neck and urethra should be completely mobilized from the pubic bone after completion of the dissection to allow passage of the calibrated cuff sizer. This passage is facilitated by passing a curved renal pedicle clamp around the bladder neck to grasp the cuff sizer, which is then replaced with the proper-sized cuff (Fig. 43.7B). Occasionally, a suprameatal incision for direct vision of the anterior aspect of the urethra and bladder neck is made if scar tissue is especially dense.

The catheter is then removed and the cuff sizer passed circumferentially around the bladder neck. The appropriately sized cuff is

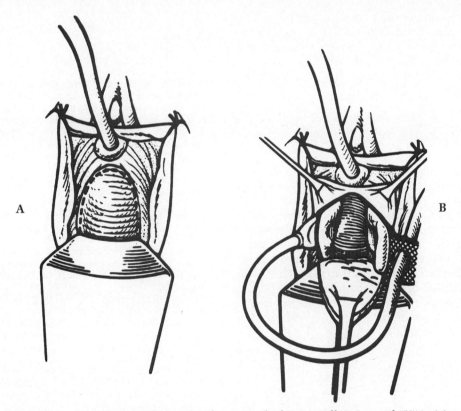

Figure 43.7. Transvaginal technique for placement of sphincter cuff. **A.** Inverted "U" incision in anterior vaginal wall. **B.** Passage of cuff around bladder neck.

inserted and snapped in position. A cystourethroscopy can be performed at this stage to ensure proper location of the cuff below the ureteric orifices and to exclude inadvertent intraoperative damage to the trigonal area of the bladder.

A small transverse lower abdominal incision is made on the ipsilateral side to where the pump will be placed, approximately 0.5 inches above the symphysis, and deepened down to the rectus fascia. The balloon can then be inserted in one of two ways. A rectus muscle splitting is performed to allow access to the retropubic space. A space is bluntly dissected in the retropubic area to accommodate the balloon. The tubing from the cuff is then passed from the vagina superiorly to exit through the lower abdominal incision using a tubing passer much as one would pass the needle carrier in a Pereyra-type bladder suspension. A space is then bluntly dissected in the ipsilateral labium majorum, and the pump is placed with the aid of an extended nasal speculum. Excess tubing is excised, and the appropriate connections are made as indicated on the color-coded tubing.

The vaginal and abdominal incision is then closed in the routine fashion, and a 14F indwelling catheter is reinserted for urinary drainage and the placement of a vaginal packing.

Postoperative Care

The catheter and vaginal pack (placed at the end of the transvaginal approach) are removed on the first postoperative day. The patient receives antibiotics for 1 week, and the device is left deactivated for 6–12 weeks. During this period, the collateral circulation should be reestablished to allow primary healing of tissues at the cuff site. This has the added benefit of eliminating immediate postoperative pump manipulation, an inherent discomfort for the patient in this early postoperative period.

Results

The results of both the abdominal approach (3–5, 8, 9) and the transvaginal approach (6, 7, 10) show comparable success with greater than 90% of patients socially continent. The success is attributed to appropriate patient selection, judicious use of antibiotics, and primary deactivation (Fig. 43.2).

Conclusions

There is a group of female patients who have persistent or recurring urinary incontinence after previous successful surgical correction of a displaced vesicourethral junction. This incontinence appears to be secondary to poor function of the urinary sphincteric mechanism. The AUS is a reliable substitute for this mechanism, allowing for unobstructed urination and offering an alternative to the various types of sling procedures. The incidence of reoperation for a cuff leak and pressure atrophy has decreased significantly after the introduction of the surface-treated narrow-back cuff. Either an abdominal or transvaginal approach can be used successfully to insert the device.

REFERENCES

1. Timm GW. An implantable incontinence device. J Biomed 1971;4:213.
2. Scott FB, Bradley WE, Timm GW. Treatment of urinary incontinence by an implantable prosthetic sphincter. Urology 1973;1:252–259.
3. Light JK, Scott FB. Management of urinary incontinence in women with the artificial urinary sphincter. J Urol 1985;134:476–478.
4. Donovan MG, Barrett DM, Furlow WL. Use of the artificial urinary sphincter in the management of severe incontinence in females. Surg Gynecol Obstet 1985;161:17–20.
5. Light JK. Abdominal approach for implantation of the AS800 artificial urinary sphincter in females. Neurourol Urodyn 1988;7:603–612.
6. Appell RA. Technique and results in the implantation of the artificial urinary sphincter in women with type III stress urinary incontinence by a vaginal approach. Neurourol Urodyn 1988;7:613–619.
7. Hadley HR. The artificial sphincter in the female. Probl Urol 1991;5:123–133.
8. Diokno AC, Hollander JB, Alderson TP. Artificial urinary sphincter for recurrent female urinary incontinence: indications and results. J Urol 1987;137:778–780.
9. Parulkar BC, Barrett DM. Application of the AS-800 artificial sphincter for intractable urinary incontinence in females. Surg Gynecol Obstet 1990;171:131–138.
10. Abbassian A. A new operation for insertion of the artificial urinary sphincter. J Urol 1988;140:512–513.

CHAPTER 44

Selection of Surgical Procedures for the Treatment of Stress Urinary Incontinence

W. Glenn Hurt

Since 1900, over 150 different surgical procedures have been recommended for the cure of stress urinary incontinence (SUI). This attests to the fact that no one operation is capable of curing all patients. It also suggests that physicians who undertake surgical treatment of the condition should be adept at performing more than one continence procedure. The selection of the surgical approach and of the operative procedure should be determined by clinical and urodynamic findings and not restricted by a surgeon's familiarity with a single procedure.

From a surgical standpoint, there are two types of SUI. One type of SUI is due to hypermobility of the urethrovesical junction in women who have an otherwise normal urethral sphincter mechanism. This type of SUI is referred to as "anatomic" SUI. A second type of SUI is due to a damaged urethral sphincter mechanism. This type of SUI is referred to as being due to intrinsic sphincter deficiency (ISD). It may or may not be associated with hypermobility of the urethrovesical junction.

In women with pure anatomic SUI, when there is a sudden increase in intraabdominal pressure, the urethrovesical junction descends, placing the urethral sphincter mechanism at an anatomic disadvantage and permitting the sudden and involuntary escape of a spurt of urine coincident with the acme of the increase in intraabdominal pressure. Most women with SUI have anatomic SUI. They need to have their hypermobile urethrovesical junction elevated to its original retropubic position and maintained in that position when there are sudden increases in intraabdominal pressure. If this is done, and if posterior rotational descent of the trigone and base of their bladder is preserved and their urethral sphincter mechanism is not damaged, their SUI can be cured. Almost all operations commonly performed for the cure of SUI are operations designed to correct anatomic SUI. In such cases, the choice of operative approach and procedure may be determined by clinical findings.

In women with SUI due to ISD, there is a loss of urine because of a damaged urethral sphincter mechanism. The coaptive forces of the urethra have been weakened. Often, their urethra has been destroyed to such an extent that it is merely a fixed and functionless drainpipe. Treatment of SUI due to ISD depends on improving coaptation of the proximal urethral lumen or partial obstruction of the urethrovesical junction. SUI due to ISD is more difficult to cure than anatomic SUI. Of all the surgical procedures recommended for the cure of SUI, those most likely to restore continence in women with ISD are a retropubic colposuspension when there is hypermobility of the urethrovesical junction and periurethral bulk injections, a suburethral sling urethropexy, or an artificial sphincter when there is limited mobility of the urethrovescial junction.

Vaginal Approach

SUI may be treated by the vaginal approach when it is associated with a significant degree of pelvic organ prolapse. The vaginal approach is more likely to be successful in the treatment of primary SUI. For best results, this approach requires healthy vaginal tissues, adequate vaginal caliber and depth, and mobility of the urethrovesical junction.

In 1913, Kelly (1) emphasized the vaginal approach in the treatment of SUI when he recommended the layering of two or three mattress sutures beneath the bladder neck. His suture technique was designed to tighten and reconstruct the "sphincter muscle." In 1937, Kennedy (2) recommended a two-layer plication of the proximal two thirds of the urethra and subsequent plication of the "voluntary sphincter." Although these operations may be effective in reducing funneling of the proximal urethra, they are limited in the extent to which they elevate and stabilize the urethrovesical junction. Despite this, the Kelly and Kennedy procedures are for many surgeons the treatment of choice for all cases of SUI. The 5-year objective cure rate for these operations has been reported to be about 40% (3). Efforts have been made to improve the cure rate by suburethral placement of a bulbocavernosus fat pad or a portion of the pubococcygeus muscle, suburethral plication of the pubourethral ligaments, or the placement of suspending sutures into the periosteum of the retropubis. Currently, the addition of one of the "needle" procedures appears to be the most predictable method of further elevating and stabilizing the urethrovesical junction when performing an anterior colporrhaphy.

The first needle procedure was introduced by Pereyra in 1959. Since that time, the initial procedure has undergone many modifications by Pereyra and others (4, 5). Today, the most effective and durable of the needle procedures is one that gathers up the endopelvic fascia and incorporates a bite of the anterior vaginal wall on either side of the urethrovesical junction. The Raz modification (5) of the Pereyra procedure is recommended. Permanent suture material should be used for suspension of the urethrovesical junction.

When performing a needle procedure, urethrocystoscopy is done to verify ureteral function, to be sure that no sutures have been placed through the bladder or urethra, and, by some, to determine the proper elevation of the urethrovesical junction. As stated above, a needle suspension of the urethrovesical junction is easily performed at the time of anterior colporrhaphy. It can also be used for prophylaxis against postoperative SUI and for additional support to the anterior vaginal wall in patients who have procidentia or posthysterectomy vaginal vault prolapse and who demonstrate SUI when their prolapse is reduced. A needle suspension of the urethrovesical junction has an initial SUI cure rate of 80–85%; however, recent reports document that these procedures tend to fail over time and the 5-year cure rate is about 45% (3).

Abdominal Approach

The current "gold standard" for the treatment of pure anatomic SUI is the abdominal retropubic urethropexy or colposuspension. It may be used to treat primary and recurrent SUI when there are good vaginal tissues, adequate vaginal caliber and depth, and hypermobility of the urethrovesical junction. A prophylactic retropubic colposuspension might be performed to prevent postoperative SUI in women undergoing abdominal sacrocolpopexy, abdominoperineal resection, or radical vulvectomy.

In 1949, Marshall, Marchetti, and Krantz (6) recommended that an abdominal retropubic vesicourethral suspension be performed for the cure of recurrent SUI. They established the importance of the abdominal retropubic approach and of elevation and stabilization of the urethrovesical junction in the cure of SUI. In 1961, Burch (7) reported a modification of the Marshall-Marchetti-Krantz (MMK) procedure for the correction of stress incontinence, cystocele, and prolapse (7). Burch placed three sutures in the perivaginal fascia on either side of the bladder neck and used them to suspend the anterior vaginal wall and the urethrovesical junction from Cooper's ligaments. This operation is recommended for women with primary and recurrent anatomic SUI.

The advantages of the Burch colposuspension over the original MMK urethropexy are as follows: it avoids urethral damage by dissection or suture placement; it uses an easily located and dependable structure (Cooper's ligament) for the suspension of the anterior vaginal wall; it corrects anterior vaginal wall prolapse; it avoids the placement of cystopexy sutures, which may contribute to urethral funneling and inhibit posterior rotational descent of the trigone and base of the bladder; and it should not be associated with an infrequent complication of the MMK procedure, osteitis pubis.

Experience has shown that prophylactic obliteration of the cul-de-sac of Douglas by a Moschcowitz or Halban procedure will reduce the incidence of enteroceles, which complicate some MMK or Burch procedures. The long-term cure rate of a Burch procedure will be improved if permanent suture material is used for the suspension. This is especially true if there is "bow-stringing" because of the failure of the anterior vaginal wall to come into direct contact with the retrosymphysis and Cooper's ligaments. The 5-year cure rate for SUI treated by a Burch colposuspension is approximately 80% (3). Thus, the cure rate as a result of this procedure appears to hold up well over time.

It is inevitable that readers will inquire about the role of the "paravaginal repair" for treating SUI. The vaginal approach to the paravaginal repair was first described by White in 1909 (8). The vaginal paravaginal repair has not been recommended for the treatment of SUI. More recently, the abdominal paravaginal repair has been popularized by Richardson et al. (9) and by Baden and Walker (10). It should be noted that in 1961, Burch tried attaching the perivaginal fascia on either side of the bladder neck to the "white line of the pelvis." He found the procedure gave "an excellent anatomical result" but stopped using the white line as the point of fixation because "it holds the sutures poorly" (7). In a more recent publication, Shull and Baden (11) state that in performing an abdominal paravaginal repair, they recommend that sutures be "placed through Cooper's ligament and tied, not to elevate the repair but to offer a safety mechanism should any of the stitches in the tendinous arch not hold." All authors who advocate the para-

vaginal repair emphasize the importance of case selection. It is a procedure primarily designed to repair lateral vaginal support defects that contribute to prolapse of the lower two thirds of the anterior vaginal wall. If a patient has a cystourethrocele and the cystourethrocele is the cause of her SUI, correction of the cystourethrocele may correct her urinary incontinence. At this time, there are no objective studies reporting on the long-term cure rate of SUI that has been treated by a paravaginal repair.

Periurethral Bulk Injections

Periurethral bulk injections of sterile nonpyrogenic purified bovine dermal glutaraldehyde cross-linked collagen ("gax collagen") are being used in the treatment of urinary incontinence due to ISD (12). Other injectables such as fat, blood, and a variety of synthetics have been used for periurethral bulking, but for a variety of reasons they have not received approval. Periurethral bulk injections are recommended for patients who have a Valsalva leak point pressure of less than 65 cm H_2O, water, low urethral closure pressure, normal anatomic relationships, and limited mobility of the urethrovesical junction. Detrusor instability that is unresponsive to medical therapy is a relative contraindication to the procedure. The short-term cure or improved rate after repeated periurethral injections is reported to be about 70%.

Periurethral bulk injections are considered a therapeutic alternative for patients who might otherwise be candidates for a suburethral sling or an artificial sphincter. It is also useful in the elderly and in high-risk patients with urogenital atrophy, minimal urethral mobility, and no significant prolapse or detrusor instability. The injections can be done in the office setting using local anesthesia. Complications are rare; the most significant are collagen sensitivity, transient urinary retention, and urinary tract infection.

Suburethral Sling

Until recently, suburethral slings were only recommended for the treatment of recurrent SUI in patients who had failed at least one abdominal retropubic procedure. Clinical findings suggesting the need for a suburethral sling included a scarred inadequate vagina, a "functionless" urethra, a persistently open vesical neck (type III incontinence), and lower urethral closure pressure (less than 20 cm H_2O) (13). More recently, it has been suggested that there are patients with primary SUI who have a congenitally short urethra or an abnormally low urethral closure pressure who are more likely to be cured by using a suburethral sling as the primary procedure. The complications (voiding dysfunction, bladder outlet obstruction, urethral erosion, vaginal erosion) associated with suburethral slings cause many surgeons to continue to restrict its use to patients with recurrent SUI and little or no evidence of detrusor instability. The sling should stabilize and support, but not unduly elevate and obstruct, the urethrovesical junction. The cure rate of recurrent SUI treated by a suburethral sling is approximately 85–90%. There are, however, a significant number of postoperative complications. These procedures may be less successful when performed in women with ISD and no mobility of the urethrovesical junction. Extensive urethrolysis may improve the cure rate under such a circumstance.

Artificial Urinary Sphincter

The artificial urinary sphincter can be used to treat recurrent intractable urinary incontinence due to ISD. Its use should be considered for patients with an anatomically intact lower urinary tract whose only other alternative is urinary diversion. Selected patients with a small capacity bladder and detrusor instability may be candidates for augmentation cystoplasty and artificial sphincter placement.

American Medical Systems supplies the only artificial urinary sphincter that is currently available. It is being placed in females by both the abdominal and the vaginal approach. It may be difficult to adjust the cuff pressure to prevent SUI without causing some urethral injury. The complications currently associated with the artificial urinary sphincter preclude its use by most surgeons treating even the most difficult cases of urinary incontinence.

REFERENCES

1. Kelly HA. Incontinence of urine in women. Urol Cut Rev 1913;17:291–293.
2. Kennedy WT. Incontinence of urine in the female, the urethral sphincter mechanism, damage of function, and restoration of control. Am J Obstet Gynecol 1937;34:576–589.
3. Elia G, Bergman A. Prospective randomized comparison of three surgical procedures for stress urinary incontinence: five year follow-up. Neurourol Urodyn 1994;13:498–500.
4. Pereyra AJ, Lebherz TB, Growdon WA, Powers JA. Pubourethral supports in perspective: modified Pereyra procedure for urinary incontinence. Obstet Gynecol 1982;59:643–648.
5. Raz S. Modified bladder neck suspension for female stress incontinence. J Urol 1981;17:82–84.
6. Marshall VF, Marchetti AA, Krantz KE. The correction of stress incontinence by simple vesicourethral suspension. Surg Gynecol Obstet 1949;88:509–518.
7. Burch JC. Urethrovaginal fixation to Cooper's ligament for correction of stress incontinence, cystocele, and prolapse. Am J Obstet Gynecol 1961;81:281–290.
8. White GR. Cystocele: a radical cure by suturing lateral sulci of vagina to white line of pelvic fascia. JAMA 1909;53:1707–1710.
9. Richardson AC, Edmonds PB, Williams NL. Treatment of stress urinary incontinence due to paravaginal fascial defect. Obstet Gynecol 1981;57:357–362.
10. Baden WF, Walker T. Urinary stress incontinence: evolution of paravaginal repair. Female Patient 1987;12:89–93.
11. Shull BL, Baden WF. A six-year experience with paravaginal defect repair for stress urinary incontinence. Am J Obstet Gynecol 1989;160:1432–1440.
12. Appell RA. Collagen injection for urinary incontinence. Urol Clin North Am 1994;21:177–182.
13. Summitt RL Jr, Bent AE, Ostergard DR, Harris TA. Suburethral sling procedure for genuine stress incontinence and low urethral closure pressure. A continued experience. Int Urogynecol J 1992;3:18–21.

CHAPTER 45

Prevention and Management of Complications after Continence Surgery

Richard C. Bump and Geoffrey W. Cundiff

Every surgeon recognizes that any surgical procedure can result in immediate and delayed postoperative complications. Many of the most severe complications are related to the patient's preexisting medical disorders, to anesthetic risks and reactions, and to restrictions in mobility imposed by postoperative discomfort or paraphernalia. Procedures performed to restore urinary continence are not spared these communal surgical risks, although they are not addressed in this chapter. Conversely, there are a number of rare and unique complications specific to individual continence procedures. Most of these problems are addressed in the several chapters concerning needle (Chapter 40), retropubic (Chapter 39), and sling procedures (Chapter 42); anterior colporrhaphy; and the artificial sphincter (Chapter 43). Although some of these problems are mentioned here, the major intent of this chapter is to concentrate on a series of continence surgery complications that transcend specific procedures. These include retropubic space hematoma, infectious and inflammatory complications, lower urinary tract injuries, postoperative retention, suprapubic catheter complications, and detrusor instability after continence surgery.

Retropubic Space Hematoma

The retropubic space is a potential space bounded by the undersurface of the rectus muscles and pubic bone anteriorly and the anterior vaginal wall, urethra, and bladder posteriorly. The space is occupied by varying amounts of fatty and areolar tissue in loose apposition to the surrounding structures. A rich thin-walled perivesical venous plexus is found under the fat, overlying the bladder and vaginal wall (1–3). The space is broadly developed and exposed, predominantly by blunt dissection in virginal cases, during the performance of exclusive transabdominal continence procedures such as the Marshall-Marchetti-Krantz (MMK) vesicourethropexy, Burch colposuspension, and paravaginal defect repair. During abdominal-vaginal needle urethropexy and sling procedures, the space is entered from the vagina by perforating the endopelvic fascia lateral to the urethra and is less extensively developed (4–6). The major complications encountered as a result of these incursions include bleeding, hematoma formation, and bacterial contamination, which can transform a hematoma into a retropubic abscess. Less common postoperative complications include clinically significant accumulations of serum or urine.

PREVENTION

Hemorrhage from the rich perivesical venous plexus can be considerable during an abdominal colposuspension. This is particularly true if an extensive defatting of the paravaginal fascia is performed in an effort to promote fibrosis and fixation of the vaginal wall to the retropubis. The use of permanent rather than absorbable suture material largely obviates the need for such extensive defatting. Relatively minor variations in technique can help minimize disruption of these veins. We find that precisely exposing the retropubic space and vaginal wall from lateral to medial, as is recommended for exposure of paravaginal defects (3), usually eliminates vascular disruption and significant bleeding during these procedures. Using this lateral approach, it is often possible to isolate and ligate vessels if disruption is unavoidable. Hemostatic vascular clips may also prove invaluable in avoiding or controlling troublesome bleeding (3, 7, 8). Another indispensable adjunctive piece of equipment is the long extension for the electrocautery. It is particularly useful to control bleeding from veins that run along the inner surface of the superior pubic ramus (3).

Using these techniques usually results in a completely hemostatic retropubic space. As a result, in recent years we have largely abandoned the routine use of retropubic drainage. However, if residual oozing of blood is observed after all suspending sutures are tied, retropubic placement of a pliable suction drainage system is a wise precaution (2, 8). An active drainage system is less likely to serve as a wick to contaminate the space and also evacuates blood more efficiently than a passive drain. We advocate the use of sterile dressings, antiseptic ointment, and sterile technique when manipulating the drain sites. Finally, the drain should be removed promptly when drainage becomes negligible and serous. Using these techniques during and after an exclusive abdominal route continence procedure, a retropubic hematoma should be an exceptional complication (8). Because accumulation of blood is the major risk factor for retropubic abscess formation after these procedures, an abscess should be an even rarer occurrence.

With combined abdominal-vaginal needle procedures, direct attempts at hemostasis and retropubic space drainage are not possible because of the blind, although limited, dissection of the space. As long as the retropubic dissection is performed intimately against the retropubis, significant disruption of the venous plexus is unlikely. However, contamination of the space with vaginal organisms is unavoidable during dissection and ligature passage. This bacterial contamination, rather than the accumulation of blood, is the major risk factor for retropubic cellulitis and abscess after these procedures. Measures to minimize these risks are considered in the section on infectious complications.

MANAGEMENT

The only effective management technique for a retropubic hematoma is prevention. Small noninfected collections of blood are probably quite common and likely resorb spontaneously. It is only when these collections become infected that they are clinically important. The management of the infected hematoma/abscess is considered in the next section.

Infectious and Inflammatory Complications

RETROPUBIC ABSCESS

The development of a postoperative abscess has two basic prerequisites: an accumulation of blood or serum to serve as a culture medium and the introduction of bacteria into the culture medium (9). The major tactics developed to prevent abscess formation are aimed at eliminating the prerequisites: maximize hemostasis during the procedure, drain the operative site to prevent accumulation of the culture medium if hemostasis is not optimal, and eliminate or minimize bacterial contamination of the operative site, usually through the use of short courses of prophylactic antibiotics. Both drainage and prophylaxis have proven successful in reducing the incidence of cuff infections after hysterectomy (10). Although neither approach has been prospectively validated in continence surgery, both tactics, alone and in combination, are used. Techniques for the control of retropubic space bleeding and for postoperative drainage of the space have already been considered. Although studies demonstrating the efficacy of antibiotic prophylaxis during continence surgery are lacking, we generally favor single-dose perioperative antibiotic prophylaxis with a first-generation cephalosporin (cefazolin, 1 g intravenously), the same prophylaxis we use with vaginal hysterectomy (11). It must be emphasized that the scientific evidence supporting prophylaxis of such procedures is retrospective and conflicting (12, 13), and well-designed prospective studies are needed. Furthermore, respected authorities are divided in their opinions regarding the use of prophylactic antibiotics (5, 14–16) in such cases or make no mention of their use (1, 2, 4, 17, 18).

Other elements of operative technique may diminish contamination of the abdominal operative site during combined abdominal-vaginal cases. These include the use of a separate clean instrument set for the abdominal incision and closure and use of a clean ligature carrier or fascial clamps for each passage through the rectus fascia and retropubic space. Operators should change gloves to avoid contamination of the abdominal incision after operating in the vaginal field. Finally, we recommend only monofilament permanent suture material for needle suspensions because of concerns over the ability of multifilament braided suture to harbor a larger inoculum of vaginal bacteria. Removal of multifilament suture has been reported in several patients due to chronic refractory infections and foreign body reactions as late as 2 years after surgery.

Despite best efforts at prevention, there is still a small risk of retropubic abscess formation after abdominal and abdominal-vaginal urethropexies. The incidence of this complication is difficult to estimate because many reports of surgical procedures do not enumerate operative complications. Of those that do, most do not specifically mention retropubic space abscess or infection among their complications (18–25). Consequently, it would seem that such occurrences are extremely rare when using the preventative techniques described above. Stanton et al. (2) reported one retropubic abscess among 40 (2.3%) women undergoing Burch colposuspensions. Two reports regarding abdominal-vaginal needle procedures performed without antibiotic prophylaxis had a 7% incidence (7 of 98 and 6 of 80) of retropubic space "infections or draining cellulitis" (5, 12).

An abscess should be suspected when persistent fever, tenderness, pain, and irritative symptoms are encountered postoperatively.

The bimanual pelvic-abdominal examination often reveals a tender mass in the retropubic area. Purulent drainage might be noted around a suprapubic bladder catheter. An abdominal or vaginal ultrasound examination should objectively confirm the lesion. Once the diagnosis is established, prompt surgical drainage and broad spectrum antibiotic coverage should be instituted. As discussed in the next section, the decision to retain or remove a permanent foreign body used to perform the surgery is difficult and must be individualized.

FOREIGN BODY COMPLICATIONS

Complications due to the presence of a permanent foreign body in an operative site are related either to enhanced invasiveness and persistence of infections or to noninfectious foreign body reactions. The foreign bodies most commonly left permanently in place after continence surgery include suture material, synthetic bands for some sling procedures, synthetic endopelvic fascia bolsters and anterior rectus fascia pledgets for various needle procedures, artificial urinary sphincters, and polytetrafluoroethylene (Teflon) paste used for periurethral injection (26). Polytetrafluoroethylene has been largely replaced by Contigen® for periurethral injections. Contigen®, a highly purified glutaraldehyde cross-linked bovine dermal collagen, is biocompatible and biodegradable. It elicits a minimal inflammatory response that causes a replacement of bovine collagen by the patient's own collagen. As opposed to other foreign bodies, the concern with collagen is its immunogenicity, and this can be addressed by preoperative skin testing to exclude patients with an immunological response (27).

The significant problem of a bacterial infection in an operative site occupied by a foreign body was already mentioned. When the bulk of the material and the magnitude of the infection are both substantial, effective management mandates the removal of the foreign body in addition to appropriate drainage and antibiotic therapy. This is particularly true with the artificial sphincter and most synthetic sling materials.

The overall incidence of infection with the artificial sphincter is 2–6%, with most infections resulting in pump or cuff erosions (28–30). Most series report a preponderance of male patients and do not separate complications by sex. It is likely that the female infection and erosion incidence is somewhat higher. When infection is apparent with the artificial sphincter, the sphincter must be removed promptly; reimplantation should be delayed for several months until all local inflammation has resolved (30).

Foreign body reactions represent a chronic granulomatous inflammatory response to a nondigestible irritant (31). Such reactions can occur in response to any of the permanent materials already described. In a report on the Stamey procedure by Mundy (32), 4 of 25 (16%) patients had Dacron rectus fascia pledgets removed because of chronic inflammation. In another report on the same procedure, 2 of 25 knitted Marlex pledgets were removed at 3 and 5 months after surgery, and a vaginal bolster of the same material became inflamed 19 months after surgery (21). Because the foreign body is incorporated into the granulomatous reaction, resolution of the reaction requires removal of the foreign body.

Pubovaginal sling procedures for stress incontinence can be performed with autologous fascia (most commonly, anterior rectus fascia or fascia lata) or with synthetic inorganic materials such as polyethylene (Mersilene gauze), polypropylene (Marlex mesh), reinforced Silastic, or polytetrafluoroethylene (Gore-tex patch). Proponents of organic slings cite the avoidance of infection with subsequent poor healing and erosion, necessitating sling removal, as their major advantage to synthetic slings (18). Rejection rates of up to 21% have been reported for synthetic slings (18, 33). In contrast, several series that followed women from 6 months to 16 years after surgery revealed no synthetic sling removals for infection (14, 34–36). Animal experiments comparing Gore-tex with Marlex mesh in the reconstruction of infected abdominal walls suggest that the porous structure of Gore-tex should allow infected slings to be treated, in-situ, with antibiotics (37). However, histological studies of polytetrafluoroethylene slings removed for tissue rejection revealed gram-positive cocci in the patch interstices despite the use of antibiotics (33). Certainly, if an acute infection does not respond rapidly to or recurs rapidly after

antibiotic therapy, removal of the sling would seem most prudent. Fortunately, removal of a sling does not necessarily compromise the success of the original procedure. A continence rate of 74% has been reported after removal of 23 Gore-tex slings for tissue reaction (33).

OSTEITIS PUBIS AND PYOGENIC ARTHRITIS

Osteitis pubis is a self-limiting nonbacterial inflammation of the symphysis pubis that can follow trauma, childbirth, prolonged running and kicking exercise, and pelvic surgery (38). Although it can occur in any of these circumstances, in urogynecology it most commonly follows the MMK procedure, presumably because of the placement of the suspending sutures into the periosteum of the superior pubic ramus or the perichondrium of the pubic symphysis. In a comprehensive review of 56 articles on the MMK procedure representing 2712 individual procedures, Mainprize and Drutz (39) found that the overall frequency of osteitis pubis was 2.5%. Although self-limiting, the syndrome can be quite distressing to the patient, resulting in incapacitating symptoms for weeks to months (39, 40). The abrupt onset of symptoms generally occurs between 1 week and several months after surgery. The patient notes burning pelvic and groin that is aggravated by climbing stairs, coughing or sneezing, walking, and getting in and out of bed. Signs include tenderness of the symphysis, pain on pelvic compression, thigh adductor spasm, limitation of abduction, and a waddling gait. The erythrocyte sedimentation rate is elevated. Initial radiographic studies are often normal; lytic changes and a "moth-eaten" appearance develop after several weeks (38, 41).

Treatment of osteitis pubis initially includes bed rest and nonsteroidal antiinflammatory drugs. Narcotic analgesia and systemic corticosteroid administration may be helpful in resistant cases (38, 41). Antibiotics are not part of therapy if there is no evidence of frank infection. However, differentiating osteitis pubis from the much rarer conditions of pyogenic arthritis or osteomyelitis may be difficult. Needle biopsy of the symphysis and culture of aspirate may be necessary to distinguish the two conditions. Physical therapy with diathermy or hydrotherapy may also be beneficial. Recalcitrant cases may require direct injections with steroids with or without local anesthetic agents; infrequently, joint fusion may be necessary (4, 40). One report of three patients described dramatic responses to heparinization and suggested that pubic thrombosis may be involved in the pathogenesis of the condition (40).

Pyogenic arthritis and pubic bone osteomyelitis can also occur after pelvic operations and have been described after the MMK procedure (38). As noted above, signs, symptoms, and radiographic findings are virtually identical to osteitis pubis, except for signs of overt bacterial infection. If the diagnosis is made immediately, intravenous antibiotic therapy may be adequate, although consideration should be given to removal of suture material used for the urethropexy. In chronic or advanced cases, surgical drainage and debridement is required in addition to antibiotic therapy (38).

URINARY TRACT INFECTIONS

Significant bacteriuria after continence surgery is quite common. Such infection is directly and primarily related to the type and duration of catheter drainage of the bladder. The most effective way of preventing catheter-associated urinary tract infection is to avoid prolonged continuous transurethral catheterization (42, 43). If such catheterization cannot be avoided, efforts should be directed toward postponement of the inevitable bacteriuria, treatment of symptomatic bacteriuria, and surveillance for the management of significant complications of bacteriuria (43).

The two techniques primarily used to avoid continuous transurethral catheterization are suprapubic catheterization and intermittent catheterization. Both techniques have been shown to significantly decrease the risk of bacteriuria. In a study of stress incontinent women undergoing the Pereyra procedure, 17% of 24 women with suprapubic catheters developed significant bacteriuria, compared with 63% of 27 women with transurethral Foley catheters (44). Most infections in both groups developed within 5 days. In another report comparing transure-

thral to suprapubic catheterization after general surgical procedures, 11 of 18 (61%) women with urethral catheters but none of 15 with suprapubic catheters became infected, with a mean catheterization time of 5 days (45). When it becomes obvious that the postoperative patient will require bladder drainage for a prolonged period of time, intermittent catheterization is the preferred technique. Even with prolonged use, the proportion of patients able to maintain sterile urine with aseptic intermittent catheterization varies between 45 and 90%. With clean intermittent self-catheterization, the proportion is 39–65% (42). The incidence of urinary tract infection with the latter technique is less than half that observed with indwelling catheters (43).

Before the introduction of closed drainage systems in the 1950s, the risk of urinary tract infection from transurethral catheterization was exceptionally high. Half of patients were infected with the first day of catheterization, and virtually all were infected within 4 days (42, 43). The fact that a meticulously maintained closed drainage system can decrease the infection incidence to 5–10% per day underscores the importance of intraluminal entry of organisms into the bladder (43). However, the further fact that even the best closed system cannot prevent infections confirms that extraluminal entry is ultimately unavoidable. Still, trying to fastidiously preserve a closed system can postpone the inevitable with chronic catheterization and avoid many infections in acute short-term catheterization. Important aspects of such a system include the following:

1. Avoid disconnecting the catheter from the drainage bag for any reason. If a urine specimen is needed, collect it by piercing the catheter obliquely with a small gauge needle to aspirate the urine (42).
2. Use a drainage bag with an incorporated urometer. The urometer is believed to break the urine column between the bag and catheter, thereby decreasing the chance of bladder colonization if the bag becomes colonized (43).
3. Have medical personnel and/or the patient handle the bag drainage port with care; avoid touching the distal end of the drainage tube to other surfaces (43).

4. Keep the drainage bag below the level of the bladder to prevent retrograde flow of urine.
5. Never clamp a transurethral catheter and only clamp a suprapubic catheter as part of a voiding trial before anticipated catheter removal.

Although these factors are stressed primarily with transurethral catheters, they also apply to suprapubic tubes. In addition, we advocate maintaining sterile techniques with respect to dressing changes and inspection of the suprapubic catheter insertion site to minimize the risk of nosocomial extraluminal contamination.

Two controversial methods to prevent bacteriuria are bladder irrigation and systemic antibiotics. The sum of evidence regarding antibiotic or antiseptic irrigation of indwelling catheters does not support the value of the practice in postponing bacteriuria (43). This is likely related to the fact that irrigation represents yet another breach of the closed system. Systemic antibiotic therapy can postpone infections but is likely of value only if the catheter is removed after a relatively short period of time (less than 5 days) (43). The advantage of this effect is diminished by the fact that in many patients, short-term catheter-associated bacteriuria resolves spontaneously once the catheter is removed. Although short courses of antibiotics can clear catheter-associated bacteriuria, infections typically recur a few days after discontinuing antibiotics if the catheter is still in place (45). Long-term therapy in the face of long-term catheterization does not prevent bacteriuria but does favor the emergence of resistant organisms (43, 45).

Any treatment scheme of catheter-associated urinary tract infection must acknowledge that sterile urine cannot be maintained indefinitely with the catheter in place. Thus, there is no rationale for the treatment of asymptomatic bacteriuria. Antibiotic therapy is indicated only if the patient becomes symptomatic. Systemic evidence of infection, such as high fever or signs of pyelonephritis or bacteremia, should prompt a search for other infectious complications and for catheter or ureteral obstruction. Bacteremia is relatively uncommon, occurring in only 2–4% of catheterized bacteriuric patients (43). However, if such signs are due to infection of the urinary tract, parenteral antibiotic therapy is appropriate (43). Symptoms of localized bladder infection, most commonly lower abdominal pain and/or bladder spasms (detrusor instability), often respond to short courses of oral antibiotics. The requisite adjunct to antibiotic therapy in the cure of all such infections is discontinuation of the indwelling catheter as soon as possible.

Urinary Tract Injuries

Surgical injury to the lower urinary tract is described with virtually every continence procedure. Such injuries have been described with 3–6% of Burch colposuspensions (21, 25), with 1–7% of needle-type urethropexies (4, 12, 19, 20), and with 1.6% of MMK procedures (39). The risk of injury can be minimized but not eliminated with experience and attention to the details of the technique. More importantly, the risk of unrecognized injury can be virtually eliminated with careful assessment of the integrity of the lower urinary tract during and after the performance of the procedure.

Injury to the bladder and urethra can occur during the dissection of these structures from the overlying rectus muscles and pubic bone as the space of Retzius is developed during abdominal retropubic procedures. It can also occur when the space is entered or when the ligature carrier is passed during Pereyra- and Stamey-type procedures. Such injuries are especially likely when there is extensive scarring in the retropubic space due to previous continence surgery. Ureteric injuries are a particular concern with the Burch colposuspension procedure. They are most likely to occur during placement of suspending sutures at or just above the urethrovesical junction if the lateral edge of the bladder has been inadequately dissected and defined (8). Although the risk of damage to the bladder and ureters during laparoscopic retropubic urethropexies is not adequately defined, these structures may be at greater risk during such minimally invasive procedures because of the absence of tactile assessment. The degree of variation in laparoscopic approaches might also increase the rate of urogenital injury for these procedures as a whole, when compared with the relatively uniform approach to open retropubic urethropexies. Ureteral injury, especially kinking and obstruction, is also a concern in surgical correction of severe degrees of uterovaginal prolapse, with the greatest danger to the ureters occurring during the closure of the cul-de-sac and plication of the uterosacral ligaments.

There are several techniques that can help prevent unrecognized urinary tract injuries. The instillation of a small amount of contrast material (30–50 mL) into the bladder at the start of the dissection will make any breach of the bladder obvious. Although irrigation fluid stained with indigo carmine or methylene blue dye is commonly used, we prefer the use of sterile infant's formula in this situation. The latter is always readily available in any hospital with a newborn nursery, is easily distinguishable from normal body fluids, and will not stain tissues like blue dyes. This last quality makes the repair of any injury easier. Finally, reserving blue dye for systemic administration, renal excretion, and ureteric evaluation facilitates separate evaluation of bladder and ureteric integrity during surgery.

The performance of a controlled high extraperitoneal cystotomy during abdominal retropubic procedures is another excellent technique to avoid more serious bladder, ureteral, or urethral injuries. Some authorities advocate cystotomy to avoid injury and to ensure proper suture placement in every such procedure (22). Certainly, such a cystotomy is invaluable as the initial step in repeat retropubic procedures, in which significant scarring is often encountered.

We advocate examination of the urethra, bladder, and ureters at the conclusion of every continence or prolapse correction surgical procedure. This can be done either via cystotomy, urethrocystoscopy, or suprapubic teloscopy. When continence surgery is performed in the supine position, valuable operative time is lost by repositioning and prepping for transurethral cystoscopy. In this situation, if significant cystoscopic findings are encountered, the abdomen must be reopened for surgical correction. Suprapubic teloscopy avoids these disadvantages and provides an excellent view of the bladder and

ureters. In terms of operating time and morbidity, suprapubic teloscopy compares favorably with the alternatives of open cystotomy, dissection of ureters, or transurethral cystoscopy (46). Inserting a three-way transurethral catheter during preparation for the supine procedure in anticipation of teloscopy allows convenient bladder distension for the procedure. The technique is described in detail in Chapter 13.

During direct visualization, if suture perforation is visualized, the suture can be immediately removed and replaced. Ureteral integrity is assessed by the administration of indigo carmine only after all suspension or plication sutures have been tied. Excretion of dye should be observed from both ureteral orifices. It is self-evident that preoperative bilateral ureteric competence (by intravenous pyelography, ultrasonography, or cystoscopy) should have been demonstrated. Observation of ureteral spill is facilitated by the instillation of 150 mL of 10% glucose into the bladder before cystoscopy (47). The increased density of this solution compared with the urine allows the blue urine to rise from the ureteral orifices through the 10% glucose. Thus, pooling of the dyed urine in the base of the bladder is avoided, and independent assessment of each ureter is quite easy. Ureteral visualization is usually not possible with a zero-degree transurethral endoscope because of elevation of the urethrovesical junction after sutures are tied. We found the 30-degree microhysteroscope ideal in this situation. It has the added advantage of simplicity and ready availability in most gynecological operating rooms. If bilateral spill is not observed, sutures should be removed, and ureteral function should be reassessed. If spill is observed and ureteric or ureterovesical kinking was due only to imperfect suture placement, no further intervention is likely necessary. Ureteral catheterization for 5–7 days may be considered in some such situations (48). If a more extensive injury is suspected or if spill is not observed, ureteral catheterization and direct ureteral inspection is necessary. If the injury has extensively damaged and devitalized the ureter (an extremely uncommon occurrence with continence surgery), excision of the damaged section and ureteroureterostomy or ureteroneocystotomy should be performed (49).

When bladder injury and laceration are identified, careful two-layer closure should be performed. Only absorbable suture material should be used for any suture line that is likely to be in contact with urine because of the risk of stone formation. Chromic catgut suture is still considered the material of choice, especially for the first simple, running, full-thickness layer of the closure (50, 51). The bulk of suture material within the lumen of the bladder should be minimized by using 2-0 or 3-0 suture, and knots should be tied on the extraluminal surface (51). Bladder decompression should be maintained for 10–14 days after injury (8, 50, 51). This can be accomplished with a transurethral catheter and/or a suprapubic tube. If significant intravesical bleeding is anticipated, a 30–32F suprapubic Malecot catheter is desirable to prevent obstruction with clots (50). When a controlled surgical cystotomy is performed extraperitoneally and repair is accomplished without tension, such prolonged decompression is not likely necessary. As long as the retropubic space is drained adequately, the catheter in such cases can often be managed as it is following comparable continence procedures without cystotomy, and voiding trials can begin 5–7 days postoperatively.

Postoperative Urinary Retention

Immediate postoperative retention, an inability to effectively empty the bladder on the initial attempt to void after surgery, is the most common of all complications after continence surgery. The precise incidence of this complication is difficult to determine because there is no standard definition for acute retention and because many authors omit reference to this particular complication when reporting their results. It would appear that retention depends on the procedure and the way it is performed as well as on the patient and her preoperative voiding mechanism.

No continence procedure is immune to the risk of immediate postoperative retention. The risk after various procedures varies among reports citing the same procedure. The incidence is 13–35% after Pereyra- and Stamey-type procedures (5, 12, 19, 20), 16–24% after the MMK procedure (4, 19, 24), and 16–25% after the Burch colposuspension (21, 52, 53). With sling procedures performed in patients with recurrent genuine stress incontinence (GSI) with irreparably poor local support tissues (18) and in patients with low urethral closure pressure (14), short-term retention is nearly universal. In two reports totaling 187 such patients, catheterization was required from 10 to 270 days, with mean catheterization times of 29 and 60 days (14, 18). It is clear that sling procedures in such patients must significantly increase urethral resistance if they are to cure disabling incontinence. This attempt to increase urethral resistance often results in functional obstruction.

Successful continence surgery permanently reconstructs anatomic relationships between the bladder and urethra, resulting in a unique stress continence mechanism whereby the urethra and urethrovesical junction are compressed during increases in abdominal pressure by the momentary descent of more mobile posterior and superior pelvic viscera (54–56). This stress-activated obstructive sphincteric mechanism may be activated by variable degrees of stress, depending on the degree of correction or overcorrection of urethrovesical junction support. Thus, the surgeon who aggressively elevates the urethrovesical junction by design for whatever reason is more likely to create retention than one who is less aggressive. Studies of acute (6 weeks to 6 months) and chronic (up to 12 years) voiding dysfunction after continence surgery demonstrated that procedures that aggressively support the bladder neck and result in extreme preferential stress pressure transmission to the urethra are more likely to cause new emptying phase dysfunction (57, 58). Likewise, the patient whose preoperative voiding mechanism depends heavily on Valsalva with minimal detrusor activity will activate her new sphincteric mechanism when she uses her former voiding mechanism. Thus, women who have normal preoperative uroflow parameters and void with good detrusor contractions are unlikely to experience postoperative retention. Patients with prolonged voiding patterns, those without demonstrable detrusor contractions, and those who void with Valsalva are more likely to require prolonged catheterization (53, 59). The risk of prolonged retention is particularly significant after surgery to correct incontinence or severe degrees of prolapse in elderly women, many of whom have deceptively precarious lower urinary tract function before surgery.

There are a number of techniques that can facilitate management of postoperative urinary retention. These include the use of a suprapubic catheter and intermittent self-catheterization, instruction on new voiding mechanisms, and the administration of pharmacological agents. Even more important than these postoperative management techniques is preoperative anticipation of the problem in a particular patient. This allows a realistic and frank discussion of the complication and enables the patient to make an informed decision regarding the proposed surgery. Some high-risk patients are unwilling or unable to trade self-catheterization for protective garments, and they should be given the option of sharing in this decision.

Suprapubic drainage has been shown to be associated with significantly earlier restoration of normal bladder function after continence surgery when compared with transurethral drainage (44). This may be because the suprapubic catheter interferes less with bladder and urethral function because urethral trauma is avoided or because voiding trials are easier for the hospital staff to perform. When it is necessary for a patient to go home with a catheter for a brief time, the suprapubic tube also allows self-monitoring of voiding trials and residual urine measurements not possible with an indwelling Foley catheter. When retention is prolonged beyond 1 or 2 weeks, we train the patient in the technique of clean intermittent self-catheterization. Patients whose sphincteric status demands frankly obstructive surgery are instructed on self-catheterization preoperatively. Their suprapubic tubes are discontinued as soon as possible postoperatively, usually before discharge from the hospital.

It is important to explain to the patient that successful voiding after surgery may require a change in her voiding mechanism. She should understand that bearing down to force her urine out will activate her new sphincteric mechanism. Instead, she should be encouraged to initiate voiding by relaxing the pelvic floor. This is often facilitated by having the patient attempt to void in a warm sitz bath initially.

Pharmacological manipulation is sometimes beneficial in some cases of postoperative retention. Diazepam (Valium) has a relaxant effect on striated muscle through its polysynaptic inhibitory action (60). In addition, its well-known anxiolytic effect through its depressant action on the brainstem reticular system can also benefit many patients who are unable to void after surgery. Diazepam in doses of 2–10 mg, one to three times daily, has been shown to be more effective than bethanechol (Urecholine) in these circumstances (61). Bethanechol in high doses can increase bladder tone but does not generally stimulate a coordinated voiding pattern (60). The muscarinic action of systemically administered bethanechol can effect detrusor contractions, but its nicotinic activity can stimulate preganglionic sympathetic and parasympathetic activity. This results in increased alpha-adrenergic activity of the urethra and bladder neck (smooth muscle contraction) when these agents are used to stimulate detrusor activity. The intravesical instillation of prostaglandin F_{2a} has been shown to decrease acute urinary retention after vaginal hysterectomy (62). It has also been shown to improve voiding function on the day of instillation in women who were unable to micturate 3 days after continence surgery (63). The role of such instillations in the management of postoperative retention is not yet established.

The most dramatic response to prolonged postoperative retention is surgical takedown and revision of the surgical repair often with extensive urethrolysis. This is an infrequent occurrence, performed in only 2.9% of 170 consecutive fascia lata sling procedures in the series reported by Beck et al. (18). Complete take-down of repairs may relieve obstruction and retention at the cost of recurrence of incontinence. One suggested alternative to this with the sling procedure is the interposition of a vaginal patch to lengthen the sling and relieve bladder neck obstruction while preserving the integrity of the sling (64). A "loop-loosening" procedure under local anesthesia to successfully treat postoperative urinary retention after the Stamey procedure, without creating recurrent incontinence, has also been described (65).

Complications of Suprapubic Catheterization

Suprapubic catheterization affords distinct benefits when compared with transurethral catheterization with respect to the risk of infection and to the resumption of normal voiding postoperatively. In addition, many patients who have experienced both types of bladder drainage voice a distinct preference for the suprapubic route (45). However, as with any other invasive procedure, suprapubic catheters and their insertion are not completely free of complications. Relatively minor, although aggravating, complications include kinking and obstruction of the tubes, dislodging of the catheter due to difficulty in fixation to the abdominal skin, breakage of the catheter, and catheter-associated detrusor instability (66, 67).

The most serious recurring complication is bowel perforation at the time of insertion of the catheter, which can occur both with suprapubic stab and transurethral insertion techniques (68–70). This risk can be minimized by distending the bladder with at least 400 mL of fluid, placing the patient in steep Trendelenburg, and inserting the catheter no more than 3 cm above the pubic symphysis. We usually insert the suprapubic catheter under direct cystoscopic visualization when the bladder and ureters are examined at the conclusion of the continence procedure. Visualization of the insertion helps to confirm proper orientation and final positioning of the catheter. During insertion, attention to the pressure on the trocar and depth of trocar insertion are important to avoid bladder base damage. Nonetheless, perforations have been described despite such precautions, especially if bowel is fixed in the anterior pelvis as a result of prior surgery.

Bowel perforation should be suspected if the patient has unexplained lower abdominal pain, fever, or peritoneal signs after surgery. Third spacing and regression of bowel function have been reported as subtle signs of bowel perforation (70). Radiographic evidence of a pneumoperitoneum after vaginal repair without opening of the cul-de-sac is pathognomonic for bowel perforation. Often the diagnosis is entertained only after bowel contents drain around the catheter site (69). A further risk to transperitoneal insertion of the catheter, even if bowel injury does not occur, is intraperitoneal leakage of urine after the catheter is removed. Finally, an extremely rare but life-threatening complication of suprapubic catheter use is necrotizing fasciitis in high-risk (diabetic) patients who develop inflammation at the insertion site (71). Immediate and extensive surgical debridement to well-vascularized margins is the foundation of therapy of this condition. Broad-spectrum antibiotic coverage should also be instituted.

Detrusor Instability After Continence Surgery

The complication of persistent or recurrent GSI after continence surgery is addressed in Chapter 47. At least as distressing to the patient and the surgeon alike, however, is the development of urgency incontinence and detrusor instability postoperatively. Six to 20% of women with pure GSI will develop detrusor instability for the first time after continence surgery (25, 53, 72, 73). Women who have mixed incontinence (combined GSI and detrusor instability) have a 40–45% risk of persistent detrusor instability postoperatively (74, 75). In most cases, the continence procedure has been a technical success, achieving both stabilization of the anatomy and correction of the pressure transmission defects. However, the woman who exchanges the loss of a spurt of urine with physical activity before surgery for the loss of a stream of urine with the sensation of uncontrollable urgency after surgery understandably does not consider her surgery successful. There are four major circumstances that can result in detrusor instability after continence surgery: (a) the original incontinence was due to detrusor instability; (b) the development of detrusor instability is unrelated to the surgery or to preexisting detrusor instability; (c) local irritative lesions are created by the surgery; and (d) surgery overcorrected urethrovesical junction support.

An indefensible but avoidable cause of detrusor instability after continence surgery is the failure to establish the correct cause of the patient's incontinence before surgery. The presence of mixed incontinence should be appreciated before therapy is started. In such a situation, it is usually best to attempt nonsurgical treatment of the detrusor instability component first. Although there are individual situations where surgery may be performed as initial therapy, the mixed nature of the problem should be known, and the increased risk of postoperative detrusor instability should be acknowledged by the surgeon and the patient alike. On the other hand, continence surgery plays no role in treatment of incontinence due to pure detrusor instability. It is always incumbent upon the physician to prove that the patient does not have detrusor instability before surgery. The fact that there is a 6–20% de novo risk of detrusor instability developing after surgery makes this particularly important. When a patient develops detrusor instability after surgery, the only way to prove it was not present before surgery is to have specifically tested for it preoperatively.

Surgery for GSI does not prevent the later unrelated development of detrusor instability. For this prospect to be tenable, the onset of the detrusor instability should be temporally distant from the surgery. In addition, urinary control should have been acceptable during the interim.

Local irritative lesions in and around the lower urinary tract can result in the loss of volitional suppression of detrusor activity. As already noted in this chapter, a number of acute and chronic irritations can result from continence surgery. These include acute inflammation related to surgical trauma, suture material, and the drainage catheter and bacterial infections of the bladder. A careful assessment for infection is always the initial step in the management of postoperative detrusor instability. When instability and infection persist despite adequate antimicrobial therapy, the bladder should be examined for the presence of a foreign body (suture material) as an ongoing source for the irritation. Examination of the bladder and urethra at the conclusion of surgery will obviate this complication. When pharmacological therapy of detrusor instability is necessary, we prefer oxybutynin (Ditropan). This agent is a cholinergic blocker and direct smooth muscle relaxant that also has local anesthetic activity. This last characteristic makes it particularly useful in patients with discomfort and detrusor instability due to surgical irritation, infection, or catheters.

There is accumulating evidence that surgical overcorrection of anatomic support of the urethrovesical junction may cause detrusor instability. Women who develop persistent detrusor instability after continence surgery have been shown to have pressure transmission ratios (PTRs) substantially above 100%, a finding that is associated with significant stress-induced obstruction of the urethra (57, 58). Such women also have significantly higher PTRs than women who have normal continence after surgery or women who develop detrusor instability without prior surgery. Surgeons (75) who achieve PTRs over 100% with the Burch colposuspension report much higher de novo detrusor instability rates than surgeons (25) who achieve PTRs under 100% with the same procedure (27% versus 6%). If a surgical procedure overcorrects urethrovesical junction support, as manifested by preferential urethral pressure transmission (PTRs over 100%) rather than equal pressure transmission, urethral obstruction is likely more profound and may not require significant stress activation. Such relative obstruction may result in detrusor instability. Further support for the role of partial obstruction in the genesis of postoperative detrusor instability is the demonstration of decreased urine flow rates and increased residual urine volumes in such women (57, 76). The development of detrusor instability in men with partial bladder obstruction from prostatic enlargement and in animals after experimental outflow obstruction (77) also supports this hypothesis.

It has been our experience that postoperative detrusor instability due to support overcorrection is more refractory to bladder retraining than detrusor instability that does not follow surgery. Patients experiencing the former nearly always require pharmacological suppression of their detrusor activity. Furthermore, they often need to remain on such therapy indefinitely. Anticholinergic and smooth muscle relaxant therapy does pose some risk of urinary retention in these circumstances. Such patients should be instructed in intermittent self-catheterization before starting such agents. As is the case with patients who develop prolonged retention after continence surgery, women whose detrusor instability is prolonged and refractory to tolerable medical therapy may need take-down and revision of their surgical repair. In our limited experience, the reversibility of instability observed in animals after release of obstruction (77) is also seen in women.

REFERENCES

1. Tanagho EA. Colpocystourethropexy: the way we do it. J Urol 1976;116:751–753.
2. Stanton SL, Williams JE, Ritchie D. The colposuspension operation for urinary incontinence. Br J Obstet Gynaecol 1976;83:890–895.
3. Shull BL. How I do the abdominal paravaginal repair. J Pelvic Surg 1995;1:43–49.
4. Pereyra AJ, Lebherz TB, Growdon WA, Powers JA. Pubourethral supports in perspective: modified Pereyra procedure for urinary incontinence. Obstet Gynecol 1982;59:643–648.
5. Muzsnai D, Carrillo E, Dubin C, Silverman I. Retropubic vaginopexy for correction of urinary stress incontinence. Obstet Gynecol 1982;59:113–118.
6. Wheeless CR. Goebell-Stoeckel fascia lata sling operation for urinary incontinence. In: Atlas of pelvic surgery. Philadelphia: Lea & Febiger, 1988:125–135.
7. Spirtos NM, Ballard CA. The use of vascular clips to minimize blood loss in colpourethropexy. Surg Gynecol Obstet 1987;165:419–420.
8. Stanton SL. Surgery of urinary incontinence. Clin Obstet Gynaecol 1978;5:83–108.
9. Swartz, WH, Tanaree P. Suction drainage as an alternative to prophylactic antibiotics for hysterectomy. Obstet Gynecol 1975;45:305–310.
10. Swartz WH, Tanaree P. T-tube suction drainage and/or prophylactic antibiotics: a randomized study of 451 hysterectomies. Obstet Gynecol 1976;47:665–670.
11. Soper DE, Yarwood RL. Single-dose antibiotic prophylaxis in women undergoing vaginal hysterectomy. Obstet Gynecol 1987;69:879–882.
12. Backer MH Jr, Probst RE. The Pereyra procedure: favorable experience with 200 operations. Am J Obstet Gynecol 1976;125:346–351.
13. Drutz HP, Sousan L. Prophylactic use of antibiotics in combined abdominovaginal Marlex sling procedures for correction of recurrent urinary stress incontinence. Can J Surg 1986;29:377–379.
14. Horbach NS, Blanco JS, Ostergard DR, Bent AE, Cornella JL. A suburethral sling procedure with polytetrafluoroethylene for the treatment of genuine stress incontinence in patients with low urethral closure pressure. Obstet Gynecol 1988;71:648–652.
15. Leach GE, Raz S. Modified Pereyra bladder neck suspension after previously failed anti-incontinence surgery. Urology 1984;23:359–362.
16. Stamey TA. Endoscopic suspension of the vesical neck for urinary incontinence in females. Ann Surg 1980;192:465–471.
17. McGuire EJ, Lytton B. Pubovaginal sling procedure for stress incontinence. J Urol 1978;119:82–84.
18. Beck RP, McCormick S, Nordstrom L. The fascia lata sling procedure for treating recurrent genuine stress incontinence of urine. Obstet Gynecol 1988;72:699–703.
19. Loughlin KR, Gittes RF, Klein LA, Whitmore WF III. The comparative medical costs of 2 major procedures available for the treatment of stress urinary incontinence. J Urol 1982;127:436–438.
20. Green DF, McGuire EJ, Lytton B. A comparison of endoscopic suspension of the vesical neck versus anterior urethropexy for the treatment of stress urinary incontinence. J Urol 1986;136:1205–1207.
21. Pow-Sang JM, Lockhart JL, Suarez A, Lansman H, Politano VA. Female urinary incontinence: preoperative selection, surgical complications and results. J Urol 1986;136:831–833.
22. Lee RA, Symmonds RE, Goldstein RA. Surgical complications and results of modified Marshall-Marchetti-Krantz procedure for urinary incontinence. Obstet Gynecol 1979;53:447–450.
23. Park GS, Miller EJ Jr. Surgical treatment of stress urinary incontinence: a comparison of the Kelly plication, Marshall-Marchetti-Krantz, and Pereyra procedures. Obstet Gynecol 1988;71:575–579.
24. Parnell JP II, Marshall VF, Vaughan ED Jr. Management of recurrent urinary stress incontinence by the Marshall-Marchetti-Krantz vesicourethropexy. J Urol 1984;132:912–914.
25. van Geelen JM, Theeuwes GM, Eskes TKAB, Martin CB Jr. The clinical and urodynamic effects of anterior vaginal repair and Burch colposuspension. Am J Obstet Gynecol 1988;159:137–144.
26. Malizia AA, Reiman HM, Myers RP, et al. Migration and granulomatous reaction after periurethral injection of polytef (Teflon). JAMA 1984;251:3277–3281.
27. Appell RA. Periurethral injections. In: Hurt WG, ed. Urogynecologic surgery. Gaithersburg: Aspen, 1992:140–142.
28. Fishman IJ, Shabsigh R, Scott FB. Experience with the artificial urinary sphincter model AS800 in 148 patients. J Urol 1989;141:307–310.
29. Goldwasser B, Furlow WL, Barrett DM. The model AS800 artificial urinary sphincter: Mayo Clinic experience. J Urol 1987;137:668–671.
30. Nurse DE, Mundy AR. One hundred artificial sphincters. Br J Urol 1988;61:318–325.
31. Robbins SL, Cotran RS, Kumar V. Inflammation and repair. In: Pathologic basis of disease. 3rd ed. Philadelphia: Saunders, 1984:64–65, 80–81.
32. Mundy AR. A trial comparing the Stamey bladder neck suspension procedure with colposuspension for the treatment of stress incontinence. Br J Urol 1983;55:687–690.
33. Bent AE, Ostergard DR, Zwick-Zaffulo M. Tissue reaction to expanded polytetrafluoroethylene

suburethral sling for urinary incontinence: clinical and histological study. Am J Obstet Gynecol 1993;169:1198–1204.

34. Morgan JE, Farrow GA. Recurrent stress urinary incontinence in the female. Br J Urol 1979;49: 37–42.

35. Bryans FE. Marlex gauze hammock sling operation with Cooper's ligament attachment in the management of recurrent urinary stress incontinence. Am J Obstet Gynecol 1979;133:292–294.

36. Morgan JE, Farrow GA, Stewart FE. The Marlex sling operation for the treatment of recurrent stress urinary incontinence: a 16-year review. Am J Obstet Gynecol 1985;151:554–556.

37. Brown GL, Richardson JE, Malangoni MA, Tobin GR, Ackerman D, Polk HC Jr. Comparison of prosthetic materials and abdominal wall reconstruction in the presence of contamination and infection. Ann Surg 1985;201:705–711.

38. Gamble JG, Simmons SC, Freedman M. The symphysis pubis: anatomic and pathologic considerations. Clin Ortho Rel Res 1986;203:261–272.

39. Mainprize TC, Drutz HP. The Marshall-Marchetti-Krantz procedure: a critical review. Obstet Gynecol Surv 1988;43:724–729.

40. Merimsdy E, Canetti R, Firstater M. Osteitis pubis: treatment by heparinisation. Br J Urol 1981; 53:154–156.

41. Lee RA. Surgical procedures for recurrent stress incontinence. In: Buchsbaum HJ, Schmidt JD, eds. Gynecologic and obstetric urology. Philadelphia: Saunders, 1982:307–317.

42. Khanna OP. Nonsurgical therapeutic modalities. In: Krane RJ, Siroky MB, eds. Clinical neurourology. Boston: Little, Brown, 1979:159–196.

43. Warren JW. Catheter-associated urinary tract infections. Infect Dis Clin North Am 1987;1: 823–854.

44. Bergman A, Matthews L, Ballard CA, Roy S. Suprapubic versus transurethral bladder drainage after surgery for stress urinary incontinence. Obstet Gynecol 1987;69:546–549.

45. Sethia KK, Selkon JB, Turner CM, Kettlewell MG, Gough MH. Prospective randomized controlled trial of urethral versus suprapubic catheterization. Br J Surg 1987;74:624–625.

46. Timmons MC, Addison WA. Suprapubic teloscopy: extraperitoneal intraoperative technique to demonstrate ureteral patency. Obstet Gynecol 1990;75:137–139.

47. Lin BL, Iwata Y. A modified cystoscopy to evaluate unilateral traumatic injury of the ureter during pelvic surgery. Am J Obstet Gynecol 1990;162: 1343–1344.

48. Pettit PD. Double-J ureteral catheters in gynecologic surgery. Obstet Gynecol 1989;75:536–540.

49. Podratz KC, Angerman NS, Symmonds RE. Complications of ureteral surgery in the nonradiated patient. In: Delgada G, Smith JP, eds. Management of complications in gynecologic oncology. New York: Wiley, 1982:113–149.

50. Maxted W. Complications of bladder surgery and cystoscopy. In: Delgado G, Smith JP, eds. Management of complications in gynecologic oncology. New York: Wiley, 1982:151–162.

51. Williams TJ. Abdominal hysterectomy, myomec-

tomy, presacral neurectomy, and surgery of ovarian malignancy with management of bladder injury and attention to thromboembolic disease. In: Ridley JH, ed. Gynecologic surgery: errors, safeguards, salvage. 2nd ed. Baltimore: Williams & Wilkins, 1981:35–39.

52. Galloway NTM, Davies N, Stephenson TP. The complications of colposuspension. Br J Urol 1987;60:122–124.

53. Lose G, Jorgensen L, Mortensen SO, Molsted-Pedersen L, Kristensen JK. Voiding difficulties after colposuspension. Obstet Gynecol 1987;69: 33–37.

54. Hertogs K, Stanton SL. Lateral bead-chain urethrocystography after successful and unsuccessful colposuspension. Br J Obstet Gynaecol 1985; 92:1179–1183.

55. Hertogs K, Stanton SL. Mechanism of urinary continence after colposuspension: barrier studies. Br J Obstet Gynaecol 1985;92:1184–1188.

56. Beck RP, McCormick S. Treatment of urinary stress incontinence with anterior colporrhaphy. Obstet Gynecol 1982;59:269–274.

57. Bump RC, Fantl JA, Hurt WG. Dynamic urethral pressure profilometry pressure transmission ratio determinations after continence surgery: understanding the mechanism of success, failure, and complications. Obstet Gynecol 1988; 72:870–877.

58. Bump RC, Hurt WG, Elser DM, et al. and the Continence Program for Women Research Group. Cough pressure transmission predicts urinary tract function in women soon after bladder neck surgery. Neurourol Urodyn 1995;14:431–432.

59. Bhatia NN, Bergman A. Urodynamic predictability of voiding following incontinence surgery. Obstet Gynecol 1984;63:85–91.

60. Crane JK, Bump RC. Drug therapy for urologic disorders. In: Rayburn WF, Zuspan FP, eds. Drug therapy in obstetrics and gynecology. 2nd ed. Norwalk, CT: Appleton-Century-Crofts, 1986: 419–433.

61. Stanton SL, Cardozo LD, Kerr-Wilson R. Treatment of delayed onset of spontaneous voiding after surgery for incontinence. Urology 1979;13: 494–496.

62. Jaschevatzky OE, Anderman S, Shalit A, Ellenbogen A, Grunstein S. Prostaglandin F_{2a} for prevention of urinary retention after vaginal hysterectomy. Obstet Gynecol 1985;66:244–247.

63. Tammela T, Kontturi M, Kaar K, Lukkarinen O. Intravesical prostaglandin F_2 for promoting bladder emptying after surgery for female stress incontinence. Br J Urol 1987;60:43–46.

64. Ghoniem GM, Elgamasy A-N. Simplified surgical approach to bladder outlet obstruction following pubovaginal sling. J Urol 1995;154:181–183.

65. Araki T, Takamotot H, Hara T, Fujimoto H, Yoshida M, Katayama Y. The loop-loosening procedure for urination difficulties after Stamey suspension of the vesical neck. J Urol 1990;144: 319–322.

66. Broberg C. Catheter drainage after gynecologic surgery: a comparison of methods. Am J Obstet Gynecol 1984;149:18–21.

67. Drutz HP, Khosid HI. Complications with Bon-

anno suprapubic catheters. Am J Obstet Gynecol 1984;149:685–686.

68. Morse RM, Spirnak JP, Resnick MI. Iatrogenic colon and rectal injuries associated with urological intervention: report of 14 patients. J Urol 1988;140:101–103.

69. Noller KI, Pratt JH, Symmonds RE. Bowel perforation with suprapubic cystotomy: report of two cases. Obstet Gynecol 1976;48:675–695.

70. Cundiff G, Bent AE. Suprapubic catheterization complicated by bowel injury. Int J Urogynecol 1995;6:110–113.

71. Bearman DM, Livengood CH III, Addison WA. Necrotizing fasciitis arising from a suprapubic catheter site. J Reprod Med 1988;33:411–413.

72. Cardozo LD, Stanton SL, Williams JE. Detrusor instability following surgery for genuine stress incontinence. Br J Urol 1979;51:204–207.

73. Kujansuu E. Urodynamic analysis of successful and failed incontinence surgery. Br J Gynaecol Obstet 1983;21:353–360.

74. Sand PK, Bowen LW, Ostergard DR, Brubaker L, Panganiban R. The effect of retropubic urethropexy on detrusor stability. Obstet Gynecol 1988;71:818–822.

75. Langer R, Ron-El R, Newman M, Herman A, Caspi E. Detrusor instability following colposuspension for urinary stress incontinence. Br J Obstet Gynaecol 1988;95:607–610.

76. Awad SA, Flood HD, Acker KL. The significance of prior anti-incontinence surgery in women who present with urinary incontinence. J Urol 1988; 140:514–517.

77. Lindner P, Mattiasson A, Perssons L, Uvelius B. Reversibility of detrusor hypertrophy and hyperplasia after removal of infravesical outflow obstruction in the rat. J Urol 1988;140: 652–656.

CHAPTER 46

Bladder Dysfunction after Intraabdominal or Vaginal Surgery

Eckhard Petri

Introduction

The close proximity of the lower urinary tract to the female genital tract makes urological complications one of the most common types after gynecological surgery (Table 46.1). Some of these are the direct result of urological injury at the time of surgery and are apparent either perioperatively or very early in the postoperative period. Other complications only become apparent with the passage of time, although some are due to operation trauma (1).

The incidence of urinary tract problems ranges from a 0.1% incidence of ureteric lesions after vaginal hysterectomy to a 70% incidence of urinary tract infections after colporrhaphy. The frequency of iatrogenic problems is important for the informed consent; in Germany, 8–10% of all legally accepted malpractice cases are related to gynecologists, and urinary tract problems comprise a major part of these.

Ureteric lesions pose problems for the gynecologist because their low frequency leads to a lack of experience with their recognition and treatment. On the other hand, problems like perioperative bladder drainage, urinary tract infection, the pros and cons of antibiotic prophylaxis, voiding dysfunction after radical surgery, and procedures for the treatment of urinary incontinence are everyday problems.

Etiology of Postoperative Voiding Difficulties

Bladder dysfunction is a frequent complication after gynecological surgery. Many patients are unable to void after an operation, irrespective of the type of procedure (i.e., vaginal, abdominal, or combined) performed. There are a variety of reasons for this difficulty.

Local causes of postoperative urinary retention include pain associated with attempts to void caused by edema around the bladder neck and urethra induced by general dissection or infection of the bladder. Also, many patients experience difficulty in voiding because of their reluctance or inability to void in a bedpan, on a public ward, or from an unnatural horizontal position.

Micturition can also be inhibited by a number of drug-related causes. Drugs can have an effect on the ability to void either because of their pharmacological influence on the central control of micturition or because of their effect on the interaction of cholinergic and adrenergic receptors of the bladder. Both agents used in surgical anesthesia and the medications and treatments administered postoperatively can affect the ability to void. Atropine, neuroleptics, and various muscle relaxants can have an initial parasympatholytic effect; anesthetics such as ketamine or enflurane can produce a reactive sympathicotonia. Both effects will produce a functional bladder neck obstruction. Analgesics administered postoperatively can decrease sensitivity of the thalamocortical pain tracts, reducing perception of the urge to void. Finally, vigorous intravenous hydration in the postoperative period can result in polyuria, which in combination with the relative loss of sensitivity of the bladder might lead to overdistension.

The type of operation performed can affect voiding in the postoperative period. Surgery done to enhance outflow resistance (e.g., colposuspension, sling procedure, or anterior repair) can produce varying degrees of retention.

Finally, many patients suffer from a variety of diseases, such as diabetes, drug abuse, or occult myelodysplasia, that are known to cause voiding disturbances. The stress and trauma of surgery may exacerbate this preexisting urological condition or cause urinary symptoms to appear de novo (2).

Radical Surgery

The causes of disorders of the lower urinary tract after radical pelvic surgery range from calculated injuries to the pelvic nerves and postural changes of the bladder in an empty pelvic cavity to accidental lesions caused by inadequate postoperative bladder drainage and urinary tract infection.

Most nerves from the pelvic plexus supplying the bladder pass over and around the vagina. Therefore, it is apparent that any operation that involves excision of the paracervical and paravaginal web of retroperitoneal tissue will interrupt at least some portion of the bladder innervation (Fig. 46.1). Some fibers pass around the lateral aspect of the vagina; however, it is evident that unless the dissection is carried fairly deeply toward the rectum (sacrouterine web), complete interruption is unlikely. It is also evident that in the operation as usually performed, this is the only site at which the parasympathetic nerves to the bladder enter the field of dissection. Complete interruption of the parasympathetic innervation can take place during abdominoperineal resection of the rectum and in posterior exenteration. In these cases, additional lesions to the somatic pudendal nerve may occur. In summary, the anatomic and functional trauma to the lower urinary tract in cancer surgery is highly related to the degree of radicalness (Tables 46.2 and 46.3).

Local causes, drug effects, and the type of operation, as described above, can all produce retention of urine after radical hysterectomy. In addition, direct nerve lesions, changes in blood supply, and lymphatic drainage play decisive roles in bladder dysfunction. Removing all connective tissue and vessels of the pelvis together with the lymph nodes leads to an interruption of lymphatic drainage. Postoperative edema and temporary interference with the nervous control result in a stiffness of the bladder wall, thus producing overflow incontinence. Given that an adequate "cancer operation" requires excision of a margin of healthy tissue around the tumor, it is difficult to see how direct

Table 46.1. Bladder Dysfunction after Gynecological Surgery

	Abdominal Hysterectomy[a] (%)	Vaginal Hysterectomy[b] (%)	Radical Hysterectomy with Lymphadenectomy[c] (%)
Stress incontinence	37	36	37
Urge incontinence			
Motor	25	24	11
Sensory	4	2	4
Overflow incontinence	2	1	8
Underactive detrusor function	10	4	41
Infravesical obstruction			
Mechanical	2	2	11
Functional	1	5	15

[a]N = 131.
[b]N = 157.
[c]N = 112.

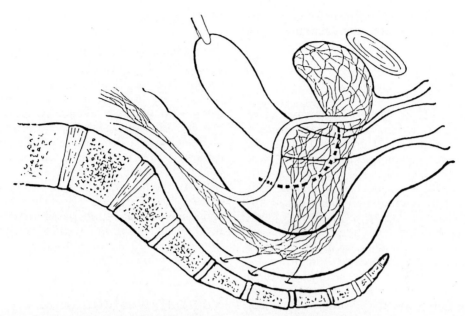

Figure 46.1. Distortion of relationships of ureter and pelvic plexus by traction during radical hysterec- tomy. Interrupted line indicates portion of plexus usually excised.

damage to the pelvic nerves and plexuses can be completely avoided during radical pelvic surgery. As demonstrated by Mundy (3), it would appear that the pelvic parasympa- thetic nerves and the pelvic plexus are far more vulnerable during rectal operations than during uterine operations. During radi- cal hysterectomy, the risk of damage to the pelvic nerves is small because the nerves are positioned well posteriorly and the bulk of the plexus lies below the cardinal ligament. This ligament contains some nerve fibers from the plexus; however, this part of the broad ligament is usually preserved during surgery. Only if the cardinal ligaments or an unusually long cuff of the upper vagina is removed is the field of excision likely to involve the plexus (Table 46.3).

Postoperative voiding disorders secondary to functional outlet obstruction are usually treated by insertion of a transurethral cath- eter. The catheter may be left in place for a variable period of time (6–60 days), depend- ing on the surgeon's preference and how soon normal micturition can resume. Known com- plications of catheterization include urethri- tis and ascending infection, which usually occur within 2–3 days after insertion of the catheter, and these can potentiate voiding difficulties by producing pain and edema.

Table 46.2. Bladder Dysfunction Depending on How Radical the Surgery (N = 202)

Procedure	Days of Drainage (mean ± SD)
Te-Linde	8.3 ± 2.3
Wertheim-Meigs	13.7 ± 4.1
Schauta	14.7 ± 8.1
Posterior exenteration	18.5 ± 5.0

Voiding problems may also result from over- distension caused by persistent residual urine (without desire to void because of the sensory loss) or from repeated catheteriza- tion to detect residual urine (4).

It has been postulated for a long time that the postoperative phase includes a period of bladder hypertonicity, which appears when the catheter is removed. This has been dem- onstrated by simple cystometry, and it has been suggested that the denervation of the detrusor muscle is responsible. Modern cys- tourethrography using microtip transducers seems to prove, however, that this is an artifact (5).

Thus, the causes of micturition disorders after radical pelvic surgery are multifactorial and include surgical lesions to nerve, blood vessels, and lymphatics; dislocation of the bladder into the wound cavity; and iatro-

genic lesions caused by repeated catheterization during the postoperative period.

Incidence

The actual incidence of postoperative
bladder dysfunction is difficult to determine.
The great number of surgical modifications,
new discussions on lesser or greater radical
surgery (6, 7), radical vaginal techniques still
in use (8–10), different forms of preoperative
or postoperative radiation therapy, and different types of intraoperative management,
together with the small numbers of patients
reviewed in most studies, make objective
comparison of the literature difficult.

Differentiation between postoperative data
and long-term results is necessary. There are
only a few prospective studies (11–13) or
controlled series. Preoperative assessment of
subjective micturition problems and urodynamic data are necessary to bring postoperative problems into correct perspective. Christ
and Gunselmann (12) performed a controlled
prospective study with preoperative urodynamic assessment that indicated preexisting
bladder dysfunction in 10 of 35 patients.
Most published data deal with subjective
complaints and would need exact confirmation (Table 46.4).

Prevention

To reduce the frequency of bladder dysfunction after radical pelvic surgery, detailed
preoperative examination of the urinary tract
is necessary. Efficient drainage of wound
cavities (to remove blood and lymph and to
prevent adhesions and infection) and the
bladder plays a decisive role. Suprapubic
catheterization is the preferred method of
bladder drainage because it allows better
patient tolerance, a decreased incidence of
urinary tract infection, an early return to
spontaneous micturition, possible control of
residual urine without further catheterization, and avoidance of urethral trauma and
discomfort (Fig. 46.2).

Vaginal or Abdominal Incontinence Surgery

Because behavior of the sphincteric
muscles of the pelvic floor has a pivotal
influence on the nature of bladder activity,
the two principal functions of the bladder—
storage and evacuation—can be viewed as
the natural consequence of neuromuscular
reflexes controlling the pelvic floor musculature (14). Many patients present with mixed

Table 46.3. Incidence of Urinary Tract Symptoms Depending on How Radical the Surgery

Procedure	Incontinence (%)	Diminished Sensation (%)	Follow-up
Wertheim-Meigs	10	27	Postoperatively
	4	18	1 year postoperatively
Latzko (ultraradical)	21	90	Postoperatively
	27	45	1 year postoperatively

Modified from Manzl J, Marberger F, Hetzel H, Klammer J, Geir W, Dapunt O. Funkitionelle Störungen des unteren Harntraktes nach Radikaloperationen des Kollumkarzinoms. Geburtsh Frauenheilkd 1981; 41:145–150.

Table 46.4. Incidence of Urinary Tract Symptoms After Radical Pelvic Surgery

Study	Vesical Dysfunction (%)	Incontinence (%)	Diminished Sensation (%)
Lewington (1956) (16)	43	28	34
Fraser (1966) (17)	59	24	22
Schmid and Baumann (1967) (18)	70	41	15 (postoperation)
	38		5 (2 y postoperation)
Ralph et al. (1988) (13)	81	52	48
		44 (preoperation)	

From Petri E. The effect of radical hysterectomy on micturition. In: General gynecology. Carnforth: Parthenon.

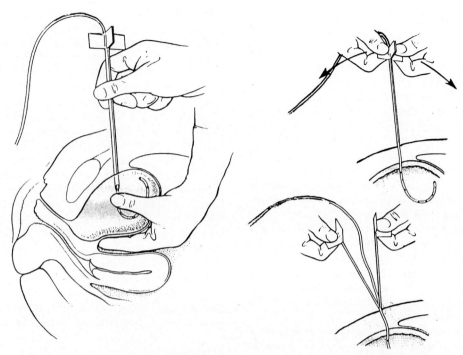

Figure 46.2.   Insertion of suprapubic catheter during laparotomy for bladder drainage.

complaints involving not only persistent or de novo stress-induced urinary leakage but also associated irritative voiding symptoms. Persistent voiding difficulties might either be caused by iatrogenic outflow obstruction or by vesical hypotonia.

Postoperative stress incontinence must first be considered as a true postoperative complication, but it can also be caused by inexpertly performed surgery or by an inappropriate antiincontinence procedure. Other complicating factors include obesity, chronic respiratory tract problems, and scar tissue formation as a result of multiple pelvic procedures. A particular complicating factor, often related to multiple surgical procedures, is the so-called "drainpipe" urethra or "frozen urethra." In this condition, the urethral wall is so heavily scarred that the urethra becomes a rigid tube and is no longer able to function as a sphincter-active pliable conduit (1). In this situation, any standard procedure is doomed to failure, and implantation of an artificial sphincter is probably all that can be offered.

Thorough pre- and postoperative urodynamic and radiographic investigations have

Table 46.5.   Cure Rate After Incontinence Surgery and Postoperative Voiding Dysfunction

	Success Rate (%)	Voiding Dysfunction (%)
Vaginal route		
Anterior repair	52–59	12–17
Puborectalis sling	50–75	0–15
Lyo-dura-sling	56–88	24–39
Abdominal route		
MMK	56–78	11–16
Cowan/Morgan	87	59
Burch	82–95	12–38

From Eberhard J, Schär G. Beziehunger zwischen Miktionsbeschwerden und tonometrischen Ver änderungen im Urethraprofil nach Inkontinenzoperationen. Arch Gynecol Obstet 1989; 245:751–753; and author's own data.

shown a negative correlation between the success rates of incontinence procedures and iatrogenic voiding difficulties (Table 46.5). Pure vaginal approaches result in voiding difficulties in 0–24% but demonstrate failure rates of 50% or more in an objective follow-up. Different forms of colposuspension, however, might have cure rates of 90% but can result in obstructed voiding and postoperative urge incontinence in 30–60% of cases.

Treatment

After determining whether a patient's voiding dysfunction results from excessive facilitation or inhibition of either the detrusor or the sphincter or both, one can apply appropriate therapy to this physiological dysfunctional activity. Effective drainage of the bladder is one of the prerequisites of treatment. The advantages of suprapubic drainage over transurethral catheterization have already been discussed. Suprapubic catheterization is preferred in all patients requiring bladder drainage for more than 48 hours. Therefore, all types of antiincontinence procedures as well as radical pelvic surgery are clear indications for suprapubic bladder drainage. The low incidence of urinary tract infection associated with suprapubic drainage results in reduced costs for antibiotic treatment.

Adjuvant pharmacotherapy seems to be of limited value because it produces severe side effects at effective dosages and, in most cases, does not treat the underlying problem. Assuming that periurethral edema, hematoma, and swelling of the bladder neck and the bladder base area is the cause of micturition problems after most antiincontinence procedures, it seems much more reasonable to administer antiinflammatory agents rather than specific antimicrobial agents. It is important to realize that after surgery, even after radical surgery for gynecological cancer, dysfunction decreases during the first postoperative months. This decrease, as well as the psychological support provided and the patient's awareness of having escaped cancer or having resolved her problems with incontinence, leads 80–90% of all patients to say that they are largely satisfied with their condition, despite demonstrable dysfunction at 1 year after surgery.

Summary

Vaginal or abdominal surgery in the small pelvis places the lower urinary tract at considerable risk of injury or dysfunction. Although intraoperative lesions of the ureter or bladder are rare, urinary problems continue to be the most significant complication after radical hysterectomy and antiincontinence surgery. Damage to pelvic nerves in radical surgery, interruption of blood supply and lymphatic drainage secondary to extensive preparation during vaginal procedures, and scar tissue formation in the periurethral space in all antiincontinence procedures result in various bladder disturbances. The therapeutic regimen cannot be decided schematically but must be influenced by clinical findings and urodynamic data. In most patients, if good bladder drainage is established postoperatively, bladder function and continence mechanisms will recover within the first month. If, despite suprapubic drainage and adjuvant antiinflammatory pharmacotherapy, adequate voiding cannot be established, then specific drugs (see Chapter 19), bladder retraining (see Chapter 34), or, in selected patients, bladder stimulation therapy or implantation of an artificial sphincter or a magnetic device may be useful.

REFERENCES

1. Mundy AR. Urological complications and how to cope. In: Stanton SL, ed. Principles of gynaecological surgery. London: Springer, 1987:245–256.
2. Petri E, Frohneberg D. Peritherapeutisches blasenmanagement. In: Petri E, ed. Gynäkologische urologie. Stuttgart: Thieme, 1996:91–100.
3. Mundy AR. An anatomical explanation for bladder dysfunction following rectal and uterine surgery. Br J Urol 1982;54:501–506.
4. Manzl J, Marberger F, Hetzel H, Klammer J, Geir W, Dapunt O. Funkytionelle Störungen des unteren Harntraktes nach Radikaloperationen des Kollumkarzinoms. Geburtsh Frauenheilkd 1981; 41:145–150.
5. Asmussen M, Miller A. Clinical gynaecological urology. London: Blackwell Scientific Publications, 1983:4.
6. Ober KG. Die abgestufte Therapie des Zervixkarzinoms. Geburtsh Frauenheilkd 1978;38: 671–684.
7. Burghardt E. Zur Frage der sogenannten konservativen Behandlung des atypischen Zervixepithels. Geburtsh Frauenheilkd 1981;41:330–334.
8. Barclay DI, Roman-Lopez JJ. Bladder dysfunction after Schauta hysterectomy. Am J Obstet Gynecol 1975;123:519–526.
9. Fischer W, Selig V, Lamm D. Fortschritte bei der Verhütung und Bekämpfung urologischer Komplikationen des Zervixkarzinoms. Zentralbl Gynaekol 1978;100:1320–1331.
10. Pflüger H, Nürnberger N, Kupka S, Leodolter S, Wagner G, Diagnostik and Therapie postoperativer Blasenentleerungsstörungen nach gynäkologischer Radikaloperation. Gynaekol Rdsch 1980;20(Suppl 2):191–194.
11. Seski JC, Diokno AC. Bladder dysfunction after

radical abdominal hysterectomy. Am J Obstet Gynecol 1977;128:643–651.

12. Christ F. Gunselmann W. Untersuchungen zur Urodynamik von Harnblase and Harnröhre nach Zervixkrebsoperationen. Geburtsh Frauenheilkd 1980;40:610–618.

13. Ralph G, Tamussino K, Lichtenegger W. Urodynamics following radical abdominal hysterectomy for cervical cancer. Arch Gynecol Obstet 1988;243:215–220.

14. Schmidt RA. Post-operative voiding dysfunction. In: Stanton SL, Tanagho EA, eds. Surgery of female incontinence, 2nd ed. London: Springer, 1986:259–266.

15. Petri E. The effect of radical hysterectomy on micturition. In: General gynecology. Carn-

forth, UK: Parthenon, 1990:219–225.

16. Lewington W. Disturbances of micturition following Wertheim hysterectomy. J Obstet Gynaecol Br Emp 1956;63:861–864.

17. Fraser AC. The late effects of Wertheim's hysterectomy of the urinary tract. Br J Obstet Gynaecol 1966;73:1002–1007.

18. Schmid I, Baumann U. Blasenkomplikationen nach abdominaler erweiterter Hysterekomie mit Lymphonodektomie und Nachbestrahlung. Geburtsh Grauenheilkd 1967;24:354–369.

19. Eberhard J, Schär G. Beziehunge zwischen Miktionsbeschwerden und tonometrischen Veränderungen im Urethraprofil nach Inkontinenzoperationen. Arch Gynecol Obstet 1989;245:751–753.

CHAPTER 47

Misadventures in the Surgical Management of Genuine Stress Incontinence

Hilary J. Cholhan and Donald R. Ostergard

Introduction

Surgery continues to be the most widely accepted and curative treatment for genuine stress incontinence (GSI). However, a patient is at times treated surgically for urinary incontinence, only to experience early recurrence or exacerbation of her preoperative condition. This is often devastating to the patient, who already may have been socially incapacitated by her incontinence before surgery. It is thus incumbent on the clinician to approach the preoperative evaluation and management of the patient with urinary incontinence in a meticulous manner.

Once GSI has been proven urodynamically and treated surgically, what constitutes successful cure? This can be viewed from the perspective of the clinician/urodynamicist and the patient. From the urodynamicist's standpoint, success is often viewed in purist terms; namely, the absence of urinary leakage with correction of pressure equalization in the face of stress as evidenced by urethral closure pressure profilometry after surgery and technically by maintenance of the bladder neck and proximal urethra in their "normal" intraabdominal sphere. From the patient's perspective, success may mean reestablishment of total continence or an amelioration of the incontinence that she had experienced before surgery. Of note, both parties would deem the surgical treatment further complicated if bladder instability

were to develop de novo, with eventual reappearance of incontinence. Avoidance of pitfalls is paramount in achieving the successful cure of GSI via surgical correction.

Preoperative Evaluation

Before consideration of surgical treatment for urinary incontinence, it is imperative to make an objective diagnosis of GSI. Most studies revealed that reliance on a history of stress-induced incontinence can be misleading. Although the symptom of stress incontinence is a sensitive detector of GSI (approaching 100%), it is not very specific (65.2%) (1). Rarely do the history and physical examination provide sufficient information to arrive at an accurate diagnosis of GSI. They merely direct the clinician to further investigation. It has become increasingly apparent that the unequivocal diagnosis of GSI should be objectively demonstrated via urodynamic testing. A hasty diagnosis of GSI may be either erroneous or may obscure other confounding diagnoses, which may impair the successful cure of the incontinent patient (2).

The critical factor involved in the prevention of untoward postoperative sequelae, including recurrence of incontinence, is the knowledge and anticipation of potential complications. For instance, a patient may have GSI in conjunction with bladder instability. The latter may be of such severity that it precludes surgical correction of GSI, because surgery may exacerbate the existing detrusor instability (DI) postoperatively (3). Interestingly, antiincontinence surgery may, on the other hand, improve preexisting DI in upward of 30–55% of patients with a mixed incontinence picture (4). At present, however, no factor or combination of factors has been uncovered that can predict how DI will be affected or precipitated by surgery in a given patient. Persistence is important in attempting to elicit involuntary bladder contractions during cystometrograms via an assortment of provocative maneuvers, including positional changes, Valsalva maneuver, cough, heel-bouncing, the sound of running water, and having the patient splash her hands in a basin of warm water. It may not be possible to reproduce involuntary bladder contractions in the laboratory setting; therefore, if the patient's history is suggestive of an unstable bladder, the investigator must persevere and repeat the cystometrogram during subsequent office visits. Thus, the diagnosis of GSI is crucial, but perhaps confirming the presence or absence of bladder instability and judging its severity is even more critical.

Uroflowmetry is useful primarily as a screening test to define a subset of patients who may experience voiding difficulties after incontinence surgery, thus necessitating prolonged postoperative bladder catheterization. The determination of residual urine is also important to rule out chronic retention with or without overflow incontinence. Bhatia and Bergman (5) demonstrated that patients with inadequate or absent bladder contractions (less than 15 cm H_2O) and abnormal voiding patterns before surgery, corroborated by both simultaneous urethrocystometry and uroflowmetry, ought to be prepared by the clinician to expect prolonged catheterization after surgery.

Cystourethroscopy is a major adjunct in the preoperative investigation of the incontinent female. Indeed, it would be embarrassing to have operated on a patient whose stress-related incontinence was precipitated by an undiagnosed urethral diverticulum, "drainpipe" urethra, ectopic ureter, or a fistula, which may leak intermittently. All these conditions can simulate GSI.

Invaluable data regarding the functional/ anatomic urethral lengths, maximum urethral closure pressure, pressure equalization with cough, and pressure transmission ratios are generated by multichannel urodynamic testing, which includes urethral pressure profilometry. This information is required when deciding which procedure would be of most benefit to the patient. For example, many patients with low maximum urethral closure pressure have undergone transabdominal retropubic urethropexy (6). For many of these patients, cure has not resulted from the surgery, and they may have fared better with a suburethral sling procedure. However, without multichannel urodynamic testing, the presence of low maximum urethral closure pressure would not have been detected preoperatively.

One of the more difficult questions confronting urogynecologists is whether all incontinent patients should undergo exhaustive multichannel urodynamic evaluation. The issue is particularly salient considering the growing number of patients who would require such testing, the expensive equipment and trained personnel required, and the recent fiscal constraints on medical expenditure. Comprehensive investigation is strongly recommended because surgery in inappropriately selected candidates can result in outright failure, exacerbation of the existing condition, or premature recurrence (7). The cost of resolving these complications would likely be several times greater than that of the preoperative evaluation. Table 47.1 illustrates our investigative approach to the female incontinent patient.

Table 47.1. Preoperative Evaluation of the Incontinent Patient

History
  24-hour urinary voiding diary
  Current medications
  Patient self-evaluation (prioritizing of urinary problems)
Physical examination
  Screening neurological examination of sacral segments
  Pelvic examination
Urodynamic evaluation
  Cotton swab test
  Urethrocystoscopy
  "Stress" test
  (multichannel urodynamic studies)

Table 47.2.   Medical Conditions that May Impair Success of GSI Surgery

Systemic disease
  Diabetes mellitus or insipidus
  Steroid-dependent disease (i.e., Cushing's disease/syndrome)
  Psychogenic polydypsia
Extensive pelvic irradiation
Nutritional deprivation
  Anorexia nervosa
  Unsupervised/starvation dieting
Chronic respiratory disease
Coagulopathy[a]
Chronic anticoagulant therapy[a]
Obesity

[a]May predispose to hematoma formation.

The anticipation of potential postoperative complications that may hinder the success of incontinence surgery is essential (Table 47.2). The preoperative evaluation of the patient with GSI includes a detailed review of the patient's medical history, including current medications. Many prescription medications have been found to decrease intraurethral pressure and either cause or contribute to the stress incontinence (see Chapter 19). The primary objective of a thorough preoperative evaluation is to optimize the patient's condition before surgery and to prepare her for all possible postoperative events from both the physiological and psychological standpoints.

Surgical Technique

CHOICE OF SUTURE MATERIAL

With the exception of the anterior colporrhaphy, where delayed-absorbable sutures have replaced the traditional chromic catgut, permanent monofilament material is the optimal choice for sutures used in the surgical correction of GSI. Incontinence surgery is intended to provide long-lasting support to the proximal urethra-bladder base unit while endogenous reparative processes (i.e., scarification) are completed. Although synthetic, delayed-absorbable sutures (glycolipid acid copolymer and polydioxanone) maintain nearly 50% of their original tensile strength by the 28th postoperative day, their rate of complete absorption is quite variable (ranging from 40–90 days) and relatively unpredictable (8). Permanent material is biologically inert and, therefore, offers long-lasting strength and a decreased risk of host reaction. Furthermore, monofilament sutures do not promote bacterial invasion and infection.

The use of the suburethral sling procedure mandates not only a choice of suture material but a choice of sling material. In the past, the use of endogenous tissue, including fascia lata, rectus fascia, and round ligaments, was commonplace. The major drawback of this option was the harvesting of a sufficient quantity and quality of sling material. Obtaining fascia lata involves a second incision, which becomes another source of postoperative pain to the patient and risks potential complications at the site of the incision (i.e., infection).

Synthetic materials are not devoid of problems. Mersilene gauze and Marlex mesh are resistant to antibiotic therapy should infection take root. Furthermore, if sling removal is required, these materials have extensive ingrowth of the patient's scar tissue, making removal difficult. More recently, the Gore-Tex (polytetrafluoroethylene [PTFE]) soft-tissue patch (W.L. Gore and Associates, Inc.), fashioned into an appropriate sling shape, has been used with exceptionally good results. This material satisfies most of the requisites of an ideal sling material, including inertness, porosity, strength, and malleability.

Inertness results in a decreased inflammatory response. Porosity permits ingrowth of natural connective tissue elements, which has the advantage of augmentation of the inherent strength and memory of the Gore-Tex material. The conformability and softness of the Gore-Tex material makes it easy to work with, less irritating to the urethra and bladder base, and resistant to twisting and rolling. However, recently, Bent et al. (9) reported a 23% reaction or removal rate due to host rejection of the PTFE sling graft. This high complication rate might dissuade us from continued usage of PTFE. Complete resolution of vaginal granulation tissue and continued maintenance of stress continence after removal in most patients may allow the PTFE patch to survive, albeit in a more limited role.

CAVEATS IN SURGICAL TECHNIQUE

Correct placement of sutures; the amount of tension placed on these sutures and slings; and the avoidance of trauma to blood vessels, nerves, and urinary structures are extremely important in incontinence surgery. In reestablishing the once-normal pelvic anatomic relationships, it is paramount not to interfere with the urethra, per se. Thus, sutures placed in the paravaginal supportive tissue must be a relatively safe distance from the urethra. In the transabdominal retropubic urethropexy, we recommend that the two pairs of sutures be placed parallel to the urethra (i.e., in the vicinity of the midurethra and at the level of the urethrovesical junction). The urethrovesical junction is delineated by placing gentle downward traction on an indwelling transurethral Foley catheter and palpating the inflatable balloon.

Adequate bites of paravaginal tissue must be taken to prevent inadvertent tearing out of the sutures. When elevating the vaginal wall to a fixed structure (e.g., Cooper's ligament, periosteum pubis, symphyseal cartilage), it is important not to hoist the elevated structure overzealously because this may precipitate immobility of the bladder base or cause outflow obstruction. The objective is to have the nonabsorbable sutures act as "struts," permitting the endogenous scarification process to afford permanent support.

Careful retropubic dissection and satisfactory exposure aids in avoidance of the aberrant obturator vein and injury to the ureters, bladder, and urethra. Intraoperative bleeding in the richly vascular retropubic space is not uncommon and must be controlled with vascular clips, electrocoagulation, or suture ligation. Often, tension created when tying the "antiincontinence" sutures sufficiently controls oozing. Unrecognized or unaddressed bleeding predisposes to hematoma formation and/or infection, unfortunately an all-too-common postoperative complication. Osteitis pubis occurs with a frequency of less than 5% in patients who undergo the Marshall-Marchetti-Krantz procedure. This process may lead, however, to significant morbidity and suffering to the patient and is difficult to eradicate.

The transvaginal retropubic urethropexy presents similar dilemmas. First, usage of absorbable material for the suspensory sutures carries a higher risk of surgical failure as reported recently by Korn (10) and Bergman and Elia (11). Also, overzealous elevation of the paravaginal tissue can commonly result in outflow obstruction and DI. An uncommon sequela is neuropraxia (weakness, hyperesthesia) of the obturator nerve branches; this is presumably the result of wide passage of the needles, which may transiently irritate or permanently injure these nerve branches. Miyazaki and Shook (12) recently described a similar phenomenon developing with ilioinguinal nerve entrapment. Performance of intraoperative cystourethroscopy must be strongly encouraged in conjunction with any antiincontinence procedure. Direct visualization of the bladder from within rules out injury to this organ. In addition, during the sling procedure, cystoscopy allows assessment of the ureteral orifices and their function (ejection of intravenously administered indigo carmine dye) to be certain that the free arms of the sling have not impinged on the ureters. Urethroscopy permits examination of the urethrovesical junction to ensure placement of desired tension on the sling.

SPECIAL CONSIDERATIONS

Obesity

Many gynecological surgeons insist that their obese patients lose a predetermined amount of weight before considering antiincontinence surgery. It has been shown that obesity causes chronically elevated intraabdominal pressures, which may compromise the success of an antiincontinence procedure. Weight reduction may be difficult for the patient, and rapid weight loss could compromise the patient's nutritional status and postoperative healing.

For markedly obese women, we modify our surgical techniques. First, we avoid transvaginal needle suspension procedures, if at all possible. Second, in performing the Burch colposuspension procedure, we substitute Prolene mesh for the usual PTFE sutures. A 2 × 2 cm mesh graft is attached to the vaginal fascia and Cooper's ligament on each side with PTFE sutures. The mesh is used in the hope of promoting increased scarification and a larger surface area over which to distribute the supporting tension over the paravaginal fascia.

Pregnancy

Pregnancy after successful antiincontinence surgery is not an uncommon situation
today, particularly with delayed childbearing. As mentioned previously, vaginal delivery is an important contributing factor in the
development of GSI. Therefore, it can be
assumed that vaginal delivery might jeopar-
dize the long-term success of antiincontinence surgery. Careful patient counseling in
preparation for childbirth ought to include
consideration of delivery by cesarean section; however, ultimately the patient will
decide on the mode of delivery, as long as she
understands the potential ramifications of
her choice. Furthermore, antiincontinence
surgery should be delayed until the patient
has completed childbearing.

Convalescent Period

The peri- and postoperative periods may
be punctuated by a number of complications
(Table 47.3).

Because urogynecological surgery often
entails concurrent suprapubic and vaginal
approaches, predisposing to inevitable con-

Table 47.3. General Risk Factors for GSI Surgery

Preoperative
  Advanced age
  Chronic illness
    Chronic systemic illness
    Chronic pulmonary disease
    Steroid therapy, protracted
  Malignant disease
  Poor nutritional status
Intraoperative
  Improper selection of
    Technique
    Suture/sling materials
  Overzealous elevation of urethrovesical
    junction
Postoperative
  Increased intraabdominal pressure
    Nausea/vomiting/retching
    Coughing
    Constipation
    Premature exertion
  Incisional site complications
    Wound infection/abscess
    Granuloma formation
    Sinus tract

tamination of the abdominal surgical field
with bacteria from the lower genital tract no
matter what precautions are taken, infection
continues to be a potential problem of concern. It has now become common practice to
use prophylactic intraoperative antibiotics to
minimize this risk of infection (13).

Most gynecological infectious disease specialists advocate the use of antibiotics with a
broad spectrum of activity to provide coverage against the potentially pathogenic bacteria most commonly found in the lower genital tract. Ideally, the goal would be to reduce
the inoculum load (i.e., count) and to prevent
the overgrowth of any particular species of
bacteria. The closest approximation to this
ideal goal is the choice of an antimicrobial
agent that possesses a spectrum of activity
against the bacteria most likely to initiate an
infection. First- or second-generation cephalosporins have been proven highly effective
in this role.

Usage of prophylactic antibiotics should
not, however, underplay the importance of
the surgeon's role in the meticulous handling
of tissues, achievement of total hemostasis,
obliteration of dead space, and avoidance of
contamination of the abdominal field.

As with all gynecological surgery in which
general inhalation anesthesia is used, prevention of pulmonary atelectasis is vital.
This becomes especially important in antiincontinence surgery, where severe coughing
causes impingement on the newly reconstructed site that buttresses the bladder neck
and the proximal urethra. Much the same can
be said for the avoidance of constipation and
the attendant straining that frequently accompanies this condition. Stool softeners
should be prescribed in the immediate postoperative period.

Before reestablishment of normal bladder
function after antiincontinence surgery, continuous bladder drainage via catheterization
is used. This, too, predisposes to infection of
the lower urinary tract. The suprapubic catheter is preferred because, unlike the transurethral catheter, it does not predispose to colonization of the lower urinary tract via ascent
of bacterial biofilm. The suprapubic catheter
allows greater flexibility in monitoring the
resumption of bladder function when measuring the voided and residual volumes.
Strict adherence to relative inactivity in the
first 3 months after surgery is of utmost

importance. Strenuous activities must be avoided, but brisk walking is permitted. In our experience, 3 months affords ample time for recuperation and for the healing process to be completed.

Summary

In the last 25 years, urogynecology has progressed from the time when a patient's complaints of urinary leakage resulted in the performance of the standard anterior colporrhaphy to the present more scientific and objective approach to the diagnosis and management of GSI.

To optimize the potential for successful surgical management of GSI, it is important to demonstrate objectively the presence of this condition, select the appropriate antiincontinence procedure and suture/sling material, evaluate the patient's presurgical medical condition and encourage the patient to maintain relative inactivity during the postoperative period of convalescence. The individualization of the therapeutic strategy, combined with a meticulous approach, should result in fewer misadventures in the surgical management of GSI in the future.

REFERENCES

1. Sand PK, Hill RC, Ostergard DR. Incontinence history as a predictor of detrusor instability. Obstet Gynecol 1988;71:257–260.
2. Thiede HA, Saini VD. Urogynecology: comments and caveats. Am J Obstet Gynecol 1987;157:563–568.
3. Karram MM, Bhatia NN. Management of coexistent stress and urge urinary incontinence. Obstet Gynecol 1989;73:4–7.
4. Sand PK, Bowen LW, Ostergard DR, et al. The effect of retropubic urethropexy on detrusor instability. Obstet Gynecol 1988;71:818–822.
5. Bhatia NN, Bergman A. Use of preoperative uroflowmetry and simultaneous urethrocystometry for predicting risk of prolonged postoperative bladder drainage. Urology 1986;28:440–445.
6. Sand PK, Bowen LW, Panganiban R, Ostergard DR. The low pressure urethra as a factor in failed retropubic urethropexy. Obstet Gynecol 1987;69:399–402.
7. Thiede HA. Urodynamic laboratory evaluation needed by all patients before surgery for genuine stress incontinence. Obstet Gynecol Rep 1989;1:354–360.
8. Sanz LE. Wound management: technique and suture material. In: Sanz LE, ed. Gynecologic surgery. Oradell, NJ: Medical Economics, 1988:21–38.
9. Bent AE, Ostergard DR, Zwick-Zaffuto M. Tissue reaction to expanded polytetrafluoroethylene suburethral sling for urinary incontinence: clinical and histologic study. Am J Obstet Gynecol 1993;169:1198–1204.
10. Korn AP. Does use of permanent suture material affect outcome of modified Pereyra procedure? Obstet Gynecol 1994;83:104–107.
11. Bergman A, Elia G. Three surgical procedures for genuine stress incontinence: five-year follow up of a prospective randomized study. Am J Obstet Gynecol 1995;173:66–71.
12. Miyazaki F, Shook G. Ilioinguinal nerve entrapment during needle suspension for stress incontinence. Obstet Gynecol 1992;80:246–248.
13. Faro S. Antibiotic prophylaxis. Obstet Gynecol Clin North Am 1989;16:2;279–289.

CHAPTER 48

Periurethral Bulking Agents

Rodney A. Appell and J. Christian Winters

Urinary incontinence may originate at the level of the bladder or the urethra. In evaluating patients for the use of intraurethral injections as a treatment of urinary incontinence, it is essential to identify the cause(s) of incontinence to recommend appropriate therapy. Intraurethral injections benefit patients with incontinence occurring at the level of the urethra. Incontinence occurring at the level of the urethra may be due to anatomic displacement of a normally functioning urethra (anatomic genuine stress urinary incontinence [GSI]) in females or intrinsic incompetence of the urethral closure mechanism (intrinsic sphincteric dysfunction [ISD]) in females or males. Patients with ISD commonly have had a previous surgical procedure on or near the urethra, a sympathetic neurological injury, or myelodysplasia. Female patients with GSI have normal urethral function but hypermobility of the bladder neck and proximal urethra resulting from a deficiency in pelvic support. These patients benefit from a bladder neck elevation and stabilization. Patients with ISD have poor urethral function and require procedures to increase outflow resistance. Bladder neck suspension procedures will fail in these patients due to the poor urethral function, and these patients require pubovaginal sling procedures, artificial urinary sphincters, or periurethral injections.

In patients with ISD, the presence or absence of anatomic support will assist in directing future management. At present, patients with a lack of anatomic support (hypermobility) and ISD are better treated with sling procedures or artificial urinary sphincters. Patients with a fixed well-supported urethra in association with ISD are excellent candidates for periurethral injec-

tion. During the multicenter investigation of collagen in the treatment of ISD, the patients selected with anatomic (type II) incontinence did not fair well (1, 2). Therefore, the recommendation currently is to perform intraurethral or periurethral injections on patients with a poorly functioning urethra (ISD) and good anatomic support. However, recent data suggest that intraurethral injections may be used for selected patients with GSI (3).

Evaluation and Patient Selection

When obtaining a history from patients with urinary incontinence, it is important to elucidate previous surgery or an underlying neurological disorder. Also, the activity precipitating urinary leakage is important. Patients who leak in the supine position, have bed wetting, or leak with a sensation of urinary urgency do not have GSI and need to be investigated for bladder instability and/or ISD. In females, the physical examination is essential to ascertain if concomitant urogenital prolapse and urethral hypermobility are present. The cotton swab test with an angle of greater than 30 degrees signifies urethral hypermobility (4).

Urodynamic studies are performed to evaluate possible bladder causes of incontinence (instability, decreased contractility/ overflow) and to evaluate urethral function. Tests of urethral function may be performed using leak point pressures or urethral pressure profiles. An abdominal leak point pressure is the abdominal pressure required to drive urine through the urethra. This corresponds to urethral opening pressure, and low urethral opening pressure implies minimal urethral resistance and poor urethral function. Therefore, low abdominal leak point pressures are required to elicit leakage per urethra in patients with ISD. The abdominal leak point pressure (Valsalva leak point pressure [VLPP]) is obtained with the patient straining while the bladder is filled at incremental volumes of 50 mL beginning at 150 mL and followed to 300 mL. The patient is asked to strain, and the pressure is recorded at which urine leaks through the sphincteric mechanism. Leakage can be identified either by direct vision or by radioflouroscopic assessment of contrast during a videourodynamic procedure. VLPP of less than 60 cm H_2O signifies poor or absent urethral function. These measurements have been shown to correlate with urethral pressure profiles and are less variable and easier to perform (5). Videourodynamics are urodynamic studies performed in conjunction with radiographic analysis of the bladder. The presence of an open bladder neck with the bladder at rest in the absence of a detrusor contraction implies the presence of ISD. Patients who have undergone multiple surgical procedures, have mixed incontinence, or have neurogenic bladders benefit greatly from videourodynamic procedures. At present, the ideal patient for periurethral injections is a patient with poor urethral function, normal bladder capacity, and good anatomic support. A clear advantage of injectables in ISD is the attainment of increased urethral closing function with only minor increases in urethral closing pressure. Patients with minimal hypermobility and high leak point pressures or elderly less active females with anatomic incontinence may be considered for periurethral injections as well; however, it is wise to reserve this therapy for patients in this population who represent a surgical risk or have a more limited mobility.

Contraindications to periurethral injections include active urinary tract infection, untreated detrusor instability, and known hypersensitivity to the injected agent. Patients who are to have intraurethral injections of collagen must undergo skin testing 1 month before the procedure to determine whether hypersensitivity to the material is present (6). In the Gax collagen multicenter trial, 4% of the female patients exhibited hypersensitivity during skin testing (7).

Injectable Materials

The ideal material for periurethral injection is one that is easily injected, biocompatible, and causes little or no inflammatory reaction. Also, the substance should elicit no immunogenic response. There should be no migration of the injected material, and it should maintain its bulking effect for a long period of time. Many agents have been used as injectables for urinary incontinence, ranging from sclerosing agents to autologous blood (8, 9). Currently, the most widely used agent is cross-linked bovine collagen. Collagen (Contigen™) received approval from the U.S. Food and Drug Administration for the treatment of ISD in male and female patients in September 1993. Autologous fat has gained acceptance in females who demonstrated hypersensitivity to collagen, although results have not been as satisfactory (10). Polytetrafluoroethylene (PTFE) paste was removed from the U.S. marketplace because of concerns over its migration and safety (11), despite being proven as an effective method of treatment for urinary incontinence with no reports of untoward sequelae in human beings (12). For this reason, PTFE is currently undergoing trials in direct comparison with Contigen™ aiming toward reapproval for the treatment of ISD in females. These agents may be injected safely under local anesthesia, allowing potential use in patients considered poor surgical risks.

PTFE PASTE (URETHRIN™)

This is a sterile mixture of PTFE micropolymer particles, glycerine and polysorbate. PTFE particles stimulate an ingrowth of fibroblasts at the injection site, become encapsulated, and produce a permanent bolstering effect (12). These particles elicit a chronic foreign body reaction with granuloma formation. Documented evidence of particle migration and granuloma formation has raised concerns about the use of this material (11).

AUTOLOGOUS FAT

As a periurethral bulking agent, fat has several advantages: availability, biocompatibility, and obtainability. Fat integrates as a graft; however, a significant portion of the injected material is reabsorbed and replaced by inflammation and fibrosis with connective tissue producing the final bulk effect (10). The high degree of absorption is the major limitation in using fat as an injectable agent. There is no evidence of migration of the injected fat particles.

GLUTARALDEHYDE CROSS-LINKED BOVINE COLLAGEN (CONTIGEN™)

This agent is both biocompatible and biodegradable. It is a sterile nonpyrogenic bovine dermal collagen cross-linked with glutaraldehyde and dispersed in a phosphate-buffered physiological saline. The cross-linking process improves the integrity of the material for the injection by increasing its resistance to collagenase and decreasing the antigenicity of the collagen. A minimal inflammatory response has been associated with the injection of collagen, and no granuloma formation or foreign body reaction is present. Also, no foreign body reaction occurs. Contigen™ begins to degrade in approximately 12 weeks; however, in this period of time, neovascularization and the deposition by fibroblasts of host collagen occurs within the implant. The collagen completely degrades within 10–19 months (13). There are no reports of particle migration of the collagen material (14).

SILICONE POLYMERS

Macroplastique™ or Bioplastique™ are textured silicone macroparticles suspended within a hydrogel. The hydrogel is rapidly absorbed by the host tissue; however, the macroimplant becomes fixed in position by encapsulation. The particle size is greater than 100 µm, which inhibits migration (15). Henly et al. (15) compared migratory and histological tendencies of solid silicone macrospheres to smaller silicone particles in dogs. Nuclear imaging revealed small particles dissipated throughout the lung, kidney, brain, and lymph nodes at 4 months. One episode of large particle migration to the lung occurred without associated inflammation, and an x-ray analysis confirmed that the particles were silicone. Initial clinical trials demonstrated the potential of this substance for the treatment of ISD and GSI; however, migration has been documented to be a problem with even large particle injections, and the use of this material will likely be limited in the United States (16).

Technique of Injection

The technique of injection of material is not difficult; however, it is essential to perform precise placement of the material to ensure an optimal result. The injection can be performed either suburothelially through a needle placed directly through a cystoscope (transurethral injection) or periurethrally with a spinal needle inserted percutaneously and positioned in the urethral tissues in the suburothelial space observing the manipulation cystoscopically (17).

Although men are injected predominantly by the transurethral approach, females are injected by either transcystoscopic implantation of a needle into the suburothelium (18) or by placement of a spinal needle inserted percutaneously along the wall of the urethra while observing the delivery of the material directly by urethroscopy (17). Also, indirect visualization by ultrasound has been described as useful in the precise localization of the injection (19). Recently, Neal et al. (20) introduced a technique to facilitate periurethral needle placement using methylene blue mixed with local anesthesia, enabling the surgeon to place the implant more accurately. There is certainly a learning curve with any technique chosen that ultimately results in using less injectable material to attain continence. We describe the technique of injection in females using collagen, as this is currently the most widely used injectable substance. After this, we make additional comments concerning the alterations of techniques in the injection of other injectable materials.

TECHNIQUE OF INJECTION IN THE FEMALE PATIENT

Women may be injected by way of a transcystoscopic technique (18) or a periurethral approach (17). We prefer the periurethral approach, as this minimizes intraurethral bleeding and extravasation of the injectable substance. With either approach, the woman is placed in the lithotomy position; the introitus is anesthetized with 20% topical benzocaine and the urethra is anesthetized with topical 2% lidocaine jelly. After this, a local injection of 1% plain lidocaine is performed periurethrally at the 3 and 9 o'clock positions using 2–4 mL on each side.

Panendoscopy is performed with a 0- or 30-degree lens, and a 22-gauge spinal needle with the obturator in place is positioned periurethrally at the 4 or 8 o'clock position with the bevel of the needle directed toward the lumen. The needle is then advanced into the urethral muscle in the lamina propria in an entirely suburothelial plane. Once the needle is positioned in the lamina propria, it usually advances with very little force. The needle may also be placed at the 6 o'clock position, and again needle placement is fully observed endoscopically. Bulging of the tip of the needle against the lining of the urethra is observed during advancement of the needle to ensure its proper placement. When the needle tip is properly positioned just below the bladder neck, the material is injected until swelling is visible on each side, creating the appearance of occlusion of the urethral lumen. Once the urethra is approximately 50% occluded, the needle is removed and reinserted on the opposite side, and additional material is injected until the urethral mucosa coapts in the midline creating the endoscopic appearance of two lateral prostatic lobes (Fig. 48.1).

The technique and approaches chosen for the injection of PTFE for urinary incontinence are similar to the Contigen™ injection with the exception of the depth of penetration of the needle. As stated previously, the needle placement for the injection of Contigen™ is suburothelially just behind the urethra mucosa. However, if the needle is placed too superficially for PFTE injection, the material may perforate and extrude into the urethral lumen, which can be problematic because the PFTE is sometimes difficult to remove. Therefore, when performing a PFTE injection, the needle is inserted at a 45-degree angle, which allows deposition of the material 1 cm below the urethral mucosa.

This allows the adequate bulk-enhancing effect, minimizing the possibility of a perforation and extrusion of the injected Teflon into the urethra.

The technique of injection of autologous fat is divided into two phases: harvesting the fat and periurethral injection of the fat. There are multiple technique variations to harvest autologous fat ranging from aspiration with a large bore needle to liposuction (21, 22). We use the Tulip fat harvesting and injection system to obtain autologous fat that consists of an injection cannula to inject a lactated Ringer/lidocaine injection solution into the subcutaneous fat. After this, a liposuction cannula is inserted into a 60-mL syringe that is locked in the suction position. With a gentle rocking motion to and fro through the infiltrated lower abdomen, 20–30 mL of fat is obtained. A 60-mL transferring adapter adds additional saline solution to the syringe, and with a rocking motion the fat is cleansed with saline. The bloody saline is discarded and the process is repeated until the saline is clear. This provides golden-brown fat. The syringe is placed upright and the fat is allowed to settle. The excess saline is discarded and the fat is then transferred to a luer lock syringe for periurethral injection through an 18-gauge needle. The second phase of autologous fat injection is similar to the injection of collagen in both needle placement and depth of needle placement.

Postoperative Care

Perioperative antibiotic coverage is continued for 3 days after the procedure. Most patients are able to void easily after the procedure; however, if retention does develop, clean intermittent catheterization is begun with a 12 or 14F catheter. Indwelling catheters are avoided in patients undergoing collagen and fat injection because this promotes molding of the material around the catheter. Although usually unnecessary, if long-term catheterization is needed, suprapubic cystotomy should be performed in these patients.

Patients are contacted 2 weeks after the procedure to determine their continence status. Repeat injections are scheduled 1 month later as necessary.

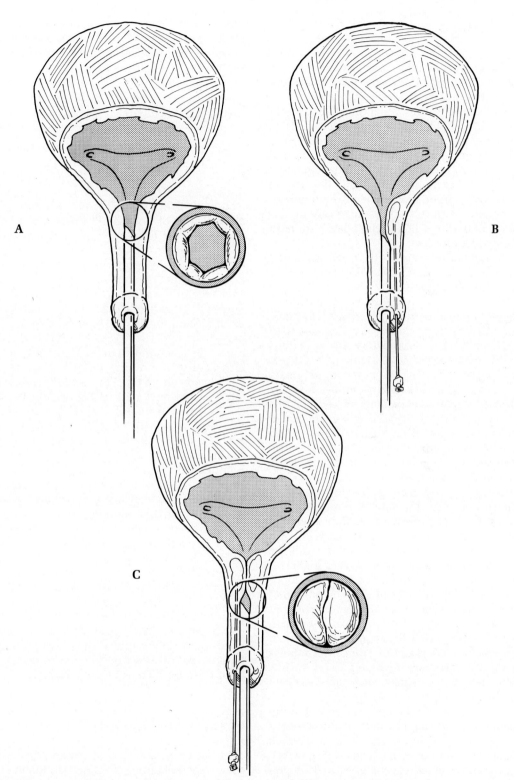

Figure 48.1. **A.** Diagram of cystoscopic view of bladder neck before injection. **B.** Diagram of periure- thral needle placement. **C.** Diagram of completed bladder neck coaptation.

Results

Many studies have been extensively reviewed for efficacy and safety of PTFE by the Department of Technology Assessment of the American Medical Association (23). It was concluded that PTFE is a reasonably effective treatment for incontinence and technically easy to perform, but because of migration of particles and granuloma formation, the safety of the product remains uncertain despite the absence of reports of untoward sequellae in human beings. A study is currently underway comparing PTFE with collagen for both safety and efficacy.

In the multicenter North American Study Group clinical trial with Contigen™ (7), in 137 female patients with ISD, 96.4% were dry at 1 year follow-up. In 17 patients with hypermobility of the sphincteric complex, 82.3% were improved or dry. Females with ISD required approximately 2.5 injections with an average of 24.3 mL of collagen. Stricker and Haylen (24) noted an 82% success rate of the injection of collagen in the first 50 Australian patients to receive this therapy. Although the success and efficacy of collagen implantation for females with ISD has been reproduced in several series, debate exists about the efficacy of collagen material in patients with type II or anatomic stress urinary incontinence. A recent study by Herschorn et al. (3) reported equal success rates among patients with type II or anatomic stress incontinence and patients with ISD; however, the number of injections and the amount of material injected were higher in patients with anatomic urinary incontinence. It has also been documented that elderly female patients with anatomic incontinence do well with the injections of collagen material (25). The overall results with periurethral injections of collagen in females with ISD compare favorably with results obtained using slings and the artificial sphincter (26).

With respect to the application of autologous fat injection for urinary incontinence, a report of 12 patients with ISD proclaimed 83% were improved subjectively; however, this improvement rate appeared to drop precipitously at 1 year (27). Therefore, although autologous fat injections seem to work reasonably well for ISD, the long-term follow-up needs to be assessed, as it appears that autologous fat undergoes a rapid rate of reabsorption because of its high water content.

Complications

The perioperative complications associated with periurethral injections are uncommon. The rate of urinary retention in patients undergoing PTFE injections is approximately 20–25% (12). In the multicenter U.S. clinical trial of Contigen™ injections, transient retention developed in approximately 15% of patients (7). Irritative voiding symptoms develop in approximately 20% of patients after the injection of PTFE but resolve after several days (28). With the Contigen™, only 1% of patients experienced irritative voiding symptoms and 5% developed a urinary tract infection (7). After PTFE injections, the development of fever with negative blood cultures and urine cultures at a rate of 25% has been noted. This usually resolves after several days and probably indicates a mild allergic response (12). Hypersensitivity responses with Contigen™ are not a problem, as the possibility is assessed by skin testing (wheal and flare) with the more immunogenic and sensitizing non-cross-linked collagen before treatment (29). Those with a positive skin test are excluded from treatment, and this amounted to 11 of 427 patients in the multicenter U.S. study. These patients had anticollagen antibody testing and no significant anticollagen responses were found. There has been no evidence to link injections of bovine collagen with any disorder (26). Regardless of the material, the use of periurethral injections has proven to be safe, eliciting only minor complications. All complications resolve rapidly, and a serious long-term complications from the use of periurethral injections has yet to be reported.

Summary

In the properly selected patient, periurethral injections offer excellent treatment results for patients with ISD. Patients with no anatomic hypermobility and ISD appear to be

the most satisfactory candidates for periurethral injections. Contigen™ is the most
widely used injectable, because it is both
biocompatible and biodegradable. There are
no reports of particle migration with this
material, and repeat injections can be performed safely under local anesthesia. Autologous fat is an alternative in periurethral injectable particularly in patients who have
positive skin tests to the collagen material.

The treatment response in females with
these procedures is similar to surgical procedures to correct ISD, and the complications
are minimal. In selected elderly and less
mobile female patients with anatomic incontinence, recent data suggest that collagen
may be useful in this patient population. The
use of periurethral injections in the treatment
of ISD certainly has a role in the treatment of
the properly selected patient and allows
treatment of incontinence in patients who are
poor surgical candidates and may be denied
other forms of therapy.

REFERENCES

1. Appell RA. Injectables for urethral incompetence. World J Urol 1990;8:208–211.
2. McGuire EJ, Appell RA. Transurethral collagen
injection for urinary incontinence. Urology 1994;
43:413–415.
3. Herschorn S, Radomski SB, Steele DJ. Early experience with intraurethral collagen injections
for urinary incontinence. J Urol 1992;148:1797–
1800.
4. Walters MD, Shields LE. The diagnostic value of
history, physical examination, and the Q-tip cotton swab test in women with urinary incontinence. Am J Obstet Gynecol 1988;159:145–149.
5. Appell RA. Valsalva leak point pressure (LPP) vs.
urethral closure pressure profile (UPP) in the
evaluation of intrinsic sphincteric deficiency
(ISD). Int Urogynecol J 1994;5:320.
6. Appell RA. Periurethral collagen injection for
female incontinence. Probl Urol 1990;5:134–140.
7. Bard CR, Inc. PMAA submission to U.S. Food and
Drug Administration for IDE #G850010, 1990.
8. Sachse H. Treatment of urinary incontinence
with sclerosing solutions, indications, results
and complications. Urol Int 1963;15:225.
9. Appell RA. Periurethral autologous blood injections: pretest for efficacy of injectables for a given
patient? Int Urogynecol J 1994;5:323.
10. Santarosa R, Blaivas J. Building continence
with periurethal fat injections. Contemp Urol
1993;5:96.
11. Malizia AA, Reiman MM, Nyers RP, et al. Migra-

12. tion and granulomatous reaction after periurethral injection of polytef (Teflon). JAMA 1984;
251:3277–3281.
12. Politano V. Periurethral polytetrafluorethylene
injection for urinary incontinence. J Urol 1982;
127:439–442.
13. Stegman SJ, Chu S, Bensch K, et al. A light and
electron microscopic evaluation of Zyderm collagen and Zyplast implants in aging human facial
skin: a pilot study. Arch Dermatol 1987;123:1644.
14. Remacle M, Marbaix E. Collagen implants in the
human larynx: pathologic dissemination of two
cases. Arch Otolaryngol 1988;245:203–209.
15. Henly DR, Barrett DM, Weiland TL, et al. Particu-
late silicone for use in periurethral injections:
local tissue effects and search for migration. J Urol
1995;153:2039–2043.
16. Press S, Badlani G. Injection therapy for urinary
incontinence. AUA Update Series 1995;14:
14–20.
17. Appell RA. Collagen injection therapy for urinary
incontinence. Urol Clin North Am 1994;21:
177–182.
18. O'Connell HE, McGuire EJ. Transurethral collagen therapy in women. J Urol 1995;154:1463–
1465.
19. Kageyama S, Kawabe K, Susuki K, et al. Collagen
implantation for post prostatectomy incontinence: early experience with a transrectal ultrasonographically guided method. J Urol 1994;152:
1473–1475.
20. Neal D Jr, Lahaye M, Lowe D. Improved needle
placement technique in periurethral collagen injection. Urology 1995;45:865–866.
21. Cervigni M, Panei M. Periurethral autologous fat
injection for Type III stress urinary incontinence.
J Urol 1993;149:403A.
22. Ganibathi K, Leach GE. Periurethral injection
techniques. Atlas Urol Clin North Am 1994;
2:101.
23. Cole HM (ed). Diagnostic and therapeutic technology assessment (DATTA). JAMA 1993;269:
2975–2980.
24. Stricker P, Haylen B. Injectable collagen for type 3
female stress incontinence: the first 50 Australian
patients. Med J Aust 1993;158:189–191.
25. Faerber GJ. Endoscopic collagen injection therapy for elderly women with Type I stress urinary
incontinence. J Urol 1995;155:527A.
26. Appell RA. Use of collagen injections for treatment of incontinence and reflux. Adv Urol 1992;
5:145–165.
27. Santarosa RP, Blaivas JG. Periurethral injection of
autologous fat for the treatment of sphincteric
incontinence. J Urol 1994;151:607–611.
28. Schulman CC, Simon J, Wespes E, Germeau F.
Endoscopic injection of Teflon for female urinary
incontinence. Eur Urol 1988;9:246–247.
29. Appell RA, McGuire EJ, DeRidder PA, et al.
Summary of effectiveness and safety in the prospective, open, multicenter investigation of con-
tigen implant for incontinence due to intrinsic
sphincteric deficiency in females. J Urol 1994;
153:418A.

CHAPTER 49

Laparoscopic Retropubic Urethropexy: Technique and Results

Robert L. Summitt, Jr.

Introduction

Data from comparative studies of the various surgical procedures used to treat uncomplicated genuine stress urinary incontinence (GSI) have clearly shown that long-term cure rates with transabdominal retropubic urethropexies (e.g., Burch colposuspension or Marshall-Marchetti-Krantz [MMK] procedure) are higher than those obtained with endoscopic needle urethropexies or the anterior colporrhaphy (1–5). In general, the anterior colporrhaphy is rarely used today to treat GSI because of cure rates after 1 year from 36 to 45% (1, 2). However, needle urethropexies such as the modified Pereyra procedure or Stamey urethral suspension are still commonly used, particularly when combined with concomitant vaginal surgery for urogenital prolapse. Their cure rates range from 40 to 85% (3, 4).

Although 1-year cure rates as high as 85–98% have been reported for the MMK procedure and Burch colposuspension, the standard procedures require an abdominal incision, a 3- to 5-day hospital stay, and a recuperative period of 8–12 weeks. Endoscopic needle urethropexies are primarily performed via the vaginal route, using one or two small suprapubic incisions for suture placement and tying. When Loughlin et al. (5) compared the economic and short-term recuperative costs between MMK procedure and Pereyra-Stamey endoscopic suspensions performed from 1975 to 1980, a shorter hospital stay and a mean hospital cost savings of $2500 was associated with the Pereyra-Stamey procedures. Although the MMK procedure was associated with a greater mean estimated blood loss, no patient in either group required intraoperative or postoperative transfusions. In addition, there were no differences between physician charges and the incidence of complications. Bhatia and Bergman (3) compared the outcomes of 64 women who underwent either a modified Pereyra procedure or a Burch urethropexy. Similar to Loughlin et al.'s study, the Pereyra procedure had a significantly shorter operating time, but there were no differences in intraoperative blood loss (270 mL with the Pereyra versus 320 mL with the Burch urethropexy) and total hospital stay.

Recently, the union of laparoscopy with retropubic urethropexies such as the Burch procedure and MMK operation has brought the potential of minimally invasive surgery, as experienced with needle urethropexies, while maintaining the superior cure rates realized with the open transabdominal procedures. Claims of better visual exposure, earlier ambulation, shorter hospital stays, and faster resumption of normal voiding combined with three to five small incisions in the abdomen have encouraged a burgeoning demand for performing this procedure. However, few objective outcome results are currently available to judge the true success of this operation, particularly as it compares with the transabdominal approach. We review the current information available regarding the laparoscopic retropubic urethropexy, describe our own technique, and review our current short-term objective results.

Current Status of Work

In 1991, Vancaillie and Schuessler (6) were the first to describe a small series of patients who underwent a laparoscopic modification of the MMK procedure. Nine women with stress urinary incontinence underwent the procedure that used four puncture sites and placed a total of two permanent sutures to elevate the bladder neck. Of the first four patients, two required a laparotomy to complete the procedure. One case incurred a bladder injury during dissection of the retropubic space, whereas technical difficulties tying the retropubic sutures were experienced in the other. The mean postoperative stay for the seven successful cases was less than 18 hours. Only two of these seven women required transurethral catheter drainage after surgery. Although all of the patients in this study were symptomatically continent after surgery, no objective results were reported. This series of nine cases was followed in 1992 by an expanded report describing the outcomes of 22 patients (including the initial 9) (7). A third patient required a laparotomy to complete the procedure, again because of technical difficulty tying the suspension sutures. Although all patients were symptomatically continent at a mean follow-up time of 9.5 months, no objective results were reported.

Liu (8) published a series of 58 laparoscopic Burch procedures. Using a five-puncture technique, two to four sutures were used to suspend the urethrovesical junction and anterior vaginal wall to the iliopectineal line (Cooper's ligament). In all cases, a cul-de-sac obliteration was performed and, in most, a laparoscopic-assisted vaginal hysterectomy was combined. The mean operating time for the Burch procedure was 73 minutes. All patients received a suprapubic catheter, and 48 were discharged with their catheters in less than 24 hours from admission. One

intraoperative bladder injury occurred but was repaired laparoscopically. Three months after surgery, 95% of the women were symptomatically continent. Objective testing consisted of only a cough stress test, which was negative in all cases. No urodynamic testing was performed. Nezhat et al. (9) reported findings similar to those of Liu, reviewing records of 62 women who underwent laparoscopic urethropexy. By various forms and degrees of postoperative evaluation, a success rate averaging 90% was demonstrated. Again, one bladder perforation occurred.

In the only randomized prospective study of laparoscopic versus open colposuspension, Burton (10) reported results of 60 procedures. Postoperative objective findings at 6 months showed similar success rates (open, 29 of 30 [97%]; laparoscopic, 26 of 30 [87%]). However, findings at 12 months revealed statistically different success. The open technique maintained a cure rate of 97% (29 of 30), but the laparoscopic approach revealed a cure rate of only 73% (22 of 30). Both types of operations were performed with delayed-absorbable sutures, and no report of complications or postoperative recovery differences were provided.

Indications and Evaluation of Surgical Candidates

Whenever a new surgical procedure is introduced, proper selection of patients is of key importance to evaluate the true success of the operation and to avoid a high complication rate until a learning curve has been overcome. As laparoscopic retropubic urethropexy is relatively new, and to some degree still in the developmental stages, care must be taken in selecting women with stress urinary incontinence. Currently, recommended operative indications include primary GSI and recurrent GSI after an anterior colporrhaphy with an anatomic defect of the urethrovesical junction. Women are excluded if they have had a previous retropubic urethropexy, endoscopic needle suspension, or suburethral sling procedure. The degree of scarring and the required dissection of the retropubic space currently preclude the laparoscopic approach in these patients. In some instances, the bladder may need to be opened to facilitate exposure and suture placement during repeat operations. The abdomen must be open to accomplish this step. As surgeon experience improves and the laparoscopic technique is refined, this approach may eventually be used after prior failed operations for GSI.

In addition, low urethral closure pressure, found with urethral pressure profilometry, has been associated with a high risk for surgical failure using the Burch colposuspension (11, 12). This finding would also present a surgical failure risk to the laparoscopic approach. Therefore, laparoscopic retropubic urethropexy should be used cautiously in this subgroup of patients with GSI.

Procedure

As noted earlier, Vancaillie and coworkers (6, 7) used a modification of the MMK procedure via the laparoscope. Liu (8) used a modification of the Burch colposuspension. However, in 54 of 58 patients, only one suture was placed on each side of the urethra, at the level of the urethrovesical junction. Before our first laparoscopic attempts, our standard retropubic urethropexy was the Burch colposuspension using two permanent sutures on each side of the urethra, as described by Tanagho (13). This technique provides maximum cure rates for GSI while minimizing the complications which might occur with the MMK procedure. To maintain this high cure rate with the laparoscopic approach, we have made every attempt to keep the key technical steps of the operation as similar to the open transabdominal approach as possible. This has included the use of two permanent polyester sutures placed on each side of the urethra. To make the operation minimally invasive, we initially attempted to use only three trocars when possible. However, we now use a fourth suprapubic trocar that allows superior directional access to placing sutures through Cooper's ligament.

EQUIPMENT

For positioning of the patient's lower extremities, we use Allen-Universal stirrups (Allen Medical, Mayfield, OH), as they pro-

vide equal support of the entire lower extremity. A three-way 16F Foley catheter with a 30-mL balloon is used for bladder drainage and retrograde filling. Four laparoscopic trocars are used: two 10 mm in diameter and two 5 mm in diameter. The suture is 0-Ethibond (braided polyester, Ethicon, Inc., Somerville, NJ), measuring 36 inches in length with an SH needle. However, other permanent sutures such as Goretex® (W.L. Gore & Assoc., Inc., Flagstaff, AZ) or Ticron® (Davis & Geck, American Cyanamid Co., Danbury, CT) have been used. We use two different needle holders. One holds the needle at 90 degrees (Cook Ob/Gyn™, Spencer, IN) and another holds the needle at 45 degrees (J. Jamner Surgical Instruments, Inc., Hawthorne, NY). A knot pusher (Elmed, Inc., Addison, IL) with a hole in the end is used, as it prevents the suture from slipping out while tying under great tension. For postoperative bladder drainage, a Rutner percutaneous suprapubic balloon catheter (Cook Urological, Inc., Spencer, IN) is used.

TECHNICAL STEPS

The procedure is performed under general anesthesia. After adequate anesthetic induction, the patient's legs are placed in the dorsal lithotomy position using the Allen-Universal stirrups. Should cystoscopy become necessary later in the case, this positioning is most advantageous. A three-way Foley catheter is inserted after sterile preparation of the perineum and vagina. A drainage bag is attached to the larger port for urine collection during the case. At the other port, cystoscopy tubing is attached that leads to a 1000-mL bag of sterile water to which 10 mL of indigo carmine dye has been added. The bladder is initially filled with 200–300 mL of dye-colored fluid, distending the bladder to allow visualization of its contour and a margin of safety during the initial dissection of the retropubic space. This tubing is then clamped until the end of the case at which time it is opened to fill the bladder. The patient is then draped with standard laparoscopy drapes after an abdominal preparation with dilute povidone iodine.

A 10-mm trocar and laparoscope are inserted into the abdomen through an infraumbilical incision. One 10-mm trocar is placed in the left lower quadrant and a 5-mm trocar

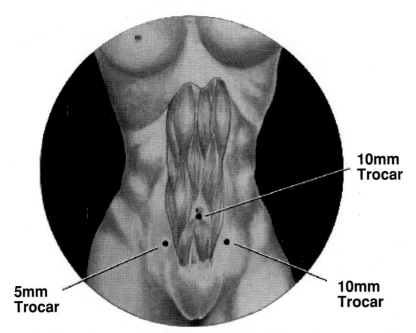

Figure 49.1. Trocar placement sites for laparoscopic retropubic urethropexy. An additional 5-mm trocar may be placed in the suprapubic location.

is placed in the right lower quadrant. Both are inserted 6–8 cm above the pubic rami, lateral to the inferior epigastric arteries (Fig. 49.1). With the patient in steep Trendelenburg, the pelvis is examined.

The retropubic space is entered by making a transverse incision in the anterior peritoneum of the abdominal wall, at least 3 cm superior to the symphysis pubis. The umbilical ligament can often serve as a landmark for proper entry into the space. Unfortunately, the ligament is not always identifiable. If the incision of the peritoneum is not made high enough, entry into the retropubic space will be too low, risking injury to the bladder or disrupting the bladder pillars, which results in significant hemorrhage. When the space is entered properly, the loose areolar tissue over the pubic symphysis and rami opens easily with scissors, exposing the bony landmarks and Cooper's ligament (Fig. 49.2). Carrying the dissection caudad, the bladder falls inferiorly, exposing the urethra and paravaginal spaces. The bladder can be emptied at this stage. Exposure of the urethra and anterior vaginal wall is improved by removing the fat from the paravaginal spaces, lateral to the urethra and urethrovesical junction. The fat can be placed in the upper abdomen or removed through the lower trocars. As an

alternative to the transperitoneal approach for opening the retropubic space, new preperitoneal balloons are available to bluntly dissect the space. Typically created as part of the subumbilical trocar, the balloon is passed into the retropubic space and inflated, expanding the space and avoiding sharp dissection or opening of the abdominal peritoneum.

With the dissection of the retropubic space complete, the 5-mm suprapubic trocar is inserted and suture placement is then performed. To minimize the amount of suture in the operative field and to avoid entanglement, each suture is passed through the vaginal wall, then Cooper's ligament, and then tied successively. Four sutures are used. A 36-inch 0-Ethibond suture on an SH needle is passed into the abdomen through the lower 10-mm trocar. The anterior vaginal wall is elevated by the surgeon's left hand while the needle holder is manipulated by the right hand. The initial suture placement is full thickness through the anterior vaginal wall, avoiding the mucosa, approximately 1 cm distal to the urethrovesical junction, 2 cm lateral to the urethra (Fig. 49.3).

After a double bite has been taken through the vagina, the needle is then passed directly lateral through Cooper's ligament (Fig. 49.4).

The angle necessary to achieve this step is often difficult to obtain. The centrally placed suprapubic trocar often provides the best angle to turn the needle holder and rotate the needle perpendicularly through the ligament. In some cases, we have placed the needle holder through the contralateral port, using an angled needle holder to drive through Cooper's ligament. With an assistant elevating the anterior vaginal wall, a surgeon's knot is tied extracorporeally and pushed down with the knot pusher. At least five throws are placed in the knot. The next suture is then passed through the anterior vaginal wall on the same side, at the level of the urethrovesical junction. It is then placed through Cooper's ligament and tied. Once two sutures have been placed on one side, the same procedural steps are completed on the contralateral side, placing the distal suture first and then the suture at the level of the urethrovesical junction. With all sutures tied and cut, the proximal urethra is elevated to an angle consistent with 0 degrees as if a cotton swab had been inserted into the urethra (Fig. 49.5).

Cystoscopy tubing to the Foley catheter is opened, filling the bladder retrograde. Once 300–400 mL have been infused, a percutaneous suprapubic catheter is inserted under laparoscopic guidance. The gas is then allowed to escape from the abdomen and the trocar sites are closed. The transurethral Foley catheter is removed before leaving the operating room.

POSTOPERATIVE MANAGEMENT

Patients are allowed to ambulate once they are alert. Voiding drills are begun on the afternoon of surgery if the patient is able to walk to the toilet. Otherwise, voiding is begun on the morning of the first postoperative day. The suprapubic catheter is removed when the patient can void at least 100 mL with each void and has residual volumes less then one fourth of the total voided volume for 24 hours. As an alternative approach, self-catheterization can be taught preoperatively and used by the patient after surgery, thus obviating the need for an indwelling catheter. This provides the eventual opportunity for making this operation an outpatient procedure.

Results

To date, our unit has performed 28 laparoscopic Burch retropubic urethropexies. All

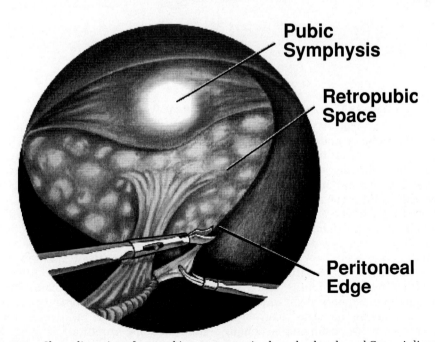

Figure 49.2. Sharp dissection of retropubic space, exposing bony landmarks and Cooper's ligament.

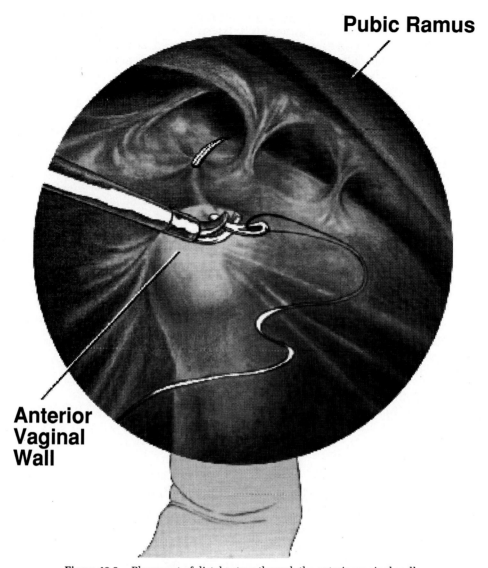

Pubic Ramus

Anterior Vaginal Wall

Figure 49.3. Placement of distal suture through the anterior vaginal wall.

have been successfully completed with no patient requiring a laparotomy. The mean operating time for all cases was 122 minutes (range 70–210). The estimated blood loss ranged from 25 to 150 mL. The mean hospital stay averaged 2.0 postoperative days (range 1–3). All patients were discharged with their suprapubic catheters removed before leaving the hospital.

Symptomatically, 27 of 28 patients (96%) were continent at least 3 months after surgery. One patient noted only slight improvement in the volume of urine lost with coughing and exercise. Postoperative cough

stress tests were consistent with symptomatic results. The mean preoperative cotton swab measure decreased from 69 degrees to a postoperative mean of 19 degrees. Postoperative urethral pressure profilometry in the sitting position with a full bladder showed the mean functional urethral length to increase minimally, from 2.4 to 2.8 cm. The mean maximum urethral closure pressure fell from 66 to 45 cm H_2O. Although 27 of 28 women have been continent upon urodynamic testing, the mean transmission ratio measured at the midfunctional urethral length only increased from 72 to 78%. Our single patient who failed the procedure had two prior anterior colporrhaphies and exhibited minimal mobility of the anterior vaginal wall during surgery. She is currently undergoing pelvic floor rehabilitation with biofeedback training in our Urogynecology Unit and is showing improvement.

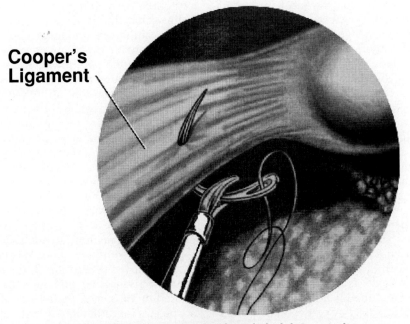

Cooper's Ligament

Figure 49.4. Needle and suture passage through the left Cooper's ligament.

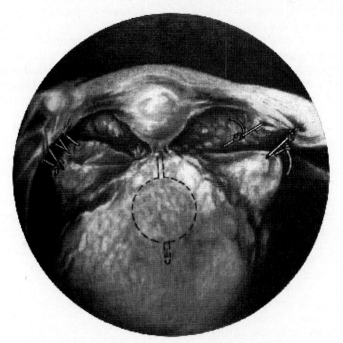

Figure 49.5. Completed laparoscopic retropubic urethropexy. The appearance is identical to the result achieved by a transabdominal (open) approach.

Conclusions

Based on our own experience and that of others, the laparoscopic retropubic urethropexy is a very feasible operation. Currently, we believe that the most important aspect of achieving success, and avoiding complications or a high failure rate, is proper selection of patients. Although our series is small, therefore making scientific conclusions impossible, factors such as previous vaginal surgery may pose a risk for failure, as we found in one of our patients. With a laparotomy, we may have achieved greater mobilization of the anterior vagina in the retropubic space and therefore a better repair. Until surgical experience with the laparoscopic approach increases, we recommend avoiding surgery in patients who have had prior retropubic procedures or endoscopic needle suspensions.

We agree that the visual exposure during the laparoscopic Burch colposuspension is excellent. With the patient in steep Trendelenburg, the bowel is removed from the operative field and the bladder falls inferiorly. Limitations of a narrow or deep abdominal incision are offset by viewing through the laparoscope. Although mean operating times are longer than those from our open cases, we expect these, and the accompanying operating room fees, to fall as surgical experience continues. One key surgical factor that we do not believe the laparoscopic approach can yet equal is the tactile dexterity that is achieved during a laparotomy. The "feel" that is necessary around the urethra and with the tying of sutures has not met our satisfaction. In scarred cases, as might be encountered with prior surgery, the ability to adequately mobilize and elevate the anterior vaginal wall and tie sutures under tension is limited.

The objective urodynamic results found with our small series is similar to those noted with open transabdominal procedures (2). We saw no significant changes in functional urethral length or urethral closure pressure after surgery. Although other studies showed significant increases in pressure transmission ratios after successful operations, our small mean increase of 8% was not significant. A larger series of cases may prove different.

There is no doubt that women undergoing laparoscopic urethropexies can ambulate earlier and with greater ease after surgery when compared with a transabdominal approach. Although claims of greater ease in postoperative voiding have been made, we believe that this is simply a function of an earlier ability to ambulate and decreased postoperative pain, allowing early initiation of voiding attempts. However, this early initiation of voiding provides the possibility of making this operation an outpatient procedure. The patient should be knowledgeable of the management of her suprapubic catheter or should be able to self-catheterize.

Shorter hospital stays may serve to decrease medical costs associated with the retropubic urethropexy when it is performed via the laparoscope. However, we do not believe that convalescence will be shortened. Avoidance of exercise, heavy lifting, and the resumption of manual labor is recommended for 8–12 weeks after a standard colposuspension to allow scarification in the retropubic space. This healing process should not be altered or shortened by the use of a laparoscope. It is important for the patient to realize that she will be not be able to return to normal activities in 2 weeks.

As more surgeons begin to perform laparoscopic retropubic urethropexies for stress urinary incontinence, it is dependent on us as scientists and clinicians to provide our patients with sound and correct information as to the benefits and risks of this new operation. The only way this is possible is to study the outcomes through randomized prospective comparative trials with standard open abdominal procedures. Until these data are available, the procedure must be used prudently. However, this operation shows great potential for providing an excellent cure rate for GSI while allowing minimal invasiveness so characteristic of laparoscopy.

REFERENCES

1. Stanton SL, Cardozo LD. A comparison of vaginal and suprapubic surgery in the correction of incontinence due to urethral sphincter incompetence. Br J Urol 1979;51:497–499.
2. van Geelen JM, Theeuwes AGM, Eskes TKAB, Martin CB. The clinical and urodynamic effects of anterior vaginal repair and Burch colposuspension. Am J Obstet Gynecol 1988;159:137–144.
3. Bhatia NN, Bergman A. Modified Burch ver-

sus Pereyra retropubic urethropexy for stress urinary incontinence. Obstet Gynecol 1985;66: 255–261.

4. Mundy AR. A trial comparing the Stamey bladder neck suspension procedure with colposuspension for the treatment of stress incontinence. Br J Urol 1983;55:687–690.

5. Loughlin KR, Gittes RF, Klein LA, Whitmore WF. The comparative medical costs of 2 major procedures available for the treatment of stress urinary incontinence. J Urol 1982;127:436–438.

6. Vancaillie TG, Schuessler W. Laparoscopic bladder neck suspension. J Laparoendosc Surg 1991; 1:169–173.

7. Albala DM, Schuessler WW, Vancaillie TG. Laparoscopic bladder neck suspension. J Endourol 1992;6:137–141.

8. Liu CY. Laparoscopic retropubic colposuspen-sion (Burch procedure): a review of 58 cases. J Reprod Med 1993;38:526–530.

9. Nezhat CH, Nezhat F, Nezhat CR, Rottenberg H. Laparoscopic retropubic cystourethropexy. J Am Assoc Gynecol Laparosc 1994;1:339–349.

10. Burton G. A randomized comparison of laparoscopic and open colposuspension. Neurourol Urodyn 1994;13:497–498.

11. Sand PK, Bowen LW, Panganiban R, Ostergard DR. The low pressure urethra as a factor in failed retropubic urethropexy. Obstet Gynecol 1987;69: 399–402.

12. Bowen LW, Sand PK, Ostergard DR, Franti CE. Unsuccessful Burch retropubic urethropexy: a case controlled urodynamic study. Am J Obstet Gynecol 1989;452–458.

13. Tanagho EA. Colpocystourethropexy: the way we do it. J Urol 1976;116:751–753.

APPENDICES

The Standardization of Terminology of Lower Urinary Tract Function

Modified from work produced by the International Continence Society
Committee on Standardization of Terminology

Introduction

The International Continence Society (ICS) established a committee for the standardization of terminology of lower urinary tract function in 1973. Five of six reports (1–6) from this committee, approved by the Society, have been published. The fifth report on quantification of urine loss was an internal ICS document that appears, in part, in this document. Pressures have not, as yet, been addressed by the ICS (see Chapter XX).

These reports are revised, extended, and collated in this monograph. The standards are recommended to facilitate comparison of results by investigators who use urodynamic methods. These standards are recommended not only for urodynamic investigations carried out on human patients but also during animal studies. When using urodynamic studies in animals, the type of any anesthesia used should be stated. It is suggested that acknowledgment of these standards in written publications be indicated by a footnote to the section "Methods and Materials" or its equivalent, to read as follows:

Methods, definitions, and units conform to the standards recommended by the International Continence Society, except where specifically noted.

Urodynamic studies involve the assessment of the function and dysfunction of the urinary tract by any appropriate method. Aspects of urinary tract morphology, physiology, biochemistry, and hydrodynamics affect urine transport and storage. Other methods of investigation such as the radiographic visualization of the lower urinary tract are useful adjuncts to conventional urodynamics. This monograph concerns the urodynamics of the lower urinary tract.

Clinical Assessment

The clinical assessment of patients with lower urinary tract dysfunction should consist of a detailed history, a frequency/volume chart, and a physical examination. In urinary incontinence, leakage should be demonstrated objectively.

HISTORY

The general history should include questions relevant to neurological and congenital abnormalities and information on previous urinary infections and relevant surgery. Information must be obtained on medication with known or possible effects on the lower urinary tract. The general history should also include assessment of menstrual, sexual, and bowel function and obstetric history.

The urinary history must consist of questions about symptoms related to both the storage and the evacuation functions of the lower urinary tract.

FREQUENCY/VOLUME CHART

The frequency/volume chart is a specific urodynamic investigation that records fluid intake and urine output per 24-hour period. The chart gives objective information on the number of voidings, the distribution of voidings between daytime and nighttime, and each voided volume. The chart can also be used to record episodes of urgency and leakage and the number of incontinence pads used. The frequency/volume chart is very useful in the assessment of voiding disorders and in the follow-up of treatment.

PHYSICAL EXAMINATION

Besides a general urological and, when appropriate, gynecological examination, the physical examination should include the assessment of perineal sensation, the perineal reflexes supplied by the sacral segments S2–S4, and anal sphincter tone and control.

Procedures Related to the Evaluation of Urine Storage

CYSTOMETRY

Cystometry is the method by which the pressure/volume relationship of the bladder is measured. All systems are zeroed at atmospheric pressure. For external transducers, the reference point is the level of the superior edge of the symphysis pubis. For catheter-mounted transducers, the reference point is the transducer itself.

Cystometry is used to assess detrusor activity, sensation, capacity, and compliance.

Before starting to fill the bladder, the residual urine may be measured. However, the removal of a large volume of residual urine may alter detrusor function, especially in neuropathic disorders. Certain cystometric parameters may be significantly altered by the speed of bladder filling (see below).

During cystometry, it is taken for granted that the patient is awake, unanesthetized, and neither sedated nor taking drugs that affect bladder function. Any variations should be specified:

1. Access (transurethral or percutaneous);
2. Fluid medium (liquid or gas);
3. Temperature of fluid (state in degrees Celsius);
4. Position of patient (e.g., supine, sitting, or standing);
5. Filling by diuresis or catheter. Filling by catheter may be continuous or incremental; the precise filling rate should be stated. When the incremental method is used, the volume increment should be stated. For general discussion, the following terms for the range of filling rate may be used:

a. Up to 10 mL/min is slow-fill cystometry ("physiological" filling);
b. 10–100 mL/min is medium-fill cystometry;
c. Over 100 mL/min is rapid-fill cystometry.

Technique

1. Fluid-filled catheter—specify number of catheters, single or multiple lumens, type of catheter (manufacturer), size of catheter;
2. Catheter tip transducer—list specifications;
3. Other catheters—list specifications;
4. Measuring equipment.

Definitions

Intravesical pressure is the pressure within the bladder. Abdominal pressure is taken to be the pressure surrounding the bladder. In current practice, it is estimated from vaginal or, less commonly, extraperitoneal pressure.

Detrusor pressure is that component of intravesical pressure that is created by forces in the bladder wall (passive and active). It is estimated by subtracting abdominal pressure from intravesical pressure. The simultaneous measurement of abdominal pressure is essential for the interpretation of the intravesical pressure trace. However, artifacts on the detrusor pressure trace may be produced by intrinsic rectal contractions.

Bladder sensation is difficult to evaluate because of its subjective nature. It is usually assessed by questioning the patient in relation to the fullness of the bladder during cystometry.

Commonly used descriptive terms include

1. First desire to void;
2. Normal desire to void (this is defined as the feeling that leads the patient to pass urine at the next convenient moment, but voiding can be delayed if necessary);
3. Strong desire to void (this is defined as a persistent desire to void without the fear of leakage);
4. Urgency (this is defined as a strong desire to void accompanied by fear of leakage or fear of pain);

5. Pain (the site and character of which should be specified). Pain during bladder filling or micturition is abnormal.

The use of objective or semiobjective tests for sensory function, such as electrical threshold studies (sensory testing), is discussed in detail below. The term "capacity" must be qualified. Maximum cystometric capacity, in patients with normal sensation, is the volume at which the patient believes he or she can no longer delay micturition. In the absence of sensation, the maximum cystometric capacity cannot be defined in the same terms and is the volume at which the clinician decides to terminate filling. In the presence of sphincter incompetence, the maximum cystometric capacity may be significantly increased by occlusion of the urethra (e.g., by Foley catheter).

The functional bladder capacity, or voided volume, is more relevant and is assessed from a frequency/volume chart (urinary diary).

The maximum (anesthetic) bladder capacity is the volume measured after filling during a deep general or spinal/epidural anesthetic, specifying fluid temperature, filling pressure, and filling time.

Compliance indicates the change in volume for a change in pressure. Compliance is calculated by dividing the volume change (ΔV) by the change in detrusor pressure ($\Delta Pdet$) during that change in bladder volume ($\Delta V / \Delta Pdet$). Compliance is expressed as mL/cm H_2O (see below).

URETHRAL PRESSURE MEASUREMENT

It should be noted that the urethral pressure and the urethral closure pressure are idealized concepts that represent the ability of the urethra to prevent leakage (see below). In current urodynamic practice, the urethral pressure is measured by a number of different techniques that do not always yield consistent values. Not only do the values differ with the method of measurement, but there is often lack of consistency for a single method. An example is the effect of catheter rotation when urethral pressure is measured by a catheter mounted transducer.

Intraluminal urethral pressure may be measured

1. At rest, with the bladder at any given volume;
2. During coughing or straining;
3. During the process of voiding (see below).

Measurements may be made at one point in the urethra over a period of time, or at several points along the urethra, consecutively forming a urethral pressure profile (UPP).

Storage Phase

Two types of UPP may be measured:

1. Resting UPP—with the bladder and subject at rest;
2. Stress UPP—with a defined applied stress (e.g., cough, strain, Valsalva).

In the storage phase, the UPP denotes the intraluminal pressure along the length of the urethra. All systems are zeroed at atmospheric pressure. For external transducers, the reference point is the superior edge of the symphysis pubis. For catheter-mounted transducers, the reference point is the transducer itself. Intravesical pressure should be measured to exclude a simultaneous detrusor contraction. The subtraction of intravesical pressure from urethral pressure produces the urethral closure pressure profile.

The simultaneous recording of both intravesical and intraurethral pressures are essential during stress urethral profilometry.

Specify

1. Infusion medium (liquid or gas);
2. Rate of infusion;
3. Stationary, continuous, or intermittent withdrawal;
4. Rate of withdrawal;
5. Bladder volume;
6. Position of patient (supine, sitting, or standing).

Technique

1. Open catheter—specify type (manufacturer), size, number, position, and orientation of side or end hole.
2. Catheter-mounted transducers—specify manufacturer, number of transducers, spacing of transducers along the catheter, orientation with respect to one another, transducer design (e.g., transducer face

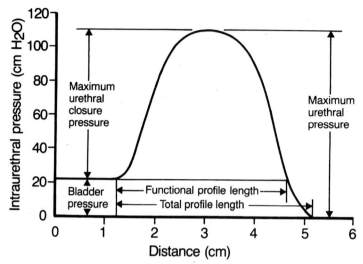

Figure AI.1. Diagram of a female UPP (static) with ICS recommended nomenclature.

depressed or flush with catheter surface), catheter diameter, and material. The orientation of the transducer(s) in the urethra should be stated.
3. Other catheters (e.g., membrane, fiber optic)—specify type (manufacturer), size, and number of channels as for microtransducer catheter.
4. Measurement technique—for stress profiles, the particular stress used should be stated (e.g., cough or Valsalva).
5. Recording apparatus—describe type of recording apparatus. The frequency response of the total system should be stated. The frequency response of the catheter in the perfusion method can be assessed by blocking the eyeholes and recording the consequent rate of change of pressure.

Definitions

The following definitions refer to profiles measured in the storage phase (Fig. AI.1).

Maximum urethral pressure is the maximum pressure of the measured profile.

Maximum urethral closure pressure is the maximum difference between the urethral pressure and the intravesical pressure.

Functional profile length is the length of the urethra along which the urethral pressure exceeds intravesical pressure.

Functional profile length (on stress) is the length over which the urethral pressure exceeds the intravesical pressure on stress.

Pressure "transmission" ratio is the increment in urethral pressure on stress as a percentage of the simultaneously recorded increment in intravesical pressure. For stress profiles obtained during coughing, pressure transmission ratios can be obtained at any point along the urethra. If single values are given, the position in the urethra should be stated. If several pressure transmission ratios are defined at different points along the urethra, a pressure "transmission" profile is obtained. During "cough profiles," the amplitude of the cough should be stated, if possible.

Note: the term "transmission" is in common usage and cannot be changed. However, transmission implies a completely passive process. Such an assumption is not yet justified by scientific evidence. A role for muscular activity cannot be excluded.

Total profile length is not generally regarded as a useful parameter.

The information gained from urethral pressure measurements in the storage phase is of limited value in the assessment of voiding disorders.

QUANTIFICATION OF URINE LOSS

Subjective grading of incontinence may not reliably indicate the degree of abnormality. However, it is important to relate the management of the individual patients to their complaints and personal circumstances, as well as to objective measurements.

To assess and compare the results of the treatment of different types of incontinence in different centers, a simple standard test can be used to measure urine loss objectively in any subject. To obtain a representative result, especially in subjects with variable or intermittent urinary incontinence, the test should occupy as long a period as possible; yet, it must be practical. The circumstances should approximate to those of everyday life yet should be similar for all subjects to allow meaningful comparison. On the basis of pilot studies performed in various centers, an internal report of the ICS (5th) recommended a test occupying a 1-hour period during which a series of standard activities was carried out. This test *can* be extended by further 1-hour periods if the result of the first 1-hour test was not considered representative by either the patient or the investigator. Alternatively, the test can be repeated after having filled the bladder to a defined volume.

The total amount of urine lost during the test period is determined by weighing a collecting device such as a nappy, absorbent pad, or condom appliance. A nappy or pad should be worn inside waterproof underpants or should have a waterproof backing. Care should be taken to use a collecting device of adequate capacity.

Immediately before the test begins, the collecting device is weighed to the nearest gram.

Typical Test Schedule

1. Test is started without the patient voiding;
2. Preweighed collecting device is put on and first 1-hour test period begins;
3. Subject drinks 500 mL sodium-free liquid within a short period (maximum 15 min) and then sits or rests;
4. Half hour period: subject walks, including stair climbing equivalent to one flight up and down;
5. During the remaining period, the subject performs the following activities:
   a. Standing up from sitting, 10 times;
   b. Coughing vigorously, 10 times;
   c. Running on the spot for 1 minute;
   d. Bending to pick up small object from floor, 5 times;
   e. Wash hands in running water for 1 minute.

6. At the end of the 1-hour test, the collecting device is removed and weighed;
7. If the test is regarded as representative, the subject voids, and the volume is recorded;
8. Otherwise, the test is repeated, preferably without voiding.

If the collecting device becomes saturated or filled during the test, it should be removed, weighed, and replaced by a fresh device. The total weight of urine lost during the test period is taken to be equal to the gain in weight of the collecting device(s). In interpreting the results of the test, it should be borne in mind that a weight gain of up to 2 g may be due to weighing errors, sweating, or vaginal discharge. The activity program may be modified according to the subject's physical ability. If substantial variations from the usual test schedule occur, this should be recorded so that the same schedule can be used on subsequent occasions.

In principle, the subject should not void during the test period. If the patient experiences urgency, then he or she should be persuaded to postpone voiding and to perform as many of the activities in number 5 as possible to detect leakage. Before voiding, the collection device is removed for weighing. If inevitable voiding cannot be postponed, the test is terminated. The voided volume and the duration of the test should be recorded. For subjects not completing the full test, the results may require separate analysis or the test may be repeated after rehydration.

The test result is given as grams urine lost in the 1-hour test period in which the greatest urine loss is recorded.

Additional Procedures

Additional procedures intended to give information of diagnostic value are permissible provided they do not interfere with the basic test. For example, additional changes and weighing of the collecting device can give information about the timing of urine loss: the absorbent nappy may be an electronic recording nappy so that the timing is recorded directly.

Specify

1. Collecting device;
2. Physical condition of subject (ambulant, chairbound, bedridden);
3. Relevant medical condition of subject;
4. Relevant drug treatments;
5. Test schedule.

In some situations, the timing of the test (e.g., in relation to the menstrual cycle) may be relevant.

Findings

Record weight of urine lost during the test (in the case of repeated tests, greatest weight in any stated period). A loss of less than 1 g is within experimental error, and the patients should be regarded as essentially dry. Urine loss should be measured and recorded in grams.

Statistics

When performing statistical analysis of urine loss in a group of subjects, nonparametric statistics should be used because the values are not normally distributed.

Procedures Related to the Evaluation of Micturition

MEASUREMENT OF URINARY FLOW

Urinary flow may be described in terms of rate and pattern and may be continuous or intermittent. Flow rate is defined as the volume of fluid expelled via the urethra per unit time. It is expressed in mL/s.

Specify

1. Voided volume;
2. Patient environment and position (supine, sitting, or standing);
3. Filling
   a. By diuresis (spontaneous or forced: specify regimen);
   b. By catheter (transurethral or suprapubic);
4. Type of fluid.

Technique

1. Measuring equipment;
2. Solitary procedure or combined with other measurements.

Definitions

1. Continuous flow (Fig. AI.2)

Voided volume is the total volume expelled via the urethra.

Maximum flow rate is the maximum measured value of the flow rate.

Average flow rate is voided volume divided by flow time. The calculation of average flow rate is only meaningful if flow is continuous and without terminal dribbling.

Flow time is the time over which measurable flow actually occurs.

Time to maximum flow is the elapsed time from onset of flow to maximum flow.

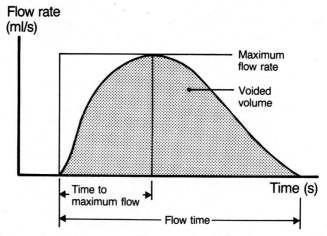

Figure AI.2. Diagram of a continuous urine flow recording with ICS recommended nomenclature.

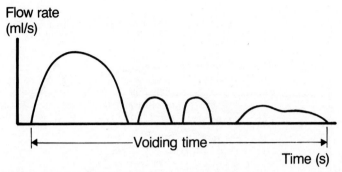

Figure AI.3. Diagram of an interrupted urine flow recording with ICS recommended nomenclature.

The flow pattern must be described when flow time and average flow rate are measured.

2. Intermittent flow (Fig. AI.3)

The same parameters used to characterize continuous flow may be applicable if care is exercised in patients with intermittent flow. In measuring flow time, the time intervals between flow episodes are disregarded.

Voiding time is total duration of micturition (i.e., includes interruptions). When voiding is completed without interruption, voiding time is equal to flow time.

BLADDER PRESSURE MEASUREMENTS DURING MICTURITION

The specifications of patient position, access for pressure measurement, catheter type, and measuring equipment are as for cystometry (see above).

Definitions

Opening time is the elapsed time from initial rise in detrusor pressure to onset of flow. This is the initial isovolumetric contraction period of micturition (Fig. AI.4). Time lags should be taken into account. In most urodynamic systems, a time lag occurs equal to the time taken for the urine to pass from the point of pressure measurement to the uroflow transducer.

The following parameters are applicable to measurements of each of the pressure curves: intravesical, abdominal, and detrusor pressure.

Premicturition pressure is the pressure recorded immediately before the initial isovolumetric contraction.

Opening pressure is the pressure recorded at the onset of measured flow.

Maximum pressure is the maximum value of the measured pressure.

Pressure at maximum flow is the pressure recorded at maximum measured flow rate.

Contraction pressure at maximum flow is the difference between pressure at maximum flow and premicturition pressure. Postmicturition events (e.g., after contraction) are not well understood and so cannot be defined as yet.

PRESSURE-FLOW RELATIONSHIPS

In the early days of urodynamics, the flow rate and voiding pressure were related as a "urethral resistance factor." The concept of a resistance factor originates from rigid tube hydrodynamics. The urethra does not generally behave as a rigid tube as it is an irregular and distensible conduit whose walls and surroundings have active and passive elements and hence influence the flow through it. Therefore, a resistance factor cannot provide a valid comparison between patients.

There are many ways of displaying the relationships between flow and pressure during micturition, and an example is suggested in the ICS 3rd Report (Fig. AI.5). As yet, available data do not permit a standard presentation of pressure/flow parameters.

When data from a group of patients are presented, pressure/flow relationships may be shown on a graph as illustrated in Figure AI.5. This form of presentation allows lines of demarcation to be drawn on the graph to separate the results according to the problem being studied. The points shown in Figure AI.5 are purely illustrative to indicate how the data might fall into groups. The group of equivocal results might include

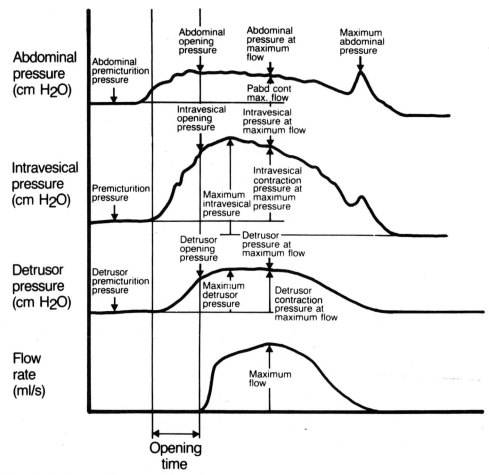

Figure AI.4. Diagram of a pressure-flow recording of micturition with ICS recommended nomenclature.

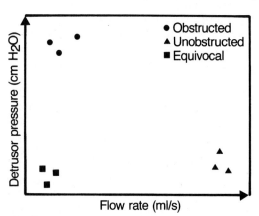

Figure AI.5. Diagram illustrating the presentation of pressure flow data on individual patients in three groups of three patients: obstructed, equivocal, and unobstructed.

either an unrepresentative micturition in an obstructed or an unobstructed patient or underactive detrusor function with or without obstruction. This is the group that invalidates the use of "urethral resistance factors."

URETHRAL PRESSURE MEASUREMENTS DURING VOIDING

The voiding urethral pressure profile (VUPP) is used to determine the pressure and site of urethral obstruction.

Pressure is recorded in the urethra during voiding. The technique is similar to that used in the UPP measured during storage (the resting and stress profiles, see above).

Specify

As for UPP during storage, see above.

Accurate interpretation of the VUPP depends on the simultaneous measurement of intravesical pressure and the measurement of pressure at a precisely localized point in the urethra. Localization may be achieved by placing a radiopaque marker on the catheter, which allows the pressure measurements to be related to a visualized point in the urethra.

This technique is not fully developed, and a number of technical as well as clinical problems need to be solved before the VUPP is widely used.

RESIDUAL URINE

Residual urine is defined as the volume of fluid remaining in the bladder immediately after the completion of micturition. The measurement of residual urine forms an integral part of the study of micturition. However, voiding in unfamiliar surroundings may lead to unrepresentative results, as may voiding on command with a partially filled or overfilled bladder. Residual urine is commonly estimated by the following methods:

1. Catheter or cystoscope (transurethral, suprapubic);
2. Radiography (excretion urography, micturition cystography);
3. Ultrasonics;
4. Radioisotopes (clearance, gamma camera).

When estimating residual urine, the measurement of voided volume and the time interval between voiding and residual urine estimation should be recorded. This is particularly important if the patient is in a diuretic phase. In the condition of vesicoureteric reflux, urine may reenter the bladder after micturition and may falsely be interpreted as residual urine. The presence of urine in bladder diverticula after micturition presents special problems of interpretation; a diverticulum may be regarded either as part of the bladder cavity or as outside the functioning bladder.

The various methods of measurement each have limitations as to their applicability and accuracy in the various conditions associated with residual urine. Therefore, it is necessary to choose a method appropriate to the clinical problems. The absence of residual urine is usually an observation of clinical value, but it does not exclude infravesical obstruction or bladder dysfunction. An isolated finding of

residual urine requires confirmation before being considered significant.

Procedures Related to the Neurophysiological Evaluation of the Urinary Tract During Filling and Voiding

ELECTROMYOGRAPHY

Electromyography (EMG) is the study of electrical potentials generated by the depolarization of muscle. The following refers to striated muscle EMG. The functional unit in EMG is the motor unit. This is comprised of a single motor neuron and the muscle fibers it innervates. A motor unit action potential is the recorded depolarization of muscle fibers that results from activation of a single anterior horn cell. Muscle action potentials may be detected either by needle electrodes or by surface electrodes.

Needle electrodes are placed directly into the muscle mass and permit visualization of the individual motor unit action potentials.

Surface electrodes are applied to an epithelial surface as close to the muscle under study as possible. Surface electrodes detect the action potentials from groups of adjacent motor units underlying the recording surface.

EMG potentials may be displayed on an oscilloscope screen or played through audio amplifiers. A permanent record of EMG potentials can only be made using a chart recorder with a high frequency response (in the range of 10 kHz).

EMG should be interpreted in the light of the patient's symptoms, physical findings, and urological and urodynamic investigations.

General Information

Specify.
1. EMG (solitary procedure, part of urodynamic or other electrophysiological investigation);
2. Patient position (supine, standing, sitting, or other);

3. Electrode placement
   a. Sampling site (intrinsic striated muscle of the urethra, periurethral striated muscle, bulbocavernosus muscle, external anal sphincter, pubococcygeus, or other)—state whether sites are single or multiple, unilateral or bilateral. Also state number of samples per site.
   b. Recording electrode—define the precise anatomic location of the electrode. For needle electrodes, include site of needle entry, angle of entry, and needle depth. For vaginal or urethral surface electrodes, state method of determining position of electrode.
   c. Reference electrode position.
4. Note: ensure that there is no electrical interference with any other machines (e.g., x-ray apparatus).

Technical Information

Specify.
1. Electrodes
   a. Needle electrodes
      (i)   Design (concentric, bipolar, monopolar, single fiber, other)
      (ii) Dimensions (length, diameter, recording area)
      (iii) Electrode material (e.g., platinum)
   b. Surface electrodes
      (i)   Type (skin, plug, catheter, other)
      (ii) Size and shape—electrode material
      (iii) Mode of fixation to recording surface
      (iv) Conducting medium (e.g., saline, jelly)
2. Amplifier (make and specifications)
3. Signal processing (data: raw, averaged, integrated, or other)
4. Display equipment (make and specifications to include method of calibration, time base, full-scale deflection in microvolts, and polarity).
   a. Oscilloscope
   b. Chart recorder
   c. Loudspeaker
   d. Other
5. Storage (make and specifications)
   a. Paper
   b. Magnetic tape recorder
   c. Microprocessor
   d. Other
6. Hard copy production (make and specifications)
   a. Chart recorder
   b. Photographic/video reproduction of oscilloscope screen
   c. Other

EMG Findings

1. Individual motor unit action potentials—normal motor unit potentials have a characteristic configuration, amplitude, and duration. Abnormalities of the motor unit may include an increase in the amplitude, duration, and complexity of waveform (polyphasicity) of the potentials. A polyphasic potential is defined as one having more than five deflections. The EMG findings of fibrillations, positive sharp waves, and bizarre high-frequency potentials are thought to be abnormal.
2. Recruitment patterns—in normal subjects, there is a gradual increase in "pelvic floor" and "sphincter" EMG activity during bladder filling. At the onset of micturition, there is complete absence of activity. Any sphincter EMG activity during voiding is abnormal unless the patient is attempting to inhibit micturition. The finding of increased sphincter EMG activity during voiding, accompanied by characteristic simultaneous detrusor pressure and flow changes is described by the term detrusor-sphincter dyssynergia. In this condition, a detrusor contraction occurs concurrently with an inappropriate contraction of the urethral and or periurethral striated muscle.

NERVE CONDUCTION STUDIES

Nerve conduction studies involve stimulation of a peripheral nerve and recording the time taken for a response to occur in the muscle innervated by the nerve under study. The time taken from stimulation of the nerve to the response in the muscle is called the "latency." Motor latency is the time taken by the fastest motor fibers in the nerve to conduct impulses to the muscle and depends on conduction distance and the conduction velocity of the fastest fibers.

General Information

Also applicable to reflex latencies and evoked potentials—see below.

Specify.

1. Type of investigation
   a. Nerve conduction study (e.g., pudendal nerve);
   b. Reflex latency determination (e.g., bulbocavernosus);
   c. Spinal evoked potential;
   d. Cortical evoked potential;
   e. Other.
2. Is the study a solitary procedure or part of urodynamic or neurophysiological investigations?
3. Patient position and environmental temperature, noise level, and illumination.
4. Electrode placement—define electrode placement in precise anatomic terms. The exact interelectrode distance is required for nerve conduction velocity calculations.
   a. Stimulation site (penis, clitoris, urethra, bladder neck, bladder, or other);
   b. Recording sites (external anal sphincter, periurethral striated muscle, bulbocavernosus muscle, spinal cord, cerebral cortex, or other);
      When recording spinal evoked responses, the sites of the recording electrodes should be specified according to the bony landmarks (e.g., L4). In cortical evoked responses, the sites of the recording electrodes should be specified as in the International 10 to 20 system (5). The sampling techniques should be specified (single or multiple, unilateral or bilateral, ipsilateral or contralateral, or other).
   c. Reference electrode position;
   d. Grounding electrode site—ideally this should be between the stimulation and recording sites to reduce stimulus artefact.

Technical Information

Also applicable to reflex latencies and evoked potentials—see below.

Specify.

1. Electrodes (make and specifications). Describe separately stimulus and recording electrodes as below:
   a. Design (e.g., needle, plate, ring, and configuration of anode and cathode where applicable);
   b. Dimensions;
   c. Electrode material (e.g., platinum);
   d. Contact medium.
2. Stimulator (make and specifications)
   a. Stimulus parameters (pulse width, frequency, pattern, current density, electrode impedance in killiohms. Also define in terms of threshold, e.g., in case of supramaximal stimulation).
3. Amplifier (make and specifications)
   a. Sensitivity (mV-uV);
   b. Filters—low pass (Hz) or high pass (kHz);
   c. Sampling time (ms).
4. Average (make and specifications)
   a. Number of stimuli sampled.
5. Display equipment (make and specifications to include method of calibration, time base, full-scale deflection in microvolts, and polarity)
   a. Paper;
   b. Magnetic tape recorder;
   c. Microprocessor;
   d. Other.
6. Hard copy production (make and specification)
   a. Chart recorder;
   b. Photographic/video reproduction of oscilloscope screen;
   c. XY recorder;
   d. Other.

Description of Nerve Conduction Studies

Recordings are made from muscle, and the latency of response of the muscle is measured. The latency is taken as the time to onset of the earliest response.

1. To ensure that response time can be precisely measured, the gain should be increased to give a clearly defined takeoff point. (Gain setting at least 100 µV/div and using a short time base, e.g., 1–2 ms/div.)
2. Additional information may be obtained from nerve conduction studies if, when using surface electrodes to record a compound muscle action potential, the amplitude is measured. The gain setting must be reduced so that the whole response is

displayed, and a longer time base is recommended (e.g., 1 mV/div and 5 ms/div). Because the amplitude is proportional to the number of motor unit potentials within the vicinity of the recording electrodes, a reduction in amplitude indicates loss of motor units and therefore denervation. (Note: A prolongation of latency is not necessarily indicative of denervation.)

REFLEX LATENCIES

Reflex latencies require stimulation of sensory fields and recordings from the muscle contracts reflexly in response to the stimulation. Such responses are a test of reflex arcs, which are comprised of both afferent and efferent limbs and a synaptic region within the central nervous system. The reflex latency expresses the nerve conduction velocity in both limbs of the arc and the integrity of the central nervous system at the level of the synapse(s). Increased reflex latency may occur as a result of slowed afferent or efferent nerve conduction or due to central nervous system conduction delays.

General Information and Technical Information

The same technical and general details apply as discussed above under Nerve Conduction Studies.

Description of Reflex Latency Measurements

Recordings are made from muscle, and the latency of response of the muscle is measured. The latency is taken as the time to onset of the earliest response.

To ensure that response time can be precisely measured, the gain should be increased to give a clearly defined takeoff point. (Gain setting at least 100 µV/div and using a short time base, e.g., 1–2 msec/div.)

EVOKED RESPONSES

Evoked responses are potential changes in central nervous system neurons resulting from distant stimulation, usually electrical. They are recorded using averaging techniques. Evoked responses may be used to test the integrity of peripheral, spinal, and central

nervous pathways. As with nerve conduction studies, the conduction time (latency) may be measured. In addition, information may be gained from the amplitude and configuration of these responses.

General Information and Technical Information

See above under Nerve Conduction Studies.

Description of Evoked Responses

Describe the presence or absence of stimulus evoked responses and their configuration.
   Specify.
1. Single or multiphasic response;
2. Onset of response—defined as the start of the first reproducible potential. Because the onset of the response may be difficult to ascertain precisely, the criteria used should be stated;
3. Latency to onset—defined as the time (ms) from the onset of stimulus to the onset of response. The central conduction time relates to cortical evoked potentials and is defined as the difference between the latencies of the cortical and the spinal evoked potentials. This parameter may be used to test the integrity of the corticospinal neuraxis;
4. Latencies to peaks of positive and negative deflections in multiphasic responses (Fig. AI.6). P denotes positive deflections, N denotes negative deflections. In multiphasic responses, the peaks are numbered

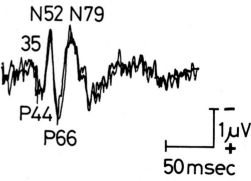

Figure AI.6. Multiphasic evoked response recorded from the cerebral cortex after stimulation of the dorsal aspect of the penis. The recording shows the conventional labeling of negative (N) and positive (P) deflections with the latency of each deflection from the point of stimulation in milliseconds.

consecutively (e.g., P1, N1, P2, N2...) or according to the latencies to peaks in milliseconds (e.g., P44, N52, P66...);

5. The amplitude of the responses is measured in µV.

SENSORY TESTING

Limited information of a subjective nature may be obtained during cystometry by recording such parameters as the first desire to micturate, urgency, or pain. However, sensory function in the lower urinary tract can be assessed by semiobjective tests by the measurement of urethral and/or vesical sensory thresholds to a standard applied stimulus such as a known electrical current.

General Information

Specify.

1. Patient's position (supine, sitting, standing, other);
2. Bladder volume at time of testing;
3. Site of applied stimulus (intravesical, intraurethral);
4. Number of times the stimulus was applied and the response recorded. Define the sensation recorded (e.g., the first sensation or the sensation of pulsing);
5. Type of applied stimulus
   a. electrical current—it is usual to use a constant current stimulator in urethral sensory measurement.
   (i) State electrode characteristics and placement as in section on EMG;
   (ii) State electrode contact area and distance between electrodes, if applicable;
   (iii) State impedance characteristics of the system;
   (iv) State type of conductive medium used for electrode/epithelial contact. Note: topical anesthetic agents should not be used;
   (v) Stimulator make and specifications;
   (vi) Stimulation parameters (pulse width, frequency, pattern, duration, current density).
   b. Other (e.g., mechanical, chemical).

Definition of Sensory Thresholds

The vesical/urethral sensory threshold is defined as the least current that consis-

tently produces a sensation perceived by the subject during stimulation at the site under investigation. However, the absolute values will vary in relation to the site of the stimulus, the characteristics of the equipment, and the stimulation parameters. Normal values should be established for each system.

Classification of Urinary Tract Dysfunction

The lower urinary tract is composed of the bladder and urethra. They form a functional unit and their interaction cannot be ignored. Each has two functions: the bladder to store and void and the urethra to control and convey. When a reference is made to the hydrodynamic function or to the whole anatomic unit as a storage organ—the vesica urinaria—the correct term is the bladder. When the smooth muscle structure known as the m. detrusor urinae is being discussed, the correct term is detrusor. For simplicity, the bladder/detrusor and the urethra will be considered separately so that a classification based on a combination of functional anomalies can be reached. Sensation cannot be precisely evaluated but must be assessed. This classification depends on the results of various objective urodynamic investigations. A complete urodynamic assessment is not necessary in all patients. However, studies of the filling and voiding phases are essential for each patient. The bladder and urethra may behave differently during the storage and micturition phases of bladder function; therefore, it is most useful to examine bladder and urethral activity separately in each phase.

Terms used should be objective, definable, and, ideally, applicable to the whole range of abnormality. When authors disagree with the classification presented below or use terms that have not been defined here, their meaning should be made clear.

Assuming the absence of inflammation, infection, and neoplasm, lower urinary tract dysfunction may be caused by

1. Disturbance of the pertinent nervous or psychological control system;
2. Disorders of muscle function;
3. Structural abnormalities.

Urodynamic diagnoses based on this classification should correlate with the patient's symptoms and signs. For example, the presence of an unstable contraction in an asymptomatic continent patient does not warrant a diagnosis of detrusor overactivity during storage.

THE STORAGE PHASE

Bladder Function During Storage

This may be described according to

1. Detrusor activity;
2. Bladder sensation;
3. Bladder capacity;
4. Compliance.

Detrusor Activity.   In this context, detrusor activity is interpreted from the measurement of detrusor pressure (Pdet). Detrusor activity may be normal or overactive.

In normal detrusor function, during the filling phase, the bladder volume increases without a significant rise in pressure (accommodation). No involuntary contractions occur despite provocation. A normal detrusor so defined may be described as "stable."

Overactive detrusor function is characterized by involuntary detrusor contractions during the filling phase, which may be spontaneous or provoked and which the patient cannot completely suppress. Involuntary detrusor contractions may be provoked by rapid filling, alterations of posture, coughing, walking, jumping, and other triggering procedures. Various terms have been used to describe these features, and they are defined as follows. The unstable detrusor is one that is shown objectively to contract, spontaneously or on provocation, during the filling phase while the patient is attempting to inhibit micturition. Unstable detrusor contractions may be asymptomatic or may be interpreted as a normal desire to void. The presence of these contractions does not necessarily imply a neurological disorder. Unstable contractions are usually phasic in type (Fig. AI.7*A*). A gradual increase in detrusor pressure without subsequent decrease is best regarded as a change of compliance (Fig. AI.7*B*).

Detrusor hyperreflexia is defined as overactivity due to disturbance of the nervous control mechanisms. The term detrusor hy-

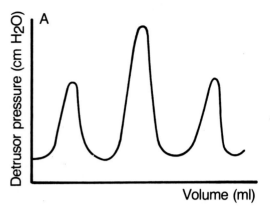

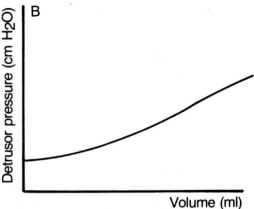

Figure AI.7. Diagrams of filling cystometry to illustrate (**A**) typical phasic unstable detrusor contraction and (**B**) the gradual increase of detrusor pressure with filling characteristic of reduced bladder compliance.

perreflexia should only be used when there is objective evidence of a relevant neurological disorder. The use of conceptual and undefined terms such as hypertonic, systolic, uninhibited, spastic, and automatic should be avoided.

Bladder Sensation.   Bladder sensation during filling can be classified in qualitative terms (see Cystometry, above) and by objective measurement (see Sensory Testing, above). Sensation can be classified broadly as follows:

1. Normal;
2. Increased (hypersensitive);
3. Reduced (hyposensitive);
4. Absent.

Bladder   Capacity.   See   Cystometry, above.

Compliance.   This is defined as $\Delta V/\Delta p$ (see Cystometry, above). Compliance may change during the cystometric examination and is variably dependent on a number of factors, including

1. Rate of filling;
2. The part of the cystometrogram curve used for compliance calculation;
3. The volume interval over which compliance is calculated;
4. The geometry (shape) of the bladder;
5. The thickness of the bladder wall;
6. The mechanical properties of the bladder wall;
7. The contractile/relaxant properties of the detrusor.

During normal bladder filling, little or no pressure change occurs; this is termed "normal compliance." However, at the present time, there is insufficient data to define normal, high, and low compliance.

When reporting compliance, specify

1. The rate of bladder filling;
2. The bladder volume at which compliance is calculated;
3. The volume increment over which compliance is calculated;
4. The part of the cystometrogram curve used for the calculation of compliance.

Urethral Function During Storage

The urethral closure mechanism during storage may be normal or incompetent. The normal urethral closure mechanism maintains a positive urethral closure pressure during filling even in the presence of increased abdominal pressure. Immediately before micturition, the normal closure pressure decreases to allow flow.

An incompetent urethral closure mechanism is defined as one that allows leakage of urine in the absence of a detrusor contraction. Leakage may occur whenever intravesical pressure exceeds intraurethral pressure (genuine stress incontinence) or when there is an involuntary fall in urethral pressure. Terms such as "the unstable urethra" await further data and precise definition.

Urinary Incontinence

Urinary incontinence is involuntary loss of urine that is objectively demonstrable and a social or hygienic problem. Loss of urine through channels other than the urethra is extraurethral incontinence.

Urinary incontinence denotes

1. A symptom;
2. A sign;
3. A condition.

The symptom indicates the patient's statement of involuntary urine loss. The sign is the objective demonstration of urine loss. The condition is the urodynamic demonstration of urine loss.

Symptoms. Urge incontinence is the involuntary loss of urine associated with a strong desire to void (urgency). Urgency may be associated with two types of dysfunction:

1. Overactive detrusor function (motor urgency);
2. Hypersensitivity (sensory urgency).

Stress incontinence is the symptom indicated by the patient's statement of involuntary loss of urine during physical exertion. "Unconscious" incontinence is incontinence that may occur in the absence of urge and without conscious recognition of the urinary loss.

Enuresis means any involuntary loss of urine. If it is used to denote incontinence during sleep, it should always be qualified with the adjective "nocturnal."

Postmicturition dribble and continuous leakage denote other symptomatic forms of incontinence.

Signs. The sign stress incontinence denotes the observation of loss of urine from the urethra synchronous with physical exertion (e.g., coughing). Incontinence may also be observed without physical exercise. Postmicturition dribble and continuous leakage denote other signs of incontinence. Symptoms and signs alone may not disclose the cause of urinary incontinence. Accurate diagnosis often requires urodynamic investigation in addition to careful history and physical examination.

Conditions. Genuine stress incontinence is the involuntary loss of urine occurring when, in the absence of a detrusor contraction, the intravesical pressure exceeds the maximum urethral pressure.

Reflex incontinence is loss of urine due to detrusor hyperreflexia and/or involuntary urethral relaxation in the absence of the sensation usually associated with the desire to micturate. This condition is only seen in patients with neuropathic bladder/urethral disorders.

Overflow incontinence is any involuntary loss of urine associated with overdistension of the bladder.

THE VOIDING PHASE

The Detrusor During Voiding

During micturition, the detrusor may be

1. Acontractile;
2. Underactive;
3. Normal.

The acontractile detrusor is one that cannot be demonstrated to contract during urodynamic studies. Detrusor areflexia is defined as acontractility due to an abnormality of nervous control and denotes the complete absence of centrally coordinated contraction. In detrusor areflexia due to a lesion of the conus medullaris or sacral nerve outflow, the detrusor should be described as decentralized, not denervated, because the peripheral neurons remain. In such bladders, pressure fluctuations of low amplitude, sometimes known as "autonomous" waves, may occasionally occur. The use of terms such as atonic, hypotonic, autonomic, and flaccid should be avoided.

The term detrusor underactivity should be reserved as an expression describing detrusor activity during micturition. Detrusor underactivity is defined as a detrusor contraction of inadequate magnitude and/or duration to bring about bladder emptying with a normal time span. Patients may have underactivity during micturition and detrusor overactivity during filling.

With normal detrusor contractility, normal voiding is achieved by a voluntarily initiated detrusor contraction that is sustained and can usually be suppressed voluntarily. A normal detrusor contraction will result in complete bladder emptying in the absence of obstruction. For a given detrusor contraction, the magnitude of the recorded pressure rise will depend on the degree of outlet resistance.

Urethral Function during Micturition

During voiding, urethral function may be

1. Normal;
2. Obstructive
   a. Overactivity;
   b. Mechanical.

The normal urethra opens to allow the bladder to be emptied. Obstruction due to urethral overactivity occurs when the urethral closure mechanism contracts against a detrusor contraction or fails to open at attempted micturition. Synchronous detrusor and urethral contraction is detrusor/urethral dyssynergia. This diagnosis should be qualified by stating the location and type of the urethral muscles (striated or smooth) that are involved. Despite the confusion surrounding "sphincter" terminology, the use of certain terms is so widespread that they are retained and defined here. The term detrusor/external sphincter dyssynergia or detrusor-sphincter dyssynergia describes a detrusor contraction concurrent with an involuntary contraction of the urethral and/or periurethral striated muscle. In the adult, detrusor sphincter dyssynergia is a feature of neurological voiding disorders. In the absence of neurological features, the validity of this diagnosis should be questioned. The term detrusor/bladder neck dyssynergia is used to denote a detrusor contraction concurrent with an objectively demonstrated failure of bladder neck opening. No parallel term has been elaborated for possible detrusor/distal urethral (smooth muscle) dyssynergia.

Overactivity of the urethral sphincter may occur during voiding in the absence of neurological disease and is termed dysfunctional voiding. The use of terms such as "nonneurogenic" or "occult neuropathic" should be avoided.

Mechanical obstruction is most commonly anatomical (e.g., urethral stricture).

Using the characteristics of detrusor and urethral function during storage and micturition, an accurate definition of lower urinary tract behavior in each patient becomes possible.

Units of Measurement

In the urodynamic literature, pressure is measured in cm H_2O and *not* in mm Hg. When Laplace's law is used to calculate tension in the bladder wall, it is often found

Table AI.1. Units of Measurement

Quantity	Acceptable Unit	Symbol
Volume	Milliliter	mL
Time	Second	s
Flow rate	Milliliters/second	mL/s
Pressure	Centimeters of water^a	cm H_2O
Length	Meters or submultiples	m, cm, mm
Velocity	Meters/second or submultiples	m/s, cm/s
Temperature	Degrees Celsius	°C

^{a}The SI unit is the pascal (Pa), but is only practical at present to calibrate our instruments in cm H_2O. One centimeter of water pressure is approximately equal to 100 pascals (1 cm H_2O = 98.07 Pa = 0.098 kPa).

Table AI.2. List of Symbols

Basic Symbols		Urological Qualifiers		Value	
Pressure	P	Bladder	ves	Maximum	max
Volume	V	Urethra	ura	Minimum	min
Flow rate	Q	Ureter	ure	Average	ave
Velocity	v	Detrusor	det	Isovolumetric	isv
Time	t	Abdomen	abd	Isotonic	ist
Temperature	T	External stream	ext	Isobaric	isb
Length	l			Isometric	ism
Area	A				
Diameter	d				
Force	F				
Energy	E				
Power	P				
Compliance	C				
Work	W				
Energy per unit volume	e				

Examples: $P_{det,max}$ = maximum detrusor pressure; e_{ext} = kinetic energy per unit volume in the external stream.

that pressure is then measured in dyne/cm^2. This lack of uniformity in the systems used leads to confusion when other parameters, which are a function of pressure, are computed, for example, "compliance" (contraction force/velocity) and so on. From these few examples, it is evident that standardization is essential for meaningful communication. Many journals now require that the results are given in SI units. This section is designed to give guidance in the application of the SI system to urodynamics and defines the units involved. The principal units to be used are listed above (Table AI.1).

Symbols

It is often helpful to use symbols in a communication. The system in Table AI.2 has been devised to standardize a code of symbols for use in urodynamics. The rationale of the system is to have a basic symbol representing the physical quantity with qualifying subscripts. The list of basic symbols largely conforms to international usage. The qualifying subscripts relate to the basic symbols for commonly used urodynamic parameters.

REFERENCES

1. Abrams P, Blaivas JG, Stanton SL, et al. Sixth report on the standardisation of terminology of lower urinary tract function. Procedures related to neurophysiological investigations: electromyography, nerve conduction studies, reflex latencies, evoked potentials and sensory testing. Scand J Urol Nephrol 1986;20:161–164.
2. Bates P, Bradley WE, Glen E, et al. First report on the standardisation of terminology of lower urinary tract function. Urinary incontinence. Procedures related to the evaluation of urine storage—cystometry, urethral closure pressure profile, units of measurement. Br J Urol 1976;48:39–42.
3. Bates P, Glen E, Griffiths D, et al. Second report on the standardisation of terminology of lower urinary tract function. Procedures related to the evaluation of micturition—flow rate, pressure

measurement, symbols. Br J Urol 1977;49:
207–210.

4. Bates P, Bradley WE, Glen E, et al. Third report on
the standardisation of terminology of lower urinary tract function. Procedures related to the
evaluation of micturition: pressure flow relationships, residual urine. Br J Urol 1980;52:348–350.

5. Jasper HH. Report to the committee on the methods
of clinical examination in electroencephalogra-
phy. Electroencephalogr Clin Neurophysiol 1958;
10:370–375.

6. Bates P, Bradley WE, Glen E, et al. Fourth report on
the standardisation of terminology of lower urinary tract function. Terminology related to neuromuscular dysfunction of lower urinary tract. Br J
Urol 1981;53:333–335.

Pharmacology of the Lower Urinary Tract ▮▮

Table AII.1. Drugs Stimulating the Parasympathetic Nervous System

Generic Name	Trade Name
Ambenonium	Mytelase
Carbachol	Carcholin, Isoptocarbachol
Echothiophate	Phospholine
Edrophonium	Tensilon
Demecarium	Humorsol
Isoflurophate	Floropryl
Methacholine	Mecholyl
Pilocarpine	Pilocar
Pralidoxime	Protopam
Pyridostigmine	Mestinon

Table AII.2. Drugs Inhibiting the Parasympathetic Nervous System

Generic Name	Trade Name
Adiphenine	Trasentine
Alverine	Profenil, Spacolin
Anisotropine	Valpin
Atropine	—
Belladonna extract	—
Carbofluorene	Pavatrine
Clidinium	Quarzan, Librax
Cyclopentolate	Cyclogyl
Diphemanil	Prantal
Ethaverine	Neopavrin
Eucatropine	Euphthalmine
Glycopyrrolate	Robinul
Hexocyclium	Tral
Homatropine hydrobromide	—
Homatropine methylbromide	Mesopin, Homapin, Novatrin, Malcotran
Hyoscyamine sulfate	Levsin
Isometheptene	Octin, Isometene
Mepenzolate	Cantil
Methixene	Trest
Methscopolamine bromide	Pamine
Methylatropine nitrate (Atropine methylnitrate)	Metropine
Oxyphenonium	Antrenyl
Papaverine	Cerespan, Ethaquine, Laverin, Neopavrin, Pap-Kaps, Pavabid, Pavacap, Pavacen, Pavarine, Pavatest, Paveril, Vasal, Vasospan

Table AII.2. (Continued)

Generic Name	Trade Name
Pentapiperium	Antrenyl; Quilene
Penthienate	Monodral
Pipenzolate	Pital
Piperidolate	Dactil
Poldine	Nacton
Scopolamine	—
Thihexinol	Sorboquel
Thiphenamil	Trocinate
Tincture of belladonna	—
Tricyclamol	Elorine
Tridihexethyl	Pathilon
Tropicamide	Mydriacyl
Valethamate	Murel

Table AII.3. Drugs Inhibiting the Parasympathetic Nervous System: Combined Preparations

Belbarb	Levsin with Phenobarbital
Belladenal	Milpath
Bellergal	Nolamine
Bentyl with phenobarbital	Pamine
Butibel	Pathibamate
Cantil with phenobarbital	Pathilon with Phenobarbital
Chardonna	Phenobarbital and Belladonna
Combid	Pro-Banthine with Dartal
Daricon-PB	
Donnalate	Pro-Banthine with Phenobarbital
Donnatal	
Donphen	Prydonnal
Enarax	Robinul-PH
Histalet	Sidonna
Hybephen	Valpin-PB
Kinesed	Trasentine-Phenobarbital
Kolantyl	

Table AII.4. Drugs Affecting the Sympathetic and Parasympathetic Nervous System: Ganglionic Blockers

Generic Name	Trade Name
Azamethonium	Pendiomide
Chlorisondamine	Ecolid
Hexamethonium	—
Mecamylamine	Inversine
Pentolinium	Ansolysen
Sparteine	Spartocin, Tocosamine
Trimethaphan	Arfonad
Trimethidinium	Ostensin

Table AII.5. Drugs Inhibiting the Sympathetic Nervous System: Adrenergic Neuron Blockers

Generic Name	Trade Name
Alseroxylon	Rauwiloid, Rautensin
Bethanidine	Esbatal
Bretylium	Darenthin
Debrisoquin	Declinax
Deserpidine	Harmonyl
Guanadrel	—
Guanethidine	Ismelin
Guanoclor	Vatensol
Guanoxan	Envacar
Hydralazine	Apresoline
Methyldopa	Aldomet
Methyldopate	Aldomet Ester
Nialamide	—
Pargyline	Eutonyl
Rauwolfia	Hyperloid, Raudixin, Rauja, Raulfin, Rautina, Rauval, Venibar
Rescinnamine	Cinatabs, Moderil
Reserpine	Lemiserp, Rau-Sed, Resercen, Reserpoid, Rolscrp, Sandril, Serpasil, Sertina, Vio-Serpine
Syrosingopine	Singoserp
Tranylcypromine	—
Veratrum alkaloids	Unitensen, Veralba, Veriloid, Vertavis

Table AII.6. Drugs Inhibiting the Sympathetic Nervous System: Combined Preparations

Aldoclor	Oreticyl
Aldoril	Pentoxyglon
Besertal	Protalba-R
Butiserpazide	Rauvera
Butiserpine	Rautrax
Diupres	Rauzide
Diutensen	Rauwiloid with Veriloid
Enduronyl	
Esimil	Regroton
Eutron	Ruhexatal with Reserpine
Exna-R	
Hydromox-R	Renese-R
Hydropres	Salutensin
Maxitate with Rauwolfia	Sandril with Pyronil
	Serpasil-Esidrix
Metatensin	Singoserp-Esidrix
Naquival	Theobarb-R
Nembu-Serpin	Theominal RS
Neo-Slowten	Vertavis-Phen
Nyomin	Vertina

Table AII.7. Drugs Affecting the Sympathetic Nervous System: Alpha Adrenergic Blockers

Generic Name	Trade Name
Azapetine	Ilidar
Dihydroergotoxine	Hydergine
Ergot alkaloids	—
Phenothiazines	(Various, see Table AII.13)
Phentolamine	Regitine
Piperoxan	Benodaine
Tolazoline	Priscoline

Table AII.8. Drugs Affecting the Sympathetic Nervous System: Beta Adrenergic Blockers

Generic Name	Trade Name
Acebutolol	Sectral
Atenolol	Tenormin
Betaxolol	Betoptic
Carteolol	Cartrol
Esmolol	Brevibloc
Labetalol	Trandate, Normodyne
Levobunolol	Betagan
Metoprolol	Lopressor
Nadolol	Corgard
Penbutolol	Levatol
Pindolol	Visken
Propranolol	Inderal
Timolol	Blocadren

Table AII.9. Drugs Affecting the Sympathetic Nervous System: General Adrenergic Stimulators

Generic Name	Trade Name
Adrenalone	Kephrine
Aminorex[a]	—
—	Aranthol
Benzphetamine	Didrex
Chlorphentermine	Pre-Sate
Clortermine	Voranil
Cyclopentamine	Clopane
Deoxyepinephrine	Epinine
Dextroamphetamine	Dexedrine
Diethylpropion	Tenuate, Tepanil
Epinephrine	—
Ethylnorepinephrine	Bronkephrine
Fenfluramine	Pondimin
Hydroxyamphetamine	Paredrine
Isometheptene	Octin
Levamphetamine	Ad-Nil, Amodril, Cydril, Maigret
Mazindol	Sanorex
Methamphetamine	Desoxyn

Continued.

Table AII.9. *(Continued)*

Generic Name	Trade Name
Mephentermine	Wyamine
Methylaminoheptane	Oenethyl
Methylhexamine	Forthane
Naphazoline	Privine
Oxymetazoline	Afrin
Phedrazine[a]	—
Phendimetrazine	Dietrol, Plegine
Phenmetrazine	Preludin
Phentermine	Ionamin, Wilpowr
Pholedrine	Paredrinol
Propylhexedrine	Benzedrex
Pseudoephredrine	Sudafed, Ro-Fedrin
Racephedrine	—
Synephrine[a]	—
Tenaphtoxaline[a]	—
Tetrahydrozoline	Tyzine
Tramazoline	—
Tuaminoheptane	Tuamine
Tymazoline[a]	Pernazene
Xylometazoline	Otrivin

[a]Not available in the United States.

Table AII.10. **Drugs Affecting the Sympathetic Nervous System: Combined Preparations**

Actifed-C Expectorant	Glynazan/EP
Acutuss	Hyadrine
Acutuss Expectorant with Codeine	Hydryllin with Racephedrine Hydrochloride
Aerolone Compound	Iso-Tabs
Amesec	Isuprel Compound
Amodrine	Luasmin
Asbron	Luftodil
Ayrcap	Lufyllin-EP
Ayr Liquid	Marax
Bihisdin	Nasocon
Brondilate	Nebair
Bronkometer	Neospect
Bronkosol	Neo-Vadrin
Bronkotabs	Norisodrine with
Calcidrine Syrup	Calcium Iodide
Cerose Expectorant	Novalene
Chlor-Trimeton Expectorant with Codeine	Numal NTZ
Citra	Orthoxine and Aminophylline
Colrex Compound	Phyldrox
Copavin	ProDecadron
Copavin Compound	Pyracort
Coricidin Nasal Mist	Pyraphed
Co-Xan	Quadrinal
Dainite	Synophedal
Dainite-KI	Tedral

Table AII.10. *(Continued)*

Deltasmyl	Tedral-25
Duo-Medihaler	Tedral Anti-H
Duovent	Thalfed
Dylephrine	Triaminicin
Ephed-Organidin	Tri-Isohalant
Ephedrine and Chlorcyclizine	Ulogesic
Ephedrine and Nembutal	Ulominic
Ephedrine and Seconal Sodium	Verequad
Ephoxamine	

Table AII.11. **Drugs Affecting the Sympathetic Nervous System: Alpha Adrenergic Stimulators**

Generic Name	Trade Name
Amidephrine[a]	—
Cyclopentamine	Clopane
Dopamine[a]	Intropin
Etafedrine[a]	—
Ethylphenylephrine[a]	Effortil
Hydroxyamphetamine	Paredrine
Metaraminol	Aramine
Methamphetamine	Desoxyn, Efroxine, Methedrine, Norodin, Synodrox
Methoxamine	Vasoxyl
Methylhexaneamine	Forthane
Nordefrin[a]	Cobefrin
Norepinephrine	Levarterenol
Novadral[a]	—
Phenylephrine	Neo-Synephrine, Isophrin, Synasal, Alcon-Efrin, Biomydrin, Isohalant Improved
Phenylpropanolamine	Dexatrim Accutrim Accutrol Dy-a-diet Capsule Prolamine Phenoxine Appedrine
Phenylpropylmethylamine	Vonedrine
Propylhexedrine	Benzedrex
Tyramine[a]	—

[a]Not available in the United States.

Table AII.12. Drugs Affecting the Sympathetic Nervous System: Beta Adrenergic Stimulators

Generic Name	Trade Name
Albuterol[a]	Proventil, Ventolin
Bamethan[a]	—
Chlorprenaline	—
Dioxethedrine	—
Etafedrine	—
Ethylnorepinephrine[a]	Bronkephrine
Hydroxyephedrine[a]	—
Isoetharine	Bronkosol
Isoproterenol	Aludrine, Isuprel, Norisodrine
Methoxyphenamine	Orthoxine
Nylidrin	Arlidin
Protokylol	Caytine
Salbutamol[a]	—
Soterenol[a]	—
Terbutaline	Bricanyl

[a]Not available in the United States.

Table AII.13. Drugs Affecting the Autonomic Nervous System: Drugs Causing Retention

Generic Name	Trade Name
Acetophenazine	Tindal
Amitriptyline	Elavil
Amphotericin B	Fungizone
Benztropine	Cogentin
Biperiden	Akineton
Bromodiphenhy-dramine	Ambodryl
Brompheniramine	Dimetane
Butaperazine	Repoise
Carbinoxamine	Clistin
Carphenazine	Proketazine
Chlorpheniramine	Chlor-Trimeton, Histaspan, Teldrin
Chlorphenoxamine	Systral, Phenoxene
Chlorpromazine	Thorazine
Chlorprothixene	Taractan
Cycrimine	Pagitane
Deanol	Deaner
Desipramine	Norpramin, Pertofrane
Dexbrompheniramine	Disomer
Dexchlorpheniramine	Polaramine
Dimethindene	Forhistal, Triten
Diphenhydramine	Benadryl
Diphenylpyraline	Diafen, Hispril
Doxepin	Adapin, Sinequan
Doxylamine	Decapryn
Droperidol	Inapsine
Ethopropazine	Parsidol
Fluphenazine	Prolixin, Permitil
Haloperidol	Haldol
Imipramine	Tofranil, Presamine
Isocarboxazid	Marplan

Table AII.13. *(Continued)*

Generic Name	Trade Name
Mesoridazine	Serentil
Mepazine	—
Metaxalone	Skelaxin
Methapyrilene	Histadyl
Methdilazine	Tacaryl
Methylphenidate	Ritalin
Methysergide	Sansert
Molindone	Moban
Nortriptyline	Aventyl
Orphenadrine	Norflex
Perphenazine	Trilafon
Phenelzine	Nardil
Phenindamine	Thephorin
Piperacetazine	Quide
Pipradrol	Meratran
Prochlorperazine	Compazine
Procyclidine	Kemadrin
Promazine	Sparine
Promethazine	Phenergan
Protriptyline	Vivactil
Pyrilamine	—
Rotoxamine	Twiston
Thiopropazate	Dartal
Thioridazine	Mellaril
Thiothixene	Navane
Tranylcypromine	Parnate
Trifluoperazine	Stelazine
Triflupromazine	Vesprin
Trihexyphenidyl	Artane, Pipanol, Tremin
Trimeprazine	Temaril
Tripelennamine	Pyribenzamine
Triprolidine	Actidil

Table AII.14. Drugs Affecting the Autonomic Nervous System: Drugs Causing Miscellaneous Urologic Symptoms

Generic Name	Trade Name	Mixtures
Frequency		
Iron Sorbitex	Jectofer	Etrafon
Dantrolene	Dantrium	Triavil
Incontinence		
Estrogens		
Hydroxystil-bamidine		
Urgency		
Disodium Edetate	Endrate	
Frequency, Retention and Incontinence		
Levodopa	Bendopa, Dopar, Larodopa, Levodopa	
Levopropoxy-phene	Novrad	

Table AII.15. Calcium-channel Blockers

Verapamil
Nifedipine
Nimodipine
Diltiazem
Gallopamil[a]
Tiapamil[a]
Fostedil[a]
Nitrendipine[a]
Nimodipine[a]
Nisoldipine[a]
Nicardipine[a]
Felodipine[a]
Cinnarizine[a]
Flunarizine[a]
Lidoflazine[a]
Perhixiline[a]
Bepridil[a]

[a]Investigational in Europe only.

Data Recording Forms for Urogynecology

URG-DATA BASE SYSTEM
URODYNAMICS AND GYNECOLOGIC UROLOGY
HISTORY

DONALD R. OSTERGARD, M.D.
WOMEN'S HOSPITAL
MEMORIAL HOSPITAL MEDICAL CENTER
UNIVERSITY OF CALIFORNIA IRVINE
2801 ATLANTIC AVENUE, P.O. BOX 1428
LONG BEACH, CA 90801 (213) 595-3824

FORM 1A
Page 1

DATE _____

CHART NO. _____

PATIENT NO. _____

NAME _____   _____
Last   First

INSTRUCTIONS TO PATIENT: Check the box if your answer is "YES"

1. Have you had treatment for urinary tract disease, such as: (Please check) stones ☐, kidney disease ☐, infections ☐, tumors ☐, injuries ☐?

2. Have you ever had paralysis ☐, polio ☐, multiple sclerosis ☐, a stroke ☐, back pain ☐, syphilis ☐, diabetes ☐, pernicious anemia ☐? (If yes, check proper ones).

3. Have you had an operation on your spine ☐, brain ☐, or bladder ☐?

4. Have you had a bladder infection during the last year? ☐

5. If yes, did it occur more than twice during the last year? ☐

6. Did the bladder infection follow intercourse at any time? ☐

7. Is your urine ever bloody? ☐

8. Have you ever been treated by urethral dilatation? ☐

9. If yes: when? _____ How many times? _____

10. Did urethral dilatation help you? ☐

11. Did you have trouble holding urine as a child? ☐

12. As a child, did you wet the bed? ☐

13. If yes, at what age did you stop? _____

14. Do you wet the bed now? ☐

15. What is the volume of urine you usually pass? (Please check) Large ☐, medium ☐, small ☐, very small ☐

16. Do you notice any dribbling of urine when you stand after passing urine? ☐

17. Do you lose urine by spurts during severe coughing ☐, sneezing ☐, or vomiting ☐?

18. If yes, in which position(s) does it occur? (Please check) Standing ☐, sitting ☐, laying down ☐

19. Do you lose urine without coughing, sneezing or vomiting? ☐

20. If yes, when does it occur? (Please check) walking ☐, running ☐, straining ☐, laying down ☐, any change of position ☐, after intercourse ☐, during intercourse ☐?

21. When you are passing urine, can you usually stop the flow? ☐

22. Did your urine difficulty start during pregnancy ☐, or after delivery of an infant ☐? (If yes, check proper one).

23. Did it follow an operation? ☐

24. If yes, check the type of operation:
☐ Hysterectomy (removal of womb), through the abdomen.
Radical ☐
☐ Hysterectomy (removal of womb), through the vagina.
☐ Removal of a tumor through the abdomen.
☐ Vaginal repair operation.
☐ Suspension of the uterus or bladder.
☐ Cesarean section.
☐ Other (describe) _____

25. Did it follow X-ray treatment? ☐

26. If your menstrual periods have stopped, did the menopause make your condition worse? ☐

27. Do you lose control and pass a large amount of urine when you cough ☐, sneeze ☐, laugh ☐, lift ☐, strain ☐, vomit ☐, during intercourse ☐, after intercourse ☐?

28. Do you have difficulty holding urine if you suddenly stand up after sitting or lying down? ☐

29. Do you find it necessary to wear protection because you get wet from the urine you lose? ☐

30. If yes, at what age did you start using this protection? _____

31. When do you wear protection? (Please check) occasionally ☐, all the time ☐, only during the day ☐, only at night ☐.

32. Is your urinary problem bad enough that you would request surgery to fix it? ☐

33. List all medications you are now taking and duration of use of each medication (include contraceptives):

CODE	MEDICATION	DURATION OF USE

34. When you lose your urine accidentally, are you ever unaware that it is passing? ☐

35. Do you always have an uncomfortably strong need to pass urine before you empty your bladder? ☐

36. Do you lose urine before reaching the toilet? ☐

37. If yes, is this urine loss painful? ☐

38. Do you have to hurry to the toilet or can you take your time? (Please check) hurry ☐, take time ☐.

39. Can you overcome the uncomfortably strong need to pass urine? (Please check) usually ☐, occasionally ☐, rarely ☐.

40. Do you have an uncomfortably strong need to pass urine with a full bladder? ☐

© 1978 DONALD R. OSTERGARD, MD

Form 1A, Page 1. History (English).

URG-DATA BASE SYSTEM
URODYNAMICS AND GYNECOLOGIC UROLOGY
HISTORY

DONALD R. OSTERGARD, M.D.
WOMEN'S HOSPITAL
MEMORIAL HOSPITAL MEDICAL CENTER
2801 ATLANTIC AVENUE, P.O. BOX 1428
LONG BEACH, CA 90801 (213) 595-3824

Form 1A
Page 2

DATE _____
CHART NO. _____
PATIENT NO. _____

NAME _____ _____
Last   First

INSTRUCTIONS TO PATIENT: Please check the box if your answer is "YES"

41. Do you have an uncomfortably strong need to pass urine without a full bladder? ☐

42. How many times do you void during the night after going to bed? _____

43. How many times do you void during the first hour after going to bed? _____

44. Does an uncomfortably strong need to pass urine wake you up? ☐

45. Are you usually awake and simply pass urine while up? ☐

46. After passing urine, can you usually go back to sleep? ☐

47. How much fluid do you usually drink before going to bed? _____ cups.

48. Do you have discomfort in the area above or to the side of your bladder? ☐

49. Do you have pain while you pass your urine? ☐

50. Is it painful during the entire time you pass urine? ☐

51. Is it painful only at the end of passing urine? ☐

52. Do you always feel that your bladder is empty after passing urine? ☐

53. Do you usually have painful passing of urine after intercourse? ☐

54. Do you need to pass urine more frequently after intercourse? ☐

55. Does your bladder discomfort stop completely after passing urine? ☐

56. How often do you pass urine during the day? Every _____ hours.

57. Is it necessary for you to pass urine frequently? ☐

58. Does the sound, the sight, or the feel of running water cause you to lose urine? ☐

59. Do you need to pass urine more frequently when riding in a car? ☐

60. Is your clothing slightly damp ☐, wet ☐, soaking wet ☐, or do you leave puddles on the floor ☐?

61. Is your loss of urine a continual drip so that you are constantly wet? ☐

62. Are you ever suddenly aware that you are losing or are about to lose control of your urine? ☐

63. How often does this occur? _____ / Day _____ / Week

64. Do you usually have difficulty starting your urine stream? ☐

65. Do you find it frequently necessary to have your urine removed by means of a catheter because you are unable to pass it? ☐

FAMILY UROLOGY HISTORY

Does (did) your natural mother, sister, aunt or grandmother have problems with urine loss as a child or an adult? ☐

	Mother	Sister	Aunt	GrandMother
Did she have surgery to correct this problem?	☐	☐	☐	☐
Did she wear a pad to protect against urine loss?	☐	☐	☐	☐
At what age did her problem start?	_____	_____	_____	_____
How old were you when her problem started?	_____	_____	_____	_____
Did she wet the bed as a child?	☐	☐	☐	☐
At what age did she stop?	_____	_____	_____	_____

SUMMARY:

In the space below please summarize your urine problem(s) as briefly as possible:

_____
_____
_____
_____
_____
_____
_____
_____

Form 1A, Page 2. History (English).

DATOS BASICOS DEL SISTEMA
GINECO-UROLOGICO
HISTORIA GINECOUROLOGICA

DONALD R. OSTERGARD, M.D.
WOMEN'S HOSPITAL
MEMORIAL HOSPITAL MEDICAL CENTER
UNIVERSITY OF CALIFORNIA IRVINE
2801 ATLANTIC AVENUE, P.O. BOX 1428
LONG BEACH, CA 90801 (213) 595-3824

Form 1B
Pagina 1

FECHA_____
CHART NO. _____
PATIENT NO. _____

NOMBRE _____   _____
                    ULTIMO   PRIMERO

| INSTRUCCIONES A LA PACIENTE: Favor de chequear (marcar) el cuadro si contesta sí. |

1. ¿ Ha tenido usted tratamiento para enfermedades de las vías urinarias, como: piedras ☐, enfermedad de los riñones ☐, infecciones ☐, tumores ☐, lesiones ☐? (favor de marcar donde corresponda).

2. ¿ Ha tenido usted alguna vez parálisis ☐, polio ☐, multiple sclerosis ☐, serias lesiones en la espalda ☐, embolia ☐, sifílis ☐, diabetes ☐, anemia perniciosa ☐ (favor de marcar donde corresponda).

3. ¿ Ha tenido un operación en la espina ☐, el cerebro ☐, la vejiga ☐? (Favor de marcar donde corresponda).

4. ¿ Ha tenido usted infección en la vejiga durante el año pasado? ☐

5. ¿ Si contesta sí, occurrió ésto mas de dos veces durante el año pasado? ☐

6. ¿ La infección de la vejiga ocurrió después de tener relaciones íntimas en alguna ocasión? ☐

7. ¿ Tiene usted sangre en la orina a veces? ☐

8. ¿ Ha recibido usted tratamiento de dilatación de la uretra? ☐

9. ¿ Si contesta sí, cuando? _____
¿ cuantas veces? _____

10. ¿ Le ayudó la dilatación de la uretra? ☐

11. ¿ Tuvo usted dificultad en detener la orina cuando era niña? ☐

12. ¿ Cuando niña, mojaba usted la cama?

13. ¿ Si contesta sí, a qué edad se le quitó el problema de mojar la cama? _____ años

14. ¿ Moja usted la cama ahora? ☐

15. ¿ Que es la cantidad de orina que usted pasa usualmente? (Por favor marque) mucho ☐, regular ☐, poco ☐, muy poquito ☐

16. ¿ Nota usted un goteo de orina al levantarse después de haber orinado? ☐

17. ¿ Pierde usted orina repentinamente al toser fuerte ☐, estornudar ☐, vomitar ☐?

18. ¿ Si lo anterior sucede, en que posición o posiciones occure? (Favor de marcar donde corresponda) de pie ☐, sentada ☐, acostada ☐.

19. ¿ Pierde usted orina sin toser ☐, estornudar ☐, o vomitar ☐? (Favor de marcar donde corresponda).

20. ¿ Si indique que sí cuando occure? Andando ☐, corriendo ☐, haciendo fuerza ☐, acostada ☐, en cambio de posición ☐, despues de relaciones sexuales ☐, durante el acto sexual ☐.

21. ¿ Cuando esta usted orinando generalmente puede contenerse y dejar de orinar? ☐

22. ¿ Cuando empezó su problema de las vías urinarias? durante el embarzo ☐, después del nacimiento de su nene ☐?

23. ¿ Empezo su problema después de una operación? ☐

24. ¿ Si contesta sí, que operación fue:
☐ Historectomía (extirpacion de la matríz) operación abdomina (Radical ☐)
☐ Historectomía (extirpación de la matríz) operación vaginal
☐ Extirpación de un tumor, operación abdominal
☐ Operación de reparación vaginal
☐ Suspensión del útero o la vejiga
☐ Cesarea
Otro operación (Describa) _____

25. ¿ Empezo su problema después del tratamiento de radiología? ☐

26. ¿ Si ya no menstrua usted, la menopausia ha empeorado su padecimiento? ☐

27. ¿ Pierde usted control de la orina cuando tose ☐, estornuda ☐, ríe ☐, levanta algo ☐, hace algun esfuerzo o vomita ☐, después de relaciones sexuales ☐, durante el acto sexual ☐?

28. ¿ Tiene usted dificultad deteniendo la orina si usted de repente se levanta después de haber estado sentada o acostada? ☐

29. ¿ Tiene usted que usar algo de protección porque se moja siempre con la orina que pierde? ☐

30. ¿ Si usa protección a que edad empezó usted a usarlo? _____

31. ¿ Cuando usa usted proteción? (Favor de marcar donde corresponda). Algunas veces ☐, Siempre ☐, Durante el día ☐, Durante la noche ☐.

32. ¿ Es su problema de las vías urinarias lo suficientemente serio que usted desea recurrir a la cirugia para corregirlo? ☐

33. ¿ Favor de hacer una lista de las medicinas que usted esta tomando ahora? (incluyendo pastillas anticonceptivas).

Coda	Medicina	Tiempo del uso

34. ¿ Cuando pierde usted la orina accidentalmente, se da usted cuenta de que esta orinando? ☐

© 1978 DONALD R. OSTERGARD, MD

Form 1B, Page 1. History (Spanish).

DATOS BASICOS DEL SISTEMA
GINECO-UROLOGICO
HISTORIA GINECOUROLOGICA

DONALD R. OSTERGARD, M.D.
WOMEN'S HOSPITAL
MEMORIAL HOSPITAL MEDICAL CENTER
UNIVERSITY OF CALIFORNIA IRVINE
2801 ATLANTIC AVENUE, P.O. BOX 1428
LONG BEACH, CA 90801 (213) 595-3824

Form 1B
Pagina 2

FECHA_____
CHART NO._____
PATIENT NO._____

NOMBRE_____, _____
ULTIMO   PRIMERO

INSTRUCCIONES A LA PACIENTE: Favor de chequear (marcar) el cuadro si contesta sí.

35. ¿ Tiene usted siempre un deseo incontrolable de orinar antes de vaciar la vejiga? ☐

36. ¿ Pierde usted orina antes de

37. ¿ Si contesta sí, esta pérdida de la orina le causa dolor? ☐

38. ¿ Tiene usted que apurarse para llegar al baño ☐ o puede usted demorarse ☐ (favor de marcar donde corresponda).

39. ¿ Puede usted sobreponerse el deseo incontrolable y fuerte de orinar? Usualmente ☐, Algunas veces ☐, Rara vez ☐. (Favor de marcar donde corresponda).

40. ¿ Tiene usted una necesidad poderosa e incomoda de orinar con la vejiga llena? ☐

41. ¿ Tiene usted necesidad poderosa e incomoda de orinar con la vejiga vacia? ☐

42. ¿ Cuantas veces se levanta usted de la cama en la noche para orinar? _____ veces.

43. ¿ Cuantas veces orina usted durante la primera hora después de acostarse? _____ veces.

44. ¿ Siente usted un deseo de orinar tan fuerte e incomodo que la despierta? ☐

45. ¿ Esta usted generalmente despierta y solo orina cuando esta levantada? ☐

46. ¿ Después de orinar puede usted generalmente volverse a dormir? ☐

47. ¿ Que cantidad de líquido toma usted generalmente antes de acostarse? _____ tazas.

48. ¿ Tiene usted algun malestar en el área arriba o al lado de la vejiga? ☐

49. ¿ Tiene usted dolor al orinar? ☐

50. ¿ Tiene usted dolor durante todo el tiempo en que esta orinado? ☐

51. ¿ Siente usted dolor solamente al terminar de orinar? ☐

52. ¿ Siempre se siente que su vejiga esta vacia después de haber pasado la orina? ☐

53. ¿ Tiene usted dolor al orinar después de haber tenido relaciones íntimas? ☐

54. ¿ Siente usted la necesidad de orinar mas frecuentemente después de tener relaciones íntimas? ☐

55. ¿ La incomodidad que siente usted desaparece completamente de la vejiga después de orinar? ☐

56. ¿ Cuántas veces orina usted durante el día? cada _____ horas.

57. ¿ Es necesario para usted orinar frecuentamente? ☐

58. ¿ Cuando usted ve, oye o toca agua corriendo, ésto le causa perder la orina? ☐

59. ¿ Siente usted deseos de orinar mas frecuentemente cuando viaja en automovil? ☐

60. ¿ Esta su ropa humeda ☐, mojada ☐, empapada ☐, o deja usted charcos en el suelo ☐? (Favor de marcar donde corresponda).

61. ¿ La pérdida de orina que usted tiene consiste en un goteo constante que la mantiene mojada? ☐

62. ¿ Esta usted alguna vez sin darse cuenta de que esta a punto de perder orina o de perder el control sobre la facultad de orinar?

63. ¿ Con que frecuencia ocurre lo anterior? _____ /día _____ /semana.

64. ¿ Tiene usted generalmente dificultad en comenzar a orinar? ☐

65. ¿ Con frecuencia necesita usted que le saquen la orina por medio de un tubo debido a que no puede orinar? ☐

HISTORIA UROLOGICA DE LA FAMILIA

¿ Tienen (o tenían) su madre natural, su hermana, su tía o su abuela problemas con la pérdida de la orina cuando era nina o adulta?
(Si contesta sí, favor de contestar lo siguiente.)

	MADRE	HERMANA	TIA	ABUELA
¿ Le operaron para corregir el problema?	☐	☐	☐	☐
¿ Usaba toalla sanitaria para protejerse de la pérdida de la orina?	☐	☐	☐	☐
¿ A que edad empezó su problema de la orina?	_____	_____	_____	_____
¿ Cuantos años tuvo ud. cuando ella empezó su problema?	_____	_____	_____	_____
¿ Mojaba la cama cuando era niña?	☐	☐	☐	☐
¿ A que edad dejó de mojar la cama?	_____	_____	_____	_____

RESUMEN

En el espacio abajo, por favor describa en pocas palabras su problema de la orina. _____
_____
_____
_____
_____
_____

© 1978 DONALD R. OSTERGARD, MD

Form 1B, Page 2. History (Spanish).

I HISTORY

Age _____ LMP _____ Weight _____

Gravida _____ Para _____ Abortions _____

Age of Menarche _____ Age of Menopause _____

Menopausal Status: Pre ☐   Peri ☐   Post ☐

Hysterectomy ☐ _____ Anterior Repair ☐ _____

RPU ☐ Type: _____

Other Positive History _____

II SUMMARY OF MEDICAL HISTORY and SELF EVALUATION

☐ Dysuria _____ + ☐ Freq. q. _____ hrs. ☐ Urgency _____ +

☐ Nocturia x _____   Incontinence ☐ Stress _____ +

☐ Post Void Fullness _____ +   ☐ Urge _____ +

III NEUROLOGICAL EVALUATION   Normal ☐   Normal Except for ☐

Rectal Evaluation (check if abnormal)

Contractions—Voluntary ☐   with Cough ☐   With hold ☐

Tone: Normal ☐   Abnormal ☐

Reflexes (check if abnormal)

Babinski Present ☐

☐ DTR's: Pattellar ☐   Ankle ☐

Proprioception ☐

Sensory: L5 ☐   S1 ☐   S2 ☐   S3 ☐   S4 ☐   Abnormal on
Motor: L5 ☐   S1 ☐   S2 ☐   S3 ☐   S4 ☐   Right ☐   Left ☐

Other: _____

IV PHYSICAL EXAMINATION   Normal ☐

	MILD	MODERATE	SEVERE
Cystocele	☐	☐	☐
Rectocele	☐	☐	☐
Urethral Displacement	☐	☐	☐
Enterocele	☐	☐	☐

Caruncle ☐   Fistula ☐ Type:

Other Positive Findings:

	NORMAL	DESCRIBE IF ABNORMAL
Vulva	☐	
Vagina	☐	
Urethra	☐	
Cervix	☐	
Fundus	☐	
Adnexa	☐	

V Q-TIP TEST

Resting Angle + ☐ – ☐ _____ °

Straining Angle + ☐ – ☐ _____ °

Change from Horizontal _____ °

VI UROFLOWMETRY

VII UROLOG

VII UROLOG	Flow Rate (cc / sec) Maximum / Mean	
FREQUENCY	Urine Volume (cc) In / Voided	
Day	Flowtime (sec)	
Night	Time to Maximum Flow (sec)	
VOLUME	Residual Urine (cc)	
Day	Normal Voiding for patient?	YES ☐ NO ☐
Night	Interpretation	N ☐ AB ☐
	Describe:	

URG-DATA BASE SYSTEM
URODYNAMICS AND
GYNECOLOGIC UROLOGY
INITIAL HISTORY AND
PHYSICAL EXAMINATION

FORM 2

DONALD R. OSTERGARD, M.D.
ALFRED E. BENT, M.D.
WOMEN'S HOSPITAL
MEMORIAL MEDICAL CENTER
OF LONG BEACH
UNIVERSITY OF CALIFORNIA, IRVINE
2880 ATLANTIC AVE., #130
LONG BEACH, CA 90806
(213) 595-3824

Name _____
        FIRST   LAST

Urine C&S Negative ☐   Positive ☐   DATE _____

DRUG ALLERGIES   CHART NO. _____

PATIENT NO. _____

VIII URETHRAL CALIBRATION

Calibration to _____ F   Dilatation to _____ F

IX DIAGNOSIS   Normal ☐

X X-RAYS   VCUG ☐   TRATNER ☐   IVP ☐   UTZ ☐

XI MEDICATIONS   None ☐

CODE	DRUG	DOSE	FREQ.	DUR / TREATMENT	RX'D
	Nitrofurantoin	50 mg.	tid	3 days	
	Vaginal Estrogen	—	qod	Indefinite	
	Pyridium	100 mg.	tid	3 days prn	

XII COMMENTS

TREATMENT PLAN:

RETURN APPOINTMENT:

Other Studies: Dictated ☐

©1987 DONALD R. OSTERGARD, M.D.

_____ M.D.

Form 2. Initial history and physical examination.

URG-DATA BASE SYSTEM
URODYNAMICS AND GYNECOLOGIC UROLOGY
URODYNAMICS VISIT SUMMARY

DONALD R. OSTERGARD, M.D.
WOMEN'S HOSPITAL
MEMORIAL HOSPITAL MEDICAL CENTER
UNIVERSITY OF CALIFORNIA IRVINE
2801 ATLANTIC AVENUE, P.O. BOX 1428
LONG BEACH, CA 90801 (213) 595-3824

New ☐
Returning ☐
Postpartum _____ Weeks

FORM 3
PAGE 1

DATE: _____
CHART NO. _____
PATIENT NO. _____

NAME _____
Last   First
CHECKED BOXES INDICATE APPLICABLE OR POSITIVE RESPONSES

I INTERVAL HISTORY LMP _____ **CYCLE DAY NO.** _____

Dysuria: ☐ _____ +   Freq ☐ q _____ hrs.   Urgency ☐ _____ +
Nocturia: ☐ x _____   Incontinence: Stress ☐ _____ +
Post Void Fullness ☐ _____ +   Urge ☐ _____ +

II CURRENT MEDICATIONS   None ☐

CODE	DRUG*	DOSE	FREQ.	DUR. OF USE	SUBJECTIVE RESPONSE**
					1___5___10
					1___5___10
					1___5___10

*includes contraceptives
**< 5 = worse, 5 = no response, > 5 = better, 10 = cured

III SUBJECTIVE RESPONSES TO PREVIOUS TREATMENTS   None ☐

TREATMENT	RESPONSE	COMMENTS
Dilatation	1___5___10	
	1___5___10	

IV UROFLOWMETRY

		†SPONT.	†INST.
Voiding Mechanism	Vesical Contraction	░░░	☐
	Urethra	░░░	‡R☐ C☐ / NC☐
	Voluntary Strain	░░░	☐
Flow Rate (cc/sec) Maximum/Mean		/	/
Urine Volume (cc) In/Voided		/	/
Flowtime (sec)			
Time to Maximum Flow (sec)			
Residual Urine (cc)		░░░	
Maximum Intravesical Pressure (cm/H$_2$0)		░░░	
Resistance = P/F^2		░░░	
Time: UP↓ to VP↑ (sec)		░░░	⊞ ⊟
Normal Voiding for patient?		YES☐ NO☐	YES☐ NO☐
Interpretation		N ☐ Ab ☐	N ☐ Ab ☐

V ELECTROMYOGRAPHIC STIMULATION

Anal Sphincter response to urethral stimulation:
Normal ☐   Abnormal ☐   Latency _____ Msec
Perineal Relaxation:
No Effect ☐   Response: Abolished ☐   Decreased ☐
Interpretation: Normal ☐   Abnormal ☐

VI NEUROLOGICAL EVALUATION   Normal ☐   Check if Abnormal

Bulbocavernosus ☐   Anal ☐ : Right ☐   Left ☐
Voluntary Rectal Contraction ☐

VII URODYNAMICS: UCPP AND URETHROVESICAL PRESSURE DYNAMICS

	SUPINE EMPTY			SUPINE FULL			SITTING FULL														CONTROL			STRETCH RESPONSE						UNITS
Length Functional																																CM
Total																																
Pressure Closure																																CM
Total																																H$_2$0
Distance 0 → Max																																CM
Max → 0																																
UCPP Closure Area																																CM²
Urethral P + EMG	P	D	E	P	D	E	P	D	E	P	D	E	P	D	E	P	D	E	P	D	E							††
Rectal Tighten																																
Hold Urine																																CM
Strain																																H$_2$0
Cough																																
Pressure Equalization																																
Cough Profile	⊞		⊟	⊞		⊟	⊞		⊟	⊞		⊟	⊞		⊟	⊞		⊟	⊞		⊟							
Intravesical Pressure																																CM H$_2$0
Urethral Instability																																

† SPONTANEOUS/INSTRUMENTED   ‡ R = RELAXES   C = CONTRACTS   NC = NO CHANGE   †† E = EMC RESPONSE / P/D = PROXIMAL/DISTAL URETHRA

1980 DONALD R. OSTERGARD, MD

Form 3, Page 1.   Visit summary (urodynamics).

FORM 3
PAGE 2

URG-DATA BASE SYSTEM
URODYNAMICS AND GYNECOLOGIC UROLOGY
URODYNAMICS VISIT SUMMARY

DONALD R. OSTERGARD, M.D.
WOMEN'S HOSPITAL
MEMORIAL HOSPITAL MEDICAL CENTER
UNIVERSITY OF CALIFORNIA IRVINE
2801 ATLANTIC AVENUE, P.O. BOX 1428
LONG BEACH, CA 90801 (213) 595 3824

DATE: _____
CHART NO. _____
PATIENT NO. _____

Name: _____

              FIRST   LAST

CHECKED BOXES INDICATE APPLICABLE OR POSITIVE RESPONSE.

VIII CYSTOMETRICS and EMG — H₂O

VOLUME	FIRST SENSATION	_____ cc	_____ cc
	FULLNESS	_____ cc	
	MAXIMUM	_____ cc	_____ cc
VOLUNTARY VOIDING	Inhibited		
TERMINAL CONTRACTION	Uninhibited		
None ☐		_____ cmH₂0	_____ cmH₂0
Urethral Sphincter Response	Relaxes	†P. †E.	P. E.
	Contracts	P. E.	P. E.
	No Change	P. E.	P. E.
Pressure Change (cmH₂0)		⊞ ⊟	⊞ ⊟
Time From UP↓ to VP↑ (sec)		⊞ ⊟	⊞ ⊟
Anal Sphincter Response	Relaxes	E.	E.
	Contracts	E.	E.
	No Change	E.	E.
OTHER VESICAL CONTRACTIONS	Inhibited	☐ cmH₂0	☐ cmH₂0
None ☐	Partial Inhib.	☐	☐
	Uninhibited	☐	☐
Spontaneous			
Induced by:	Jolt		
	Cough		
	Filling		
Bladder Volume		_____ cc	_____ cc
Urethral Sphincter Response	Relaxes	P. E.	P. E.
	Contracts	P. E.	P. E.
	No Change	P. E.	P. E.
Pressure Change (cmH₂0)		⊞ ⊟	⊞ ⊟
Time From UP↓ to VP↑ (sec)		⊞ ⊟	⊞ ⊟
Anal Sphincter Response	Relaxes	E.	E.
	Contracts	E.	E.
	No Change	E.	E.

†P = Pressure Response   E = EMG Response

IX TREATMENT PROCEDURES   None ☐

☐ Anesthesia: Local ☐   Topical ☐

                Previous   Present

☐ Calibration To _____ _____ F   Bleeding ☐
   Dilation To _____ _____ F   Pain ☐

Cryosurgery ☐:   Polyps ☐   Caruncle ☐

X LABORATORY

Urine C&S ordered ☐:
          Neg ☐   Pos ☐ on _____ (date)

XI XRAYS   VCUG ☐   TRATNER ☐   UTZ ☐   IVP ☐

XII CONSULTATIONS REQUESTED: CYSTOSCOPY ☐

Psychiatry ☐   Urology ☐   Neurology ☐   EMG ☐   Other ☐

XIII DIAGNOSIS codes: No Change ☐

1. _____
                            Code: _____

2. _____
                            Code: _____

3. _____
                            Code: _____

4. _____
                            Code: _____

COMMENTS AND RECOMMENDATIONS

XI MEDICATIONS   None ☐

Code	Drug	Dose	Freq.	Duration/Treatment	Rx'd
	Nitrofurantoin	50 mg	tid	3 days	
	Vaginal Estrogen		god	indefinite	
	Pyridium	100 mg	tid	3 days/prn	

DICTATED ☐

RETURN APPOINTMENT DATE _____ MD

Form 3, Page 2.   Visit summary (urodynamics).

URG-DATA BASE SYSTEM

URODYNAMICS AND GYNECOLOGIC UROLOGY

RETURN VISIT SUMMARY   FORM 5

DONALD R. OSTERGARD, M.D.
ALFRED E. BENT, M.D.
2880 ATLANTIC AVE. #130
LONG BEACH, CA 90806
(213) 595-3824

Name_____

        Last   First   Date

CHECKED BOXES INDICATE APPLICABLE OR POSITIVE RESPONSES

I INTERVAL HISTORY LMP_____ CYCLE DAY NO._____

Dysuria: ☐ _____ +   Freq ☐ q _____ hrs.   Urgency ☐ _____ +

Nocturia: ☐ x _____   Incontinence: Stress ☐ _____ +

Post Void Fullness ☐ _____ +   Urge ☐ _____ +

VI SUPINE H$_2$O CYSTOMETRY

1st Sensation _____; Fullness _____   YES ☐

Max Volume _____   Vesical Contraction;   NO ☐

VII STANDING H$_2$O CYSTOMETRY | Flowrate: cc/min | N ☐

1st Sensation	cc	Vesical Contraction None	
Fullness	cc	☐ Inhibited ☐ Uninhibited	
Maximum	cc	Pressure	CM H$_2$O
Position		Induced by Filling	

II CURRENT MEDICATIONS   None ☐

CODE	DRUG*	DOSE	FREQ.	DUR. OF USE	SUBJECTIVE RESPONSE**
					1 ___ 5 ___ 10
					1 ___ 5 ___ 10
					1 ___ 5 ___ 10

*includes contraceptives

** <5=worse   5=no response   >5=improved   10=no symptoms

III SUBJECTIVE RESPONSES TO PREVIOUS TREATMENTS   None ☐

TREATMENT	RESPONSE	COMMENTS
☐ Dilatations	1 _____ 5 _____ 10	
	1 _____ 5 _____ 10	

IV UROFLOWMETRY

NOT DONE ☐	Flow Rate (cc/sec) Maximum/Mean	
	Urine Volume (cc) In/Voided	
	Flowtime (sec)	
	Time to Maximum Flow (sec)	
	Residual Urine (cc)	
	Normal Voiding for patient?	YES ☐ NO ☐
	Interpretation	N ☐ Ab ☐

VIII DIAGNOSIS

IX X-RAYS   VCUG ☐   TRATNER ☐   IVP ☐   UTZ ☐

X MEDICATIONS   None ☐

Code	Drug	Dose	Freq.	Dur/Treatment	Rx'd
	Nitrofurantoin	50 mg	tid	3 days	
	Vaginal Estrogen	–	qod	indefinite	
	Pyridium	100 mg	tid	3 days prn	

XI COMMENTS

V CYSTO URETHROSCOPY   Anesthesia: Topical ☐ Local ☐ None ☐

Urethro - Vesical Junction	Partial Closure	Closes	No Change	Opens
Response to Hold	☐	☐	☐	☐
Response to Cough	☐	☐	☐	☐
Response to Valsalva	☐	☐	☐	☐

Mobility   Fixed ☐   Minimal ☐   Moderate ☐   Extreme ☐

Palpation of Urethra with Scope in Place: Normal ☐   Diverticula ☐

Description Normal ☐	Bladder Trigone	UV Junction	URETHRA		
			Proximal	Mid	Distal
Red	☐	☐	☐	☐	☐
Granular	☐	☐	☐	☐	☐
Shaggy, Fronds	☐	☐	☐	☐	☐
Polyps	☐	☐	☐	☐	☐
Cysts	☐	☐	☐	☐	☐
Exudate	☐	☐	☐	☐	☐
Diverticulum	☐	☐	☐	☐	☐
Paleness	☐	☐	☐	☐	☐
	☐	☐	☐	☐	☐

☐ Photo Roll No.   ☐ Video Tape No.

CYSTOSCOPY   WNL ☐   URETERS   WNL ☐

TREATMENT PLAN:

RETURN VISIT:

Other Studies: Dictated ☐

_____ M.D.

Form 4A.   Visit summary (routine).

URG-DATA BASE SYSTEM
URODYNAMICS AND GYNECOLOGIC UROLOGY
RETURN VISIT SUMMARY

DONALD R. OSTERGARD, M.D.
WOMEN'S HOSPITAL
MEMORIAL HOSPITAL MEDICAL CENTER
UNIVERSITY OF CALIFORNIA IRVINE
2801 ATLANTIC AVENUE, P.O. BOX 1428
LONG BEACH, CA 90801 (213) 595-3824

New ☐   FORM 4
Returning ☐
Postpartum _____ Weeks
DATE: _____
CHART NO. _____
PATIENT NO. _____

NAME _____ _____
　　　　　　　Last　　　　　　　　　　　First

CHECKED BOXES INDICATE APPLICABLE OR POSITIVE RESPONSES

I INTERVAL HISTORY LMP _____ **CYCLE DAY NO.** _____

Dysuria: ☐ ____ +　　Freq ☐　q ____ hrs.　Urgency ☐ _____ +
Nocturia: ☐ x ____　　Incontinence:　Stress ☐ _____ +
Post Void Fullness ☐ _____ +　　　　Urge ☐ _____ +

II CURRENT MEDICATIONS　　　None ☐

CODE	DRUG*	DOSE	FREQ.	DUR. OF USE	SUBJECTIVE RESPONSE**
					1___5___10
					1___5___10
					1___5___10

*includes contraceptives
**< 5 = worse 5 = no response > 5 = improved 10 = no symptoms

III SUBJECTIVE RESPONSES TO PREVIOUS TREATMENTS　　None ☐

TREATMENT	RESPONSE	COMMENTS
☐ Dilatations	1___5___10	
	1___5___10	

IV UROFLOWMETRY

		†SPONT.	†INST.
Voiding Mechanism	Vesical Contraction	▨	☐
	Urethra	▨	+R☐ C☐ NC☐
	Voluntary Strain	▨	☐
Flow Rate (cc/sec) Maximum/Mean		/	/
Urine Volume (cc) In/Voided		/	/
Flowtime (sec)			
Time to Maximum Flow (sec)			
Residual Urine (cc)			
Maximum Intravesical Pressure (cm/H$_2$0)			
Resistance = P/F²		▨	
Time: UP↓ to VP↑ (sec)		⊞ ⊟	
Normal Voiding for patient?		YES☐ NO☐	YES☐ NO☐
Interpretation		N☐ Ab☐	N☐ Ab☐

COMMENTS:

V URETHROSCOPY:　　Anesthesia: Topical ☐　Local ☐

Urethro vesical Junction	Closes	No Change	Opens
Response to Hold	☐	☐	☐
Response to Cough	☐	☐	☐
Response to Valsalva	☐	☐	☐

Mobility:　Fixed ☐　Minimal ☐　Moderate ☐　Extreme ☐
Palpation of Urethra with Scope in Place:　Normal ☐　Diverticula ☐

Description	Bladder Trigone	UV Junction	URETHRA Proximal	Mid	Distal
Red	☐	☐	☐	☐	☐
Granular	☐	☐	☐	☐	☐
Shaggy, Fronds	☐	☐	☐	☐	☐
Polyps	☐	☐	☐	☐	☐
Cysts	☐	☐	☐	☐	☐
Exudate	☐	☐	☐	☐	☐
Diverticulum	☐	☐	☐	☐	☐
Paleness	☐	☐	☐	☐	☐
	☐	☐	☐	☐	☐

☐ Photo Roll No.　　　☐ Video Tape No.

VI TREATMENT PROCEDURES　　None ☐

Anesthesia:　Local ☐　Topical ☐
　　　　　　　　　Previous　　　　Present
☐　Calibration To _____ _____ F　Bleeding ☐
　　Dilation To _____ _____ F　Pain ☐

Cryosurgery ☐ (See Form 5)　　Polyps ☐　　Caruncle ☐

VII LABORATORY

Urine C&S ordered ☐ :
Negative ☐　Positive ☐　on _____ (date)

VIII XRAYS　VCUG ☐　　UTZ ☐　　TRATNER ☐　　IVP ☐

IX CONSULTATIONS REQUESTED:　　CYSTOSCOPY ☐

Psychiatry ☐　Urology ☐　Neurology ☐　EMG ☐　Other ☐

X DIAGNOSIS codes:　　No Change ☐

1. _____
　　　　　　　　　　　　　　　　　Code: _____
2. _____
　　　　　　　　　　　　　　　　　Code: _____

XI MEDICATIONS　　None ☐

Code	Drug	Dose	Freq.	Dur/Treatment	Rx'd
	Nitro Furantoin	50 mg.	tid	3 days	
	Vaginal Estrogen			Indefinite	
	Pyridium	100 mg	tid	3 days prn	

Dictated ☐

© 1980 DONALD R. OSTERGARD, MD

+R = RELAXES　C = CONTRACTS　NC = NO CHANGE　RETURN APPOINTMENT DATE _____ MD.
† = SPONTANEOUS/INSTRUMENTED

Form 4B.　Visit summary (return).

URG-DATA BASE SYSTEM
URODYNAMICS AND GYNECOLOGIC UROLOGY
MISCELLANEOUS SPECIAL EVALUATIONS

DONALD R. OSTERGARD, M.D.
WOMEN'S HOSPITAL
MEMORIAL HOSPITAL MEDICAL CENTER
UNIVERSITY OF CALIFORNIA IRVINE
2801 ATLANTIC AVENUE, P.O. BOX 1428
LONG BEACH, CA 90801 (213) 595-3824

FORM 5

NAME _____ , _____
Last   First

DATE: _____
CHART NO. _____
PATIENT NO. _____

CHECKED BOXES INDICATE APPLICABLE OR POSITIVE RESPONSE

SPECIAL EVALUATIONS

☐ Ice Water Test
_____ cc Introduced into Bladder
Time to Expulsion _____ sec. _____ No Expulsion ☐
Maximum Bladder Pressure _____ cm H_2O
Subjective Sensation:
None ☐ Mild ☐ Moderate ☐ Severe ☐
Interpretation: Normal ☐ Abnormal ☐

CRYOSURGERY

	Bladder Trigone	UV Junction	URETHRA Proximal	URETHRA Mid	URETHRA Distal
Temp. °C	_____ °C	_____ °C	_____ °C	_____ °C	_____ °C
TIME	_____ sec	_____ sec	_____ sec	_____ sec	_____ sec
	_____ sec	_____ sec	_____ sec	_____ sec	_____ sec
	_____ sec	_____ sec	_____ sec	_____ sec	_____ sec

☐ Propantheline Test ☐ Bethanechol Test
☐ Phentolamine Test (minutes after injection: _____)
☐ Pudendal Block (minutes after injection: _____)
☐ Alpha Stimulation Test _____

NOTES

		Baseline	15 min	30 min	Units
Pulse/BP		/	/	/	
UCPP (Empty)	Max. Pressure				cmH$_2$O
	Closing Pressure				cmH$_2$O
	Functional Length				cm
UCPP (Full)	Max. Pressure				cmH$_2$O
	Closing Pressure				cmH$_2$O
	Functional Length				cm
Cystometry	1st Desire Vol				cc
CO$_2$ ☐	Fullness Volume				cc
H$_2$O ☐	Capacity				cc
	Uninhibited Contr.	YES☐ NO ☐	YES☐ NO ☐	YES☐ NO ☐	
Uroflow	Voiding pressure				cmH$_2$O
	Maximum Flow				cc/sec
	Voided Volume				cc
	Resistance				

Therapeutic Benefit Anticipated   yes ☐   no ☐

COMMENTS:

Form 5. Miscellaneous special evaluations.

URG-DATA BASE SYSTEM
URODYNAMICS AND GYNECOLOGIC UROLOGY
PATIENT'S RESPONSE CHART

DONALD R. OSTERGARD, M.D.
WOMEN'S HOSPITAL
MEMORIAL HOSPITAL MEDICAL CENTER
UNIVERSITY OF CALIFORNIA IRVINE
2801 ATLANTIC AVENUE, P.O. BOX 1428
LONG BEACH, CA 90801 (213) 595-3824

Form 6A

DATE _____
CHART NO. _____
PATIENT NO. _____

NAME _____ , _____
Last   First

INSTRUCTIONS

You are under treatment for your urinary complaints. We are anxious to learn more from you regarding your urinary problem and any change which may occur. We are also interested in any other symptom that is currently present or may develop in your general condition. The accurate completion of this form will enable us to help you in the best way possible. Below is a list of symptoms. Each is followed by 4 columns with dates marked at the top. On the date indicated, please circle the correct choice for each item.

THE NUMBERS REFER TO THESE PHRASES:

0 - NONE
1 - A LITTLE
2 - SOME
3 - QUITE A BIT
4 - UNBEARABLE

Reporting Date	_____	_____	_____	_____
Number of capsules this date	_____	_____	_____	_____
1) Nausea	0 1 2 3 4	0 1 2 3 4	0 1 2 3 4	0 1 2 3 4
2) Vomiting	0 1 2 3 4	0 1 2 3 4	0 1 2 3 4	0 1 2 3 4
3) Diarrhea	0 1 2 3 4	0 1 2 3 4	0 1 2 3 4	0 1 2 3 4
4) Loss of appetite	0 1 2 3 4	0 1 2 3 4	0 1 2 3 4	0 1 2 3 4
5) Dryness of mouth	0 1 2 3 4	0 1 2 3 4	0 1 2 3 4	0 1 2 3 4
6) Dizziness	0 1 2 3 4	0 1 2 3 4	0 1 2 3 4	0 1 2 3 4
7) Weakness	0 1 2 3 4	0 1 2 3 4	0 1 2 3 4	0 1 2 3 4
8) Change of vision	0 1 2 3 4	0 1 2 3 4	0 1 2 3 4	0 1 2 3 4
9) Sleeplessness	0 1 2 3 4	0 1 2 3 4	0 1 2 3 4	0 1 2 3 4
10) Sleepiness	0 1 2 3 4	0 1 2 3 4	0 1 2 3 4	0 1 2 3 4
11) Palpitations	0 1 2 3 4	0 1 2 3 4	0 1 2 3 4	0 1 2 3 4
12) Trembling	0 1 2 3 4	0 1 2 3 4	0 1 2 3 4	0 1 2 3 4
13) Nervousness	0 1 2 3 4	0 1 2 3 4	0 1 2 3 4	0 1 2 3 4
14) Tension	0 1 2 3 4	0 1 2 3 4	0 1 2 3 4	0 1 2 3 4
15) Depression	0 1 2 3 4	0 1 2 3 4	0 1 2 3 4	0 1 2 3 4
16) Uncomfortably strong need to pass urine	0 1 2 3 4	0 1 2 3 4	0 1 2 3 4	0 1 2 3 4
17) Burning when passing urine	0 1 2 3 4	0 1 2 3 4	0 1 2 3 4	0 1 2 3 4
18) Sensation of continued need to pass urine after emptying bladder	0 1 2 3 4	0 1 2 3 4	0 1 2 3 4	0 1 2 3 4
19) Loss of urine with coughing or straining	0 1 2 3 4	0 1 2 3 4	0 1 2 3 4	0 1 2 3 4
20) Loss of urine before reaching toilet	0 1 2 3 4	0 1 2 3 4	0 1 2 3 4	0 1 2 3 4
21) Lower abdominal pressure	0 1 2 3 4	0 1 2 3 4	0 1 2 3 4	0 1 2 3 4
22) Lower abdominal pain	0 1 2 3 4	0 1 2 3 4	0 1 2 3 4	0 1 2 3 4
25) Backache	0 1 2 3 4	0 1 2 3 4	0 1 2 3 4	0 1 2 3 4
24) Painful intercourse	0 1 2 3 4	0 1 2 3 4	0 1 2 3 4	0 1 2 3 4
25) Indicate number of headaches in last 24 hours.	_____	_____	_____	_____
26) Indicate number of hours between times you pass urine.	_____	_____	_____	_____
27) Indicate number of times you pass urine at night.	_____	_____	_____	_____
28) Indicate number of times you pass urine during first hour after going to bed.	_____	_____	_____	_____
PHYSICIAN USE ONLY:				
LMP _____ Cycle Day	_____	_____	_____	_____

© 1978 DONALD R. OSTERGARD, MD

Form 6A. Patient's response chart (English).

**DATOS BASICOS DEL SISTEMA GINECO –
UROLOGICO
HOJA DE REPUESTAS DE LA PACIENTE**

DONALD R. OSTERGARD, M.D.
WOMEN'S HOSPITAL
MEMORIAL HOSPITAL MEDICAL CENTER
UNIVERSITY OF CALIFORNIA IRVINE
2801 ATLANTIC AVENUE, P.O. BOX 1428
LONG BEACH, CA 90801 (213) 595-3824

Form 6B

FECHA: _____
CHART NO. _____
PATIENT NO. _____

Nombre _____

INSTRUCCIONES

Usted esta bajo tratamiento para su padecimiento de las vías urinarias. Estamos deseosos de conocer más a fondo los detalles de su problema de las vías urinarias y estar al tanto de cualquier cambio que pueda ocurrir. Estamos tambien interesados en cualquier otro síntoma que esta presente en estos momentos o puede desarrollarse en su estado general. El llenar esta forma con exactitud nos ayudará a atender a usted en la mejor forma posible. Cada uno de estos, tiene 4 columnas con fechas marcadas arriba. En la fecha indicada, por favor haga un circulo en la contestación correcta para cada síntoma.

LOS NUMEROS SE REFIEREN A ESTAS FASES:

0 - NINGUNA
1 - UN POCO
2 - ALGO
3 - BASTANTE
4 - INAGUANTABLE

1) Nausea	0 1 2 3 4	0 1 2 3 4	0 1 2 3 4	0 1 2 3 4
2) Vómito	0 1 2 3 4	0 1 2 3 4	0 1 2 3 4	0 1 2 3 4
3) Diarrea	0 1 2 3 4	0 1 2 3 4	0 1 2 3 4	0 1 2 3 4
4) Pérdida de apetito	0 1 2 3 4	0 1 2 3 4	0 1 2 3 4	0 1 2 3 4
5) Boca seca	0 1 2 3 4	0 1 2 3 4	0 1 2 3 4	0 1 2 3 4
6) Mareos	0 1 2 3 4	0 1 2 3 4	0 1 2 3 4	0 1 2 3 4
7) Debilidad	0 1 2 3 4	0 1 2 3 4	0 1 2 3 4	0 1 2 3 4
8) Problemas de la vista	0 1 2 3 4	0 1 2 3 4	0 1 2 3 4	0 1 2 3 4
9) Falta de sueño	0 1 2 3 4	0 1 2 3 4	0 1 2 3 4	0 1 2 3 4
10) Exceso de sueño	0 1 2 3 4	0 1 2 3 4	0 1 2 3 4	0 1 2 3 4
11) Palpitaciones	0 1 2 3 4	0 1 2 3 4	0 1 2 3 4	0 1 2 3 4
12) Temblor	0 1 2 3 4	0 1 2 3 4	0 1 2 3 4	0 1 2 3 4
13) Nerviosidad	0 1 2 3 4	0 1 2 3 4	0 1 2 3 4	0 1 2 3 4
14) Tensión	0 1 2 3 4	0 1 2 3 4	0 1 2 3 4	0 1 2 3 4
15) Depresión	0 1 2 3 4	0 1 2 3 4	0 1 2 3 4	0 1 2 3 4
16) Deseo incontrolable de orinar	0 1 2 3 4	0 1 2 3 4	0 1 2 3 4	0 1 2 3 4
17) Ardor al orinar	0 1 2 3 4	0 1 2 3 4	0 1 2 3 4	0 1 2 3 4
18) Sensación de necesidad de seguir orinando aun después de haber vaciado la vejiga	0 1 2 3 4	0 1 2 3 4	0 1 2 3 4	0 1 2 3 4
19) Perdida de orina al toser	0 1 2 3 4	0 1 2 3 4	0 1 2 3 4	0 1 2 3 4
20) Pérdida de orina antes de llegar al baño	0 1 2 3 4	0 1 2 3 4	0 1 2 3 4	0 1 2 3 4
21) Presión en la región púbica	0 1 2 3 4	0 1 2 3 4	0 1 2 3 4	0 1 2 3 4
22) Dolor en la parte inferior del abdomen	0 1 2 3 4	0 1 2 3 4	0 1 2 3 4	0 1 2 3 4
23) Dolor de espalda	0 1 2 3 4	0 1 2 3 4	0 1 2 3 4	0 1 2 3 4
24) Dolor al tener relaciones intimas	0 1 2 3 4	0 1 2 3 4	0 1 2 3 4	0 1 2 3 4
25) Indique cuantos dolores de cabeza en las últimas 24 horas	_____	_____	_____	_____
26) Indique cada cuantas horas tiene que orinar	_____	_____	_____	_____
27) Cuantas veces orina en la noche?	_____	_____	_____	_____
28) Indique el número de veces que orina durante la primera hora después de que va a la cama	_____	_____	_____	_____
Para el Medico Solamente: LMP _____ Cycle Day _____	_____	_____	_____	_____

© 1978 DONALD R. OSTERGARD. MD

Form 6B. Patient's response chart (Spanish).

URG - DATA BASE SYSTEM
URODYNAMICS AND GYNECOLOGIC UROLOGY
RADIOLOGIC PROCEDURES

DONALD R. OSTERGARD, M.D.
WOMEN'S HOSPITAL
MEMORIAL HOSPITAL MEDICAL CENTER
UNIVERSITY OF CALIFORNIA IRVINE
2801 ATLANTIC AVENUE, P.O. BOX 1428
LONG BEACH, CA 90801 (213) 595-3824

NAME _____ , _____   DATE _____
        First   Last   CHART NO. _____
                                             PATIENT NO. _____

DYNAMIC CYSTOURETHROGAPHY

Volume of contrast used: _____ cc.   Supine or scout films: Reflux ☐   Diverticula ☐
                                                                             Bladder ☐
                                                                             Urethra ☐

VIEW	NON-STRAIN	STRAIN
AP (Erect with catheter)	Cystocele ☐ Funneling ☐ Vesical Neck Displacement _____ cm Other: _____	Cystocle ☐ Funneling ☐ Vesical Neck Displacement _____ cm Other: _____

Lateral (erect with catheter)	Describe:
	   Urethral
	      Displacement ☐
	      Cystocele ☐
	      Funneling ☐
	Other: _____
		UV angle: no change ☐
		             flattens ☐
		Vesical neck Displacement: _____ cm
		Urethral Displacement ☐
		Cystocele ☐
		Other: _____

Oblique (erect without catheter)	Describe: _____	Response to cough: True SI ☐ Delayed urine loss ☐ Other: _____

VOIDING CYSTOURETHROUGRAPHY

Urethral Appearance
  Normal ☐
  Abnormal ☐
Obstruction
  Yes ☐
  No ☐

URETHROGRAM

Normal ☐
Diverticula ☐   Number _____
Location: Normal ☐
           Distal ☐
           Proximal ☐

Diagnosis: _____

Comments: _____

Code _____ _____ _____

_____ M.D.

© 1978 DONALD R. OSTERGARD, MD

Form 7. Radiologic procedures.

VOIDING DIARY/UROLOG

This chart is a record of your voiding (urinating) and leakage (incontinence) of urine. Please complete this according to the following instructions prior to your visit to our office. Choose a *24 hour* period to keep this record when you can conveniently measure every voiding, and begin your record with the first voiding on arising as in the sample below.

EXAMPLE

(1) Time	(2) Amount voided	(3) Activity	(4) Leak Volume	(5) Urge Present	(6) Amount/Type of Intake
6:45 A.M.	550 cc	Awakening			
7:00		Turned on H$_2$O	2	Yes	2 cups coffee 6 oz OJ

(1) Record the time of all voidings, leakage, and intake of liquids.

(2) Measure all intake and output in *cc* or *oz*.

(3) Describe the activity you were performing at the time of leakage. If you were not actively doing anything, record whether you were sitting, standing, or lying down.

(4) Estimate the amount of leakage according to the following scale:

    1 = damp, few drops only;

    2 = wet underwear or pad;

    3 = soaked or emptied bladder.

(5) If the urge to urinate accompanied (or preceded) the urine leakage, write YES. If you felt no urge when the leakage occurred, write NO.

(6) Record the amount and type of *all liquid* intake in either cc or oz (1 cup = 8 oz = 240 cc).

Form 8A. Voiding diary/urolog instruction sheet.

VOIDING DIARY

Time	Amount Voided	Activity	Leak Volume	Urge Present	Amount/Type of Intake

Form 8B. Urolog.

URG-DATA BASE SYSTEM
URODYNAMICS AND GYNECOLOGIC
UROLOGY PATIENT SUMMARY

DONALD R. OSTERGARD, M.D.
WOMEN'S HOSPITAL
MEMORIAL HOSPITAL MEDICAL CENTER
UNIVERSITY OF CALIFORNIA IRVINE
2801 ATLANTIC AVENUE, P.O. BOX 1428
LONG BEACH, CA 90801 (213) 595-3824

Form 9

DATE _____
CHARTNO. _____
PATIENT NO. _____

NAME _____ Last / _____ First

I. PATIENT DATA

Address _____ Tel. No. ( ) _____
Birthdate _____ Marital Status: M☐ S☐ D☐ P☐ W☐   Race: W☐ N☐ S☐ O☐ AI☐
Also Known as _____ Soc. Sec. No. _____
Spouse: Name _____ Address _____
_____ Tel. No. ( ) _____

Person who will always be aware of patient's whereabouts—Relationship: _____
Name _____ Address _____
_____ Tel. No. ( ) _____

Referred by Physician
Name _____ Address _____
_____ Tel. No. ( ) _____

DATE	VISIT SUMMARY (One line per visit)		INITIALS
		Urine C&S ☐	

SPECIAL NOTES:

© 1978 DONALD R. OSTERGARD, MD

Form 9. Patient summary.

INDEX

Page numbers followed by *f* denote figures; those followed by *t* denote tables.